BOARDS
and
WARDS

FOURTH EDITION

BOARDS
and
WARDS

FOURTH EDITION

Carlos Ayala, MD, FACS
Adjunct Assistant Professor of Surgery
Uniformed Services University Health Sciences (USUHS)
Chief of Facial Plastic Surgery
Department of Otolaryngology, Head & Neck Surgery
Landstuhl Regional Medical Center
Landstuhl, Germany

Brad Spellberg, MD, FIDSA
Associate Professor of Medicine
Divisions of General Internal Medicine
and Infectious Diseases
Harbor-UCLA Medical Center
Torrance, California

. Wolters Kluwer | Lippincott Williams & Wilkins
Health

Philadelphia • Baltimore • New York • London
Buenos Aires • Hong Kong • Sydney • Tokyo

Acquisitions Editor: Charles W. Mitchell
Managing Editor: Kelley A. Squazzo
Marketing Manager: Jennifer Kuklinski
Designer: Holly McLaughlin
Compositor: Maryland Composition/ASI

Fourth Edition

Library of Congress Cataloging-in-Publication Data

Ayala, Carlos, MD.
  Boards and wards / Carlos Ayala, Brad Spellberg. —4th ed.
    p. ; cm.
  Rev. ed. of: Boards and wards. 3rd ed. 2006.
  Includes bibliographical references and index.
  ISBN 978-0-7817-8743-7
  1. Medicine—Examinations, questions, etc. I. Spellberg, Brad. II. Boards and wards.
III. Title.
  [DNLM: 1. Clinical Medicine—Examination Questions. WB 18.2 A973b 2006]
  R834.5.B63 2009
  610.76—dc22

                                                          2008055647

DISCLAIMER

Care has been taken to confirm the accuracy of the information present and to describe
generally accepted practices. However, the authors, editors, and publisher are not responsible for errors or omissions or for any consequences from application of the information
in this book and make no warranty, expressed or implied, with respect to the currency,
completeness, or accuracy of the contents of the publication. Application of this information in a particular situation remains the professional responsibility of the practitioner; the
clinical treatments described and recommended may not be considered absolute and uni-
versal recommendations.

The authors, editors, and publisher have exerted every effort to ensure that drug selection
and dosage set forth in this text are in accordance with the current recommendations and
practice at the time of publication. However, in view of ongoing research, changes in
government regulations, and the constant flow of information relating to drug therapy
and drug reactions, the reader is urged to check the package insert for each drug for any
change in indications and dosage and for added warnings and precautions. This is particularly important when the recommended agent is a new or infrequently employed drug.

Some drugs and medical devices presented in this publication have Food and Drug
Administration (FDA) clearance for limited use in restricted research settings. It is the responsibility of the health care provider to ascertain the FDA status of each drug or device
planned for use in their clinical practice.

To purchase additional copies of this book, call our customer service department at **(800)
638-3030** or fax orders to **(301) 223-2320**. International customers should call **(301)
223-2300**.

Visit Lippincott Williams & Wilkins on the Internet: http://www.lww.com. Lippincott Williams
& Wilkins customer service representatives are available from 8:30 am to 6:00 pm, EST.

Dedicated to my wife and family, Teresa, Juancarlos, and Yasmin, and to all those who strive to be competent, caring, and compassionate physicians.

Carlos Ayala, MD

To all the interns manning the front lines of our hospitals, and to all the MS IVs who will soon know their pain.

Brad Spellberg, MD

Abbreviations

↑ (↑↑)	Increases/High (Markedly Increases/Very High)
↓ (↓↓)	Decreases/Low (Markedly Decreases/Very Low)
→	Causes/Leads to/Analysis shows
⊕	Positive
1°/2°	Primary/Secondary
Abd	Abdominal
BP	Blood Pressure
Bx	Biopsy
c/o	complain of
CA	Carcinoma
CBC	Complete Blood Count
CN	Cranial Nerve
CNS	Central Nervous System
CT	Computed Tomography Scan
Cx	Culture
CXR/X-ray	Chest X-ray/X-ray
Dx/DDx	Diagnosis/Differential Diagnosis
dz	Disease
EKG	Electrocardiogram
GI	Gastrointestinal
H&P	History and Physical
HA	Headache
HIV	Human Immunodeficiency Virus
HTN	Hypertension
Hx/FHx	History/Family History
ICP	Intracranial Pressure
I&D	Incision and Drainage
infxn	Infection
ICU	Intensive Care Unit
IV	Intravenous
IVIG	Intravenous Immunoglobulin
Lab/Labs	Laboratory/Laboratory Tests/Results
N or Nml	Normal
PE	Physical Exam or Pulmonary Embolus
pt(s)	Patient(s)
Px	Prognosis
RBC	Red Blood Cell
Rx	Prescription/Indicated Drug
q#	Every #
Si/Sx/aSx	Sign/Symptom/Asymptomatic
subQ	Subcutaneous
Tx	Treatment/Therapy
Utz	Ultrasound
WBC	White Blood Cell

Preface

Scutted-out medical students and exhausted interns have no time to waste studying for the USMLE Steps 2 and 3 exams. That's where we come in. We cover all the major fields of medicine tested on the USMLE exams: Internal Medicine, Surgery, Obstetrics-Gynecology, Pediatrics, Family Medicine, Psychiatry, Neurology, Dermatology, Radiology, Emergency Medicine, and Medical Ethics/Law. However, in contrast to most review texts, we have targeted each chapter toward clinicians *who are not going into that field of medicine*. Thus, Family Medicine is written for surgeons, Obstetrics-Gynecology is written for psychiatrists, Internal Medicine is written for pediatricians, and so on.

None of you surgeons out there want to spend the 5 minutes you have before nodding off to sleep learning Dermatology for the USMLE Step 2 or 3 exam! Rather, you need a concise review, broad in content but lacking extensive detail, to jar your memory of testable concepts you long ago learned and forgot. Don't waste your precious waking hours poring over voluminous review texts! Remember, sleep when you can sleep. During those few minutes before dozing off in the call room, use a text written by colleagues and designed to help you breeze through subjects you have little interest in and have forgotten most of, but in which you need the most review. Like you, we know and live by the old axiom: study 2 months for the USMLE Step 1 exam, 2 days for the Step 2 exam, and bring a number 2 pencil to the Step 3 exam!

We welcome any feedback you may have about *Boards and Wards*. Please feel free to contact the authors with your comments or suggestions. You can email us at Boards_Wards@yahoo.com or write us at

Boards and Wards
c/o Lippincott Williams & Wilkins
351 W. Camden Street
Baltimore, MD 21201

Finally, we would also like to thank all the medical students and residents and attendings who have reviewed this new edition and provided their suggestions and comments.

Third Edition Contributors

Joseph Rosales
Ming-Sing Si
Eric Daniels
Griselda Gutierrez
Beatriz Mares
Pedro Cheung
Charles Lee
Michael Gentry

Fourth Edition Contributors

Ryan Blenker, MD
James T. Kwiatt, MD
Jay Mepani, MD
Benjamin M. Schneeberger, MD

List of Tables

1.1 Hypertension Definitions and Treatment Indication 1
1.2 Causes of Secondary Hypertension 2
1.3 Medical Treatment of Hypertension 3
1.4 Angina Treatment 4
1.5 Initiation of Therapy for Hypercholesterolemia 4
1.6 Treatment by Risk Stratification of Unstable Angina 6
1.7 Risk Stratification for Acute Coronary Syndrome 7
1.8 Cardiomyopathy 31
1.9 Summary of Major Murmurs 32
1.10 Physical Examination Differential Diagnosis for Murmurs . . 33
1.11 Duke Criteria for Endocarditis Diagnosis 36
1.12 Five Mechanisms of Hypoxemia 38
1.13 Chronic Obstructive Pulmonary Disease 40
1.14 Diagnosis and Treatment of Restrictive Lung Disease 42
1.15 Lab Analysis of Pleural Effusions 43
1.16 Parenchymal Lung Cancers 46
1.17 Mediastinal Tumors 48
1.18 Community Acquired Pneumonia 53
1.19 Comparison of Inflammatory Bowel Disease 59
1.20 Congenital Hyperbilirubinemia 59
1.21 Hepatitis Diagnosis and Treatment 62
1.22 Ascites Differential Diagnosis 64
1.23 Causes of Portal Hypertension 66
1.24 Laboratory Characteristics of Acute Renal Failure 68
1.25 Renal Tubular Acidosis 70
1.26 Nephrotic Glomerulopathies 72
1.27 Systemic Glomerulonephropathies 73
1.28 Nephritic Glomerulonephropathies 74
1.29 Urinalysis in Primary Glomerular Diseases 75
1.30 Differential Diagnosis of Male Gonadal Disorders 83
1.31 Genetic Hypogonadism 84
1.32 Multiple Endocrine Neoplasia Syndromes 89
1.33 Diagnosis and Treatment of Primary Bone Neoplasms 92
1.34 α-Thalassemia 112
1.35 β-Thalassemia 113
1.36 Hypoproliferative Anemias 115

1.37 Hemolytic Anemias 116
1.38 Causes of Platelet Destruction (Thrombocytopenia) 118
1.39 Labs in Platelet Destruction 118
1.40 Hypercoagulable Diseases 119
1.41 Myeloproliferative Diseases 120
1.42 Empiric Antibiotic Treatment of Specific Infections 125
1.43 Hypokalemia 127
1.44 Hyperkalemia 127
2.1   Common Electrolyte Disorders 138
2.2   Risk of Viral Infection from Blood Transfusions 142
2.3   Goldman Cardiac Risk Index 144
2.4   Glasgow Coma Scale 150
2.5   Differential Diagnosis of Shock 151
2.6   Correction of Defect in Shock 151
2.7   Body Surface Area in Burns 153
2.8   Neck Mass Differential Diagnosis 154
2.9A Right Upper Quadrant Differential Diagnosis 159
2.9B Right Lower Quadrant Differential Diagnosis 160
2.9C Left Upper Quadrant Differential Diagnosis 161
2.9D Left Lower Quadrant Differential Diagnosis 161
2.9E Midline Differential Diagnosis 162
2.10 Hernia Definitions 165
2.11 Ranson's Criteria 171
2.12 Knee Injuries 201
2.13 Intracranial Hemorrhage 203
2.14 CNS Malignancy 207
3.1   Teratogens 220
3.2   US Food and Drug Administration Drug Categories 221
3.3   Height of Uterus by Gestational Week 222
3.4   Types of Pregnancy-Induced Hypertension 227
3.5   Bishop Score 239
3.6   Types of Abortions 244
3.7   Comparison of Placenta Previa and Placental Abruption . . . 245
3.8   Phases of the Menstrual Cycle 250
3.9   Risks and Benefits of Oral Contraceptives 251
3.10 Alternatives to Oral Contraceptives 252

3.11 Differential Diagnosis of Vaginitis 255
3.12 Differential Diagnosis of Hirsutism and Virilization 260
3.13 Ovarian Neoplasms 267
4.1 Development Milestones 271
4.2 Tanner Stages 271
4.3 The ToRCHS 272
4.4 Viral Exanthems 274
4.5 Pediatric Upper Respiratory Disorders 278
4.6 Pediatric Painful Limp 286
4.7 Types of Juvenile Rheumatoid Arthritis 289
4.8 Differential Diagnosis of Neonatal Jaundice
     by Time of Onset 291
4.9 Pediatric Toxicology 305
5.1 Summary of Headaches 309
5.2 Treatment of Headache 311
5.3 Causes of Vertigo 313
5.4 Sinusitis 316
5.5 Pharyngitis 318
5.6 Diarrheas 322
5.7 Infectious Causes of Diarrhea 325
5.8 Sexually Transmitted Diseases 327
5.9 Low Back Pain Red Flags 334
6.1 DSM-IV Classifications 343
6.2 Prognosis of Psychiatric Disorders 344
6.3 Pharmacologic Therapy for Depression 345
6.4 Diagnosis of Psychotic Disorders 348
6.5 Antipsychotic Drugs 349
6.6 Antipsychotic-Associated Movement Disorders 350
6.7 Specific Personality Disorders 354
6.8 Drug Intoxications and Withdrawal 363
6.9 Sleep Stages 366
7.1 Presentation of Stroke 369
7.2 Cerebrospinal Fluid Findings in Meningitis 372
7.3 Empiric Therapy for Meningitis by Age 373
7.4 Bacterial Meningitis 373
7.5 Encephalitis 375
7.6 Seizure Therapy 379

7.7 Dementia versus Delirium 380
8.1 Use of Topical Steroids 390
8.2 Skin Cancer 408
8.3 Neurocutaneous Syndromes (Phakomatoses) 412
8.4 Fungal Cutaneous Disorders 422
9.1 Palpebral Inflammation 428
9.2 Red Eye 430
9.3 Eye Related Trauma 440
9.4 Ophthalmic Medications 442
10.1 Common Radiologic Studies 446
10.2 Common Radiologic Findings 448
12.1 Biostatistics 471
12.2 Sample Calculation of Statistical Values 473
12.3 Ethical/Legal Terms 475
12.4 Interviewing Techniques 479

Contents

Abbreviations v

Preface vii

List of Tables xi

1. Internal Medicine 1
   Cardiology 1
   Pulmonary 37
   Gastroenterology and Hepatology 56
   Nephrology 68
   Endocrinology 77
   Musculoskeletal 89
   Hematology 109
   Empiric Antibiotic Treatment for Specific Infections 124

2. Surgery 136
   Fluid and Electrolytes 136
   Blood Product Replacement 137
   Perioperative Care 143
   Trauma 147
   Burns 152
   Neck Mass Differential 154
   Surgical Abdomen 156
   Esophagus 157
   Gastric Tumors 164
   Hernia 164
   Hepatic Tumors 166
   Gallbladder 167
   Exocrine Pancreas 170
   Small Intestine 173
   Colon 175
   Rectum and Anus 182
   Breast 184
   Urology 192
   Orthopedics 196
   Neurosurgery 200
   Vascular Diseases 209

3. Obstetrics and Gynecology 219
   Obstetrics 219
   Gynecology 248

4. Pediatrics 270
   Development 270
   Infections 270

Respiratory Disorders 270
Musculoskeletal 285
Metabolic 290
Genetic and Congenital Disorders 292
Trauma and Intoxication 301
Adolescence 305

5. Family Medicine 308
Headache 308
Ears, Nose, and Throat 308
Outpatient Gastrointestinal Complaints 319
Urogenital Complaints 325
Common Sports Medicine Complaints 332
Nutrition 338
Hoarseness 341

6. Psychiatry 343
Introduction 343
Mood Disorders 344
Psychosis 347
Anxiety Disorders 349
Personality Disorders 353
Somatoform and Factitious Disorders 356
Child and Adolescent Psychiatry 358
Abuse of Drugs 363
Miscellaneous Disorders 365
Sleep 366

7. Neurology 369
Stroke 369
Infection and Inflammation 372
Demyelinating Diseases 374
Metabolic and Nutritional Disorders 376
Seizures 378
Degenerative Diseases 379

8. Dermatology 383
Terminology 383
Topical Steroids 390
Infections 390
Common Disorders 394
Cancer 407
Neurocutaneous Syndromes (Phakomatoses) 407
Blistering Disorders 407
Vector-Borne Diseases 417

Parasitic Infections 418
Fungal Cutaneous Disorders 422

9. Ophthalmology 424
Eyes 424

10. Radiology 445
Helpful Terms and Concepts 445
Common Radiologic Studies 446
An Approach to a Chest X-Ray 446
Common Radiologic Findings 447

11. Emergency Medicine 463
Toxicology 463
Fish and Shellfish Toxins 465
Bites and Stings 467
ENT Trauma 468

12. Ethics/Law/Clinical Studies 471
Biostatistics 471
Study Types 472
Calculation of Statistical Values 473
Law and Ethics 476
Doctoring 478
Health Care Delivery 481

Appendix 484

Questions 496

Answers 531

Index 555

1. INTERNAL MEDICINE

I. Cardiology

A. **HTN (Table 1.1)**

1. **Causes**

   a. 95% of all HTN is idiopathic, called **"essential HTN"**

   b. Most of 2° HTN causes can be divided into three organ systems and drugs **(Table 1.2)**

2. **Malignant HTN**

   a. Can be hypertensive urgency or emergency

   b. Hypertensive urgency

      (1) High BP (e.g., systolic >200 or diastolic >110, but numbers vary depending upon source) **without evidence of end-organ damage**

      (2) Tx = oral BP medications with goal of slowly reducing BP over several days—does not require admission to hospital

   c. Hypertensive emergency

      (1) Defined as severe HTN with evidence of end-organ compromise (e.g., encephalopathy, renal failure, congestive heart failure [CHF]/ischemia)

      (2) Si/Sx = mental status changes, papilledema, focal neurologic findings, anuria, chest pain, evidence of CHF (e.g., lower extremity edema, elevated jugular venous pressure [JVP], rales on pulmonary exam), or microangiopathic hemolytic anemia (hemolysis with schistocytes on smear)

      (3) **This is a medical emergency and immediate Tx is needed**

Table 1.1	Hypertension Definitions and Treatment Indication	
Condition	**BP**	**Tx**
Nml	<120/80	• None
PreHTN	120/80–139/89	• Medication if cardiac or renal dz or diabetes • Diet and exercise otherwise
Stage I HTN	140/90–159/99	• Medication
Stage II HTN	≥160/100	• Medication—typically more than 1

Table 1.2 Causes of Secondary Hypertension

Cardiovascular	• Aortic regurgitation causes **wide pulse pressure** • Aortic coarctation causes HTN in arms with ↓ **BP in legs**
Renal	• **Glomerular dz commonly presents with proteinuria** • **Renal artery stenosis causes refractory HTN** in older men (atherosclerosis) or young women (fibromuscular dysplasia) • Polycystic kidneys
Endocrine	• Hypersteroidism, typically **Cushing's and Conn's syndromes, which cause HTN with hypokalemia** (↑ aldosterone) • Pheochromocytoma causing episodic autonomic Sx • Hyperthyroidism causing **isolated systolic HTN**
Drug induced	• Oral contraceptives, glucocorticoids, phenylephrine, NSAIDs

   (4) Tx = IV drip with nitroprusside or nitroglycerin (the latter preferred for ischemia), but **do not lower BP by more than one fourth within the first hour or the pt is at risk for complications of hypoperfusion, including stroke**
3. **HTN Tx**
   a. Lifestyle modifications first line in pts without comorbid dz
      (1) Weight loss, exercise, and quitting alcohol and smoking can each significantly lower BP independently; salt restriction may help
      (2) ↓ Fat intake to ↓ risk of coronary artery dz (CAD); HTN is a cofactor
   b. Medications (Table 1.3)
B. **Ischemic Heart Dz (CAD)**
   1. **Risk Factors for CAD**
      a. **Major risk factors (memorize these!!!)**
         (1) Diabetes (may be the most important)
         (2) Smoking
         (3) HTN
         (4) Hypercholesterolemia
         (5) FHx
         (6) Age
      b. Minor risk factors: obesity, lack of estrogen (males or postmenopausal women not on estrogen replacement), homocystinuria
      c. Smoking is the number one preventable risk factor
      d. Diabetes probably imparts the greatest risk of all of them

Table 1.3 Medical Treatment of Hypertension

Indications	1) Failure of lifestyle modifications after 6 mos to 1 yr
	2) Immediate use necessary if comorbid organ dz is present (e.g., stroke, angina, renal dz)
	3) Immediate use in emergent or urgent hypertensive states (e.g., neurologic impairment, ↑ ICP)
First-Line Drugs	
No comorbid dz	**Thiazide diuretic (proven safe and effective)**
Diabetes	**ACE inhibitors or angiotensin receptor blocker (ARB) (proven to ↓ vascular and renal dz)**
CHF	**ACE inhibitors, ARB, β-blocker, and potassium-sparing diuretic (all proven to ↓ mortality)**
Myocardial infarction	**β-blocker and ACE inhibitor** (proven to ↓ mortality)
Osteoporosis	**Thiazide diuretics** ($\downarrow Ca^{2+}$ excretion)
Prostatic	**α-blockers** (Tx HTN and benign prostatic hypertrophy concurrently) hypertrophy
Pregnancy	**α-methyldopa** (known safe in pregnancy)
Contraindications	
β-blockers	**Chronic obstructive pulmonary dz,** because of bronchospasm
β-blockers (relative)	**Diabetes,** because of alteration in insulin/glucose homeostasis and blockage of autonomic response to hypoglycemia
β-blockers	**Hyperkalemia,** because of risk of ↑ serum potassium levels
ACE inhibitors	**Pregnancy,** because of teratogenicity
ACE inhibitors	**Renal artery stenosis,** because of precipitation of acute renal failure (glomerular filtration rate-dependent on angiotensin-mediated constriction of efferent arteriole)
ACE inhibitors	**Renal failure (creatinine >1.5),** because of hyperkalemia morbidity
K^+-sparing diuretics	**Renal failure (creatinine >1.5),** because of hyperkalemia morbidity
Diuretics	**Gout,** because of causation of hyperuricemia
Thiazides	**Diabetes,** because of hyperglycemia

2. **Stable Angina Pectoris**
   a. Caused by atherosclerotic CAD, supply of blood to heart<demand
   b. Si/Sx = precordial pain radiating to left arm, jaw, back, relieved by rest and nitroglycerin, EKG → **ST depression and T-wave inversion** (see Figure 1.2R)

Table 1.4 Angina Treatment

Acute	Sublingual nitroglycerin
	• Usually acts in 1–2 min
	• May be taken up to 3 times q3- to 5-min intervals
	• If does not relieve pain after 3 doses, pt may be infarcting
Chronic Prevention	• Long-acting nitrates (e.g., isosorbide dinitrate) effective in prophylaxis
	• β-blockers ↓ myocardial O_2 consumption in stress/exertion
	• Aspirin to prevent platelet aggregation in atherosclerotic plaque
	• Quit smoking! (2 years after quitting, MI risk = nonsmokers)
	• ↓ LDL levels, ↑ HDL with diet (↓ saturated fat intake more important than actual cholesterol intake), ↑ exercise, ↑ fiber intake, stop smoking, lose weight, HMG-CoA reductase inhibitors (see Table 1.5)
Endovascular Intervention	• Percutaneous transluminal coronary angioplasty (PTCA)
	• Indicated with failure of medical management
	• Morbidity less than surgery but has up to 50% restenosis rate
	• Stent placement reduces restenosis rate to 20%–30%
	• Platelet GPIIb-IIIa antagonists further reduce restenosis rate
Surgery	• Coronary artery bypass graft (CABG)
	• Indications = failure of medical Tx, three-vessel CAD, or two-vessel dz in diabetes
	• Comparable mortality rates with PTCA after several years, except in pts with diabetes who do better with CABG

c. **Classic Sx often not present in elderly and pts with diabetes (neuropathy)**
d. Dx = clinical, based on Sx, CAD risks; confirm CAD with angiography
e. Tx (Tables 1.4 and 1.5)

Table 1.5 Initiation of Therapy for Hypercholesterolemia

Condition	Low-density Lipoprotein Goal (mg/dl)*	Low-density Lipoprotein at Drug Initiation (mg/dl)
Less than two risk factors for CAD	<160	>190
Two or more risk factors for CAD	<130	>160
With CAD or with diabetes mellitus	<100	>130

*If **low-density lipoprotein** is above goal, immediately initiate diet and exercise.

3. **Acute Coronary Syndrome (ACS)**

   a. ACS occurs when insufficient perfusion occurs to the myocardium because of obstruction in one or more coronary arteries

   b. ACS has a spectrum of severity, ranging from ischemia without infarction (unstable angina) to non-ST-elevation myocardial infarction (NSTEMI) to ST-elevation myocardial infarction (STEMI)

   c. Dx of ACS is based on H&P, EKG, and cardiac enzymes

4. **Unstable Angina**

   a. Sx similar to stable angina but occur more frequently with less exertion and/or **occurs at rest**

   b. Unstable angina is caused by transient clotting of atherosclerotic vessels; clot spontaneously dissolves before infarction occurs

   c. EKG during ischemia typically shows ST depression or T-wave inversions (Figure 1.2R)

   d. Labs: by definition cardiac enzymes are negative in unstable angina

   e. Tx is based on stratification of risk of bad outcome, defined as risk of recurrent unstable angina, infarction, or death 30 days after presentation (Table 1.6)

   f. Once a pt has ruled out for myocardial infarction (MI) with negative enzymes, the pt should undergo risk stratification (Table 1.7)

5. **NSTEMI**

   a. Sx similar to unstable angina, but pain often lasts $\geq$20 min without resolving and may only partially respond or not respond to nitroglycerin

   b. EKG similar to unstable angina (ST depression or T-wave inversions)

   c. Labs: by definition cardiac enzymes (i.e., troponin and creatine-MB [CK-MB]) are elevated, and this is how NSTEMI is Dx—both have similar sensitivities and specificities, but CK-MB normalizes 72 hr after infarction, whereas troponin remains elevated for up to 1 wk

   d. Acute Tx: see Table 1.6

6. **ST Elevation MI**

   a. Infarct usually 2° to acute plaque rupture causing thrombosis in atherosclerotic vessel

Table 1.6 Treatment by Risk Stratification of Unstable Angina*

	Low Risk	Intermediate Risk	High Risk
Defining factors	• ↑ frequency of angina compared with baseline • Rest pain <20 min	• Rest pain ≥20 min now resolved • Nocturnal angina • Pain resolved with nitroglycerin • Symmetric T-wave inversions or ST depressions <1 mm	• Rest pain ≥20 min ongoing • ST depressions ≥1 mm • + Troponon or creatine-MB (i.e., NSTEMI) • Presence of acute pulmonary edema or S_3 on examination
Tx	• Aspirin • O_2 • β-blocker • Sublingual nitroglycerin when needed	• Add longer-acting nitro drug (i.e., isosorbide dinitrate) • Consider heparin	• Add heparin or low molecular-weight heparin • Nitroglycerin drip if pain ongoing • Add GPIIb-IIIa antagonist if enzymes positive or ST depressions >1 mm • Clopidogrel can be added for NSTEMI or if stent placed during catheterization

*Defined as risk of recurrent unstable angina, MI, or death at 30 days after presentation. This list of defining factors is not all-inclusive but rather highlights the most "testable" factors on the boards. Note that ST-elevation MI does not fit into this algorithm.

    b. Si/Sx = crushing substernal pain, as per angina, but not relieved by rest, ↑ diaphoresis, nausea/vomiting, tachycardia or bradycardia, dyspnea

    c. Dx

       (1) **EKG → ST elevation and Q waves** (Figures 1.1 and 1.2S)

       (2) Enzymes: troponin I or CK-MB

       (3) Appropriate signs and symptoms with risk factors

Table 1.7 Risk Stratification for Acute Coronary Syndrome

Test	Sensitivity/ Specificity*	Comments
Stress treadmill	70%/70%	Inexpensive • Because of low sensitivity/specificity, only useful for pts with intermediate probability of having CAD
Stress echocardiogram	80%/80%	• Only form of stress test that enables visualization of valve function • Also measures ejection fraction • Can be done with exercise or pharmacologically with dobutamine—pharmacological done for people who cannot exercise but sensitivity is lower
MIBI	80%/80%	• Also measures ejection fraction • Can be done with exercise or pharmacologically with persantine—pharmacological done for people who cannot exercise but sensitivity is lower
Catheterization	95%/95%	• Gold-standard for dx • Provides an anatomical view of the coronaries and estimate of ejection fraction • Can be false negative for partial coronary lesions if the artery undergoes compensatory dilation

*Sensitivities and specificities are for finding evidence of CAD; approximate values shown—studies typically show a range of +/− 5% from values shown.

    d. Tx = re-establish vessel patency
      (1) Medical Tx = thrombolysis within 6 hr of the infarct: by using tissue plasminogen activator (**tPA**) + **heparin** (first line) or streptokinase
      (2) Percutaneous transluminal coronary—(PTCA) may be more effective—can open vessels mechanically or with local administration of thrombolytics
      (3) Coronary artery bypass graft (CABG) is longer-term Tx, rarely used for acute process

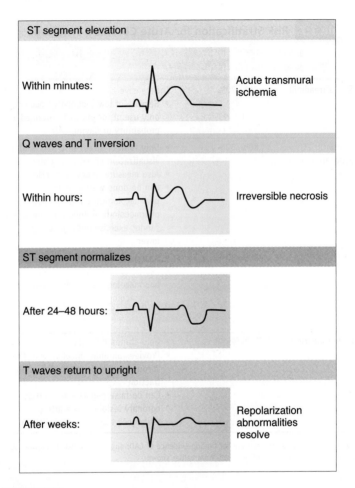

FIGURE 1.1

The changing pattern of the EKG in the affected leads during the evolution of a myocardial infarction. (Adapted from Axford JS. *Medicine.* Oxford: Blackwell Science, 1996.)

e. Adjuvant medical therapies
   (1) **Number one priority is aspirin! (proven to ↓ mortality)**
   (2) **Number two priority is β-blocker (proven to ↓ mortality)**
   (3) Statin drugs to lower cholesterol are essential **(low-density lipoprotein [LDL] must be <100 postinfarct,** proven to ↓ mortality) (see Table 1.7)

(4) Heparin should be given for 48 hr postinfarct **if tPA was used to lyse the clot** (heparin has no proven benefit if streptokinase was used or if no lysis was performed)

(5) Oxygen (O_2) and morphine for pain control

(6) Nitroglycerin to reduce both preload and afterload

(7) Angiotensin-converting enzyme (ACE) inhibitors are excellent late- and long-term Tx; ↓ afterload and prevent remodeling

(8) Exercise strengthens heart, develops collateral vessels, ↑ high density lipoprotein (HDL)

(9) STOP SMOKING!

7. **Prinzmetal's Angina**

a. Coronary artery vasospasm causing rest pain

b. Unlike true "angina," the EKG shows ST elevation with Prinzmetal's angina

c. Differentiating Prinzmetal's angina from an acute MI is challenging at first, but enzymes typically are negative, and ST elevation is only transient

d. Tx is vasodilators (nitroglycerin or calcium blocker), and pts should undergo catheterization because vasospasm often occurs at the site of an atherosclerotic lesion in the coronaries

C. **EKG Findings and Arrhythmias**

1. Basic EKG Review

a. P-QRS-T complex (Figure 1.2A)

(1) P wave is the sinus beat that precedes ventricular depolarization

(2) PR interval is the period of time between the beginning of atrial depolarization and the beginning of ventricular depolarization—nml PR interval ≤0.2 ms, which is ≤5 small boxes on the EKG

(3) Q wave is when the INITIAL part of ventricular depolarization is downward, not upward—Q wave is nonpathologic (<1 box = <0.04 ms wide), Q wave is pathologic (>1 box = >0.04 ms wide)

(4) QRS represents ventricular depolarization—nml QRS interval = <0.12 ms (3 small boxes wide)

(5) ST segment represents the beginning of ventricular repolarization—should be isoelectric (neither higher nor lower) with the PR segment

(6) T wave represents the bulk of ventricular repolarization—should be upright

Text continues on page 24

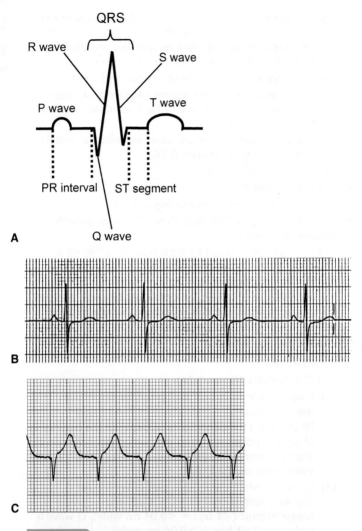

FIGURE 1.2 **P-QRS-T Complex.** *(continued)*

(A) Figure of Wave Form. (B) Nml sinus rhythm. There is a p before every QRS and a QRS after every p. There are no prolonged intervals or conduction delays. The rate is approximately 60 bpm. (C) Junctional tachycardia. Note the absence of p waves, indicating no sinus activity. Therefore the rhythm must be an escape rhythm originating at the AV junction or below. Because the complexes are narrow, this rhythm originates in the junction and not in the ventricle. The rate exceeds 100 bpm (rate is approximately 105 bpm). Therefore this is a tachycardia originating from the AV junction.

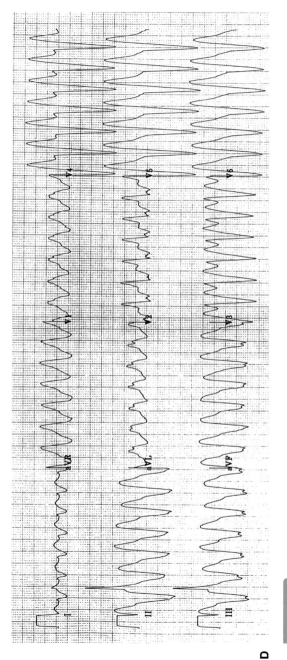

FIGURE 1.2 P-QRS-T Complex. *(continued)*

(D) Ventricular tachycardia. Note lack of p waves, and all complexes are very wide, indicating they are of ventricular origin. The rate is approximately 150 bpm, so this is ventricular tachycardia. Do not miss this on an examination! Of note, technically one cannot be certain that this is not supraventricular tachycardia with a bundle branch block, because the bundle branch block would also cause wide complexes. However, on a Step 2 or 3 examination, this EKG will always be ventricular tachycardia.

D

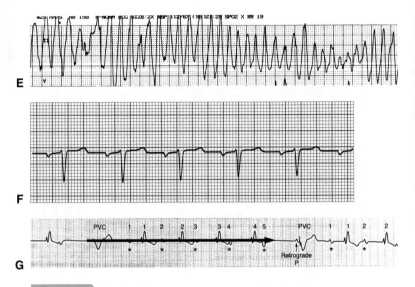

FIGURE 1.2 *(continued)*

(E) Ventricular fibrillation—torsades de pointes. The wide complexes that vary in amplitude are indicative of ventricular fibrillation. The twisting of the axis and amplitude resulting in increasing and decreasing height, like a ribbon, is consistent with torsades de pointes. **(F)** First-degree block. The rhythm is sinus, and the rate is nml. However, the interval between the **beginning** of the p wave and the beginning of the small r wave exceeds 1 large box, meaning that it is >5 mm, or 0.2 ms. This indicates first-degree block. **(G)** Second-degree, type 1 (Wenckebach) block. Note how the PR interval becomes progressively longer; that is, the p waves (marked with *asterisks*) become progressively farther apart from each corresponding QRS complex (*numbers above* refer to the same p wave and resulting QRS complex). The fifth p wave occurs during the T wave of the fourth QRS complex, and that p wave is not conducted, so there is no fifth QRS complex. The next complex that appears is actually a premature ventricular contraction (PVC, a ventricular escape beat), with a retrograde p wave in front of it (you know the p wave is retrograde because it is so close to the PVC, and because it is shaped differently from the sinus p waves before and after it). The PVC "resets" the system, and the sinus p waves take over again, with the same increasing PR interval between beats 1 and 2. Incidentally noted is the presence of a bundle branch block (note the rabbit ears in the QRS complexes—more on this to come).

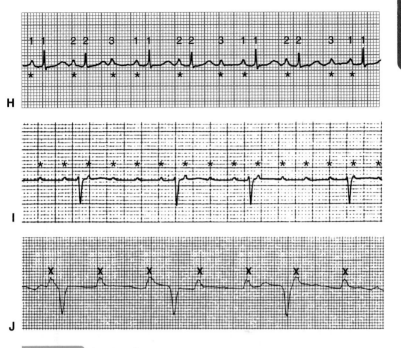

H

I

J

FIGURE 1.2 *(continued)*

(H) Second-degree, type 2 (Mobitz) block. P waves again marked by *asterisk*, and *numbers above* refer to paired p waves and QRS complexes. In contrast to Figure 1.2G, note the consistent PR intervals. However, the third p wave in each series is not conducted, resulting in a dropped beat. This is a 3:2 second-degree Mobitz block. **(I)** Third-degree block with junctional escape. Note the absence of relationship between the much faster p waves (annotated with *asterisk*) and the slower QRS complexes. By their narrow width and rate (approximately 55), the QRS rhythm is junctional escape. **(J)** Third-degree block with ventricular escape. Again there is no relationship between the p waves (annotated with *asterisk*) and the QRS complexes. Here the QRS complexes are very wide and the rate (approximately 40) is slower, indicative of a ventricular escape rhythm.

- wide QRS ~~VSP~~ V5, V6
- S V1 V2

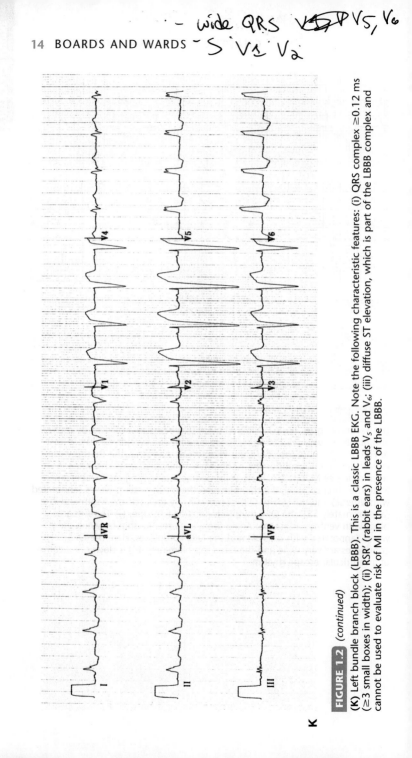

FIGURE 1.2 *(continued)*

(K) Left bundle branch block (LBBB). This is a classic LBBB EKG. Note the following characteristic features: (i) QRS complex ≥0.12 ms (≥3 small boxes in width); (ii) RSR′ (rabbit ears) in leads V_5 and V_6; (iii) diffuse ST elevation, which is part of the LBBB complex and cannot be used to evaluate risk of MI in the presence of the LBBB.

K

- wide QRS V1 V2
- S V5 V6

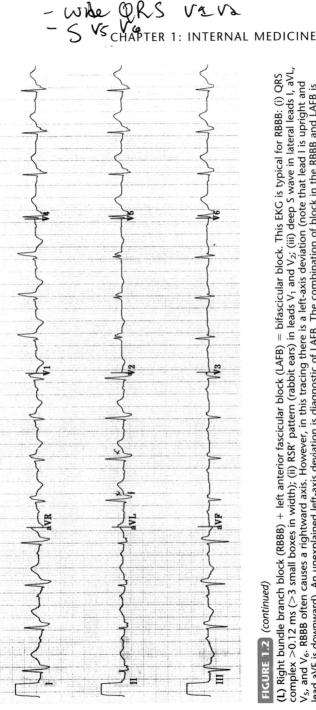

FIGURE 1.2 (continued)

(L) Right bundle branch block (RBBB) + left anterior fascicular block (LAFB) = bifascicular block. This EKG is typical for RBBB: (i) QRS complex >0.12 ms (>3 small boxes in width); (ii) RSR' pattern (rabbit ears) in leads V_1 and V_2; (iii) deep S wave in lateral leads I, aVL, V_5, and V_6. RBBB often causes a rightward axis. However, in this tracing there is a left-axis deviation (note that lead I is upright and lead aVF is downward). An unexplained left-axis deviation is diagnostic of LAFB. The combination of block in the RBBB and LAFB is known as bifascicular block.

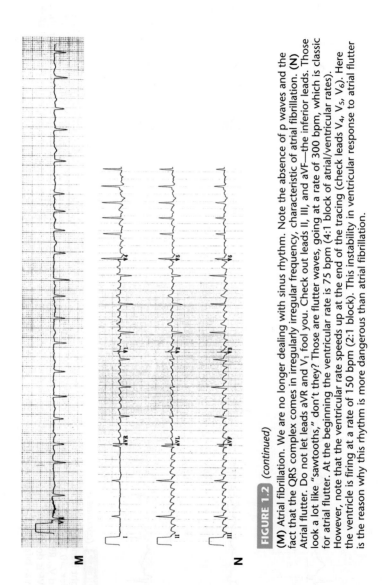

FIGURE 1.2 (continued)

(M) Atrial fibrillation. We are no longer dealing with sinus rhythm. Note the absence of p waves and the fact that the QRS complex comes in irregularly irregular frequency, characteristic of atrial fibrillation. (N) Atrial flutter. Do not let leads aVR and V₁ fool you. Check out leads II, III, and aVF—the inferior leads. Those look a lot like "sawtooths," don't they? Those are flutter waves, going at a rate of 300 bpm, which is classic for atrial flutter. At the beginning the ventricular rate is 75 bpm (4:1 block of atrial/ventricular rates). However, note that the ventricular rate speeds up at the end of the tracing (check leads V₄, V₅, V₆). Here the ventricle is firing at a rate of 150 bpm (2:1 block). This instability in ventricular response to atrial flutter is the reason why this rhythm is more dangerous than atrial fibrillation.

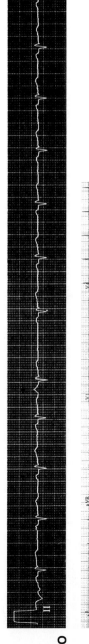

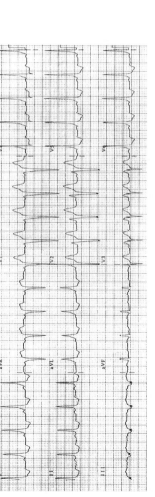

FIGURE 1.2 *(continued)*

(O) Wandering pacemaker. This rhythm strip has an interesting feature. There are three different shapes to the p waves (*asterisks*). The ventricle is being paced by three atrial pacers (probably the SA node and two ectopic pacers). But the ventricular rate is approximately 75 bpm, so this is not a tachycardia. This is a "wandering pacemaker" (slow form of multifocal tachycardia). If the rate were ≥100 bpm, this would be multifocal atrial tachycardia (MFAT). **(P)** Wolff-Parkinson-White (WPW) syndrome. The two characteristic features are shown on this tracing: (i) short PR interval (especially clear in leads I and V_1) and (ii) slurring delta wave connecting the P wave to the QRS complex (especially clear in leads I, aVR, aVL, V_4, V_5, V_6). Note also the prominent ST depressions in leads I, II, aVL, and V_4–V_6, highly concerning for anterolateral ischemia.

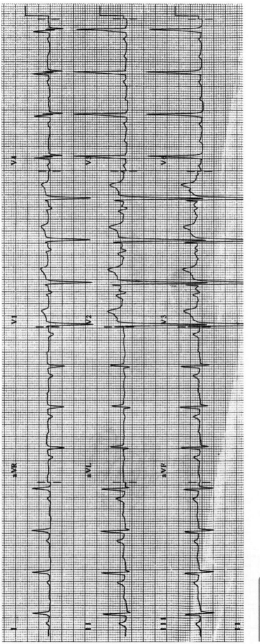

FIGURE 1.2 *(continued)*

(Q) Left ventricular hypertrophy (LVH) 1 left atrial enlargement (LAE) + right atrial enlargement (RAE). R wave in V_5 or V_6 + S wave in V_1 or $V_2 \geq 35$ mm (35 small boxes = 7 large boxes) is diagnostic for LVH. Other LVH criteria (R wave in $V_5 \geq 25$ mm; R wave in aVL ≥ 11 mm) are not present here, but any one of these criteria is diagnostic, and all do not need to be present. The P waves in lead V_1 are impressively depressed; $\geq 1 \times 1$ box depression in the P wave in lead V_1 is diagnostic for LAE. The P waves in lead II are very tall; ≥ 2.5-mm amplitude of the P wave in lead II is diagnostic for RAE.

Q

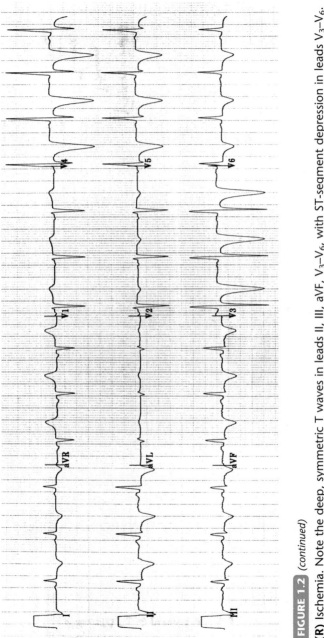

FIGURE 1.2 *(continued)*

(R) Ischemia. Note the deep, symmetric T waves in leads II, III, aVF, V_3–V_6, with ST-segment depression in leads V_3–V_6. This is highly concerning for inferior (II, III, aVF), anterior (V_3–V_4), and lateral (V_5, V_6) ischemia.

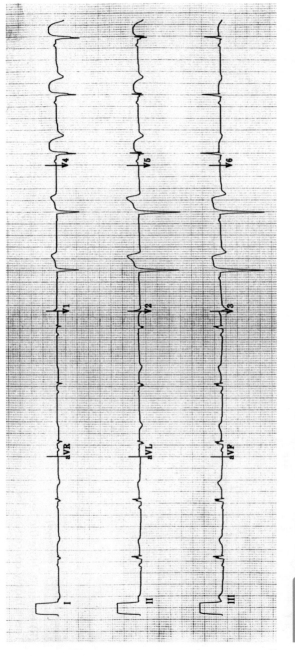

FIGURE 1.2 *(continued)*

(**S**) T-elevation myocardial infarction (STEMI). Note the prominent ST elevations in leads V_2–V_5. The shape of the ST elevations in leads V_3–V_4 is very much like a "tombstone." You can imagine the letters "RIP" being placed there. This is the classic tombstone sign of STEMI. Note also the prominent Q waves in leads V_1–V_5, demonstrating that the MI occurred a number of hours earlier.

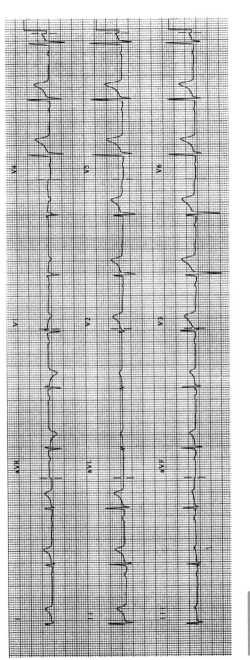

T

FIGURE 1.2 (continued)

(T) "Early repolarization" or "J-point elevation." Not all ST elevations are because of myocardial infarction. The most common cause of ST elevation on EKGs is early repolarization, which is a nml variant that typically is found in young people and in athletes. This tracing was taken from a healthy 29-year-old man. Note that the ST segments cove gently upward concavely. Draw two dots above the ST segments in leads V_2, V_4, V_5, and V_6 and you will see smiley faces staring back at you, with the dots representing the eyes and the ST segments the lips. The smiley face means no MI.

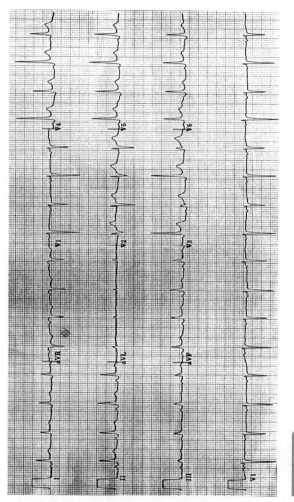

FIGURE 1.2 (continued)

(U) Acute pericarditis. This EKG has several characteristic features of acute pericarditis: (i) diffuse ST elevation; (ii) ST elevations appear more gently sloping in a concave manner—you can almost envision a "smiley face" as they curve concavely upward (in lead V_5 draw two dots above the ST segment, with the dots being the eyes and the ST segment being the lips); (iii) diffuse PR segment depressions in all leads, with reciprocal PR-segment elevation in aVR; (iv) finally, the classic finding of "electrical alternans" (check leads V_1–V_4, and the rhythm strip at the bottom, which is lead V_1), in which there is a beat-to-beat change

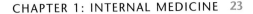

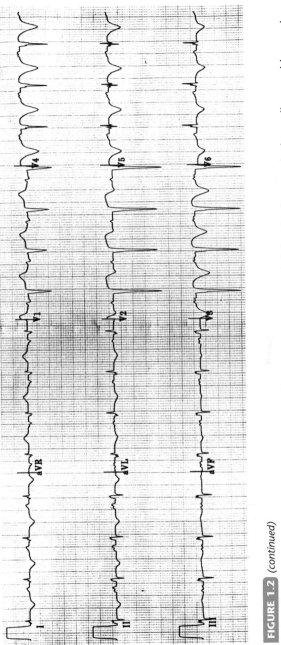

FIGURE 1.2 *(continued)*

(V) Ventricular aneurysm. Yet another cause of ST elevation is a fixed defect in the ventricular wall caused by a prior infarction. This causes the fibrosed segment of the myocardial wall to bulge outward during systole, manifested by ST-segment elevation. EKG is from the same pt whose acute STEMI was shown in Figure 1.2S. This tracing was taken 6 wk after the acute episode, when the pt presented for routine follow-up. Enzymes were checked, and there was no evidence of reinfarction, indicating the likely presence of a ventricular aneurysm, later confirmed by echocardiogram.

b. Rate
  (1) Nml sinus node rate is 60–100 bpm
  (2) Tachycardia = >100 bpm
  (3) Bradycardia = <60 bpm
c. Rhythm
  (1) Nml sinus rhythm = regular rhythm with a rate of 60 to 99 where there is a p in front of every QRS and a QRS after every p (Figure 1.2B)
  (2) Junctional rhythm
    (a) Atrioventricular (AV) node starts firing, causing **narrow QRS complexes in the absence of p waves**
    (b) Nml junctional escape rhythm has a rate of 40–60 bpm; junctional rhythm with rate >60 bpm = "accelerated junctional rhythm," junctional rhythm with rate >100 bpm = "junctional tachycardia" (Figure 1.2C)
  (3) Ventricular rhythm
    (a) Ventricle starts firing in the absence of conduction from above
    (b) **Ventricular beats have very wide QRS complexes**
    (c) Nml rate = 20–40 bpm (= ventricular escape rhythm), ventricular rhythm with rate >40 bpm = "accelerated ventricular rhythm," ventricular rhythm with rate >100 bpm = ventricular tachycardia (Figure 1.2D)
    (d) Ventricular fibrillation (v-fib) = chaotic ventricular rhythm (Figure 1.2E); **this is a medical emergency requiring immediate electrical cardioversion!**
    (e) Torsades de pointes ("twisting of the points") = special form of v-fib in which the axis of the waveforms shifts or twists over time, resulting in a ribbon-like pattern (Figure 1.2E)-associated with medications that cause QT prolongation, such as tricyclic antidepressants, antipsychotics, some antiarrhythmics (e.g., quinidine, procainamide), clarithromycin, erythromycin
  (4) Heart blocks
    (a) First-degree AV block—nml sinus rhythm with PR interval ≥0.2 ms (= 5 small boxes or 1 large box; Figure 1.2F)
    (b) Second-degree, type 1 (Wenckebach) block—PR interval elongates from beat to beat until it become so long that a beat drops (Figure 1.2G)

(c) Second-degree, type 2 (Mobitz) block—PR interval fixed, but there are regular nonconducted p waves leading to dropped beats (Figure 1.2H)

(d) Third-degree block—no relationship between p waves and QRS complexes, typically presents with junctional escape rhythm (Figure 1.2I) or ventricular escape rhythm (Figure 1.2J)

(e) Left bundle branch block (LBBB) (Figure 1.2K)
   (i) QRS complex $\geq$0.12 ms ($\geq$3 small boxes)
   (ii) RSR' (rabbit ears) in V_5 and V_6
   (iii) Diffuse ST elevation that makes it difficult to diagnose MI

(f) Right bundle branch block (RBBB) (Figure 1.2L)
   (i) QRS complex $\geq$0.12 ms ($\geq$3 small boxes)
   (ii) RSR' (rabbit ears) in V_1 and V_2
   (iii) Deep S waves in lateral leads (I, aVL, V_5, V_6)

(g) Left anterior fascicular block (LAFB)—presents with an unexplained left-axis deviation (see Figure 1.2L)

(h) Left posterior fascicular block (LPFB)—presents with an unexplained right-axis deviation

(i) Bifascicular block—RBBB + LAFB, appears like RBBB, but axis is leftward instead of rightward (see Figure 1.2L)

(5) Atrial conduction abnormalities

(a) Atrial fibrillation—irregularly irregular QRS complexes with no p waves visible (Figure 1.2M)

(b) Atrial flutter–atrial "sawtooth" pattern most prominent in inferior leads, with rate of 200–400 bpm (Figure 1.2N)

(c) Atrial ectopy
   (i) Wandering pacemaker = $\geq$3 different p waves with a ventricular rate <100 bmp (Figure 1.2O)
   (ii) Multifocal atrial tachycardia (MFAT) = $\geq$3 different p waves with a ventricular rate >100 bpm

(6) Wolff-Parkinson-White syndrome (Figure 1.2P)

(a) Caused by a "short-circuit" conducting system that bypasses the AV node and allows re-entrant ventricular tachycardia

(b) Short PR interval

(c) Delta wave, which appears like a slurring of the upstroke of the r wave

d. Axis
  (1) If leads I and aVF are upright, the axis is nml
  (2) If lead I is upright and aVF is downward, there is a left-axis deviation (axis $<-30°$)
  (3) If lead I is downward and aVF is upward, there is a right-axis deviation (axis $>90°$)
  (4) If leads I and aVF are downward, there is extreme right-axis deviation (axis $>180°$)
e. Hypertrophy
  (1) Left atrial enlargement (LAE): $>1 \times 1$ box depression in p wave in lead V_1 (Figure 1.2Q)
  (2) Right atrial enlargement (RAE): >2.5 box height of p wave in lead II (see Figure 1.2Q)
  (3) Left ventricular hypertrophy (LVH): S wave in V_1 + R wave in V_5 or $V_6 \geq 35$ mm OR R wave in V_5 or $V_6 \geq 25$ mm or R wave in lead aVL ≥ 11 mm (see Figure 1.2Q)
  (4) Right ventricular hypertrophy (RVH): R wave in $V_1 > 5$ mm
f. Ischemia/infarction
  (1) Ischemia or NSTEMI (subendocardial infarction) presents with deep symmetric T-wave inversions and/or ST depressions ≥ 1 mm (Figure 1.2R)
  (2) Transmural MI presents with ST elevations = STEMI (Figure 1.2S)
  (3) Differential diagnosis of ST elevations—must distinguish these from STEMI
    (a) Most common cause of ST elevation is "early repolarization" (i.e., "J-point elevation")—concave J point on the tracing is the gentle concave upward slope of the transition from the S wave to the ST segment (Figure 1.2T)
    (b) Pericarditis—characteristics include diffuse ST elevations, diffuse PR depressions, PR elevation in lead aVR, electrical alternans (beat-to-beat change in amplitude of R wave; Figure 1.2U)
    (c) Ventricular aneurysm—characteristics include ST elevations concerning for MI but no symptoms and enzymes negative; echocardiogram confirms the presence of the aneurysm, which occurs at the site of a prior MI (Figure 1.2V)
    (d) Prinzmetal's angina (see Section I.B.6)

2. **Atrial Fibrillation (A-fib)** (see Figure 1.2M)
   a. Most common chronic arrhythmia
   b. Etiologies include ischemia, atrial dilation (often from valve dz), surgery (or any systemic trauma), pulmonary dz, toxicity (e.g., thyrotoxicosis, alcohol intoxication, or withdrawal)
   c. Pulse is **irregularly irregular, classic descriptor of atrial fibrillation (a-fib)**
   d. Si/Sx = chest discomfort/palpitations, hypotension/syncope, tachycardia
   e. Complications = diffuse embolization, often to brain, of atrial mural thrombi
   f. Tx
      (1) Rate control with β-blockers, digoxin (not acutely), calcium blockers (e.g., verapamil and diltiazem)
      (2) Convert to nml rhythm (cardioversion) with drugs or electricity
         (a) Drug = IV procainamide (first line), sotalol, or amiodarone
         (b) Electrical → shocks of 100–200 J followed by 360 J
         (c) All pts with a-fib lasting >24 hr should be anticoagulated with warfarin (Coumadin) for 3 wk before electrical cardioversion to prevent embolization during cardioversion
      (3) If conversion to sinus rhythm does not work, treat with long-term anticoagulation unless pt has a contraindication—warfarin is first line, aspirin second

3. **Atrial Flutter** (see Figure 1.2N)
   a. Atrial tachyarrhythmia that is less stable than a-fib
   b. In flutter, the atrium beats at a **slower** rate than in fibrillation (approximately 250–350 bpm in flutter)
   c. However, the ventricular rate in flutter has the potential to go much faster than the ventricular rate in fibrillation, and flutter is considered a more dangerous, more unstable rhythm—medically slowing the atrial rate can ↑ nodal conduction resulting in an ↑ ventricular rate
   d. **The classic rhythm is an atrial flutter rate of 300 bpm with 2:1 block resulting in a ventricular rate of 150 bpm**
   e. Etiologies and Si/Sx are similar to those of a-fib
   f. Complications include syncope, embolization (as in fibrillation), ischemia, and heart failure

    g. The classic EKG finding in flutter is "sawtooth" pattern on EKG (see Figure 1.2N)

    h. Tx

      (1) For stable pts slow ventricular rate with calcium or β-blockers—avoid use of class I agents such as procainamide, which can result in ↑ ventricular rate as the atrial rate slows

      (2) Cardioversion in a nonemergent setting (e.g., pt is stable) requires anticoagulation for 3 wk prior to prevent embolization

      (3) Unstable pts require direct cardioversion, but atrial flutter is easier to convert than fibrillation, so start at 50 J

4. **Multifocal Atrial Tachycardia (MFAT)**

    a. Multiple concurrent pacemakers in the atria, also an irregularly irregular rhythm, usually found in pts with chronic obstructive pulmonary dz

    b. **EKG → tachycardia with ≥3 distinct P waves present in 1 rhythm strip** (Note: if the pt has ≥3 distinct P waves but is not tachycardic, rhythm = wandering pacemaker)

    c. Tx = verapamil; also treat underlying condition

5. **Supraventricular Tachycardia**

    a. Supraventricular tachycardia (SVT) is a "grab bag" of tachyarrhythmias originating "above the ventricle"

    b. Pacer can be in atrium or at AV junction, and multiple pacers can be active at any one time (MFAT)

    c. It can be very difficult to distinguish ventricular tachycardia from SVT if the pt also has a bundle branch block

    d. Tx depends on etiology

      (1) Correct electrolyte imbalance, ventricular rate control (digoxin, Ca^{2+}-channel blocker, β-blocker, adenosine) and electrical cardioversion in unstable pts

      (2) Attempt carotid massage in pts with paroxysmal SVT

      (3) Adenosine breaks >90% of SVT, converting it to sinus rhythm; failure to break a rhythm with adenosine is a potential diagnostic test to rule out SVT

6. **Ventricular Tachycardia (V-tach)** (see Figure 1.2D)

    a. Defined as ≥3 consecutive premature ventricular contractions (PVCs)

    b. Sustained V-tach lasts a minimum of 30 sec, requires immediate intervention because of risk for onset of v-fib (see below)

      c. If hypotension or no pulse is coexistent → defibrillate and treat as v-fib

      d. Tx depends on symptomatology

         (1) If hypotension or no pulse is coexistent → emergency electrical defibrillation, 200–300–360 J

         (2) If pt is aSx and not hypotensive, first-line medical Tx is amiodarone or lidocaine, which can convert rhythm to nml

  7. **Ventricular Fibrillation (V-fib)** (see Figure 1.2E)

      a. Si/Sx = syncope, severe hypotension, sudden death

      b. **Emergent electric countershock is the primary Tx** (very rarely precordial chest thump is effective), converts rhythm 95% of the time (200–300–360 J) if done quickly enough

      c. Second-line Tx is amiodarone or lidocaine

      d. Without Tx, natural course = total failure of cardiac output → death

D. **Congestive Heart Failure (CHF)**

  1. **Etiologies and Definition**

      a. Causes = valve dz, MI (acute and chronic), HTN, anemia, pulmonary embolism (PE), cardiomyopathy, thyrotoxicosis, endocarditis

      b. Definition = cardiac output insufficient to meet systemic demand, can have right-, left-, or both-sided failure

  2. **Si/Sx, and Dx**

      a. Left-sided failure Si/Sx due to ↓ cardiac output and ↑ cardiac pressures = **exertional dyspnea, orthopnea, paroxysmal nocturnal dyspnea,** cardiomegaly, rales, S_3 gallop, renal hypoperfusion → ↑ aldosterone production → sodium retention → ↑ total body fluid → worse heart failure

      b. Right-sided failure Si/Sx because of blood pooling "upstream" from R-heart = ↑ jugular venous pressure (JVP), dependent edema, hepatic congestion with transaminitis, fatigue, weight loss, cyanosis

      c. A-fib common in CHF, ↑ risk of embolization

      d. Dx = echocardiography that reveals ↓ cardiac output

  3. **Tx**

      a. First-line regimen = ACE inhibitor or angiotensin receptor blocker (ARB), β-blocker, diuretics (loop and potassium [K]-sparing), and digoxin

      b. If pt intolerant of ACE inhibition, use a combination of hydralazine and isosorbide dinitrate

    c. **ACE inhibitors and ARBs proven to ↓ mortality in CHF**

    d. β-blockers

       (1) **Proven to ↓ mortality**

       (2) β-blockers should NEVER be started while the pt is in active failure because they can acutely worsen failure

       (3) Add the β-blockers once the pt is diuresed to dry weight and on stable doses of other medicines

    e. **Spironolactone is proven to ↓ mortality in class IV CHF** and presumed to also ↓ mortality in milder CHF (but not yet proven to)—mechanism not entirely clear

    f. Loop diuretics (usually furosemide) are almost always used to maintain dry weight in CHF pts

    g. Digoxin does not improve mortality in CHF but does improve Sx and ↓ hospitalizations

    h. The combination of hydralazine and isosorbide dinitrate is an excellent second-line Tx for pts intolerant of ACE inhibitors because this combination has ALSO been shown to ↓ mortality in CHF; however, in head-to-head trials, the mortality benefit is less than with ACE inhibitors

    i. Beware of giving loop diuretics without spironolactone (a K^+-sparing diuretic), because in the presence of hypokalemia, digoxin can become toxic at formerly therapeutic doses—digoxin toxicity presents as **SVT with AV block and yellow vision** and can be acutely treated with antidigitalis Fab antibodies (Abs) as well as correction of the underlying potassium deficit

E. **Cardiomyopathy (Table 1.8)**

F. **Valvular Dz**

  1. **Mitral Valve Prolapse (MVP)**

    a. Seen in 7% of population; in vast majority is a benign finding in young people that is aSx and eventually disappears

    b. **Murmur: pathologic prolapse → late systolic murmur with midsystolic click (Barlow's syndrome)**, predisposing to regurgitation

    c. Dx = clinical, confirm with echocardiography

    d. Tx not required

  2. **Mitral Valve Regurgitation (MVR)**

    a. Seen in severe MVP, rheumatic fever, papillary muscle dysfunction (often 2° to MI) and endocarditis, Marfan's syndrome

    b. Results in dilation of left atrium (LA), ↑ in LA pressure, leading to pulmonary edema/dyspnea

    c. See Table 1.9 for physical findings

Table 1.8	Cardiomyopathy		
	Dilated	**Hypertrophic**	**Restrictive**
Cause	Ischemic, infectious (HIV, Coxsackie virus, Chagas' dz), metabolic, drugs (alcohol, doxorubicin, azidothymidine)	Genetic myosin disorder	Amyloidosis, scleroderma, hemochromatosis, glycogen storage dz, sarcoidosis
Si/Sx	Right and left heart failure, afib, S₃ gallop, mitral regurgitation **Systolic dz**	Exertional syncope, angina, EKG → left ventricular hypertrophy **Diastolic dz**	Pulmonary HTN, S₄ gallop, EKG → ↓ QRS voltage **Diastolic dz**
Tx	Stop offending agent, once cardiomyopathy onsets, Tx similar to CHF	Implantable cardiac defibrillator	None

  d. Dx = clinical, confirm with echocardiography
  e. Tx = ACE inhibitors, vasodilators, diuretics, consider surgery in severe dz
3. **Mitral Stenosis (MS)**
  a. Almost always because of prior rheumatic fever
  b. ↓ Flow across the mitral valve leads to left atrial enlargement (LAE) and eventually to right heart failure
  c. Si/Sx = dyspnea, orthopnea, hemoptysis, pulmonary edema, a-fib
  d. See Table 1.9 for physical findings
  e. Dx = clinical, confirm with echocardiography
  f. Tx
    (1) β-blockers to slow HR, enabling prolongation of flow of blood across the narrowed valve
    (2) Digitalis to slow ventricle in pts with a-fib
    (3) Anticoagulants for embolus prophylaxis
    (4) Surgical valve replacement for uncontrollable dz
4. **Aortic Regurgitation (AR)**
  a. Seen in endocarditis, rheumatic fever, ventricular septal defect (children), congenital bicuspid aorta, 3° syphilis, aortic dissection, Marfan's syndrome, trauma
  b. **There are three murmurs in AR** (Tables 1.9 and 1.10)

Table 1.9 Summary of Major Murmurs*

Dz	Murmur	Physical Examination
Mitral stenosis	Diastolic apical rumble and opening snap	Feel for right ventricular lift 2° to right ventricular hypertrophy
Mitral valve prolapse	Late systolic murmur with midsystolic click (Barlow's syndrome)	Valsalva → click earlier in systole, murmur prolonged
Mitral regurgitation	High-pitched apical blowing holosystolic murmur radiate to axilla	Laterally displaced point of maximum impulse, systolic thrill
Tricuspid stenosis	Diastolic rumble often confused with mitral stenosis	Murmur louder with inspiration
Tricuspid regurgitation	High-pitched blowing holosystolic murmur at left sternal border	Murmur louder with inspiration
Aortic stenosis (AS)	Midsystolic crescendo-decrescendo murmur at second right interspace, radiates to carotids and apex, with S_4 because of atrial kick, systolic ejection click	Pulsus parvus et tardus = peripheral pulses are weak and late compared with heart sounds, systolic thrill second interspace
Aortic sclerosis	Peaks earlier in systole than AS	None
Aortic regurgitation	Three murmurs: • Blowing early diastolic at aorta and left sternal border • Austin Flint = apical diastolic rumble-like mitral stenosis but no opening snap • Midsystolic flow murmur at base	Laterally displaced point of maximum impulse, wide pulse pressure, pulsus bisferiens (double-peaked arterial pulse); see text for classic physical findings
Hypertrophic subaortic stenosis	Systolic murmur at apex and left sternal border that is poorly transmitted to carotids	Murmur ↑ with standing and Valsalva

*The authors thank Dr. J. Michael Criley and Dr. Richard D. Spellberg for assistance with creation of this table.

Table 1.10	Physical Examination Differential Diagnosis for Murmurs*

Timing	Possible Dz: Differentiating Characteristics			
Midsystolic ("ejection")	**Aortic stenosis/ sclerosis:** crescendo-decrescendo, second right interspace	**Pulmonic stenosis:** second left interspace, EKG → right ventricular hypertrophy	**Any high low state → "flow murmur": aortic regurgitation** (listen for other aortic regurgitation murmurs), **A-S defect** (fixed split S_2), **anemia, pregnancy, adolescence**	
Late systolic	**Aortic stenosis:** worse dz → later peak	**Mitral valve prolapse:** apical murmur	**Hypertrophic subaortic stenosis:** murmur louder with Valsalva	
Holosystolic	**Mitral regurgitation:** radiates to axilla	**V-S defect:** diffuse across precordium	**Tricuspid regurgitation:** louder with inspiration	
Early diastolic	**Aortic regurgitation:** blowing aortic murmur	**Pulmonic regurgitation:** Graham Steell murmur		
Middiastolic	**Mitral stenosis:** opening snap, no change with inspiration	**Aortic regurgitation** (Austin Flint murmur): apical, resembles MS	**A-S defect:** listen for fixed spit S_2, diastolic rumble	**Tricuspid stenosis:** louder with inspiration
Continuous	**Patent ductus:** machinery murmur loudest in back	**Mammary soufflé:** harmless, heard in pregnancy due to ↑ flow in mammary artery	**Coarctation of aorta:** upper/lower extremity pulse discrepancy	**A-V fistula**

*The authors thank Dr. J. Michael Criley and Dr. Richard D. Spellberg for assistance with creation of this table.
A-S defect, atrial-septal defect; A-V, arterio-venous; V-S defect, ventricular-septal defect.

    c. AR has numerous classic signs

      (1) **Water-Hammer pulse** = wide pulse pressure presenting with forceful arterial pulse upswing with rapid falloff

      (2) **Traube's sign** = pistol-shot bruit over femoral pulse

      (3) **Corrigan's pulse** = unusually large carotid pulsations

      (4) **Quincke's sign** = pulsatile blanching and reddening of fingernails upon light pressure

      (5) **de Musset's sign** = head bobbing caused by carotid pulsations

      (6) **Müller's sign** = pulsatile bobbing of the uvula

      (7) **Duroziez's sign** = to-and-fro murmur over femoral artery heard best with mild pressure applied to the artery

    d. Dx = clinical, confirm by echocardiography

    e. Tx

      (1) ↓ Afterload with ACE inhibitors or vasodilators (e.g., hydralazine)

      (2) Consider valve replacement if dz is fulminant or refractory to drugs

5. **Aortic Stenosis (AS)**

    a. Frequently congenital, also seen in rheumatic fever; mild degenerative calcification = AS that is a nml part of aging

    b. Obstructive hypertrophic subaortic stenosis (OHSS)

      (1) Also called "hypertrophic obstructive cardiomyopathy"

      (2) Ventricular septum hypertrophies inferior to the valve

      (3) Stenosis because of septal wall impinging upon anterior leaflet (rarely posterior leaflet) of mitral valve during systole

    c. **Si/Sx = classic triad of syncope, angina, exertional dyspnea**

    d. Dx = clinical, confirm by echocardiography

    e. Tx is surgery for all symptomatic pts who can tolerate it

      (1) Either mechanical or bioprosthesis required; pt anticoagulated chronically after surgery

      (2) Use balloon valvuloplasty of aortic valve for poor surgical candidates

      (3) Pts need endocarditis prophylaxis prior to procedures

      (4) **NEVER give β-blockers or afterload reducers (vasodilators and ACE inhibitors) to pts with AS— peripheral vasculature is maximally constricted to**

> maintain BP, so administration of such agents can cause pt to go into shock

6. **Tricuspid and Pulmonary Valves**
   a. Both undergo fibrosis in carcinoid syndrome
   b. Tricuspid stenosis → **diastolic rumble easily confused with MS, differentiate from MS by ↑ loud with inspiration**
   c. Tricuspid regurgitation → holosystolic murmur differentiated from MS by being louder with inspiration; look for jugular and hepatic systolic pulsations
   d. Pulmonary stenosis → dz of children or in adults with carcinoid syndrome, with midsystolic ejection murmur
   e. Pulmonary regurgitation → develops 2° to pulmonary HTN, endocarditis, or carcinoid syndrome, because of valve ring widening; **Graham Steell murmur** = diastolic murmur at left sternal border, mimicking AR murmur
   f. Tx for stenosis = balloon valvuloplasty; valve replacement rarely done

7. **Endocarditis**
   a. Acute endocarditis usually is caused by *Staphylococcus aureus*
   b. Subacute dz (insidious onset, Sx less severe) usually caused by viridans group *Streptococcus* (oral flora), other *Streptococcus* spp., and *Enterococcus*
   c. Marantic endocarditis is due to CA seeding of heart valves during metastasis—very poor Px, malignant emboli → cerebral infarcts
   d. Culture-negative endocarditis is caused by hard-to-culture organisms known as the HACEK group: **H**aemophilus, **A**ctinobacillus (recently renamed *Aggregatibacter*), **C**ardiobacterium, **E**ikenella, **K**ingella
   e. Prosthetic valve endocarditis often caused by coagulase negative *S. aureus*
   f. Systemic lupus erythematosus (SLE) causes **Libman-Sacks endocarditis;** may be because of autoantibody damage of valves—usually endocarditis is aSx, but murmur can be heard
   g. Si/Sx = splenomegaly, **splinter hemorrhages** in fingernails, **Osler's nodes** (painful red nodules on digits), **Roth spots** (retinal hemorrhages with clear central areas), **Janeway lesions** (dark macules on palms/soles), conjunctival petechiae, brain/kidney/splenic abscesses → focal neurologic findings/hematuria/abd or shoulder pain
   h. Dx based upon the Duke criteria (Table 1.11)

Table 1.11	Duke Criteria for Endocarditis Diagnosis*
Major criteria	1) ⊕ Blood cultures growing common organisms
	2) ⊕ Echocardiogram or onset of new murmur (transesophageal should be used because transthoracic only 50% to 60% sensitive)
Minor criteria	1) Presence of predisposing condition (i.e., valve abnormality)
	2) Fever >38°C
	3) Embolic dz (e.g., splenic, renal, hepatic, cerebral)
	4) Immunologic phenomena (i.e., Roth spots, Osler's nodes)
	5) ⊕ Blood culture × 1 or rare organisms cultured

*Criteria positive two major or one major plus three minor, or five minor criteria are met.

    i. Tx = prolonged antibiotics, 4 to 6 wk typically required (2 wk for uncomplicated *S. viridans* endocarditis)
    j. Empiric Tx often is a combination of a vancomycin for methicillin-resistant *Staphylococcus aureus* (MRSA) and third-generation cephalosporin; then Tx is tailored based upon sensitivities of the organism cultured from blood
    k. Surgery required for: valve ring abscess, CHF from a dysfunctional valve, multiple systemic emboli occur after initiation of antibiotic Tx, if the organism is very difficult to treat (i.e., vancomycin-resistant enterococci [VRE], multidrug resistant *Pseudomonas*, *Aspergillus*, etc.), for prosthetic valve endocarditis, or if the vegetation is >1 cm in diameter

8. **Rheumatic Fever/Heart Dz**
    a. Presents usually in 5- to 15-year-old pts after group A *Streptococcus* infxn
    b. Dx = Jones criteria (two major and one minor)
    c. Major criteria (**mnemonic: J ♥ NES**)
       (1) Joints (migratory polyarthritis), responds to nonsteroidal anti-inflammatory drugs (NSAIDs)
       (2) ♥carditis (pancarditis, Carey-Coombs murmur = middiastolic)
       (3) Nodules (subcutaneous)
       (4) Erythema marginatum (serpiginous skin rash)
       (5) Sydenham's chorea (face, tongue, upper-limb chorea)
    d. Minor criteria = fever, ↑ erythrocyte sedimentation rate (ESR), arthralgia, long EKG PR interval

e. In addition to Jones criteria, need evidence of prior strep infxn by either culture or ⊕ antistreptolysin O (ASO) Ab titers

f. Tx = penicillin

G. Pericardial Dz

1. Pericardial Fluid

a. Pericardial effusion can result from any dz causing systemic edema

b. Hemopericardium is blood in the pericardial sac, often 2° to trauma, metastatic CA, viral/bacterial infxns

c. Both can lead to cardiac tamponade

(1) **Classic Beck's triad: distant heart sounds, distended jugular veins, hypotension**

(2) **Look for pulsus paradoxus, which is ≥10 mm Hg fall in BP during nml inspiration**

(3) EKG shows **electrical alternans**, which is beat-to-beat alternating height of QRS complex (see Figure 1.2U)

d. Dx = clinical, confirm with echocardiography

e. Tx = immediate pericardiocentesis in tamponade; otherwise, treat the underlying condition and allow the fluid to resorb

2. Pericarditis

a. Caused by bacterial, viral, or fungal infxns, also in generalized serositis 2° to rheumatoid arthritis (RA), SLE, scleroderma, uremia

b. Si/Sx = retrosternal pain relieved when sitting up, often following upper respiratory infxn (URI), not affected by activity or food, listen for pleural friction rub

c. **EKG → ST elevation in all leads**, also see PR depression (see Figure 1.2U)

d. Dx = clinical, confirm with echocardiography

e. Tx = NSAIDs for viral, antimicrobial agents for more severe dz, pericardiectomy reserved for recurrent dz

II. Pulmonary

A. Hypoxemia

1. DDx (Table 1.12)

$$PAO_2 = FIO_2 (P_{breath} + P_{H2O}) - (PaCO_2/R)$$

At sea level: $FIO_2 = .21$, $P_{H2O} = 47$, $P_{breath} = 760$:

$$PAO_2 = 150 - (PaCO_2/R)$$

$PaCO_2$ is measured by lab analysis of arterial blood, $R = 0.8$

Table 1.12 Five Mechanisms of Hypoxemia

Cause	PCO_2	$PA\text{-}aO_2$*	Effect of O_2	DLCO	Tx
↓ FIO_2	Nml	Nml	Positive	Nml	O_2
Hypoventilation	↑	Nml	Positive	Nml	O_2
Diffusion impairment	Nml	↑	Positive	↓	O_2
V/Q mismatch	↑ / Nml	↑	Positive	Nml	O_2
Shunt	↑ / Nml	↑	—	Nml	Reverse cause

*PAO_2 gradient (PA-a O_2) ≡ PO_2 in **a**lveoli minus PO_2 in **a**rteries.
Nml gradient = 10, ↑ by 5 to 6 per decade above age 50.

Algorithm 1.1

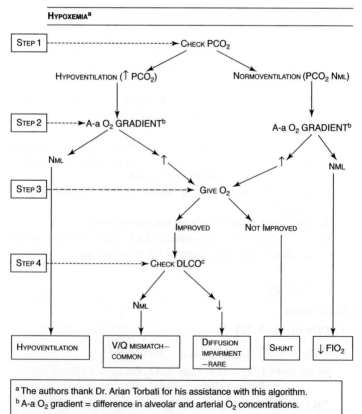

HYPOXEMIA[a]

STEP 1 - → CHECK PCO_2

HYPOVENTILATION (↑ PCO_2)   NORMOVENTILATION (PCO_2 NML)

STEP 2 - - - - - - →A-a O_2 GRADIENT[b]   A-a O_2 GRADIENT[b]

NML   ↑   ↑   NML

STEP 3 - → GIVE O_2

IMPROVED   NOT IMPROVED

STEP 4 - - - - - - - - - - - - →CHECK DLCO[c]

NML   ↓

HYPOVENTILATION | V/Q MISMATCH—COMMON | DIFFUSION IMPAIRMENT—RARE | SHUNT | ↓ FIO_2

[a] The authors thank Dr. Arian Torbati for his assistance with this algorithm.
[b] A-a O_2 gradient = difference in alveolar and arterial O_2 concentrations.
[c] DLCO = diffusion limited carbon monoxide, a measurement of diffusion capacity.

2. **Causes**
   a. Low inspired FIO_2 most often caused by high altitude
   b. Hypoventilation
      (1) Can be because hypopnea ($\downarrow$ respiratory rate) or $\downarrow$ vital capacity
      (2) Hypopnea causes = CNS dz (e.g., because of narcotics, trauma, infxn, etc.)
      (3) $\downarrow$ Vital capacity causes = chest wall neuromuscular dz (e.g., amyotrophic lateral sclerosis, kyphoscoliosis, etc.), airflow obstruction (e.g., sleep apnea), or any parenchymal lung dz
      (4) **Hallmark of hypoventilation is an elevation in carbon dioxide**
   c. Diffusion impairment
      (1) Causes = $\uparrow$ diffusion path (fibrosis) or $\downarrow$ blood transit time through lung ($\uparrow$ cardiac output, anemia)
      (2) Hallmark = $\uparrow$ carbon monoxide diffusing capacity (DLCO)
   d. Ventilation–perfusion (V/Q) inequality causes = PE, parenchymal lung dz (e.g., pneumonia)
   e. R–L shunt
      (1) Causes = pulmonary edema, atelectasis, atrial and ventricular septal defects, and chronic liver dz
      (2) **Hallmark = administration of O_2 does not completely correct the hypoxia**

3. **Presentation**
   a. Sx = tachycardia (very sensitive; primary compensation for hypoxia is to $\uparrow$ tissue blood flow), dyspnea/tachypnea
   b. Si = rales present in some pulmonary parenchymal disorders, clubbing/cyanosis (not just in lung dz but can be correlated to long-term hypoxemic states)

4. **Tx**
   a. In addition to O_2, need to correct underlying disorder
   b. O_2 can be administered by nasal cannula (NC), face mask, continuous positive airway pressure (CPAP), intubation/tracheostomy
   c. Goal of O_2 administration is to $\uparrow$ the fraction of inspired O_2 (FIO_2), which is normally 21% at sea level
      (1) General rule: 1 L/min O_2 $\uparrow$, FIO_2 by 3% (e.g., giving pt 1 L/min O_2 $\rightarrow$ FI O_2 = 24%)
      (2) NC cannot administer >40% FIO_2, even if flow rate is >7 L/min

Table 1.13 Chronic Obstructive Pulmonary Disease

Dz	Characteristics	Tx
Emphysema (pink puffer)	**Dilation of air spaces with alveolar wall destruction** • **Smoking is by far the most common cause;** α_1-antitrpsin deficiency causes **panacinar** dz • Si/Sx = hypoxia, hyperventilation barrel chest, **classic pursed lips breathing**, ↓ breath sounds • CXR → loss of lung markings and **lung hyperinflation** • Dx = clinical	• Ambulatory O_2 including home O_2 • Stop smoking! • Bronchodilators • Steroid pulses for acute desaturations
Chronic bronchitis (blue bloater)	• Defined as **productive cough on most days during ≥3 consecutive mos for ≥2 consecutive yrs** • Si/Sx = as per emphysema but **hypoxia is more severe,** plus pulmonary hypertension with right ventricular hypertrophy, distended neck veins, hepatomegaly • Dx clinical, confirmed by lung bx → ↑ Reid index (gland layer is >50% of total bronchial wall thickness)	As per emphysema, use of antibiotics very controversial
Asthma	• Bronchial hyperresponsiveness → **reversible bronchoconstriction** because of smooth muscle contraction • Usually starts in childhood, in which case it often resolves by age 12, but can start in adulthood • Si/Sx = episodic dyspnea and **expiratory wheezing, reversible with bronchodilation** • Dx = ≥10% ↑ in FEV with bronchodilator Tx • Status asthmaticus (refractory attack lasting for days, can cause death) is a major complication	• Albuterol/ Atrovent inhalers are mainstay • Add inhaled steroids for improved long-term control • Pulse with steroids for acute attacks • Intubate as needed to protect airway
Bronchiectasis	• Permanent abnormal dilation of broncholes commonly because of cystic fibrosis, chronic infxn (often tuberculosis, fungal infxn, or lung abscess), or obstruction (e.g., tumor)	• Ambulatory O_2 • Aggressive antibiotic use for frequent infxns

Table 1.13	*Continued*	
Dz	**Characteristics**	**Tx**
Bronchiectasis *(continued)*	• Si/Sx = foul breath, purulent sputum, hemoptysis, CXR → **tram-track lung markings**, CT → thickened bronchial walls with dilated airways • Dx = clinical with radiologic support	• Consider lung transplant for long-term cure

    (3) Face mask ↑ maximum FIO_2 to 50% to 60%; nonre-breather face mask = maximum FIO_2 to >60%

    (4) CPAP = tightly fitting face mask connected to generator that creates continuous positive pressure, can ↑ maximum FIO_2 to 80%

    (5) Intubation/tracheostomy = maximum FIO_2 to 100%

  d. **Remember that ↑ FIO_2 will not completely correct hypoxemia caused by R–L shunt!** (Because alveoli are not ventilated, and blood will not come in close contact with O_2)

  e. O_2 toxicity seen with FIO_2 >50% to 60% for >48 hr presents with neurologic dz and acute respiratory distress syndrome (ARDS)-like findings

B. **Chronic Obstructive Pulmonary Dz (COPD) (Table 1.13)**

  ↓ forced expiratory volume (FEV)/forced vital capacity (FVC) and Nml/↑ total lung capacity (TLC)

  (FEC at 1 sec/FVC and TLC)

C. **Restrictive Lung Dz and Pleural Effusion (Tables 1.14 and 1.15)**

  Nml/ = FEV/FVC and ↓ **TLC (Figure 1.4)**

D. **Pulmonary Vascular Dz**

  1. **Pulmonary Edema and Acute Respiratory Distress Syndrome (ARDS) (Figure 1.3)**

    a. Si/Sx = dyspnea, tachypnea, resistant hypoxia, diffuse alveolar infiltrate

    b. Differential for pulmonary edema

      (1) **If pulmonary capillary wedge pressure <12 = ARDS**

      (2) **If pulmonary capillary wedge pressure >15 = cardiogenic**

    c. Tx = O_2, diuretics, positive end-expiratory pressure (PEEP) ventilation

Table 1.14 Diagnosis and Treatment of Restrictive Lung Disease

Dz	Characteristics	Tx
↓ Lung tissue	• Causes = atelectasis, airway obstruction (tumor, foreign body), surgical excision	• Ambulate pt • Incentive spirometer to encourage lung expansion • Remove foreign body/tumor
Parenchymal dz	• Causes = inflammatory (e.g., vasculitis and sarcoidosis), idiopathic pulmonary fibrosis, chemotherapy (the **"B's": b**usulfan and **b**leomycin), amiodarone, radiation, chronic infxns (TB, fungal), and toxic inhalation (e.g., asbestos and silica) • Dx = clinical, Bx to rule out infxn	• Antibiotics for chronic infxn • Steroids for vasculitis, sarcoidosis, and toxic inhalations
Interstitial fibrosis	• Chronic injury caused by asbestos, O_2 toxicity, organic dusts, chronic infxn (e.g., TB, fungi, cytomegalovirus, idiopathic pulmonary fibrosis, and collagen-vascular dz) • CXR → **"honeycomb" lung** (Figure 1.4)	• Ambulatory O_2 • Steroids for collagen-vascular dz • Add positive end-expiratory pressure to reducee FIO_2 for O_2 toxicity
Extrapulmonary dz	• Neuromuscular dz (e.g., multiple sclerosis, kyphoscoliosis, amyotrophic lateral sclerosis, Gullain-Barré, spinal cord trauma) • ↑ Diaphragm pressure (e.g., pregnancy, obesity, ascites)	Supportive

Pleural effusion	• ↑ Fluid in the pleural space, transudative or exudative
	• Presents on CXR with bluting of the costophrenic angle and causes dullness to percussion, ↓ tactile fremitus, and ↓ breath sounds on examination
	• Transudate
	  ◊ **Low protein content**
	  ◊ Causes = CHF, nephrotic syndrome, hepatic cirrhosis
	• Exudate
	  ◊ High protein content
	  ◊ Causes = malignancy, pneumonia ("parapneumonic effusion"), collagen-vascular dz, pulmonary embolism
		Thoracentesis (see below)

Table 1.15	Laboratory Analysis of Pleural Effusions	
Study	Transudate	Exudate
Protein	≤3.0 g/dL (≤0.5 of serum)	>3.0 g/dL* (>0.5 of serum)
Lactate dehydrogenase	≤200 IU/L (≤0.6 of serum)	>200 IU/L* (>0.6 of serum)
Specific gravity	≤1.015	>1.015
pH	≥7.2	<7.2 (if ≤ 7.0 = empyema)
Gram stain	No organisms	Any organism → parapneumonic
Cell count	WBC ≤ 1000	WBC > 1000 (lymphocytes → TB)
Glucose	≥50 mg/dL	<50 mg/dL → infxn, neoplasm, collagen-vascular dz
Amylase	↑ in pancreatitis, esophageal rupture, malignancy	
Rheumatoid factor	Titer >1:320 → highly indicative for rheumatoid arthritis	
Antinuclear antibody	Titer >1:160 → highly indicative for systemic lupus erythematosus	

*Either of these findings rules out transudative effusion, rules in exudative effusion.

    d. Purpose of PEEP
      (1) Helps prevent airway collapse in a failing lung
      (2) Expands alveoli for better diffusion, resulting in maintained lung volume (↑ functional residual capacity) and ↓ shunting
 2. **Pulmonary Embolism**
    a. 95% of emboli are from leg deep venous thrombosis (DVT)
    b. Si/Sx = swollen, painful leg, sudden dyspnea/tachypnea, tachycardia, hemoptysis—**often no Sx at all; most emboli are clinically silent**
    c. Risk factors = **Virchow's triad = endothelial cell trauma, stasis, hypercoagulable states** (e.g., nephrotic syndrome, antiphospholipid syndrome, disseminated intravascular coagulation [DIC], tumor, postpartum amniotic fluid exposure,

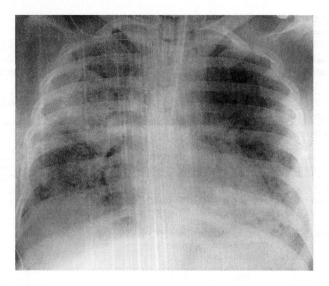

FIGURE 1.3

Adult respiratory distress syndrome (ARDS). There is widespread consolidation of the lungs. This pt had experienced extensive trauma to the limbs. (From Berg D. *Advanced clinical skills and physical diagnosis.* Oxford: Blackwell Science, 1999, with permission.)

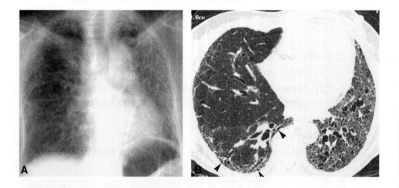

FIGURE 1.4

(A) Reticular and honeycomb pattern in a 73-year-old woman with idiopathic pulmonary fibrosis. Chest radiograph shows asymmetric fine reticular pattern with basal honeycombing. **(B)** Computed tomography shows left-sided predominant reticular abnormality with traction bronchiectasis (*white arrows*) and peripheral subpleural rows of honeycomb cysts (*black arrowheads*). (From Crapo JD, Glassroth J, Karlinsky JB, et al. *Baum's textbook of pulmonary diseases,* 7th Ed. Philadelphia: Lippincott Williams & Wilkins, 2004.)

antithrombin III deficiency, protein C or S deficiency, factor V Leiden deficiency, oral contraceptives, smoking)

    d. PE can cause lung infarctions

        (1) 75% occur in lower lobes

        (2) **Classic CXR finding is "Hampton's hump,"** a wedge-shaped opacification at distal edges of lung fields

    e. EKG findings

        (1) Classically (but rarely) $\rightarrow$ S wave in I, Q in III, inverted T in III ($S_I Q_{III} T_{III}$)

        (2) **Most common finding is simply sinus tachycardia**

    f. Dx = leg Utz to check for DVT, **spiral CT of chest and ventilation/perfusion (V/Q) scan best to rule out PE,** pulmonary angiography (criterion standard)

    g. Tx = prevention with heparin, inferior vena cava (IVC) filter, or warfarin; use tPA thrombolysis in massive PE or hemodynamic compromise

  3. **Pulmonary Hypertension**

    a. Defined as pulmonary pressure $\geq$one fourth systemic (should be one eighth)

    b. Can be active (1° pulmonary dz) or passive (2° to heart dz)

        (1) 1° dz includes idiopathic pulmonary HTN (rare, occurs in young women), chronic obstructive pulmonary dz (COPD), and interstitial restrictive dz

        (2) 2° dz seen in any heart dz, **commonly seen in HIV**

    c. Si/Sx: loud S_2, tricuspid regurgitation, EKG $\rightarrow$ right atrial enlargement, CXR $\rightarrow$ large hilar shadow

    d. Dx = clinical, confirm with heart catheterization

    e. Tx = home O_2 and try intravenous or inhaled prostacyclin

E. **Respiratory Tract CA**

  1. **Epidemiology**

    a. **Number one cause of CA deaths and second most frequent CA**

    b. Can only be seen on x-rays if >1 cm in size; usually by that time they have already metastasized, **so x-rays are not a good screening tool**

    c. Si/Sx = cough, hemoptysis, hoarseness (recurrent laryngeal nerve paralysis), weight loss, fatigue, recurrent pneumonia

  2. **Parenchymal Lung CA (Table 1.16)**

Table 1.16 Parenchymal Lung Cancers

CA	Characteristics
AdenoCA	• **Most frequent lung CA in nonsmokers** • **Presents in subpleura and lung periphery** • Presents in preexisting scars, "scar CA" • Carcinoembryonic antigen (CEA) ⊕, used to follow Tx, not for screening due to ↓ specificity
Bronchoalveolar CA	• Subtype of adenoCA **not related to smoking** • **Presents in lung periphery**
Large cell CA	• **Presents in lung periphery** • Highly anaplastic, undifferentiated CA • Poor prognosis
Squamous cell CA	• **Central hilar masses arising from bronchus** • **Strong link to smoking** • **Causes hypercalcemia because of secretion of PTHrp** (parathyroid hormone-related peptide)

Small cell (oat cell) CA	• **Usually has central hilar location**
	• **Often already metastatic at Dx, very poor Px**
	• **Strong link to smoking (99% are smokers)**
	• Associated with Lambert-Eaton syndrome
	• Causes numerous endocrine syndromes
	  ◊ Adrenocorticotropic hormone secretion (cushingoid)
	  ◊ Secretes antidiuretic hormone, causing syndrome of inappropriate antidiuretic hormone

Bronchial carcinoid tumors	• Carcinoid syndrome = serotonin (5-HT) secretion • **Si/Sx = recurrent diarrhea, skin flushing, asthmatic wheezing, and carcinoid heart dz** • Dx by ↑ 5-HIAA metabolite in urine • Tx = methysergide, a 5-HT antagonist
Lymphangioleiomyomatosis	• Neoplasm of lung smooth muscle → cystic obstructions of bronchioles, vessels, and lymph • **Almost always seen in menstruating women** • Classic presentation = **pneumothorax** • Tx = progesterone or lung transplant

3. **Other CA Syndromes**
   a. **Superior sulcus tumor (Pancoast tumor)** (Figure 1.5A)
      (1) **Horner's syndrome** (ptosis, miosis, anhydrosis) by damaging the sympathetic cervical ganglion in the lower neck (Figure 1.5B), often associated with Pancoast tumor

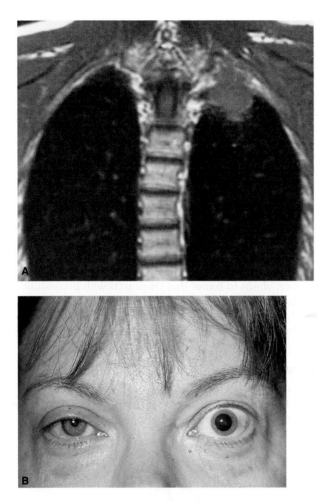

FIGURE 1.5

(A) Pancoast tumor. This CA of the lung can be seen invading the root of the neck on this coronal MRI scan (T1-weighted). **(B)** Horner's syndrome. The right eye has ptosis and miosis (compare pupil size with the dilated left pupil). (From Tasman W, Jaeger E. *The Wills eye hospital atlas of clinical ophthalmology*, 2nd Ed. Baltimore: Lippincott Williams & Wilkins, 2001).

Table 1.17	Mediastinal Tumors (Figure 1.6)	
Anterior*	**Middle**	**Posterior†**
Thymoma	Lymphoma	Neuroblastoma
Thyroid tumor	Pericardial cyst	Schwannoma
Teratoma	Bronchial cyst	Neurofibroma
Terrible lymphoma Tx = excision for all, add radiation/chemotherapy as needed		

*The four Ts.
†Neural tumors.

(2) **Superior vena cava (SVC) syndrome** = obstructed SVC → facial swelling, cyanosis, and dilation of veins of head and neck

b. Small cell CA can cause a **myasthenia gravis-like condition known as the Lambert-Eaton syndrome** because of induction of Abs to tumor that crossreacts with presynaptic calcium (Ca) channel

c. Renal cell CA metastatic to lung can cause 2° polycythemia by ectopic production of erythropoietin (EPO)

F. **Mediastinal Tumors (Table 1.17; Figure 1.6)**

G. **Tuberculosis**

 1. **1° tuberculosis (TB)**

 a. Classically affects lower lobes (bacilli deposited in dependent portion of lung during inspiration)

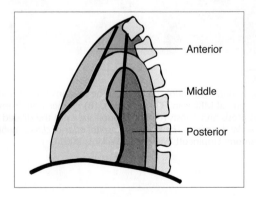

— Anterior

— Middle

— Posterior

FIGURE 1.6 **Mediastinal compartments.**

   b. Usually aSx
   c. **Classic radiologic finding is "Ghon complex"** = calcified nodule at primary focus $\oplus$ calcified hilar lymph nodes

2. **2° (Reactivation) TB**
   a. Reactivates in **apical lung** due to $\uparrow$ O_2 tension in upper lobes
   b. Si/Sx = insidious fevers, night sweats, weight loss, cough, hemoptysis, upper lobe infiltration, scarring, and/or cavities on CXR (Figure 1.7)
   c. Risk factors = HIV, imprisonment, homelessness, malnourishment, geography (immigrants from Latin America, Africa, Eastern Europe, Asia except for Japan are all high risk)

3. **Miliary (Disseminated) TB**
   a. An acute, hematogenous **dissemination involving any organ**
   b. Often in pts with immune deficiency
   c. Pts appear acutely ill and toxic on top of chronic illness
   d. CXR shows a fine, millet seedlike appearance (i.e., micronodular infiltrates) throughout all the lung fields (Figure 1.8)

4. Classic Chronic Extrapulmonary Reactivation Syndromes
   a. Pott's dz = TB of spine; presents with multiple compression fractures
   b. Scrofula = TB causing massive cervical lymphadenopathy
   c. Terminal ideal inflammation and colitis; mimicking Crohn's disease
   d. Serous dz = chronic lymphocyte-predominant effusions of pleural space, pericardial space (associated with chronic constrictive pericarditis), or peritoneum (lymphocyte-prodominant ascites)
   e. Meningitis = chronic, lymphocyte predominant pleocytosis in cerebrospinal fluid (CSF)

5. **Dx and Tx**
   a. Latent infxn
      (1) Defined by positive purified protein derivative (PPD) or interferon-γ (IFN-γ) production in peripheral blood tests (e.g., Quantiferon test)
      (2) No Si/Sx of active dz and no active dz on CXR
      (3) PPD and blood IFN-γ tests are **screening tests for latent infxn**, not Dx tests for active TB
      (4) Guidelines for interpretation of PPD
         (a) $\geq$5-mm induration is positive if the pt:
            (i) Has HIV

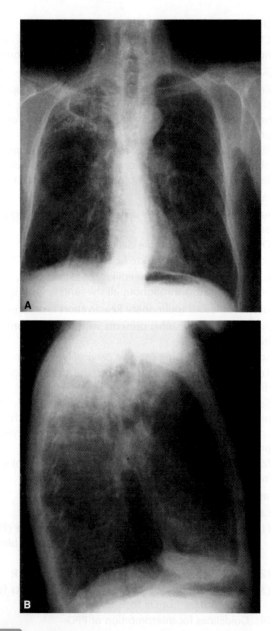

FIGURE 1.7

CXR in reactivation tuberculosis, showing hilar adenopathy and right upper lobe cavitation and scarring. (From Crapo JD, Glassroth J, Karlinsky JB, et al. *Baum's textbook of pulmonary diseases*, 7th Ed. Philadelphia: Lippincott Williams & Wilkins, 2004.)

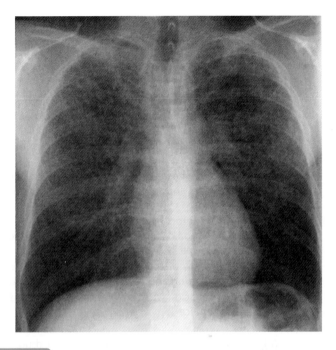

FIGURE 1.8

CXR showing miliary tuberculosis of the lung. (From Crapo JD, Glassroth J, Karlinsky JB, et al. *Baum's textbook of pulmonary diseases*, 7th Ed. Philadelphia: Lippincott Williams & Wilkins, 2004.)

        (ii) Has been in close contact with someone with active TB

        (iii) Has fibrotic changes on CXR consistent with old TB

        (iv) Is taking immunosuppressive medicines (e.g., >15 mg/day of prednisone for >1 month, cyclosporin, etc.)

    (b) ≥10-mm induration is positive if the pt:

        (i) Is a recent immigrant from a high-risk country (most developing countries)

        (ii) Is an injection drug user

        (iii) Works or resides in a prison/jail, nursing home, health care facility, or homeless shelter

        (iv) Has a chronic debilitating illness such as renal failure, CA, or diabetes mellitus

    (c) ≥15-mm induration is positive test if the pt does not meet any of the above categories

  (5) Tx of latent infxn is isoniazid × 9 mos (alternate regimens should only be given by specialists)

b. Active infxn

  (1) To reiterate a point made above: **PPD is not intended as a Dx test for active TB**—it is commonly falsely negative in pts with active dz, and a ⊕ test only indicates latent infxn, not active dz; thus, it is neither sensitive nor specific for active dz

  (2) Active infxn is Dx based on three components: clinical assessment, CXR, and sputum (or other body fluid if extrapulmonary dz is considered)

    (a) Clinical indicators of active dz include subacute/chronic cough, night sweats, weight loss, hemoptysis, etc.

    (b) CXR indicators of active dz include upper lobe infiltrates or scarring and cavitary lesions in a pt with Sx

    (c) Sputum for acid-fast staining and culture is the Dx study of choice

  (3) Tx

    (a) For routine cases, start regimen with four drugs: isoniazid, rifampin, ethambutol, and pyrazinamide

    (b) Narrow regimen based on sensitivities of culture organism

    (c) If drug resistance is a concern, start with a minimum of six drugs, at least one of which is injectable

    (d) Treat for a minimum of 6 mos for lung dz, typically longer for extrapulmonary dz

    (e) Tx should be given by specialists in TB care

H. **Pneumonia**

1. Community Acquired Pneumonia (CAP)

  a. Can affect healthy outpts or those with chronic dz

  b. See Table 1.18 for typical and atypical causes

  c. Si/Sx = cough, dyspnea, tachypnea, fever, rales on exam

  d. Dx

    (1) Dx = CXR showing pneumonia in the presence of appropriate Si/Sx

    (2) Sputum Gram stain and culture may help identify bacterial causes, enabling targeted antibiotics

Table 1.18   Community Acquired Pneumonia

Organism	Characteristics
Typical Bacterial Community Acquired Pneumonia (CAP)	
Streptococcus pneumoniae	• **Most commonly identified cause of** CAP • **Pts with HIV have 100-fold ↑ risk** • Also ↑ risk in the elderly, and in alcoholics, asplenic pts, and pts with B-cell/antibody deficiencies • Classic sign is severe shaking rigors • Can cause acutely fatal pneumonia even in otherwise healthy young pts
Hemophilus influenzae	• Less common in the era of vaccination against this bacterium
Moraxella catarrhalis	• Presents with mild to moderate CAP
Klebsiella pneumoniae	• The only Gram-negative rod that typically causes CAP • Typically presents in an alcoholic or diabetic pt • Often with hemoptysis, classically find a bulging upper lobe consolidation, often with cavitation
Staphylococcus aureus	• Not a typical cause of CAP • Can cause pneumonia during or after influenza infxn—the virus denudes the airways, allowing *S. aureus* to penetrate down to the alveolae • In some parts of the country, methicillin-resistant *S. aureus* (MRSA) is causing CAP even in pts without prior influenza
Atypical CAP *Legionella pneumonia*	• Can cause very severe CAP, requiring ICU care • A hallmark is concurrent CAP + diarrhea • Often with high lactate dehydrogenase (LDH) (>400) and low serum sodium
Mycoplasma pneumonia	• The classic cause of "walking pneumonia," mild but nagging for weeks • Classically seen in teenagers or young adults living in close quarters; e.g., college dormitory, military barracks, summer camp, etc. • Associated with cold agglutinins and hemolysis, and with erythema multiforme
Chlamydophila pneumoniae	• Typically causes mild CAP
Chlamydia psittaci	• Causes psittacosis, mild to moderate CAP • Contracted from birds (often parrots), and the birds may also show signs of illness (ruffled feathers)

(continued)

Table 1.18 *Continued*

Organism	Characteristics
Fungal Pneumonia	
Pneumocystis jiruveci	• Still called PCP (*Pneumocystis* pneumonia) • Almost always in a pt with HIV—can be seen in pts on corticosteroids • Insidious onset of dry cough/dyspnea, bilateral infiltrates, not pleural effusions, high LDH almost always seen • Dx → sputum silver stain • Tx → TMP-SMX, add prednisone if $PO_2 < 70$ or A-a gradient ≥ 35
Coccidioides immitis	• "San Joaquin Valley Fever," major risks = travel to southwest desert (e.g., California, Arizona, New Mexico, Texas), imprisonment, ↑ incidence after earthquakes • Filipinos and African American pts have ↑ rate of disseminated dz • Dx by serum antibody test • Tx = fluconazole
Histoplasma capsulatum	• Seen in the Midwest and South, particularly in the areas of the Ohio/Mississippi River Valleys • Can acquire from exposure to bat or bird dung • Typically aSx • Can cause severe reactivation dz in pts with HIV or other immune-suppressives (e.g., corticosteroids) • Tx = itraconazole or amphotericin
Blastomyces dermatiditis	• Rare cause of pneumonia, seen in areas overlapping *Histoplasma*, but a denser endemicity in the St. Lawrence River Valley in the northeast • Can cause acute, fulminant pneumonia in immunocompromised host • Can cause chronic, scarring pneumonia over years • Often associated with skin lesions • Tx = amphotericin
Cryptococcus neoformans	• Causes pneumonia in immunocompromised, often HIV or steroids • Can appear like pneumocystis pneumonia in an AIDS pt, can also cause focal consolidation, nodules, or cavities • Always perform lumbar puncture to determine if meningitis is coexistent • Tx is fluconazole or amphotericin

Table 1.18	*Continued*
Organism	**Characteristics**
Anaerobes Typically oral flora	• "Aspiration pneumonia," typically seen in pts with altered mental status, on drugs, status post seizure, etc. • Presents with foul smelling sputum, abscess seen on CXR • Tx with clindamycin or metronidazole + cephalosporin
Viral Influenza	• The most common cause of viral pneumonia • Particular problem in the elderly or immunocompromised • Initiation of amantadine, oseltamivir, or zanamavir within the first 48 hrs can shorten duration and lessen severity of dz

   (3) Blood cultures positive 10% of cases—important to check these to identify bacterial cause
   (4) Check an HIV test in all pts with CAP as a matter of routine
  e. Tx
   (1) Empiric Tx is with either:
       (a) A third-generation cephalosporin (e.g., ceftriaxone/cefotaxime) plus either doxycycline or a second-generation macrolide (e.g., clarithromycin or azithromycin); OR
       (b) Monotherapy with a respiratory fluoroquinolone (e.g., levofloxacin, moxifloxacin, gatifloxacin, gemifloxacin)
   (2) If the pt has been recently exposed to antibiotics, consider adding broader coverage for drug-resistant pathogens
   (3) Narrow Tx based on culture results
   (4) See Table 1.18 for Tx of fungal, viral, or anaerobic pneumonia
 2. Health Care Associated Pneumonia (HCAP) and Hospital Acquired Pneumonia (HAP)
  a. In contrast to CAP, the most common causes are drug-resistant Gram-negative rods (GNR), such as *Pseudomonas* and *Acinetobacter*, and MRSA
  b. Dx is also by chest x-ray, but it is critical to obtain sputum Gram stain/culture or bronchoscopy to target antibiotics to appropriate organism

    c. Tx is with broad spectrum Gram-negative and Gram-positive agents, typically vancomycin plus (ceftazidime or piperacillin-tazobactam or imipenem or meropenem, etc.)

III. Gastroenterology and Hepatology

A. **Gastroesophageal Dz**

  1. **Chronic Gastritis (Atrophic Gastritis)**

    a. Type A (fundal) = autoimmune (pernicious anemia, thyroiditis, etc.)

    b. Type B (antral) because of *Helicobacter pylori (H.p.)*, NSAIDs, herpes, cytomegalovirus (CMV)

    c. Si/Sx = usually aSx, may cause pain, nausea/vomiting, anorexia, upper GI bleeding manifested as coffee grounds emesis or hematemesis

    e. Dx = upper endoscopy

    f. *H. pylori* infxn Dx by urease breath test; can screen with serum IgG test (less expensive but less sensitive and does not necessarily indicate active infxn), can confirm with endoscopic Bx

    g. Tx depends on etiology

      (1) Tx *H. pylori* with proton pump inhibitor + 2 antibiotics (e.g., amoxicillin + clarithromycin) + bismuth compound

      (2) If drug induced, stop offending agent (usually NSAIDs), add sucralfate, H_2 blocker, or proton pump inhibitor

      (3) Pernicious anemia Tx = vitamin B_{12} replenishment

      (4) Stress ulcer (especially in ICU setting), Tx with sucralfate or H_2 blocker IV infusion

  2. **Gastric Ulcer (GU)**

    a. *H. pylori* found in 70% of Gus; 10% caused by ulcerating malignancy

    b. Si/Sx = gnawing/burning pain in midepigastrium, **worse with food intake;** if ulcer erodes into artery can cause hemorrhage and peritonitis, may be guaiac positive

    c. Dx = endoscopy with Bx to confirm not malignant, *H. pylori* testing as above

    d. Tx = mucosal protectors (e.g., bismuth, sucralfate, misoprostol), H_2 blockers or proton pump inhibitors and antibiotics for *H. pylori*

B. **Small Intestine**

1. **Duodenal Ulcer (Peptic Ulcer)**
   a. *H. pylori* found in 90% of duodenal ulcers
   b. Smoking and excessive alcohol intake ↑ risk
   c. Sx/Si = burning or gnawing epigastric pain 1 to 3 hr post-prandial, **relieved by food/antacids;** pain typically awakens pt at night; melena
   d. Dx = endoscopy, barium swallow if endoscopy is unavailable
   e. Tx = as for gastric ulcer above, quit smoking
   f. Sequelae
      (1) Upper GI bleed
         (a) Usually see hematemesis, melena, or (rarely) hematochezia if briskly bleeding ulcer
         (b) Dx with endoscopy
         (c) Tx = endoscopic coagulation or sclerosant; surgery rarely necessary
      (2) Perforation
         (a) Change in pain pattern is suspicious for perforation
         (b) Plain abd films may show free air, can perform upper GI series with water-soluble contrast (barium contraindicated)
         (c) Tx is emergency surgery

2. **Crohn's Dz (Inflammatory Bowel Dz)**
   a. GI inflammatory dz that may be infectious in nature
   b. Affects any part of GI from mouth to rectum, but usually the intestines
   c. Si/Sx = abd pain, diarrhea, malabsorption, fever, stricture causing obstruction, fistulae; see below for extraintestinal manifestations
   d. Dx = colonoscopy with Bx of affected areas → transmural, **noncaseating granulomas, cobblestone mucosal morphology, skip lesions, creeping fat on gross dissection is pathognomonic**
   e. Tx
      (1) Sulfasalazine better for colonic dz but also helps in small bowel
      (2) Steroids for acute exacerbation, but no effect on underlying dz

  (3) Immunotherapy (azathioprine and mercaptopurine)—useful in pts with unresponsive dz
  (4) Newest Tx is antitumor necrosis factor Tx, with infliximab or etanercept

3. Carcinoid Syndrome

  a. APUDoma (**a**mine **p**recursor **u**ptake and **d**ecarboxylate)
  b. Occurs most frequently in the appendix
  c. Carcinoid results from liver metastases that secrete serotonin (5-HT)
  d. Si/Sx = flushing, watery diarrhea and abd cramps, bronchospasm, right-sided heart valve lesions
  e. Dx = ↑ levels of urine 5-hydroxyindoleacetic acid (5-HIAA) (false ⊕ seen if pt eats many bananas)
  f. Tx = somatostatin and methysergide

C. Large Intestine

1. Ulcerative Colitis (Inflammatory Bowel Dz)

  a. Idiopathic autoinflammatory disorder of the colon
  b. Always starts in rectum and spreads proximal
  c. If confined to rectum = ulcerative proctitis, a benign subtype
  d. Si/Sx = bloody diarrhea, colicky abd pain, can progress to generalized peritonitis, watch for toxic megacolon
  e. Dx = colonoscopy with bx → crypt abscess with numerous polymorphonuclear leukocytes (PMNs), friable mucosal patches that bleed easily
  f. Tx depends on site and severity of dz
    (1) Distal colitis → topical mesalamine and corticosteroids
    (2) Moderate colitis (above sigmoid) → oral steroids, mesalamine, and sulfasalazine
    (3) Severe colitis → IV steroids, cyclosporine, and surgical resection if unresponsive
    (4) Fulminant colitis (rapidly progressive) → broad-spectrum antibiotics
  g. Comparison of inflammatory bowel dz (Table 1.19)

D. Liver

1. Jaundice

  a. Visible when serum bilirubin exceeds 2 mg/dL
  b. Congenital hyperbilirubinemia (Table 1.20)
  c. Hemolytic anemias
    (1) Excess production → ↑ unconjugated bilirubin

Table 1.19 Comparison of Inflammatory Bowel Disease

	Ulcerative Colitis	Crohn's Dz
Location	Isolated to colon	Anywhere in GI tract
Lesions	Contiguously proximal from colon	Skip lesions, disseminated
Inflammation	Limited to mucosa/ submucosa	Transmural
Neoplasms	Very high risk for development	Lower risk for development
Fissures	None	Extend through submucosa
Fistula	None	Frequent: can be enterocutaneous
Granulomas	None	Noncaseating are characteristic
Extraintestinal manifestations	Seen in both: • Arthritis, iritis, erythema nodosum, pyoderma gangrenosum • Sclerosing cholangitis = chronic, fibrosing, inflammation of biliary system leading to cholestasis and portal hypertension	

Table 1.20 Congenital Hyperbilirubinemia

Syndrome	Characteristics	Tx
Gilbert's	• Mild defect of glucoronyl transferase in 5% of population • Si/Sx = ↑ serum **unconjugated bilirubin** → jaundice in stressful situations, completely benign	None required
Crigler-Najjar	• Genetic deficiency of glucuronyl transferase → ↑ serum **unconjugated bilirubin** • Type 1 = severe, presents in neonates with ↑ bilirubin levels → death from kernicterus by age 1 • Type 2 = mild, pts experience no severe clinical deficits	Phenobarbital
Dubin-Johnson	• ↑ **Conjugated bilirubin** because of defective bilirubin excretion • Si/Sx = jaundice, liver turns black, no serious clinical deficits	None required
Rotor	• ↑ **Conjugated bilirubin** similar to Dubin-Johnson • Defect is in bilirubin storage, not excretion	None required

   (2) Si/Sx = as per any anemia (weakness, fatigue, etc.), others depend on etiology of hemolytic anemia (see Hematology)
   (3) Dx = $\oplus$ Coombs' test, $\downarrow$ haptoglobin, $\oplus$ urine hemosiderin
   (4) Tx depends on etiology (see Hematology)
d. Intrahepatic cholestasis (hepatocellular)
   (1) May be because of viral hepatitis or cirrhosis
   (2) May be because of drug-induced hepatitis (acetaminophen, methotrexate, oral contraceptives, phenothiazines, isoniazid [INH], fluconazole)
   (3) Dx = $\uparrow$ transaminases, liver Bx to confirm hepatitis
   (4) Tx = cessation of drugs, or supportive for viral infxn
e. Extrahepatic
   (1) Myriad causes include choledocholithiasis (but not cholelithiasis), CA of biliary system or pancreas, cholangitis, biliary cirrhosis
   (2) 1° biliary cirrhosis (see Section 3 below)
   (3) 2° biliary cirrhosis results from long-standing biliary obstruction due to any cause (e.g., cholangitis)
   (4) Sclerosing cholangitis
      (a) Primary sclerosing cholangitis is an idiopathic inflammatory condition in which bile ducts are destroyed, leading to fibrosis and hepatic cirrhosis
      (b) Strong correlation exists between primary sclerosing cholangitis and ulcerative colitis
      (c) Many pts are aSx and are diagnosed by an isolate abnormal alkaline phosphatase on laboratories
      (d) Some pts present with pruritus and jaundice
      (e) Eventually liver failure develops with transaminitis and hyperbilirubinemia
      (f) Dx made by endoscopic retrograde cholangiopancreaticoduodenoscopy (ERCP), showing "beads on a string" appearance of the bile ducts, because of strictures separated by dilated ducts
      (g) 2° sclerosing cholangitis can be because of chronic infxns (often in the setting of HIV), drugs, etc.
      (h) Tx = liver transplantation
   (5) Si/Sx of acquired jaundice = acholic stools (pale), urinary bilirubin, fat malabsorption, pruritus, $\uparrow$ serum cholesterol, xanthomas

      (6) Dx may require abd CT or ERCP to rule out malignancy or obstruction of bile pathway

      (7) Tx depends on etiology

2. **Hepatitis**

    a. General Si/Sx = jaundice, abd pain, diarrhea, malaise, fever, ↑ aspartate aminotransferase (AST), and alanine aminotransferase (ALT)

    b. Dx and Tx (Table 1.21)

3. 1° biliary cirrhosis

    a. Autoimmune disorder usually seen in women

    b. Si/Sx = jaundice, pruritus, hypercholesterolemia; **antimitochondrial Ab test is 90% sensitive**

    c. Dx = clinical ⊕ serology, confirm with bx

    d. Tx = liver transplant, otherwise supportive

4. **Cirrhosis**

    a. Most commonly because of alcoholism or chronic hepatitis B virus (HBV) or hepatitis C virus (HCV) infxn; also 1° biliary cirrhosis, other chronic hepatic dz (e.g., sclerosing cholangitis, Wilson's dz, hemochromatosis, etc.)

    b. Si/Sx = purpura and bleeding ↑ and prothrombin time (PT)/partial thromboplastin time (PTT), jaundice, ascites 2° to to ↓ albumin and portal HTN, spontaneous bacterial peritonitis, encephalopathy, asterixis

    c. Ascites differential (Table 1.22)

    d. Spontaneous bacterial peritonitis

      (1) Usually low protein ascites

      (2) Si/Sx can be very subtle, in some cases even without abd pain; fever is variable

      (3) Common organisms include *Escherichia coli*, *Klebsiella*, *Enterococcus*, and *Streptococcus pneumoniae*

      (4) Tx = ceftriaxone or cefotaxime, plus IV albumin to maintain renal perfusion pressure

    e. Encephalopathy

      (1) Because of ↑ levels of toxins, likely related to ammonia, but ammonia levels do not correlate well with encephalopathy

      (2) Flapping tremor of the wrist upon extension*

      (3) Tx of encephalopathy is to lower ammonia levels

        (a) Lactulose metabolized by bacteria, acidifies the bowel, $NH_3 \rightarrow NH_4^+$, which cannot be absorbed

        (b) Neomycin kills bacteria-making NH_3 in gut

Table 1.21 Hepatitis Diagnosis and Treatment

Type	Characteristics	Tx
Fulminant	• Complications of acute hepatitis, progresses over <4 wk • Can be 2° to viral hepatitis, drugs (isoniazid), toxins, and some metabolic disorders; e.g., Wilson's dz • Elevated prothrombin time and hepatic encephalopathy	Urgent liver transplant
Viral	• Hepatitis A virus (HAV) → fecal-oral transmission, transient flulike illness • Hepatitis B (HBV) and C (HCV) → blood transmission, HBV also sex and vertical → chronic hepatitis • 5% to 10% of HBV and >50% of HCV infxn → chronic • Dx = serologies (Figure 1.9) and ↑ alanine aminotransferase (ALT) and aspartate aminotransferase (AST) ◊ HBV surface antigen = active infxn ◊ anti-HBV surface antibody = immunity ◊ anti-HBV core antibody = exposed, not necessarily immune ◊ HBV e antigen = highly infectious ◊ HCV antibody = exposure, not immune	HAV—none HBV—interferon or antiviral (lamivudine, adefovir, entecavir) HCV—interferon plus ribavirin
Granulomatous	• Causes = TB, fungal (e.g., *Coccidioides*, *Histoplasma*), sarcoidosis, brucella, rickettsia, syphilis, leptospirosis • Dx = liver bx	Antibiotics, prednisone for sarcoidosis
Alcoholic	• Most common form of liver dz in U.S. • Si/Sx = as per other hepatitis with specific alcohol signs = palmar erythema, Dupuytren's contractures, spider angiomas, gynecomastia, caput medusae • Dx = clinical ↑ AST and ALT, and AST/ALT = 2:1 is highly suggestive	Cessation of alcohol can reverse dz if early in course; otherwise → cirrhosis and only Tx is transplant
Autoimmune	• Type I occurs in young women, ⊕ antinuclear antibody, ⊕ anti-smooth muscle Ab • Type II occurs mostly in children, linked to Mediterranean ancestry, ⊕ anti–liver-kidney-muscle (anti-LKM) antibody • Si/Sx as for any other hepatitis	Tx = prednisone ± azathioprine

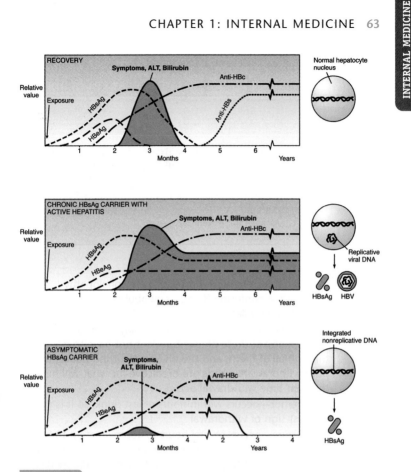

FIGURE 1.9

Typical serologic events in three distinct outcomes of hepatitis B. (*Top panel*) In most cases, the appearance of anti-HBs ensures complete recovery. Viral DNA disappears from the nucleus of the hepatocyte. (*Middle panel*) In about 10% of cases of hepatitis B, HBs antigenemia is sustained for longer than 6 mos, because of the absence of anti-HBs. Pts in whom viral replication remains active, as evidenced by sustained high levels of HBeAg in the blood, develop active hepatitis. In such cases, the viral genome persists in the nucleus but is not integrated into host DNA. (*Lower panel*) Pts in whom active viral replication ceases or is attenuated, as reflected in the disappearance of HBeAg from the blood, become aSx carriers. In these individuals, fragments of the HBV genome are integrated into the host DNA, but episomal DNA is absent. (From Rubin E, Farber JL. *Pathology*, 3rd Ed. Philadelphia: Lippincott Williams & Wilkins, 1999.)

Table 1.22 Ascites Differential Diagnosis

	Portal HTN	No Portal HTN
Serum/ascites albumin gradient (SAAG)	≥1.1 g/dL	<1.1 g/dL
Causes	Cirrhosis, alcoholic hepatitis, nephrosis, Budd-Chiari, CHF	Pancreatic dz, TB, peritoneal metastases, idiopathic
Other labs	Ascites total protein >2.5 → heart dz Ascites total protein ≤2.5 → liver dz	Amylase ↑ in pancreatic dz

(4) Watch for Wernicke-Korsakoff's encephalopathy (triad = confusion [largely confabulation], ataxia, ophthalmoplegia)

f. Alcohol withdrawal has four phases—any given pt can go through any of these phases but does not have to go through all of them, and the phases occurring during a prior withdrawal episode are predictive for what will happen the next time withdrawal occurs

(1) Tremor—occurs within hours of last drink, so it is the first sign of withdrawal

(2) Seizure—occurs several hours to approximately 48 hr after the last drink; seizures can be fatal and are best Tx with benzodiazepines, not standard antiseizure medicines

(3) Hallucinosis—occurs 48 to 72 hr after the last drink; this is NOT delirium tremens (DTs), but rather is simply auditory or tactile hallucinations, also best Tx with benzodiazepines

(4) DTs—at approximately 72 hr after the last drink, the autonomic instability that defines DTs begins with dangerous tachycardia and hypertension and can be accompanied by each of the other three phases (tremor, seizure, hallucinosis)—the autonomic instability is also best Tx with benzodiazepines

g. Tx of inpt alcoholics

(1) IV thiamine and B_{12} supplements to correct deficiency (very common)

(2) Give IV glucose, fluids, and electrolytes

(3) Correct any underlying coagulopathy

(4) Benzodiazepine for prevention and Tx of DTs

5. Hepatic Abscess

a. Caused by (in order of frequency in the US) bacteria, parasites (usually amebic) or fungal

b. Bacterial abscesses usually result from direct extension of infxn from gallbladder, hematogenous spread via the portal vein from appendicitis of diverticulitis, or via the hepatic artery from distant sources such as from a pneumonia or bacterial endocarditis

c. Organisms in pyogenic hepatic abscesses are usually of enteric origin (e.g., *E. coli*, *Klebsiella pneumoniae*, *Bacteroides*, and *Enterococcus*)

d. Amebic abscess caused by *Entoemeba histolytica*, and in the US is almost always seen in young Hispanic males

e. Si/Sx = high fever, malaise, rigors, jaundice, epigastric or right upper quadrant (RUQ) pain and referred pain to the right shoulder

f. Labs → leukocytosis, anemia, liver function tests may be nml or ↑

g. Dx = Utz or CT scan

h. Tx

(1) Antibiotics to cover anaerobes (e.g., metronidazole) + Gram negatives (e.g., ceftriaxone, piperacillin, fluoroquinolone, etc.) + *Enterococcus* (ampicillin)

(2) Percutaneous or surgical drainage

(3) For amebic abscesses (caused by *Entamoeba histolytica*) use metronidazole

i. Complications = intrahepatic spread of infxn, sepsis, and abscess rupture

j. Mortality of hepatic abscesses is 15%, higher with coexistent malignancy

6. Portal HTN

a. Defined as portal vein pressure >12 mm Hg (nml = 6–8 mm Hg)

b. Si/Sx = ascites, hepatosplenomegaly, variceal bleeding, encephalopathy

c. Can be presinusoidal, intrahepatic, or postsinusoidal in nature (Table 1.23)

Table 1.23	Causes of Portal Hypertension		Posthepatic
Prehepatic	Intrahepatic		Posthepatic
• Portal vein thrombosis • Splenomegaly • Arteriovenous fistula	• Cirrhosis • Schistosomiasis • Massive fatty change • Nodular regenerative hyperplasia	• Idiopathic portal hypertension • Granulomatous dz (e.g., tuberculosis, sarcoidosis)	• Severe right-sided heart failure • Hepatic vein thrombosis (Budd-Chiari syndrome) • Constrictive pericarditis • Hepatic venoocclusive dz

    d. Dx = endoscopy and angiography (variceal bleeding) and Utz (dilated vessels) (Figure 1.10)

    e. Tx

      (1) Acute variceal bleeding controlled by sclerotherapy

      (2) If continued bleeding, use Sengstaken-Blakemore tube to tamponade bleeding

      (3) Pharmacotherapy = IV infusion of vasopressin or octreotide

      (4) Long term → propranolol once varices are identified (↓ bleeding risk but effect on long-term survival is variable)

      (5) Decompressive shunts—most efficacious way of stopping bleeding

      (6) **Indication for liver transplant is end-stage liver dz, not variceal bleeding**

  7. Budd-Chiari syndrome

    a. Rarely congenital, usually acquired thrombosis occluding hepatic vein or hepatic stretch of inferior vena cava

    b. Associated with hypercoagulability (e.g., polycythemia vera, hepatocellular or other CA, pregnancy, etc.)

    c. Sx = acute onset of abd pain, jaundice, ascites

    d. Hepatitis quickly develops, leading to cirrhosis and portal HTN

    e. Dx = RUQ Utz

    f. Tx = clot lysis or hepatic transplant

    g. Px poor; less than one third of pts survive at 1 yr

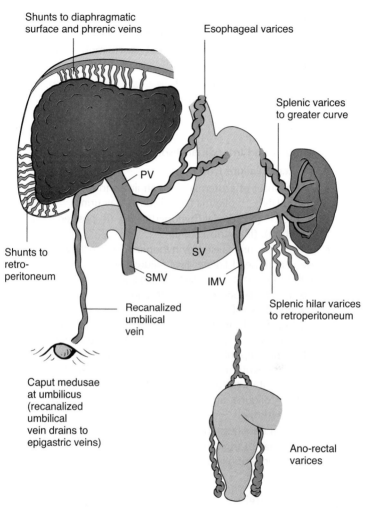

FIGURE 1.10

Sites of occurrence of portal–systemic communications in pts with portal hypertension. IMV, inferior mesenteric vein; PV, portal vein; SMV, superior mesenteric vein; SV, splenic vein.

8. Veno-occlusive dz
   a. Occlusion of hepatic venules (not large veins)
   b. Associated with graft-versus-host dz, chemotherapy, and radiation Tx
   c. Px = 50% mortality at 1 yr
   d. Tx = hepatic transplant, sometimes is self-limiting

IV. Nephrology

A. Renal Tubular and Interstitial Disorders

1. **Acute Renal Failure (ARF)**
   a. Rapid onset of azotemia (↑ creatinine and blood urea nitrogen [BUN]), ± oliguria (= <500 mL/day urine)
   b. Causes = (i) prerenal (hypoperfusion), (ii) postrenal (obstruction), (iii) intrinsic renal
   c. Prerenal failure caused by hypoperfusion because of volume depletion, heart failure, liver failure, sepsis, heatstroke (myoglobinuria), burns, or bilateral renal artery stenosis
   d. Postrenal ARF because of obstruction 2° to benign prostatic hypertrophy (BPH), bladder/pelvic tumors, calculi
   e. Intrinsic renal causes = acute tubular necrosis (ATN), which is most common; allergic interstitial nephritis (AIN); glomerulonephritis; nephrotoxin exposure; or renal ischemia (prerenal azotemia and ATN are a spectrum of dz; as the prerenal state persists the tubules become infarcted)
   f. Si/Sx = oliguria, anion gap metabolic acidosis, hyperkalemia → arrhythmias
   g. Dx from urinalysis (Table 1.24)
      (1) Urinary eosinophils suggest allergic nephritis or atheroembolic dz

Table 1.24	Laboratory Characteristics of Acute Renal Failure		
Test/Index	Prerenal	Postrenal	Renal
Urine osmolality	>500	<350	<350
Urine Sodium	<20	>40	>20
FE$_{Na}$*	<1%	>4%	>2%
Blood Urea Nitrogen/creatinine	>20	>15	<15

*FE$_{Na}$ = (Urine/Serum sodium)/(Urine/Serum creatinine).

(2) **RBC casts virtually pathognomonic for glomeru-lonephritis**

(3) Muddy brown casts in urine are typical of ATN

h. Tx

   (1) IV fluids to maintain urine output, diurese to prevent volume overload

   (2) Closely monitor electrolyte abnormalities

   (3) Indications for dialysis: recalcitrant volume overload status, critical electrolyte abnormalities, unresponsive metabolic acidosis, toxic ingestion, uremia

2. **Acute Tubular Necrosis (ATN)**

a. Most common cause of ARF, falls into the intrinsic renal category

b. ATN causes = persistent prerenal state of any cause, rhabdomyolysis → myoglobinuria, direct toxins (e.g., amphotericin, aminoglycosides, radiocontrast dyes)

c. Three phases of injury: (i) prodromal, (ii) oliguric, (iii) postoliguric

d. Tx = resolution of precipitating cause, IV fluids to maintain urinary output, monitor electrolytes, diurese as needed to prevent fluid overload

3. **Drug-Induced Allergic Interstitial Nephritis**

a. Penicillin, sulfonamides, diuretics, and NSAIDs are the most frequent causes

b. Si/Sx = pyuria, maculopapular rash, eosinophilia, proteinuria, hematuria, oliguria, flank pain, fever, eosinophiluria—**eosinophiluria is rare but is pathognomonic for either allergic interstitial nephritis (AIN) or atheroembolic dz**

c. Dx = clinical, improvement following withdrawal of offending drug can help confirm dx, but sometimes the dz can be irreversible

d. Tx = removal of underlying cause, consider corticosteroids for allergic dz

4. **Renal Tubule Functional Disorders**

a. Renal tubular acidosis (RTA) (Table 1.25)

b. Diabetes insipidus (DI)

   (1) ↓ Antidiuretic hormone (ADH) secretion (central) or ADH resistance (nephrogenic)

   (2) Si/Sx = polyuria, polydipsia, nocturia, urine specific gravity <1.010, urine osmolality (U_{osm}) ≤200, serum osmolality (S_{osm}) ≥300

Table 1.25	Renal Tubular Acidosis*	
Type	**Characteristic**	**Urinary pH**
Type I	• **Distal tubular defect** of urinary H^+ gradient • Seen in amphotericin nephrotoxicity	
Type II	• **Proximal tubule failure** to resorb HCO_3 • Classic causes include acetazolamide, nephrotic syndrome, multiple myeloma, Fanconi's syndrome	>5.5 early, then → <5.5 as acidosis worsens
Type IV	• ↓ **Aldosterone** → hyperkalemia and hyperchloremia • Usually due to ↓ secretion **(hypereninemic hypoaldosteronism)**, seen in diabetes, interstitial nephritis, NSAID use, ACE inhibitors, and heparin • Also because of aldosterone resistance, seen in urinary obstruction and sickle cell dz	<5.5

*There is no renal tubular acidosis III for historical reasons.

    (3) Central DI
        (a) 1° (idiopathic) or 2° (acquired via trauma, infarction, granulomatous infiltration, fungal or TB infxn of pituitary)
        (b) Tx = Desmopressin acetate (DDAVP) (ADH analogue) nasal spray
    (4) Nephrogenic DI
        (a) 1° dz is X-linked, seen in infants, may regress with time
        (b) 2° dz in sickle cell, pyelonephritis, nephrosis, amyloid, multiple myeloma, drugs (aminoglycoside, lithium, demeclocycline)
        (c) Tx = ↑ water intake, sodium restriction
    (5) **Dx = water deprivation test**
        (a) Hold all water, administer vasopressin
        (b) Central DI: U_{osm} after deprivation no greater than S_{osm}, but ↑ ≥10% after vasopressin given
        (c) Nephrogenic DI: U_{osm} after deprivation no greater than S_{osm}, and vasopressin does not ↑ U_{osm}
  c. Syndrome of inappropriate antidiuretic hormone (SIADH)

    (1) Etiologies

        (a) CNS dz: trauma, tumor, Guillain-Barré, hydrocephalus

        (b) Pulmonary dz: pneumonia, tumor (usually small cell CA), abscess, COPD

        (c) Endocrine dz: hypothyroidism, Conn's syndrome

        (d) Drugs: NSAIDs, antidepressants, chemotherapy, diuretics, phenothiazine, oral hypoglycemics

    (2) Dx = hyponatremia with $U_{osm} > 300$ mmol/kg

    (3) Tx

        (a) If euvolemic, water restriction is first line

        (b) If euvolemic and no response to water restriction (i.e., serum sodium does not $\uparrow$), prescribe conivaptan, which is a vasopressin receptor antagonist

        (c) If hypovolemic, prescribe nml saline

        (d) For refractory cases use demeclocycline (which causes nephrogenic diabetes insipidus, counteracting the effects of the SIADH) or hypertonic saline (3%)—**beware of central pontine myelinolysis with rapid correction of hyponatremia**

5. **Chronic Renal Failure**

  a. Always associated with azotemia of renal origin

  b. Uremia is <u>not</u> just a synonym for azotemia—uremia is a biochemical and clinical syndrome of the following characteristics

    (1) Azotemia (i.e., elevated serum creatinine and/or BUN)

    (2) Acidosis because of accumulation of sulfates, phosphates, organic acids

    (3) Hyperkalemia because of inability to excrete K^+ in urine

    (4) Fluid volume disorder (early cannot concentrate urine, late cannot dilute)

    (5) Hypocalcemia because of lack of vitamin D production

    (6) Anemia because lack of EPO production

    (7) Hypertension $2°$ to activated renin-angiotensin axis

  c. Si/Sx = anorexia, nausea/vomiting, dementia, convulsions, eventually coma, bleeding because of platelet dysfunction, fibrinous pericarditis, which can lead to tamponade

  d. Dx = renal Utz $\rightarrow$ small kidneys in chronic dz, anemia from chronic lack of EPO, diffuse osteopenia

  e. Tx = salt and water restriction, diuresis to prevent fluid overload, dialysis to correct acid–base or severe electrolyte disorders

Table 1.26   Nephrotic Glumerulopathies

Dz	Characteristics
Minimal change dz (MCD)	• Classically seen in young children • Electron microscopy shows fusion of podocyte foot processes • Tx = prednisone; dz is very responsive, Px is excellent
Focal segmental glomerulosclerosis	• Clinically similar to MCD, but occurs in adults with refractory HTN • Usually idiopathic, but heroin, HIV, diabetes, sickle cell are associated • The idiopathic variant typically presents in young, hypertensive male pts • Tx = prednisone + cyclophosphamide; dz is refractory, Px poor

Membranous glomerulonephritis	• Most common primary cause of nephritic syndrome in adults
	• Slowly progressive disorder with ↓ response to steroid Tx seen
	• Causes of this dz are numerous
	  ◊ Infxns include HBV, HCV, syphilis, malaria
	  ◊ Drugs include gold salts, penicillamine (note, both used in RA)
	  ◊ Occult malignancy
	  ◊ Systemic lupus erythematosus (10% of pts develop)
	• Tx = prednisone ± cyclophosphamide, 50% → end-stage renal failure

Membranoproliferative glomerulonephritis	• Dz has two forms
	  ◊ Type I often slowly progressive
	  ◊ Type II more aggressive, often have an autoanti-body against C3 convertase "C3 nephritic factor" → ↓ serium levels of C3
	• Tx = prednisone ± plasmapheresis or interferon-α, Px very poor

Systemic dz	See Table 1.27

B. **Glomerular Dz**
   1. **Nephrotic Syndrome**
      a. Si/Sx = proteinuria >3.5 g/day, generalized edema (anasarca), lipiduria with hyperlipidemia, marked ↓ albumin, hypercoagulation (e.g., DVT)

    b. Dx of type made by renal bx

    c. General Tx = protein restriction, salt restriction and diuretic Tx for edema, HMG-CoA reductase inhibitor for hyperlipidemia

    d. Nephrotic glomerulopathies (Table 1.26)

    e. Systemic glomerulopathies (Table 1.27)

2. **Nephritic Syndrome**

    a. Results from diffuse glomerular inflammation

    b. Si/Sx = acute onset hematuria (smoky-brown urine), $\downarrow$ glomerular filtration rate (GFR) resulting in azotemia ($\uparrow$ BUN and creatinine), oliguria, hypertension, and edema

    c. Nephritic glomerulopathies (Table 1.28)

3. **Urinalysis in primary glomerular dz (Table 1.29)**

Table 1.27	Systemic Glomerulonephropathies
Dz	**Characteristic Nephropathy**
Diabetes	• Most common cause of end-stage renal dz in U.S. • Early manifestation is microalbuminuria ◊ ACE inhibitors $\downarrow$ progression to renal failure if started early ◊ Strict glycemic and hypertensive control also $\downarrow$ progression • Bx shows pathognomonic Kimmelstiel-Wilson nodules • As dz progresses only Tx is renal transplant
HIV	• Usually seen in HIV acquired by intravenous drug abuse • Presents with focal segmental glomerulonephritis • Early Tx with antiretrovirals may help kidney dz
Renal amyloidosis	• Dx $\rightarrow$ birefringence with Congo red stain • Tx = transplant; dz is refractory and often recurrent
Lupus Type I Type II Type III Type IV Type V	 • No renal involvement • **Mesangial dz** with focal segmental glomerual pattern Tx not typically required for kidney involvement • **Focal proliferative dz** Tx = aggressive prednisone $\pm$ cyclophosphamide • **Diffuse proliferative dz;** the most severe form of lupus nephropathy Presents with a combination of nephritic/nephritic dz Classic light microscopy (LM) $\rightarrow$ wire-loop abnormality Tx = prednisone + cyclophosphamide; transplant may be required • **Membranous dz,** indistinguishable from other 1° membranous glomerulonephropathies Tx = consider prednisone, may not be required

Text continues on page 76

Table 1.28	Nephritic Glomerulonephropathies
Dz	**Characteristics**
Poststreptococcal (postinfectious) glomerulonephritis (PSGN/PIGN)	• Prototype of nephritic syndrome (acute glomerulonephritis) • Classically follows infxn with group A β-hemolytic streptococci (*S. pyogenes*) but can follow infxn by virtually any organism, viral or bacterial • Labs → urine red cells and casts, azotemia, ↓ serum C3, ↑ ASO titer (for strep infxn) • **Immunofluorescence → coarse granular IgG or C3 deposits** • Tx typically not needed; dz usually self-limiting

Crescentic (rapidly progressive) glomerulonephritis	• Nephritis progresses to renal failure within wks or mos
	• May be part of PIGN or other systemic dz
	• Goodpasture's dz
	  ◊ **Dz causes glomerulonephritis with pneumonitis**
	  ◊ **Presents with positive antiglomerula basement membrane (anti-GBM) antibody**
	  ◊ **90% pts present with hemoptysis,** only later get glomerulonephritis
	  ◊ **Classic immunofluorescence → smooth, linear deposition of IgG**
	• Tx = prednisone and plasmapheresis, minority → end-stage renal dz

Berger's dz (IgA nephropathy)	• **Most common worldwide nephropathy** • Because of IgA deposition in the mesangium • Si/Sx = recurrent hematuria with low-grade proteinuria • Whereas PIGN presents weeks after infxn, **Berger's presents concurrently or within several days of infxn** • 25% of pts slowly progress to renal failure, otherwise harmless • Tx = prednisone for acute flares, will not halt disease progression

Table 1.28 *Continued*

Dz	Characteristics
Henoch-Schönlein purpura (HSP)	• Also an IgA nephropathy, but almost always presents in children • Presents with abd pain, vomiting, hematuria, and GI bleeding • **Classic physical finding = "palpable purpura" on buttocks and legs in children** • Often follows respiratory infxn • Tx not required, dz is self-limiting
Multiple myeloma	• ↑ Production of light chains → tubular plugging by Bence-Jones proteins • 2° hypercalcemia also contributes to development of "myeloma kidney" • Myeloma cells can directly invade kidney parenchyma • Defect in nml antibody production leaves pt susceptible to chronic infxns by encapsulated bacteria (e.g., *E. coli*) → chronic renal failure • Tx is directed at underlying myeloma

Table 1.29 Urinalysis in Primary Glomerular Diseases

	Nephrotic Syndrome	Nephritic Syndrome	Chronic Dz
Proteinuria	↑↑↑↑	±	±
Hematuria	±	↑↑↑↑	±
Cells	—	⊕ RBCs ⊕ WBCs	±
Casts	**Fatty casts**	**RBC and granular casts**	**Waxy and pigmented granular casts**
Lipids	Free fat droplets, oval fat bodies	—	—

C. **Renal Artery Stenosis**
   1. **Presentation**
      a. **Classic dyad = sudden hypertension with low K^+** (pt not on diuretic)
      b. Causes are atherosclerotic plaques and fibromuscular dysplasia
      c. Fibromuscular dysplasia
         (1) Fibrous and muscular stenosis of renal artery
         (2) Causes renovascular HTN seen most commonly in women during their reproductive years
         (3) Beware of dissecting aneurysms of affected arteries
      d. Screening Dx = oral captopril induces ↑ renin
      e. Dx confirmed with angiography
      f. Tx = surgery versus angioplasty

D. **Urinary Tract Obstruction**
   1. **General Characteristics**
      a. Most common causes in children are congenital
      b. Most common causes in adults are benign prostatic hypertrophy (BPH) and stones
      c. Obstruction → urinary stasis → ↑ risk of urinary tract infxn (UTI)
   2. **Nephrolithiasis**
      a. Calcium pyrophosphate stones
         (1) 80% to 85% stones are **radiopaque**, associated with hypercalciuria
         (2) Hypercalciuria can be idiopathic or due to because of ↑ intestinal calcium absorption, ↑ 1° renal calcium excretion, or hypercalcemia
         (3) **50% associated with idiopathic hypercalciuria**
         (4) Tx = vigorous hydration, loop diuretics if necessary
      b. Ammonium magnesium phosphate stones ("struvite stones")
         (1) Second most common form of stones, are **radiopaque**
         (2) Most often because of urease ⊕ *Proteus* or *Staphylococcus saprophyticus*
         (3) Can form large staghorn or struvite calculi
         (4) Tx = directed at underlying infxn
      c. Uric acid stones
         (1) 50% of pts with stones have hyperuricemia

      (2) $2°$ to gout or ↑ cell turnover (leukemia, myeloproliferative dz)

      (3) Stones are **radiolucent**

      (4) Tx = alkalinize urine, treat underlying disorder

   d. Si/Sx of stones = urinary colic = sharp, 10/10 on the pain scale, often described as the worst pain in the pt's life, radiates from back → anterior pelvis/groin

   e. Tx = vigorous hydration, loop diuretics as needed

E. Tumors of the Kidney

  1. **Renal Cell CA**

   a. Most common renal malignancy, occurs in male smokers aged 50 to 70

   b. **Hematogenously disseminates by invading renal veins or the vena cava**

   c. Si/Sx = hematuria, palpable mass, flank pain, fever, $2°$ polycythemia

   d. Can be associated with von Hippel-Lindau syndrome

   e. Tx = resection, systemic interleukin-2 immunotherapy, poor Px

  2. **Wilms' Tumor**

   a. Most common renal malignancy of childhood, incidence peaks at 2 to 4 yr

   b. Si/Sx = palpable flank mass (often huge)

   c. Can be part of **WAGR** complex = **W**ilms' tumor, **A**niridia, **G**enitourinary malformations, mental motor **R**etardation

   d. **Also associated with hemihypertrophy of the body**

   e. Tx = nephrectomy plus chemotherapy and/or radiation

V. Endocrinology

A. Hypothalamic Pituitary Axis

  1. **Prolactinoma**

   a. Si/Sx = headache, diplopia, CN III palsy, impotence, amenorrhea, gynecomastia, galactorrhea, ↑ androgens in females → virilization

   b. **50% cause hypopituitarism, caused by mass effect of the tumor**

   c. Dx = MRI/CT confirmation of tumor

   d. Tx

      (1) First line = dopamine agonist (e.g., bromocriptine)

      (2) Large tumors or refractory → transsphenoidal surgical resection

      (3) Radiation Tx for nonresectable macroadenomas

2. **Acromegaly**

  a. Almost always because of pituitary adenoma secreting growth hormone

  b. Childhood secretion prior to skeletal epiphyseal closure → gigantism

  c. If secretion begins after epiphyseal closure → acromegaly

  d. Si/Sx = adult whose glove, ring, or shoe size acutely ↑, coarsening of skin/facial features; prognathism; voice deepening; joint erosions; peripheral neuropathies because of nerve compression

  e. Dx = ↑ insulin-like growth factor-1 and/or MRI/CT confirmation of neoplasm

  f. Tx = surgery or radiation to ablate the enlarged pituitary; octreotide (somatostatin analogue) second line for refractory tumors

B. **Diabetes**

1. **Type I Diabetes**

  a. Autoinflammatory destruction of pancreas → insulin deficiency

  b. Si/Sx = polyphagia, polydipsia, polyuria, weight loss in child or adolescent, can lead to diabetic ketoacidosis (DKA) when pt is stressed (e.g., infxn)

  c. Dx = see type II below for criteria

  d. Tx = **insulin replacement required—oral hypoglycemics will not work**

  e. Complication of type I diabetes = DKA

  f. Si/Sx of DKA = **Kussmaul hyperpnea** (deep and labored breathing), **abd pain, dehydration, ⊕ anion gap,** urine/blood ketones, hyperkalemia, hyperglycemia, mucormycosis = fatal fungal infxn seen in DKA

  g. DKA Tx

      (1) 1° Tx = **FLUIDS**

      (2) 2° = **K^+ and insulin**

      (3) 3° = **add glucose to insulin drip if pt becomes normoglycemic**—insulin is given to shut down ketogenesis, NOT to ↓ glucose, so insulin must be given until ketones are gone despite nml glucose

2. **Type II Diabetes**
   a. Peripheral insulin resistance—a metabolic dz, not autoinflammatory
   b. Usually adult onset, not ketosis prone, often strong FHx
   c. Si/Sx
      (1) Acute = dehydration, polydipsia/polyphagia/polyuria, fatigue, weight loss
      (2) Subacute = infxns (yeast vaginitis, mucormycosis, *S. aureus* boils)
      (3) Chronic (Figure 1.10)
         (a) Macrovascular = stroke, CAD
         (b) Microvascular = retinitis, nephritis
         (c) Neuropathy = ↓ sensation, paresthesias, glove-in-hand burning pain, autonomic insufficiency
   d. Dx of any diabetes (type I or II)
      (1) Random plasma glucose >200 with Sx *or*
      (2) Fasting glucose >125 twice *or*
      (3) 2-hr oral glucose tolerance test glucose >200 with or without Sx
   e. Tx
      (1) Oral hypoglycemics first line for mild to moderate hyperglycemia
      (2) Dz refractory to oral hypoglycemics requires insulin
      (3) Diet and nutrition education
      (4) ACE inhibitors slow progression of nephropathy
   f. Monitoring: glycosylated hemoglobin A_{1c} (HbA_{1c})
      (1) Because of serum half-life of hemoglobin, HbA_{1c} is a marker of the prior 3 mos of therapeutic regimen
      (2) **Tight glucose control has been shown to reduce complications and mortality in insulin-dependent diabetes mellitus (IDDM) and noninsulin-dependent diabetes mellitus (NIDDM)**, thus HbA_{1c} is a crucial key tool to follow efficacy and compliance of diabetic Tx regimens
      (3) HbA_{1c} <8 is recommended
   g. Complication = hyperosmolar hyperglycemic nonketotic coma (HHNK)
      (1) 2° to hypovolemia, precipitated by acute stress (e.g., infxn, trauma)
      (2) Glucose often >1000 mg/dL, no acidosis, ⊕ renal failure, and confusion

(3) Tx = rehydrate (may require 10 L); mortality approaches 50%

C. Adrenal Disorders

1. Cushing's Syndrome

a. Usually iatrogenic (cortisol Tx) or because of pituitary adenoma = Cushing's dz; rarely because of adrenal hyperplasia, ectopic adrenocorticotropic hormone (ACTH)/corticotropin-releasing hormone (CRH) production

b. Si/Sx (Figure 1.11) = **buffalo hump, truncal obesity, moon facies, striae,** hirsutism, hyperglycemia, hypertension, purpura, amenorrhea, impotence, acne

c. Dx = 24-hr urine cortisol and high-dose dexamethasone suppression test

d. Tx

   (1) Excision of tumor with postoperative glucocorticoid replacement

   (2) Mitotane (adrenolytic), ketoconazole (inhibits P450), metyrapone (blocks adrenal enzyme synthesis), or aminoglutethimide (inhibits P450) for nonexcisable tumors

2. Adrenal Insufficiency

a. Can be 1° (Addison's dz) or 2° ($\downarrow$ ACTH production by pituitary)

b. Addison's dz

   (1) Causes = autoimmune (most common), granulomatous dz, infarction, HIV, DIC (Waterhouse-Friderichsen syndrome)

   (2) **Waterhouse-Friderichsen** = hemorrhagic necrosis of adrenal medulla during the course of meningococcemia

   (3) Si/Sx = fatigue, anorexia, nausea/vomit, constipation, diarrhea, salt craving (pica), hypotension, **hyponatremia, hyperkalemia**

   (4) **Dx = hyperpigmentation, $\uparrow$ ACTH, $\downarrow$ cortisol response to ACTH**

c. **2° Dz → NO hyperpigmentation, $\downarrow$ ACTH, $\uparrow$** cortisol response to ACTH

d. Acute adrenal crisis

   (1) Because of stress (e.g., surgery or trauma), usually in setting of Tx chronic insufficiency or withdrawal of Tx

   (2) Can occur in pituitary apoplexy (infarction)

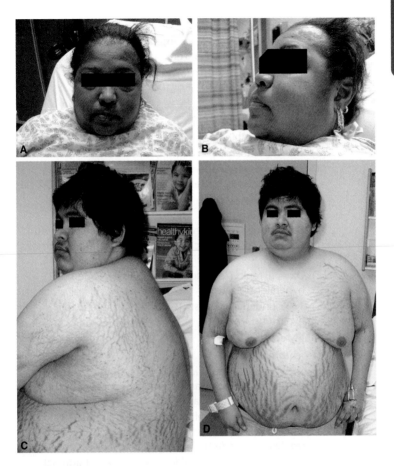

FIGURE 1.11

(A,B) Typical cushingoid "moon face" associated with excessive corticosteroid use or production. (Courtesy of Mark Silverberg, MD.) (C,D) Moon face, truncal obesity, buffalo hump, and purple striae seen here are all associated with Cushing's syndrome. (Courtesy of Bronson Terry, MD. All photos from Greenberg MI, Hendrickson RG, Silverberg M, et al. *Greenberg's text-atlas of emergency medicine.* Philadelphia: Lippincott Williams & Wilkins, 2004, with permission.)

e. Tx = cortisol replacement, ↑ replacement for times of illness or stress—**must taper replacement off slowly to allow hypothalamic-pituitary-adrenal (HPA) axis to restore itself**

3. **Adrenal Cortical Hyperfunction**
   a. 1° hyperaldosteronism = Conn's syndrome
      (1) Adenoma or hyperplasia of zona glomerulosa
      (2) Si/Sx = **HTN, ↑ Na, ↑ Cl, ↓ K, alkalosis,** ↓ renin (feedback inhibition)
      (3) Dx = ↑ aldosterone, ↓ renin, CT → adrenal neoplasm
      (4) Tx = excision of adenoma—bilateral hyperplasia → spironolactone; bilateral adrenalectomy should NOT be performed
   b. 2° hyperaldosteronism
      (1) Because of ↑ renin production 2° to renal hypoperfusion (e.g., CHF, shock, renal artery stenosis), cirrhosis, or tumor
      (2) Dx = ↑ renin (renin levels differentiate 1° versus 2° hyperaldosteronism)
      (3) Tx = underlying cause, β-blocker or diuretic for hypertension

4. **Adrenal Medulla**
   a. Pheochromocytoma
      (1) Si/Sx = HTN (episodic or chronic), **diaphoresis, palpitations,** tachycardia, headache, nausea/vomit, flushing, dyspnea, diarrhea
      (2) **Rule of 10:** 10% malignant, 10% bilateral, 10% extra-adrenal (occurs in embryologic cells that reactivate outside the adrenal gland)
      (3) Dx = ↑ urinary catecholamines, CT scan of adrenal showing neoplasm
      (4) Tx
         (a) Surgical excision after preoperative administration of α-blockers
         (b) Ca² channel blockers for hypertensive crisis
         (c) Phenoxybenzamine or phentolamine (α-blockers) for inoperable dz

D. **Gonadal Disorders**
   1. **Male Gonadal Axis (see OB-Gyn for Female Axis) (Table 1.30)**
   2. **Hypogonadism of Either Sex (Table 1.31)**

Table 1.30   Differential Diagnosis of Male Gonadal Disorders

Dz	Characteristics	Tx
Klinefelter's syndrome	• XXY chromosome inheritance, variable expressivity • Often not Dx until puberty, when ↓ virilization is noted • Si/Sx = tall, eunuchoid, with small testes and gynecomastia, ↓ testosterone, ↑ luteinizing hormone /follicle-stimulating hormone from lack of feedback • **Dx = buccal smear analysis for presence of Barr bodies**	Testosterone supplements
XYY syndrome	• Si/Sx = may have mild mental retardation, severe acne, ↑ incidence of violence and antisocial behavior • Dx = karyotype analysis	None
Testicular feminization syndrome	• Defect in the dihydrotestosterone, receptor → female external genitalia with sterile, undescended testes • Si/Sx = appear as females but are sterile and the vagina is blind-ended, testosterone, estrogen, and luteinizing hormone are all ↑ • Dx = history, physical exam, genetic testing	None
5-α-Reductase deficiency	• Si/Sx = ambiguous genitalia until puberty, then a burst in testosterone overcomes lack of dihydrotestosterone → external genitalia become masculinized, **testosterone and estrogen are nml** • Dx = genetic testing	Testosterone supplements

Table 1.31	Genetic Hypogonadism	
Dz	**Characteristics**	**Tx**
Congenital adrenal hyperplasia (CAH)	• Defects in steroid synthetic pathway causing either virilization of females or faile to virilize males • 21-α-hydroxylase deficiency causes 95% of all CAH • Severe dz presents in infancy with ambiguous genitalia and salt loss (2° to ↓↓ aldosterone) • Less severe variants → minimal virilization and salt loss, and can have Dx delayed for several years	Tx = replacement of necessary hormones
Prader-Willi syndrome	• Paternal imprinting (only gene from dad is expressed) • Si/Sx = presents in infancy with floppy baby, **short limbs,** obesity because of gross hyperphagia, nasal speech, retardation, **classic almond-shaped eyes with strabismus** • Dx = clinical or genetic analysis	None
Laurence-Moon-Biedl syndrome	• Autosomal recessive inheritance • Si/Sx = obese children, **nml craniofacies,** may be retarded, **are not short, have polydactyly** • Dx = clinical or genetic	None
Kallmann's syndrome	• Autosomal dominant hypogonadism with anosmia (cannot smell) • Due to ↓ production/secretion of gonadotropin-releasing hormone by hypothalamus • Dx by lack of circulating luteinizing hormone and follicle-stimulating hormone	Pulsatile gonadotropin-releasing hormone → virilization

E. **Thyroid**
  1. **Hyperthyroidism**
     a. Si/Sx of hyperthyroidism = tachycardia, **isolated systolic hypertension,** tremor, a-fib, anxiety, diaphoresis, weight loss with ↑ appetite, insomnia/**fatigue,** diarrhea, **exophthalmus, heat intolerance**
     b. Graves' dz
        (1) Diffuse, autoimmune goiter, causes 90% of U.S. hyperthyroid cases
        (2) Seen in young adults, is eight times more common in female pts than male pts
        (3) **Si/Sx include two findings only seen in hyperthyroid because of Graves' dz: infiltrative ophthalmopathy and pretibial myxedema**
        (4) **Infiltrative ophthalmopathy** = exophthalmus not resolving when thyrotoxicosis is cured, because of autoantibody-mediated damage (Figure 1.12)
        (5) **Pretibial myxedema**
           (a) Brawny, pruritic, nonpitting edema usually on the shins
           (b) Often spontaneously remits after mos to yrs

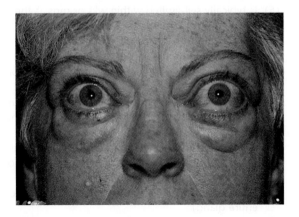

FIGURE 1.12
Exophthalmos in Grave's dz. (From Tasman W, Jaeger E. *The Wills eye hospital atlas of clinical ophthalmology*, 2nd Ed. Baltimore: Lippincott Williams & Wilkins, 2001).

      (6) Dx confirmed with thyroid-stimulating immunoglobulin (TSI) test (autoantibody binds to thyroid receptor, activating it, which is the cause of the dz)

  c. Plummer's dz (toxic multinodular goiter)

      (1) Because of multiple foci of thyroid tissue that cease responding to T_4 feedback inhibition, more common in older people

      (2) Dx = multiple thyroid nodules felt in gland, confirm with radioactive iodine uptake tests → hot nodules with cold background

  d. Thyroid adenoma because of overproduction of hormone by tumor in the gland

  e. Subacute thyroiditis (giant cell or de Quervain's thyroiditis)

      (1) Gland inflammation with spilling of hormone from the damaged gland

      (2) Can be painful (typically following a viral upper respiratory infxn) or painless (because of drug toxicity—e.g., amiodarone or lithium, or autoimmune—which can be seen postpartum)

      (3) Painful dz presents with **jaw/tooth pain,** can be confused with dental dz, ↑ erythrocyte sedimentation rate (ESR)

      (4) **Presents initially with hyperthyroidism but later turns into hypothyroidism as thyroid hormone is depleted from the inflamed gland**

      (5) Is typically self-limited within wks or mos as the viral or autoimmune cause burns itself out, so thyroid replacement is not necessary

      (6) Tx with aspirin or with cortisol in very severe dz

  f. Tx for all forms of hyperthyroidism (not necessary for subacute thyroiditis)

      (1) Propylthiouracil or methimazole induces remission in 1 mo to 2 yrs (up to 50% of time); lifelong Tx not necessary unless dz relapses

      (2) Radioiodine is first line for Graves'dz: radioactive iodine is concentrated in the gland and destroys it, resolving the diffuse hyperthyroid state

      (3) If the above Tx fail → surgical excision (of adenoma or entire gland)

  g. Thyroid storm is the most extreme manifestation of hyperthyroidism

      (1) Because of exacerbation of hyperthyroidism by surgery or infxn

(2) Si/Sx = high fever, dehydration, cardiac arrhythmias, high-output cardiac failure, transaminitis, coma, 25% mortality

(3) Tx

    (a) β-blockers and IV fluids are first priority to restore hemodynamic stability

    (b) Give propylthiouracil (PTU) to inhibit iodination of more thyroid hormone

    (c) After PTU on board, give iodine compounds, which will feedback inhibit further thyroid hormone release—make sure the PTU is on board first, or the iodine can cause an initial ↑ in hormone release before it feedback suppresses release

2. **Hypothyroidism**

    a. Causes include Hashimoto's and subacute thyroiditis

    b. Si/Sx = **cold intolerance**, weight gain, **low energy**, husky voice, mental slowness, constipation, thick/coarse hair, puffiness of face/eyelids/hands **(myxedema)**, loss of lateral third of eyebrows, prolonged relaxation phase of deep tendon reflexes (Figure 1.13)

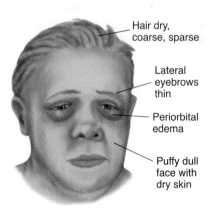

Hair dry, coarse, sparse

Lateral eyebrows thin

Periorbital edema

Puffy dull face with dry skin

FIGURE 1.13

Myxedema. The pt with severe hypothyroidism (myxedema) has a dull, puffy facies. The edema, often particularly pronounced around the eyes, does not pit with pressure. The hair and eyebrows are dry, coarse, and thinned. The skin is dry. (From Bickley LS, Szilagyi P. *Bates' guide to physical examination and history taking*, 8th Ed. Philadelphia: Lippincott Williams & Wilkins, 2003).

    c. Hashimoto's dz
        (1) Autoimmune lymphocytic infiltration of the thyroid gland
        (2) **8:1 ratio in women to men**, usually between ages of 30 and 50
        (3) **Dx confirmed by antithyroid peroxidase (TPO) or Antimicrosomal Antibodies**
        (4) Tx = lifelong synthroid
    d. Subacute thyroiditis—see E.1.f. above
    e. Myxedema coma
        (1) **The only emergent hypothyroid condition**—spontaneous onset or precipitated by cold exposure, infxn, analgesia, sedative drug use, respiratory failure, or other severe illness
        (2) Si/Sx = stupor, coma, seizures, hypotension, hypoventilation
        (3) Tx = IV levothyroxine, cortisone, mechanical ventilation

F. **Thyroid Malignancy**
    1. Solitary dominant thyroid nodule management
        a. Dx by fine-needle aspiration
        b. Surgical excision, thyroid lobectomy versus total thyroidectomy if highly suspicious for malignancy
    2. Radioactive iodine hot nodules are less likely cancerous, usually seen in elderly, soft to palpation; Utz shows cystic mass; thyroid scan shows autonomously functioning nodule
    3. Radioactive iodine cold nodule
        a. Has a greater potential of being malignant
        b. More common in women
        c. Nodule is firm to palpation, can be accompanied by vocal cord paralysis; Utz shows solid mass with calcifications
    4. Papillary CA
        a. Most common CA of thyroid
        b. Good Px, 85% 5-yr survival, spread is indolent via lymph nodes
        c. Pathologically distinguished by ground-glass Orphan Annie nucleus and psammoma bodies (with calcifications) **(NOTE: other psammoma body dz = serous papillary cystadenoCA of ovary, mesothelioma, meningioma)**
        d. Bilateral thyroid lobe spread is common
        e. Tx = surgical excision followed by radioactive iodine

Table 1.32 Multiple Endocrine Neoplasia Syndromes

Type I (Wermer's syndrome)	**The 3 (4) Ps: P**ituitary (**Pr**olactinoma most common), **P**arathyoid, **P**ancreatoma
Type IIa (Sipple's syndrome)	Pheochromocytoma, medullary thyroid CA, parathyroid hyperplasia or tumor
Type IIb (Type III)	Pheochromocytoma, medullary thyroid CA, mucocutaneous neuromas, particularly of the GI tract

5. Medullary CA
   a. Has intermediate Px
   b. CA of parafollicular "C" cells that are derived from the ultimobranchial bodies (cells of branchial pouch 5)
   c. Secretes calcitonin; can Dx and follow dz with this blood assay
6. Follicular CA commonly results in blood-borne metastases to bone and lungs
   a. Tx = surgical excision followed by radioactive iodine
7. Anaplastic CA has one of the poorest Px of any CA (0% survival at 5 yr)

G. **Multiple Endocrine Neoplasia Syndromes (Table 1.32)**

VI. Musculoskeletal

A. **Metabolic Bone Dz**
   1. **Osteoporosis**
      a. Because of **postmenopausal ($\downarrow$ estrogen),** physical inactivity, high cortisol states (e.g., Cushing's dz, exogenous), hyperthyroidism, Ca^{2+} deficiency
      b. Si/Sx = typically aSx until fracture occurs, particularly of hip and vertebrae
      c. Dx = **Dual Energy X-ray Absortiometry (DEXA) scan** showing $\downarrow$ bone density compared with general population
      d. Tx
         (1) Bisphosphonates have become first-line Tx, proven to $\downarrow$ risk of fracture and slow or stop bone degeneration
         (2) Estrogens highly effective at stimulating new bone growth and preventing fractures, but long-term side effects (i.e., CA and heart dz risks) limit their use

(3) Calcitonin particularly useful for Tx bone pain, but its effects wear off after chronic use

(4) Raloxifene and tamoxifen (selective estrogen receptor modulators) ↑ bone density but also ↑ risk for thromboembolism—role unclear

e. **Every pt with osteoporosis should take calcium to keep dietary intake ≥1.5 g/day**

2. **Rickets/Osteomalacia**

a. Vitamin D deficiency in children = rickets; in adults = osteomalacia

b. Si/Sx in kids (rickets) = **craniotabes** (thinning of skull bones), **rachitic rosary** (costochondral thickening looks like string of beads), **Harrison's groove** (depression along line of diaphragmatic insertion into rib cage), **Pigeon breast** = pectus carinatum (sternum protrusion)

c. In adults the dz mimics osteoporosis

d. Dx = x-ray → radiolucent bones, can confirm with vitamin D

e. Tx = vitamin D supplementation

3. **Scurvy**

a. Vitamin C deficiency → ↓ osteoid formation

b. Si/Sx = subperiosteal hemorrhage (painful), **bleeding gums,** multiple ecchymoses, osteoporosis, **"woody leg" from soft-tissue hemorrhage**

c. Dx = clinical

d. Tx = vitamin C supplementation

4. **Paget's Bone Dz (Osteitis Deformans)**

a. Idiopathic ↑ activity of both osteoblasts and osteoclasts, usually in elderly

b. Si/Sx = **diffuse fractures and bone pain,** most commonly involves spine, pelvis, skull, femur, tibia; **high-output cardiac failure;** ↓ hearing

c. Dx = ↑↑ **alkaline phosphatase,** ⊕ bone scans, x-rays → sclerotic lesions

d. Tx = bisphosphonates first line, calcitonin second line

e. Complications = pathologic fractures, hypercalcemia and kidney stones, spinal cord compression in vertebral dz, osteosarcoma in long-standing dz

B. **Nonneoplastic Bone Dz**

1. **Fibrous Dysplasia**

a. Idiopathic replacement of bone with fibrous tissue

b. Three types = (i) monostotic, (ii) polystotic, (iii) McCune-Albright's

c. McCune-Albright's syndrome

(1) Syndrome of hyperparathyroidism, hyperadrenalism, and acromegaly

(2) **Dx = polystotic fibrous dysplasia, precocious puberty, café-au-lait spots**

d. Tx = supportive surgical debulking of deforming defects

2. **Osteomyelitis**

a. Caused by bacterial infxn of bone; *S. aureus* most common cause, but any bacterium can cause, as can certain fungi

b. **Pts with sickle cell dz get *Salmonella*; IV drug abusers get *Pseudomonas***

c. Si/Sx = painful inflammation of bone, with chronic or recurrent periods of drainage of pus through skin

d. Dx = x-ray → **periosteal elevation, can lag onset of dz by wks**; MRI is gold-standard, can confirm with cultures of deep bone Bx

e. Tx = surgical débridement + weeks to months of antibiotics

C. **Bone Tumors**

1. Dx/Tx of primary bone neoplasms (Table 1.33)

2. Multiple myeloma

a. Malignant clonal neoplasm of plasma cells producing whole Abs (e.g., IgM, IgG, etc.), light chains only, or very rarely no Abs (just ↑ B cells)

b. Seen in pts >40 yrs; African American pts have 2:1 incidence

c. **Si/Sx = bone pain worse with movement, lytic bone lesions on x-ray** (Figure 1.14), pathologic fractures, **hypercalcemia**, renal failure, anemia, frequent infxns by encapsulated bacteria, ↓ **anion gap** (Abs positively charged, unseen cations make anion gap appear ↓)

d. **Hyperviscosity syndrome** = stroke, retinopathy, CHF, ESR >100

e. **Bence-Jones proteinuria**

f. **Urine dipsticks do NOT detect light chain protein;** can use sulfosalicylic acid test in lieu of dipstick to screen

g. Dx = 24-hr urine collection → protein electrophoresis

h. Light-chain deposition causes renal amyloidosis

i. Dx

Table 1.33	Diagnosis* and Treatment of Primary Bone Neoplasms		
Tumor	Pt Age[†]	Characteristics	Tx
Osteochondroma	<25	• Benign, usually in males • Seen at distal femur and proximal tibia	Excision
Giant cell	20–40	• Benign, epiphysical ends of long bones (>50% in knee) • X-ray → **soap bubble** sign • Often recurs after excision	Excision and local irradiation
Osteosarcoma	10–20	• Number one 1° bone malignancy • Seen at distal femur and proximal tibia • Two- to threefold ↑ alkaline phosphatase • X-ray → **Codman's triangle** = periosteal elevation because of tumor and **"sun burst" sign** = lytic lesion with surrounding speculated periostitis (Figure 1.15)	Excision and local irradiation
Ewing's sarcoma	<15	• Young boys, metastasizes very early • Si/Sx mimic osteomyelitis (Figure 1.14) • Presents with "onion skin" appearance on x-ray	Chemotherapy

*Dx all confirmed with bone bx.
[†]Peak age of onset.

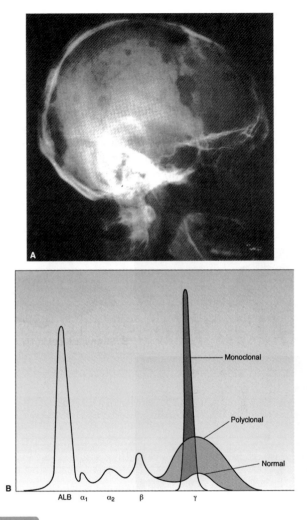

FIGURE 1.14

(A) Multiple myeloma. A radiograph of the skull shows numerous punched-out radiolucent areas. (Image from Rubin E, Farber JL. *Pathology*, 3rd Ed. Philadelphia: Lippincott Williams & Wilkins, 1999.) **(B)** Serum protein electrophoretic patterns. Abnormal serum protein electrophoretic patterns are contrasted with a nml pattern. In polyclonal hypergammaglobulinemia, which is characteristic of benign reactive processes, there is a broad-based ↑ in immunoglobulins because of immunoglobulin secretion by myriad discrete reactive plasma cells. In monoclonal gammopathy, which is characteristic of monoclonal gammopathy of unknown significance or plasma cell neoplasia, there is a narrow peak, or spike, because of the homogeneity of the immunoglobulin molecules secreted by a single clone of aberrant plasma cells. (Image from Rubin E, Farber JL. *Pathology*, 3rd Ed. Philadelphia: Lippincott Williams & Wilkins, 1999.)

(1) Serum protein and urine protein electrophoresis (SPEP and UPEP)

(2) Both → tall electrophoretic peak called "M-spike" due to ↑ Ab (Figure 1.15)

(3) SPEP → M-spike if clones make whole Ab

(4) UPEP → spike if clones make light chains only

(5) **Either SPEP or UPEP will almost always be** ⊕

(6) Dx = ⊕ SPEP/UPEP and any of **(i)** ↑ plasma cells in bone marrow, **(ii)** osteolytic bone lesions, OR **(iii)** Bence-Jones proteinuria

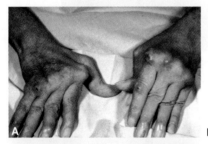

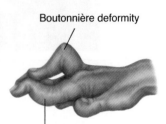

Boutonnière deformity

B Swan neck deformity

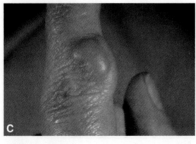

FIGURE 1.15

(A) Rheumatoid arthritis. The hands of a pt with advanced arthritis show swelling of the metacarpophalangeal joints and the classic ulnar deviation of the fingers. (Image from Rubin E, Farber JL. *Pathology*, 3rd Ed. Philadelphia: Lippincott Williams & Wilkins, 1999.) **(B)** As the arthritic process continues and worsens, the fingers may show "swan neck" deformities (i.e., hyperextension of the proximal interphalangeal joints with fixed flexion of the distal interphalangeal joints). Less common is a boutonniere deformity (i.e., persistent flexion of the proximal interphalangeal joint with hyperextension of the distal interphalangeal joint). (From Bickley LS, Szilagyi P. *Bates' guide to physical examination and history taking*, 8th Ed. Philadelphia: Lippincott Williams & Wilkins, 2003.) **(C)** Rheumatoid nodule. A pt with rheumatoid arthritis has a mass on a digit. (Image from Rubin E, Farber JL. *Pathology*, 3rd Ed. Philadelphia: Lippincott Williams & Wilkins, 1999.)

      j. Tx
        (1) Radiation given for isolated lesions, chemotherapy for metastatic dz
        (2) Bone marrow transplantation (BMT) may prolong survival
        (3) Palliative care important for pain
      k. Px poor despite Tx

D. **Arthropathies and Connective Tissue Disorders**
   1. **Rheumatoid Arthritis (RA)**
      a. Autoimmune dz of unknown etiology → **symmetric inflammatory arthritis**
      b. Female/male = 3:1, pts are commonly **HLA-DR4 ⊕**
      c. Si/Sx = **symmetric arthritis worse in morning** affecting knees, feet, metacarpophalangeal **(MCP)** and proximal interphalangeal **(PIP)** joints (Figure 1.15A), flexion contractures → ulnar deviation of digits (Figure 1.15A), swan neck and boutoniere deformity of hand (Figure 1.15B), subcutaneous nodules (present in <50% of pts) (Figure 1.15C), pleural effusions (serositis), anemia of chronic dz
      d. Labs
        (1) Rheumatoid factor (RF) = IgM anti-IgG
          (a) Present in >70% of pts with RA but may appear late in dz course
          (b) **Not specific for RA**, can be ⊕ in any chronic inflammatory state and may be present in 5% to 10% of healthy geriatric pts
        (2) ESR is elevated in >90% cases but is not specific for RA
      e. **Dx = clinical**, no single factor is sufficient
      f. Tx
        (1) NSAIDs are first line
        (2) Hydroxychloroquine second line, refractory pts → prednisone, gold salts, penicillamine, all of which cause severe side effects
        (3) Tumor necrosis factor (TNF) antagonists markedly improve symptoms, even in pts refractory to standard Tx

   2. **Systemic Lupus Erythematosus (SLE)**
      a. Systemic autoimmune disorder, female/male ratio = 9:1
      b. Si/Sx = fever, polyarthritis, skin lesions, splenomegaly, hemolytic anemia, thrombocytopenia, serositis (e.g., pleuritis and pericarditis), Libman-Sacks endocarditis, renal dz, skin rashes, thrombosis, neurologic disorders

c. Labs

(1) **Antinuclear antibody (ANA) sensitive (>98%) but not specific**

(2) **Anti–double-stranded DNA (anti–ds-DNA) Abs 99% specific**

(3) Anti-Smith (anti-Sm) Abs are highly specific but not sensitive

(4) Anti-Ro Abs are ⊕ in 50% of ANA-negative lupus

(5) Antiribosomal P and antineuronal Abs correlate with risk for cerebral involvement of lupus (lupus cerebritis)

(6) Antiphospholipid autoantibodies cause false ⊕ lab tests in SLE

   (a) **Pts with SLE frequently have false ⊕ rapid plasma regain/Venereal Dz Research Laboratory test (RPR/VDRL) tests for syphilis**

   (b) Pts with **SLE frequently have ↑ PTT (lupus anticoagulant Ab)**

      (i) PTT is falsely ↑ because the lupus anticoagulant Ab binds to phospholipid that initiates clotting in the test tube

      (ii) **Despite the PTT test and the name lupus anticoagulant Ab, pts with SLE are THROMBOGENIC because antiphospholipid Abs cause coagulation in vivo**

d. Mnemonic for SLE diagnosis: **DOPAMINE RASH**

(1) **D**iscoid lupus = circular, erythematous macules with scales (Figure 1.16)

(2) **O**ral aphthous ulcers (can be nasopharyngeal as well)

(3) **P**hotosensitivity

(4) **A**rthritis (typically hands, wrists, knees)

(5) **M**alar rash = classic butterfly macule on cheeks

(6) **I**mmunologic criteria = anti–ds-DNA, anti-Sm Ab, anti-Ro Ab, anti-La

(7) **N**eurologic changes = psychosis, personality change, seizures

(8) **E**SR rate ↑ (NOT 1 of the 11 criteria but is a frequent lab finding)

(9) **R**enal dz → nephritic or nephrotic syndrome

(10) **A**NA⊕

(11) **S**erositis (pleurisy, pericarditis)

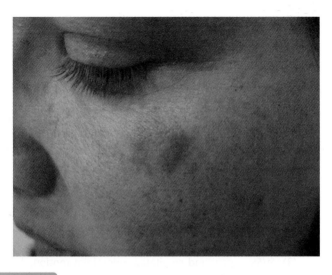

FIGURE 1.16

Circular plaque lesion of discoid lupus on the cheek.

        (12) **H**ematologic dz = hemolytic anemia,
            thrombocytopenia, leukopenia
    e. Drug-induced SLE
       (1) Drugs = procainamide, hydralazine, phenytoin,
          sulfonamides, isoniazid (INH)
       (2) **Labs → antihistone Abs,** differentiating from idiopathic
          SLE
    f. Tx = NSAIDs, hydroxychloroquine, prednisone,
      cyclophosphamide depending on severity of dz
    g. Px = variable; 10-yr survival is excellent; **renal dz is a poor
      Px indicator**
3. **Sjögren's Syndrome (SS)**
    a. Autoinflammatory disorder associated with **HLA-DR3**
    b. Si/Sx = **classic triad of keratoconjunctivitis sicca** (dry
      eyes), **xerostomia** (dry mouth), **arthritis,** usually less severe
      than pure RA
    c. Systemic Si/Sx = pancreatitis, fibrinous pericarditis, CN V
      sensory neuropathy, renal tubular acidosis, 40-fold ↑ in
      lymphoma incidence

    d. Dx = Concomitant presence of two of the triad is diagnostic, consider salivary gland Bx

    e. Labs → ANA ⊕, anti-Ro/anti-La Ab ⊕ ("SSA/SSB Abs"), 70% are RF ⊕

    f. Tx = steroids, cyclophosphamide for refractory dz

4. **Behçet's Syndrome**

    a. Multisystem inflammatory disorder that chronically recurs

    b. Si/Sx = painful oral and genital ulcers, also arthritis, vasculitis, neurologic dz

    c. Tx = prednisone during flare-ups

5. **Seronegative Spondyloarthropathy**

    a. Osteoarthritis

       (1) **Noninflammatory arthritis** caused by joint wear and tear

       (2) Most common arthritis, results in wearing away of joint cartilage

       (3) Si/Sx = pain and crepitation upon joint motion, ↓ range of joint motion, can have radiculopathy because of cord impingement

       (4) **X-ray → osteophytes (bone spurs) and asymmetric joint space loss**

       (5) Physical exam → **Heberden's nodes** (distal interphalangeal joint [DIP] swelling 2° to osteophytes) and **Bouchard's nodes** (PIP swelling 2° to osteophytes) (Figure 1.17)

       (6) **Note: RA affects MCP and PIP joints, while osteoarthritis affects PIP and DIP joints**

       (7) Tx = NSAIDs, muscle relaxants, joint replacement (third line)

       (8) **Isometric exercise to strengthen muscles around joint has been shown to improve Sx**

    b. Ankylosing spondylitis

       (1) Rheumatologic dz usually in **HLA-B27** ⊕ male pts (male/female ratio = 3:1)

       (2) Si/Sx = sacroiliitis, spinal dz → complete fusion of adjacent vertebral bodies causing **"bamboo spine" (Figure 1.18)**, uveitis, heart block

       (3) **If sacroiliac joint is not affected, it is not ankylosing spondylitis**

       (4) Dx = x-ray signs of spinal fusion and negative RF

       (5) Tx = NSAIDs and strengthening of back muscles

Radial deviation of distal phalanx

Heberden's node

Bouchard's node

Metacarpophalangeal joints uninvolved

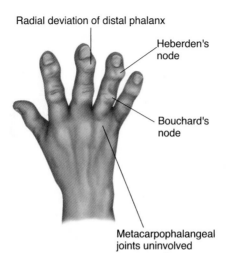

FIGURE 1.17

Osteoarthritis (degenerative joint dz). Nodules on the dorsolateral aspects of the distal interphalangeal joints (Heberden's nodes) are because of the bony overgrowth of osteoarthritis. Usually hard and painless, they affect the middle-aged or elderly pts and often, although not always, are associated with arthritic changes in other joints. Flexion and deviation deformities may develop. Similar nodules on the proximal interphalangeal joints (Bouchard's nodes) are less common. The metacarpophalangeal joints are spared. (From Bickley LS, Szilagyi P. *Bates' guide to physical examination and history taking*, 8th Ed. Philadelphia: Lippincott Williams & Wilkins, 2003.)

   c. Reiter's syndrome
     (1) Usually seen in male pts; **approximately three fourths of these pts are HLA-B27⊕**
     (2) Presents with nongonococcal **urethritis** (often chlamydial), **conjunctivitis, reactive arthritis,** and **uveitis**—mnemonic, "Can't see, can't pee, can't climb a tree"
     (3) Classic dermatologic Sx = **circinate balanitis** (serpiginous, moist plaques on glans penis) and **keratoderma blennorrhagicum** (crusting papules with central erosion, **looks like mollusk shell**)
     (4) Tx = erythromycin (for *Chlamydia* coverage) plus NSAIDs for arthritis
   d. Psoriatic arthritis
     (1) Presents with **nail pitting and DIP** joint involvement

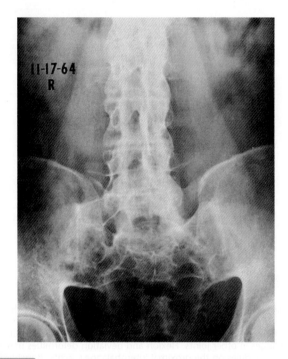

11-17-64
R

FIGURE 1.18

X-ray changes of spine (classic "bamboo spine"). (From Gold DH, Weingeist TA. *Color atlas of the eye in systemic disease*. Baltimore: Lippincott Williams & Wilkins, 2001.)

        (2) Occurs in up to 10% of pts with psoriasis

        (3) Psoriatic flares may exacerbate arthritis and vice versa

        (4) Tx = ultraviolet light for psoriasis and gold/penicillamine for arthritis

    e. Inflammatory bowel dz can cause seronegative arthritis

    f. Disseminated gonococcal infxn can cause **monoarticular** arthritis

  6. **Scleroderma (Progressive Systemic Sclerosis [PSS])**

    a. Systemic fibrosis affecting virtually every organ, female/male ratio = 4:1

    b. Skin tightening of face causing classic facial appearance (Figure 1.19)

    c. Can be diffuse dz (PSS) or more benign CREST syndrome

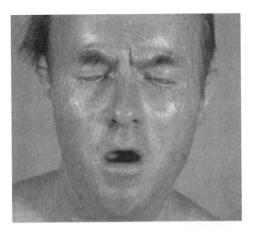

FIGURE 1.19

Classic scleroderma facies with skin tightening. (With permission from Clements PJ, Furst DE. *Systemic sclerosis*. Baltimore: Williams & Wilkins, 1996.)

    d. **Si/Sx of CREST syndrome**
        (1) **C**alcinosis = subcutaneous calcifications, often in fingers (Figure 1.20)
        (2) **R**aynaud's phenomenon, often the initial symptom
        (3) **E**sophageal dysmotility because of lower esophageal sphincter sclerosis → reflux

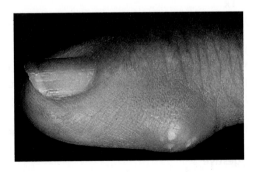

FIGURE 1.20

Calcinosis. Subcutaneous and periarticular calcium deposits may be extremely painful. (From Axford JS, Callaghan CA. *Medicine*, 2nd Ed. Oxford: Blackwell Science, 2004, with permission.)

    (4) **S**clerodactyly = fibrosed skin causes immobile digits

    (5) **T**elangiectasias occur in mouth, on digits, face, and trunk

  e. Other Sx = flexion contractures, biliary cirrhosis, lung/cardiac/renal fibrosis

  f. Labs = ⊕ ANA in 95%; anti–Scl-70 has ↓ sensitivity but ↑ specificity; anticentromere is 80% sensitive for CREST syndrome

  g. Dx = clinical

  h. Tx = immunosuppressives for palliation; none are curative

7. **Sarcoidosis**

  a. Idiopathic, diffuse dz presenting in 20s to 40s, **African American pts are three times more likely to develop than Caucasian pts**

  b. Si/Sx = **50% of pts present with incidental finding on CXR and are aSx**; other presentations include fevers, chills, night sweats, weight loss, cough, dyspnea, rash, arthralgia, blurry vision (uveitis)

  c. **CXR has several stages of dz (Figure 1.21)**

    (1) Stage I = **bilateral hilar adenopathy**

    (2) Stage II = hilar adenopathy with infiltrates

    (3) Stage III = lung involvement only

    (4) Stage IV = chronic scarring

  d. Can affect ANY organ system

    (1) CNS → CN palsy, classically CN VII (can be bilateral)

    (2) **Eye → uveitis (can be bilateral), requires aggressive Tx**

    (3) Cardiac → heart blocks, arrhythmias, constrictive pericarditis

    (4) Lung → typically a restrictive defect

    (5) GI → ↑ AST/ALT; CT → granulomas in liver, cholestasis

    (6) Renal → nephrolithiasis because of hypercalcemia

    (7) Endocrine → DI

    (8) Hematologic → anemia, thrombocytopenia, leukopenia

    (9) Skin → various rashes, including erythema nodosum

  e. Dx is clinical; **noncaseating granulomas on bx is very suggestive**

  f. Labs → 50% of pts have ↑ ACE level

  g. Tx = prednisone (first line), but 50% of pts spontaneously remit, so only Tx if (i) eye/heart involved, or (ii) dz does not remit after mos

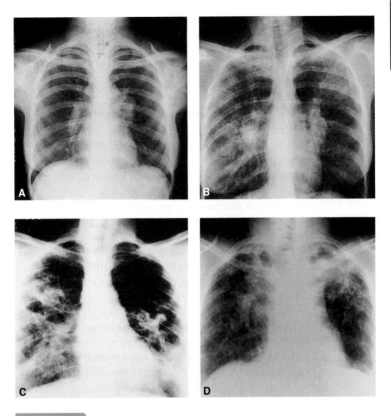

FIGURE 1.21

X-rays illustrating the different stages of sarcoidosis. **(A)** Stage I. Bilateral hilar adenopathy and paratracheal adenopathy with nml lung fields. **(B)** Stage II. Bilateral hilar adenopathy with interstitial lung field involvement. **(C)** Stage III. Lung field involvement only. **(D)** Stage IV. Severely fibrotic lungs with volume loss and cyst formation. (From Crapo JD, Glassroth J, Karlinsky JB, et al. *Baum's textbook of pulmonary diseases*, 7th Ed. Philadelphia: Lippincott Williams & Wilkins, 2004.)

8. **Mixed Connective Tissue Dz (MCTD)**
   a. Commonly onsets in women in teens and 20s
   b. Si/Sx = overlapping SLE, scleroderma, and polymyositis but **characterized by ⊕ anti-U1 RNP Ab that defines the dz**
   c. Dx = anti-U1RNP Ab
   d. Tx = steroids, azathioprine

9. **Gout**
   a. **Monoarticular arthritis** because of urate crystal deposits in joint
   b. **Gout develops after 20 to 30 yrs of hyperuricemia, often precipitated by sudden changes in serum urate levels** (gout in teens → 20s likely genetic)
   c. **Most people with hyperuricemia never get gout**
   d. ↑ Production of uric acid can be genetic or acquired (e.g., alcohol, hemolysis, neoplasia, psoriasis)
   e. Underexcretion of urate via kidney (<800 mg/dL urine urate) can be idiopathic or because of kidney dz, drugs (aspirin, diuretics, alcohol)
   f. Si/Sx of gout = painful monoarticular arthritis affecting distal joints (often first metatarsophalangeal joint = **podagra** [Figure 1.22A]); chronic dz leads to tophaceous gout with destruction of joints (Figure 1.22B)
   g. Dx = **clinical triad of monoarticular arthritis, hyperuricemia, ⊕ response to colchicine**, confirm with needle tap of joint → crystals
   h. Acute Tx = colchicine and NSAIDs (not aspirin)
   i. Px = some people never experience more than one attack; those that do → chronic tophaceous gout, with significant joint deformation (**classic rat-bite appearance to joint on x-ray—Figure 1.22C**) and toothpaste-like discharge from joint
   j. Maintenance Tx
      (1) Do not start unless pt has more than one attack
      (2) Overproducers → allopurinol (inhibits xanthine oxidase)
      (3) Underexcreters → probenecid/sulfinpyrazone
      (4) **Always start while pt still taking colchicine, because sudden ↓ in serum urate precipitates an acute attack**
   k. Pseudogout
      (1) Caused by calcium pyrophosphate dihydrate (CPPD) crystal deposition in joints and articular cartilage (chondrocalcinosis)
      (2) Mimics gout very closely; seen in persons age 60 or older; often affects larger, more proximal joints
      (3) Can be 1° or 2° to metabolic dz (hyperparathyroidism, Wilson's dz, diabetes, hemochromatosis)
      (4) Dx → microscopic analysis of joint aspirate
      (5) Tx = colchicine and NSAIDs

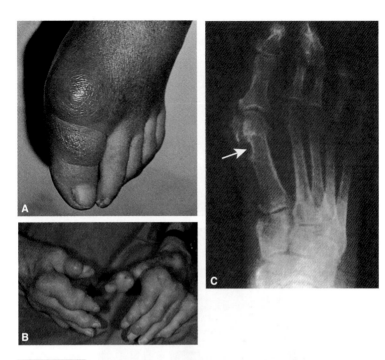

(A) Podagra of acute gout. **(B)** Chronic tophaceous gout. (Image from Rubin E, Farber JL. *Pathology*, 3rd Ed. Philadelphia: Lippincott Williams & Wilkins, 1999.) **(C)** "Rat-bite" (*white arrow*) appearance of chronic tophaceous gout on x-ray. (Reprinted with permission from Barker LR, Burton JR, Zieve, PD. *Principles of ambulatory medicine*, 4th Ed. Baltimore: Williams & Wilkins, 1995:935.)

    I. Microscopy
        (1) **Gout → needle-like negatively birefringent crystals** (Figure 1.23A)
        (2) **"P"seudogout → "P"ositively birefringent crystals** (Figure 1.23B)
  10. Septic Arthritis
     a. Monoarticular arthritis in a sexually active pt usually because of *Neisseria gonorrhea*
     b. Otherwise, the most common cause is *S. aureus,* with *Streptococcus* spp. and Gram-negative rods (GNR) less common

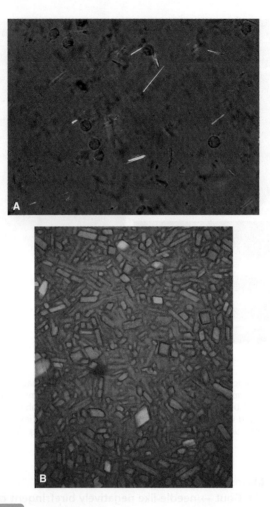

FIGURE 1.23

(A) Gout. Synovial fluid microscopy under compensated polarized light showing the slender, needle-shaped, negatively birefringent urate crystals. The axis of slow vibration is from *bottom left* to *top right*. (From Axford JS. *Medicine*. Oxford: Blackwell Science, 1996, with permission.) (B) Calcium pyrophosphate dehydrate crystals (extracted from synovial fluid), which are pleomorphic, rectangular, and weakly positively birefringent. The axis of slow vibration is from *bottom left* to *top right*. (From Axford JS. *Medicine*. Oxford: Blackwell Science, 1996, with permission.)

   c. Septic arthritis must be distinguished from gout and pseudogout, which can present similarly

   d. Dx = joint fluid Gram stain, culture, swabbing all orifices for *N. gonorrhea,* and sending fluid for crystals

   e. Joint fluid WBC count in pyogenic septic arthritis (e.g., *S. aureus, Streptococcus,* GNR) typically is >50,000; in arthritis caused by *N. gonorrhea* it is often <50,000

   f. Tx = antibiotics targeted either at *N. gonorrhea* or *Staphylococcus, Streptococcus,* and GNR depending on Gram stain and culture (GS/Cx) results

11. Polymyalgia Rheumatica

   a. Inflammatory condition that typically occurs in elderly women (age >50)

   b. Si/Sx = painful muscle tenderness in the neck, shoulders, and upper back relieved by NSAIDs or steroids

   c. Dx = demographics (elderly, typically but not exclusively female) and invariably a very high ESR (>100)

   d. Beware, often associated with temporal arteritis

   e. Tx is prednisone taper

E. Muscle Dz

1. **General**

   a. Dz of muscle are divided into two groups: neurogenic and myopathic

   b. Neurogenic dz → **distal weakness, no pain, fasciculations present**

   c. Myopathic dz → **proximal weakness, ± pain, no fasciculations**

2. **Duchenne's Muscular Dystrophy**

   a. **X-linked** lack of dystrophin

   b. Si/Sx commence at age 1 yr with **progressive proximal weakness and wasting**, ↑ creatine phosphate kinase (CPK), **calf hypertrophy**, waddling gait, Gower's maneuver (pts pick themselves off the floor by using arms to help legs)

   c. Tx = supportive

   d. Px = death occurs in 10s–20s, most often because of pneumonia

   e. Becker's dystrophy is similar but less severe dz

3. **Polymyositis and Dermatomyositis**

   a. Autoinflammatory dz of muscles and sometimes skin (dermatomyositis)

b. Female/male = 2:1; occurs in young children and geriatric populations

c. Si/Sx = symmetric weakness/atrophy of proximal limb muscles, muscle aches, dysphonia (laryngeal muscle weakness), dysphagia

d. Dermatomyositis presents with above as well as with **periorbital heliotropic** purple rash and **shawl sign** (rash over shoulders, upper back, and V-shaped around neck line); also look for **Gottron's papules** (see Figure 1.24B), which are purple papules over the DIP and MCP joints of hand, and **periungual (i.e., around the nail bed) telangiectasias**

e. Dx = ANA ⊕, ↑ creatine kinase, muscle Bx → inflammatory changes

f. Tx = steroids, methotrexate, or cyclophosphamide for resistant dz

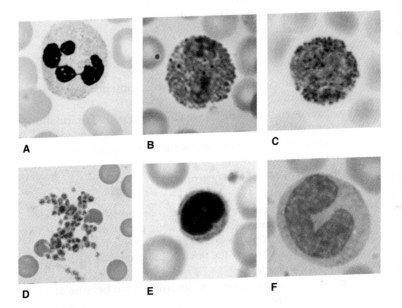

FIGURE 1.24

Nml blood cells. **(A)** Neutrophil. **(B)** Eosinophil. **(C)** Basophile. **(D)** Platelets. **(E)** Lymphocyte. **(F)** Monocyte. (From Cohen BJ, Wood DL. *Memmler's the human body in health and disease*, 9th Ed. Philadelphia: Lippincott, Williams & Wilkins, 2000, with permission.)

4. **Myasthenia Gravis (MG)**
   a. Autoantibodies block the postsynaptic acetylcholine receptor
   b. Most common in women in 20s to 30s or men in 50s to 60s
   c. **Associated with thymomas, thyroid, and other autoimmune dz (e.g., lupus)**
   d. Sx = **muscle weakness worse with use**, diplopia, dysphagia, proximal limb weakness, can progress to cause respiratory failure
   e. Dx = trial of edrophonium (so-called Tensilon test) → immediate ↑ in strength, confirm with electromyelography → repetitive stimulation ↓ action potential
   f. DDx
      (1) **Lambert-Eaton syndrome**
         (a) AutoAb to **pre**synaptic Ca channels seen with small cell lung CA
         (b) Differs from MG in that Lambert-Eaton → ↓ reflexes, autonomic dysfunction (xerostomia, impotence), and **Sx improve with muscle use (action potential strength ↑ with repeated stimulation)**
      (2) Aminoglycosides can worsen MG or induce mild MG Sx in critically ill pts
   g. Tx = anticholinesterase inhibitors (e.g., pyridostigmine) first line
      (1) Steroids, cyclophosphamide, azathioprine for ↑ severe dz
      (2) Plasmapheresis temporarily alleviates Sx by removing the Ab
      (3) Resection of thymoma can be curative

VII. Hematology (Figure 1.24)

A. **Anemia**
   1. **Microcytic Anemias (≡ MCV <80)**
      a. **Result from ↓ hemoglobin (Hb) production or impaired Hb function**
      b. Iron deficiency anemia
         (1) **NOT a Dx, must find the cause of iron deficiency**
         (2) Epidemiology
            (a) Number one anemia in the world; hookworms are the number one cause in the world
            (b) ↑ incidence in women of childbearing age 2° to menses

(c) **In the elderly it is colon CA until proven otherwise**

(d) Dietary deficiency **virtually impossible in adults, seen in children**

(3) Si/Sx = tachycardia, fatigue, pallor all from anemia, smooth tongue, brittle nails, esophageal webs, and pica all from iron deficiency

(4) Dx = ↓ **serum iron,** ↓ serum ferritin, ↑ **total iron-binding capacity (TIBC),** peripheral smear → target cells (Figure 1.25A)

(5) Tx = iron sulfate; should achieve baseline hematocrit within 2 mos

c. Sideroblastic anemia

(1) Ineffective erythropoiesis because of disorder of porphyrin pathway

(2) Etiologies = chronic alcoholism, drugs (commonly isoniazid), genetic

(3) Si/Sx as per any anemia

(4) Labs: ↑ **iron,** N/↑ TIBC, ↑ ferritin

(5) Dx = ringed sideroblasts on iron stain of bone marrow (Figure 1.25B)

(6) Tx = sometimes responsive to pyridoxine (vitamin B_6 supplements)

d. Lead poisoning

(1) Si/Sx = anemia, encephalopathy (worse in children), seizures, ataxic gait, **wrist/foot drops,** renal tubular acidosis

(2) Classic findings

(a) **Bruton's lines** = blue/gray discoloration at gum-lines

(b) **Basophilic stippling of red cells (blue dots in red cells) (Figure 1.25C)**

FIGURE 1.25

(A) Target cells on blood smear. (From Anderson SC. *Anderson's atlas of hematology.* Baltimore: Wolters Kluwer Health/Lippincott Williams & Wilkins, 2003.) **(B)** Ringed sideroblasts on Prussian blue staining of iron in bone marrow. (McClatchey KD. *Clinical laboratory medicine,* 2nd Ed. Philadelphia: Lippincott Williams & Wilkins, 2002.) **(C)** Basophilic stippling of red cells on blood smear. (From Anderson SC. *Anderson's atlas of hematology.* Baltimore: Wolters Kluwer Health/Lippincott Williams & Wilkins, 2003.)

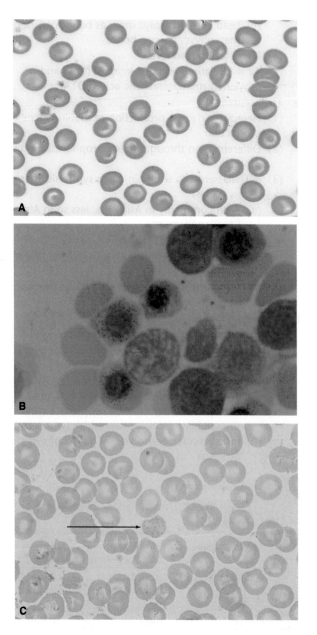

> > > (c) Lead lines on x-rays show as bands of ↑ density at
> > >   metaphyses of long bones
> >
> > (3) Dx = serum lead level
> > (4) Tx = chelation with dimercaprol (BAL) and/or
> >   ethylenediaminetetraacetic acid (EDTA)
>
> e. Thalassemias
>   (1) Hereditary dz of ↓ production of globin chains → ↓ Hb
>   production
>   (2) Differentiation through gel electrophoresis of globin
>   proteins
>   (3) α-Thalassemia (↓ α-globin chain synthesis; there are
>   four α alleles)
>   (a) Seen commonly in Asian pts, less so in African and
>   Mediterranean pts
>   (b) Characteristics (Table 1.34)
>   (4) β-Thalassemia (↓ β-globin chain synthesis; there are two
>   β alleles)
>   (a) Usually of Mediterranean or African descent
>   (b) Characteristics (Table 1.35)
> f. Sickle cell anemia (Figure 1.26)
>   (1) HbS tetramer polymerizes, causing sickling of
>   deoxygenated RBCs
>   (2) Si/Sx
>   (a) Vaso-occlusion → pain crisis, myocardiopathy,
>   infarcts of bone/CNS/lungs/kidneys, and
>   autosplenectomy because of splenic infarct → ↑
>   susceptibility to encapsulated bacteria
>   (b) **Intravascular hemolysis → gallstones in children
>   or teens**

Table 1.34 α-Thalassemia

# Alleles Affected	Dx	Characteristic	Blood Smear
4	Hydrops fetalis	Fetal demise, total body edema	Bart's γ_4 Hb precipitations
3	HbH dz	Precipitation of β-chain tetramers	Intraerythrocytic inclusions
2	α-Thalassemia minor	Usually clinically silent	Mild microcytic anemia
1	Carrier state	No anemia, aSx	No abnormalities

Table 1.35   β-Thalassemia

	Thalassemia Major (β−/β−)	Thalassemia Minor (β+/β−)
Si/Sx	Anemia develops at age 6 mos (because of the switch from fetal γ Hb to adult β), splenomegaly, frontal bossing because of extramedullary hematopoiesis, iron overload (2° to transfusions)	Typically aSx carriers
Dx	Electrophoresis ↓↓↓ HbA, ↑ HbA₂, ↑ HbF	Electrophoresis ↓ HbA, ↑ HbA₂ (γ), **N HbF**
Tx	Folate supplementation, splenectomy for hypersplenism, transfuse only for severe anemia	Avoid oxidative stress

(c) ↑ risk of aplastic anemia from parvovirus B19 infxns
(3) Dx = hemoglobin electrophoresis → HbS phenotype
(4) Tx
    (a) O₂ (cells sickle when Hb desaturates), transfuse as needed
    (b) Hydroxyurea → ↓ incidence and severity of pain crises
    (c) Pneumococcal vaccination due to ↑ risk of infxn

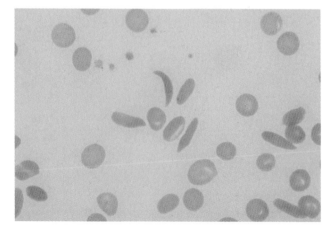

FIGURE 1.26

Sickle cell anemia on blood smear. (From Anderson SC. *Anderson's atlas of hematology.* Baltimore: Wolters Kluwer Health/Lippincott Williams & Wilkins, 2003.)

2. **Megaloblastic Anemias** ($\equiv$ MCV >100)
   a. **Results from** $\downarrow$ **DNA synthesis with nml RNA/protein synthesis**
   b. **Pathognomonic blood smear** $\rightarrow$ **hypersegmented neutrophils** (Figure 1.27)
   c. Vitamin B_{12} deficiency
      (1) Pernicious anemia is most common cause
         (a) Ab to gastric parietal cells $\rightarrow$ $\downarrow$ production of intrinsic factor (necessary for uptake of B_{12} in the terminal ileum)
         (b) Accompanied by achlorhydria and atrophic gastritis
      (2) Other causes = malabsorption becasue of gastric resection, resection of terminal ileum, or intestinal infxn by *Diphyllobothrium latum*
      (3) Si/Sx = megaloblastic anemia **with neurologic signs** = peripheral neuropathy, paresthesias, $\downarrow$ balance and position sense, **worse in legs**
      (4) **Dx = $\uparrow$ serum methylmalonic acid and $\uparrow$ homocysteine levels**—more sensitive than B_{12} levels, which may or may not be $\downarrow$
      (5) **Tx** = vitamin B_{12} high-dose oral Tx proven equivalent to parenteral

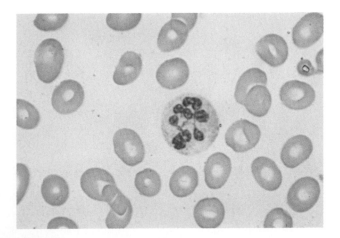

FIGURE 1.27

Hypersegmented neutrophil. (From Gold DH, Weingeist TA. *Color atlas of the eye in systemic disease.* Baltimore: Lippincott Williams & Wilkins, 2001.)

    d. Folic acid deficiency
      (1) Folic acid derived from green, leafy vegetables ("foliage")
      (2) Causes = dietary deficiency (most common), pregnancy or hemolytic anemia ($\uparrow$ requirements), methotrexate or prolonged TMP-SMX Tx (inhibits reduction of folate into tetrahydrofolate)
      (3) Si/Sx = megaloblastic anemia, no neurologic signs
      (4) Dx = **nml serum methylmalonic acid but $\uparrow$ homocysteine levels**—more sensitive than folate levels, which may or may not be $\downarrow$
      (5) Tx = oral folic acid supplementation
  3. **Normocytic Anemias**
    a. Hypoproliferative (Table 1.36)
    b. Hemolytic (Table 1.37)
B. **Coagulation Disorders**
  1. **Thrombocytopenia**
    a. Caused by splenic sequestration, stem-cell failure, or $\uparrow$ destruction
    b. Si/Sx = bleeding time $\uparrow$ at counts <50,000, clinically significant bleeds start at counts <20,000, CNS bleeds occur when counts <10,000

Table 1.36 Hypoproliferative Anemias

Dz	Characteristics	Tx
Anemia of renal failure	• $\downarrow$ Erythropoietin production by kidney • Indicates chronic renal failure	Erythropoietin
Anemia of chronic dz	• Seen in chronic inflammation (e.g., CA, TB or fungal infxn, collagen-vascular dz) • Dx = $\downarrow$ **serum iron**, Nml/$\uparrow$ ferritin, $\downarrow$ **total iron-binding capacity**	Tx underlying inflammatory dz, supportive
Aplastic anemia	• Bone marrow failure, usually idiopathic, or because parvovirus B19 (especially in sickle cell) hepatitis virus, radiation, drugs (e.g., chloramphenicol) • Dx = bone marrow Bx → hypocellular marrow	Bone marrow for severe dz, antihymocyte globulin and cyclosporine may help for mild dz

Table 1.37 Hemolytic Anemias

Dz	Characteristics	Tx
Intrinsic Hemolysis (RBC defects)		
Spherocytosis	• Autosomal dominant defect of spectrin → spherical, stiff RBCs trapped in spleen • Si/Sx = childhood jaundice and gallstones, indirect hyperbilirubinemia, Coombs' negative • Dx = clinical ⊕ peripheral smear → spherocytes	Folic acid, splenectomy for severe dz
Extrinsic Hemolysis		
Autoimmune hemolysis (IgG-mediated)	• Etiologies = idiopathic (most common), lupus, drugs (e.g., penicillin), leukemia, lymphoma • Si/Sx = rapid-onset, **speherocytes on blood smear**, ↑ indirect bilirubin, jaundice, ↓ **haptoglobin**, ↑ **urine hemosidern** • Dx = ⊕ direct Coombs' test	First line = prednisone ± splenectomy, cyclophosphamide for refractory dz
Cold-agglutinin dz (IgM-mediated)	• Most commonly idiopathic, can be because of *Mycoplasma pneumoniae* & mononucleosis mild cytomegalovirus, Epstein-Barr virus infxns • Si/Sx = anemia on exposure to cold or following upper respiratory infxns • Dx = cold-agglutinin test and indirect Coombs' test	Prednisone for severe dz, supportive for mild
Mechanical destruction	• Causes = disseminated intravascular coagulation (DIC), thrombotoc thrombocytopenic purpura (TTP), hemolytic-uremic syndrome (HUS), and artificial heart valve • Peripheral smear → schistocytes (see Figure 1.28)	Tx directed at underlying disorder

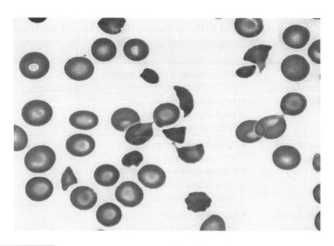

FIGURE 1.28

Schistocytes on blood smear. (From Anderson SC. *Anderson's atlas of hematology*. Baltimore: Wolters Kluwer Health/Lippincott Williams & Wilkins, 2003.)

    c. ↓ Production seen in leukemia, aplastic anemia, and alcohol (even minimal)

    d. Causes (Table 1.38)

    e. Lab values (Table 1.39)

2. **Inherited Disorders**

    a. von Willebrand factor (vWF) deficiency

      (1) **Most common inherited bleeding dz**

      (2) Si/Sx = **episodic ↑ bleeding time and ecchymoses, nml PT/PTT**

      (3) Dx = vWF levels and ristocetin–cofactor test

      (4) Tx = DDAVP (↑ vWF secretion) or cryoprecipitate for acute bleeding

    b. Hemophilia

      (1) X-linked deficiency of factor VIII (hemophilia A) or X-linked deficiency of factor IX (hemophilia B = Christmas dz)

      (2) Si/Sx = hemarthroses (bleeding into joint), ecchymoses with minor trauma, ↑ **PTT, nml PT, nml bleeding time**

      (3) Dx = ↓ factor levels

      (4) Tx = recombinant factor VIII or factor IX concentrate

3. **Hypercoagulable Dz (Table 1.40)**

Table 1.38 Causes of Platelet Destruction (Thrombocytopenia)

Dz	Characteristics	Tx
Idiopathic thrombocytopenic purpura (ITP)	• Autoantibody-mediated platelet destruction • **In children, follows upper respiratory infxn and is self-limiting; in adults it is chronic**	Steroids, IVIG, splenectomy
Thrombotic thrombocytopenic purpura (TTP)	• Idiopathic dz, often seen in HIV, can be fatal • **Pentad** = hemolytic anemia, renal failure, thrombocytopenia, fever, neurologic dz	Plasma exchange or fresh frozen plasma until dz abates, dz is fatal without Tx
Hemolytic-uremic syndrome (HUS)	• Usually in kids, often because of *E. coli* 0157:H7 • Si/Sx = acute renal failure, bloody diarrhea, abd pain, seizures, **fulminant thrombocytopenia with hemolytic anemia**	Dialysis
Disseminated intravascular coagulations (DIC)	• Seen in adenoCA, leukemia, sepsis, trauma • ↑ Fibrin split products, ↓ fibrinogen, ↑ prothrombin time/partial thromboplastin time	Directed at underlying cause
Drug-induced	• Causes = heparin, sulfonamides, valproic acid • Reverses within days of ceasing drug intake	Stop drug

Table 1.39 Labs in Platelet Destruction

Study	Autoantibody	Disseminated Intravascular Coagulation	Thrombotoc Thrombocytopenic Purpura/Hemolytic-Uremic Syndrome
Blood smear	Microspherocytes	Schistocytes (+)	**Schistocytes (+++)**
Coombs' test	⊕	—	—
Prothrombin Time /Partial Thromboplastin Time	Nml	↑	Nml /↑

Table 1.40 Hypercoagulable Diseases

1° (Inherited)	2° (Acquired)	
Antithrombin III deficiency	Prolonged immobilization	L-Asparaginase
Protein C deficiency	Pregnancy	Hyperlipidemia
Protein S deficiency	Surgery/trauma	Anticariolipin Ab
Factor V Leiden deficiency	Oral contraceptives	Lupus anticoagulant
Dysfibrinogenemia	Homocystinuria	Disseminated intravascular coagulation
Plasminogen (activator) deficiency	Malignancy (adenoCA)	Vitamin K deficiency
Heparin cofactor II deficiency	Smoking	
Homocystinemia	Nephrotic syndrome	
Factor II (prothrombin) mutation		

C. **Myeloproliferative Dz (Table 1.41)**

   1. Caused by clonal proliferation of a myeloid stem cell → excessive production of mature, differentiated myeloid cell lines

   2. All can transform into acute leukemias

   3. Thrombocytosis

      a. 1° (bone marrow disorder) versus 2° (reactive)

      b. 1° can be essential thrombocythemia but also can see a thrombocytosis in polycythemia rubra vera or chronic myelogenous leukemia—typically count is >1 million

      c. 2° or reactive thrombocytosis can be seen in any chronic inflammatory disorder, serious infxn, acute bleed, iron-deficiency anemia (mechanism unclear), or following splenectomy—typically count is < 1 million

D. **Leukemias**

   1. **Acute Lymphoblastic Leukemia**

      a. **Peak age is 3 to 4 yr;** most common neoplasm in children

      b. Si/Sx = fever, fatigue, anemia, pallor, petechiae, infxns

      c. Labs → leukocytosis, anemia, ↓ platelets, marrow bx → ↑ blasts, peripheral blood blasts are **PAS +, CALLA +, TdT +**

Table 1.41 Myeloproliferative Diseases

Dz	Characteristics	Tx
Polycythemia vera	• Rare, peak onset at 50–60 yrs, male predominance • Si/Sx = headache, diplopia, retinal hemorrhages, stroke, angina, claudication (all because of vascular sludging), early satiety, splenomegaly, gout, **pruritus after showering, plethora, basophilia** • **5% progress to leukemia, 20% to myelofibrosis**	Phlebotomy, hydroxyurea to keep blood counts low
Essential thrombocythemia	• Si/Sx = platelet count $>5 \times 10^5$ cells/ml, splenomegaly ecchymoses • Dx = rule out 2° thrombocytosis (because of iron deficiency, malignancy, etc.) • 5% progress to myelofibrosis or acute leukemia	Platelet exchange (apheresis), hydroxyurea, or anagrelide
Ideopathic myelofibrosis	• Typically affects pts ≥50 yrs • Si/Sx = massive hepatosplenomegaly, blood smear → **teardrop cells** • Dx = hypercellular marrow on Bx • Poor Px, median 5 yrs before marrow failure	Supportive (splenectomy, antibiotics, allopurinol for gout)

Chronic myelogenous leukemia (see section D.3).

    d. Tx = chemotherapy: induction, consolidation, maintenance intrathecal chemotherapy during consolidation

    e. Px = 80% cure in children (much worse in adults)

2. **Acute Myelogenous Leukemia (AML)**

    a. **Most common leukemia in adults**

    b. Si/Sx = fever, fatigue, pallor, petechiae, infxns, lymphadenopathy

    c. Labs → thrombocytopenia, peripheral blood, and marrow bx → myeloblasts that are **myeloperoxidase +, Sudan Black +, Auer Rods +**

    d. Tx

       (1) Chemotherapy → induction, consolidation (no maintenance)

       (2) All-*trans* retinoic acid used for the M3 subtype of AML, causes differentiation of blasts—beware of onset of DIC in these pts

    e. Px = overall 30% cure; bone marrow transplant (BMT) improves outcomes

3. **Chronic Myelogenous Leukemia**

    a. Presents most commonly in the 50s but can be any age

    b. Si/Sx = anorexia, early satiety, diaphoresis, arthritis, bone tenderness, leukostasis (WBC $\geq 1 \times 10^5$) → dyspnea, dizzy, slurred speech, diplopia

    c. Labs → **Philadelphia (Ph) chromosome ⊕, peripheral blood → cells of all maturational stages,** ↓ leukocyte alkaline phosphatase

    d. Ph chromosome is pathognomonic, seen in >90% of pts with CML, because of translocation of *abl* gene from chromosome 9 to *bcr* on 22

    e. Tx = imatinib mesylate (Gleevec), interferon (IFN), hydroxyurea, or BMT for blast crisis

    f. **Blast crisis = acute phase, invariably develops causing death in 3 to 6 mos; mean time to onset = 3 to 4 yrs; only BMT can prevent**

4. **Chronic Lymphocytic Leukemia**

    a. ↑ incidence with age, causes 30% of leukemias in US

    b. Si/Sx = typically aSx for many yrs, and when it eventually does become Sx pts have organomegaly, hemolytic anemia, thrombocytopenia, blood smear and marrow → nml morphology lymphocytosis of blood and marrow; **lymphocytes almost always express CD5 protein**

    c. **Tx = palliative, early Tx does NOT prolong life**

    d. Other presentations of similar leukemias

       (1) Hairy cell leukemia (B-cell subtype)

          (a) Si/Sx = characteristic hairy cell morphology (Figure 1.29A), pancytopenia

          (b) Tx = IFN-α, splenectomy

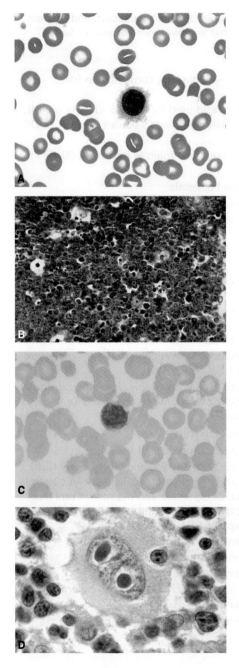

FIGURE 1.29

(A) Hairy cell leukemic cell on blood smear. (From Anderson SC. *Anderson's atlas of hematology.* Baltimore: Wolters Kluwer Health/Lippincott Williams & Wilkins, 2003.) (B) Starry sky pattern of Burkitt's lymphoma on bx. (Image from Rubin E, Farber JL. *Pathology,* 3rd Ed. Philadelphia: Lippincott Williams & Wilkins, 1999.) (C) Sézary cell of T-cell lymphoma (From Anderson SC. *Anderson's atlas of hematology.* Baltimore: Wolters Kluwer Health/Lippincott Williams & Wilkins, 2003.) (D) Reed-Sternberg cell in pt with Hodgkin's dz. Mirror-image, owl-eye nuclei contain large eosinophilic nucleoli. (Image from Rubin E, Farber JL. *Pathology,* 3rd Ed. Philadelphia: Lippincott Williams & Wilkins, 1999.)

(2) T-cell leukemias tend to involve skin, often present with erythematous rashes; some are because of human T-cell leukemia virus (HTLV)

Most Common Leukemias by Age:
Up to age 15 = ALL; age 15–39 = AML; age 40–59 ≥ AML & CML; ≥60 = CLL

E. **Lymphoma**

1. **Non-Hodgkin's Lymphoma (NHL)**
   a. Commonly seen in HIV, often in brain, teenagers get in head and neck
   b. Burkitt's lymphoma
      (1) Closely related to Epstein-Barr virus (EBV) infxns
      (2) African Burkitt's involves jaw/neck; U.S. Burkitt's involves abdomen
      (3) Burkitt's shows a classic "starry sky" pattern on histopathology, caused by spaces scattered within densely packed lymph tissue (Figure 1.29B)
   c. Cutaneous T-cell lymphoma (CTCL, mycosis fungoides)
      (1) Si/Sx = often in elderly, diffuse scaly rash or erythroderma (total body erythema), precedes clinically apparent malignancy by yrs
      (2) **Stained cells have cerebriform nuclei** (looks like cerebral gyri) (Figure 1.29C)
      (3) Leukemic phase of this dz is called "Sézary syndrome"
      (4) Tx = ultraviolet light Tx, consider systemic chemotherapy
   d. Angiocentric T-cell lymphoma
      (1) Two subtypes = nasal T-cell lymphoma (lethal midline granuloma) and pulmonary angiocentric lymphoma
      (2) Si/Sx = large mass, Bx often nonDx because of diffuse necrosis
      (3) Tx = palliative radiation, Px very poor

2. **Hodgkin's Lymphoma**
   a. Occurs in a bimodal age distribution, young men and the elderly
   b. EBV infxn is present in up to 50% of cases
   c. Si/Sx = **Pel-Epstein fevers** (fevers wax and wane over weeks), chills, night sweats, weight loss, pruritus; **Sx worsen with alcohol intake**
   d. Reed-Sternberg (RS) cells seen on Bx, **appear as binucleated giant cells ("owl eyes") or mononucleated giant cell (lacunar cell)** (Figure 1.29D)

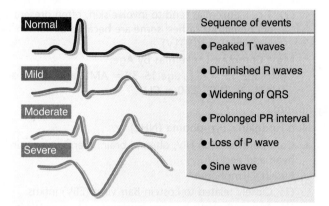

FIGURE 1.30

Hyperkalemia-related EKG changes.

    e. Tx depends on clinical staging

       (1) Stage I = 1 lymph node involved → radiation

       (2) Stage II = ≥2 lymph nodes on same side of diaphragm → radiation

       (3) Stage III = involvement on both sides of diaphragm → chemotherapy

       (4) Stage IV = disseminated to organs or extranodal tissue → chemotherapy

       (5) Chemotherapy regimens

          (a) MOPP = **m**echlorethamine, **O**ncovin (vincristine), **p**rocarbazine, **p**rednisone

          (b) ABVD = **A**driamycin (daunorubicin), **b**leomycin, **v**incristine, **d**acarbazine

VIII. Empiric Antibiotic Tx for Specific Infxns (Table 1.42)

Table 1.42 Empiric Antibiotic Treatment of Specific Infections

Dz	Micro-organisms*	Empiric Antibiotics*
Abd infxn	GNR, anaerobes	3rd gen ceph + metronidazole
Aspiration pneumonia	Mouth and throat anaerobes	3rd gen ceph + metronidazole OR clindamycin
Bites	GNR and anaerobes	amoxicillin-clavulonic acid
Brain abscess	GPC, GNR, anaerobes	3rd gen ceph + metronidazole +/− vancomycin
Bronchitis	S. pneumoniae, H. influenzae, M. catarrhalis, viruses	None, or TMP-SMX or amoxicillin
CAP	S. pneumoniae, H. influenzae, M. catarrhalis, Mycoplasma pneumoniae, Chlamydophila pneumoniae, Chlamydia psittaci, Legionella	3rd gen ceph + macrolide OR fluoroquinolone
Cellulitis	S. aureus, Group A Strep, other Strep	vancomycin
Cholangitis	GNR, anaerobes	3rd gen ceph ⊕ metronidazole
Dental infxn	Mouth anaerobs	Clindamycin
Diabetic foot	GNR, anaerobes, +/− S. aureus	(3rd gen ceph + metronidazole OR ampicillin-sulbactam) +/− vancomycin
Endocarditis	S. aureus, viridians Strep, HACEK, coag neg Staph	3rd gen ceph + vancomycin
Epididymitis and prostatitis	<35 yo → N. gonorrhea >35 yo → GNR	<35 yo → 3rd gen ceph >35 yo → 3rd gen ceph OR fluoroquinolone
Necrotizing fasciitis	Group A Strep, Clostridium, community MRSA	(Penicillin or 3rd gen ceph) + clindamycin + vancomycin
Gastroenteritis	GNR	Fluoroquinolone OR 3rd gen ceph
Urethritis	N. gonorrhea, Chlamydia trachomatis	3rd gen ceph + doxycycline
Liver abscess	GNR, anaerobes OR Entamoeba histolytica	3rd gen ceph + metronidazole OR metronidazole
Lung abscess	Mouth/throat anaerobes	3rd gen ceph + metronidazole OR clindamycin
Meningitis (adult)	S. pneumoniae, N. meningitidis, H. influenzae, Listeria	3rd gen ceph + ampicillin + vancomycin

Table 1.42 *Continued*

Dz	Microorganisms*	Empiric Antibiotics*
Meningitis (pediatric)	*E. coli, Listeria, S. pneumoniae, N. meningitides*	3rd gen ceph + ampicillin + vancomycin
Neutropenic fever	GNR, GPC	(Ceftazidime OR cefepime OR imipenem OR piperacillin-tazobactam) ± gentamicin ± vancomycin
Nosocomial pneumonia	GNR, *S. aureus*	(Ceftazidime OR cefepime OR imipenem OR piperacillin-tazobactam OR ciprofloxacin) + vancomycin
Osteomyelitis	GPC, GNR	3rd gen ceph + vancomycin
Pharyngitis	Group A Strep	Penicillin
Pelvic inflammator dz	GNR, anaerobes, *Chlamydia/Neisseria*	Clindamycin + gentamicin + doxycycline
Pyelonephritis	GNR	3rd gen ceph or gentimicin
Spontaneous bacterial peritonitis	GNR, *S. pneumoniae*	3rd gen ceph
Septic arthritis	*S. aureus, Strep spp.*, GNR	Vancomycin + 3rd gen ceph
Septic shock	GPC, GNR	Vancomycin + (3rd gen ceph OR piperacillin-tazobactam OR imipenem) +/− fluoroquinolone +/− metronidazole
Bell's palsy	Herpes simplex virus, other	Valacyclovir/acyclovir
Herpes zoster	Varicella zoster virus	Valacyclovir/acyclovir
Retinitis in HIV	Cytomegalovirus	Valganciclovir/ganciclovir
Enephalitis	Herpes simplex virus, other	Acyclovir (iv)
Oral thrush	*Candida*	Nystatin swish and swallow if just oral, fluconazole if esophageal dz

*GNR, Gram-negative rod; GPC, Gram-positive cocci; 3rd gen ceph, third-generation cephalosporin. For community acquired infxns, pseudomonal coverage is not required, and ceftriaxone or cefotaxime are the preferred third-generation cephalosporins; for nosocomial infxns, pseudomonal coverage is required and ceftazidime or cefepime (actually a fourth-generation cephalosporin) are the preferred agents.

After identification of the actual causative organism, the initial empiric tx should always be narrowed as much as possible.

Table 1.43 Hypokalemia

1. For urgent potassium (K^+) replacement give iv and oral K^+ simultaneously.
   - Give IV at 10 mEq/h through peripheral line or 20 mEq/h through central line (more rapid administration causes vessel necrosis).
   - Give oral K^+ at up to 40 mEq/h
   - Contrary to popular belief, oral K^+ ↑ serum K^+ much faster than IV (because you cannot give IV quickly)
   - Each 10 mEq oral or IV should ↑ serum K^+ by 0.1 mmol/L

2. If K^+ repeatedly falls or remains low:
   - Check pt's medications for diuretics or toxins (e.g., amphotericin) that cause K^+ wasting
   - Replete serum magnesium; nml magnesium is required for maintenance of serum K^+ levels
   - Start K^+-sparing diuretic (e.g., spironolactone) or angiotensin-converting enzyme inhibitor to help maintain K^+ levels
   - Advise to eat high K^+ food (e.g., banana)

3. Peri-MI, the K^+ should be kept >4.0 to suppress arrhythmias—be aggressive!

4. In renal failure, small doses of oral or IV K^+ will dramatically ↑ serum K^+, so be careful!

Table 1.44 Hyperkalemia

Dx

Plasma potassium >6.5 mmol/L.
Dangerous level of potassium (K^+) depends on if acute (7 ≈ 5 mmol/L) or chronic (≈6.5 mmol/L).
May be associated with muscle weakness and EKG abnormalities (e.g., widening of QRS complexes, peaked T waves, loss of the P wave).
Predominantly occurs in pts with renal failure or muscle breakdown.

Emergency Tx: Hyperkalemia Associated with EKG Abnormalities

Give:
10 mL of 10% calcium gluconate bolus IV, repeated if necessary (up to 100 mL/24 h) to stabilize myocardial cell membranes.
It does not lower potassium.
Then:
Glucose + insulin: give 50 mL of dextrose 50% with 10 units of short-acting insulin. This will lower plasma potassium for several hrs (4–6 hrs).
±05 mL 8.4% sodium bicarbonate if pH <7.4.
±Kayexalate oral or per rectum (↓ K^+ for 24 h).

Longer-Term Tx

Remove the cause.
Diet (≤60 mmol K^+/day)
Regular dialysis in renal failure.

Algorithm 1.2

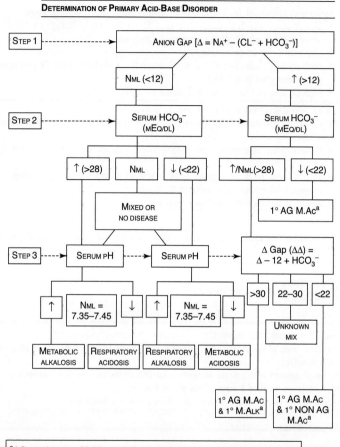

DETERMINATION OF PRIMARY ACID-BASE DISORDER

STEP 1 → ANION GAP $[\Delta = Na^+ - (Cl^- + HCO_3^-)]$

N_{ML} (<12) | ↑ (>12)

STEP 2 → SERUM HCO_3^- (mEq/dL) | SERUM HCO_3^- (mEq/dL)

↑ (>28) | N_{ML} | ↓ (<22) | ↑/N_{ML}(>28) | ↓ (<22)

MIXED OR NO DISEASE

1° AG M.Ac[a]

STEP 3 → SERUM pH → SERUM pH → Δ Gap $(\Delta\Delta)$ = $\Delta - 12 + HCO_3^-$

↑ | N_{ML} = 7.35–7.45 | ↓ | ↑ | N_{ML} = 7.35–7.45 | ↓ | >30 | 22–30 | <22

UNKNOWN MIX

METABOLIC ALKALOSIS | RESPIRATORY ACIDOSIS | RESPIRATORY ALKALOSIS | METABOLIC ACIDOSIS

1° AG M.Ac & 1° M.Alk[a] | 1° AG M.Ac & 1° NON AG M.Ac[a]

[a]AG = anion gap. M.Alk = metabolic alkalosis. M.Ac = metabolic acidosis.

Algorithm 1.3

METABOLIC ACIDOSIS

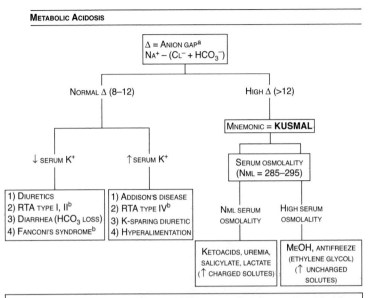

Check for compensation or the presence of a mixed disorder. Winter's formula predicts the CO_2 if there is compensation: $CO_2 = 1.5 * HCO_3^- + 8 \pm 2$. If the CO_2 is higher than expected, there is an additional acidotic process occurring. If the CO_2 is lower than expected, there is an additional alkalotic process occurring.

[a] Calculate Δ in *all* patients, regardless of pH or HCO_3^-. Mixed acidosis and alkalosis can cancel each other out, causing neutral pH. Perform the following steps to search for a mixed disorder.
1) Calculate Δ: if $\Delta \geq 12$, the disorder is a 1° anion gap acidosis
2) Calculate $\Delta\Delta = |\Delta - 12 + HCO_3^-|$: if $\Delta\Delta \geq 31$, there is also a 1° metabolic alkalosis
    if $\Delta\Delta \leq 21$, there is also a 1° nonanion gap acidosis
Example: A diabetic in ketoacidosis who is vomiting can have a 1° anion gap acidosis from the ketoacidosis and a 1° metabolic alkalosis from the vomiting. In this case, the $\Delta > 12$, the $\Delta\Delta \geq 31$. A diabetic with renal failure who presents with ketoacidosis can have a 1° anion gap and nonanion gap acidosis, with a $\Delta > 12$ and a $\Delta\Delta \leq 21$. Note that this patient may also be vomiting and either tachypneic or bradypneic from obtundation. Thus the patient may have three 1° metabolic acid-base disorders (1° AG acidosis, 1° nonAG acidosis, 1° metabolic alkaosis) and a respiratory disorder. In this case, the disorders must be discriminated clinically or by changes in status in response to therapy.
        Our thanks to Dr. Arian Torbati for his assistance with the $\Delta\Delta$ algorithm.
[b] See Section III.F for description of RTA and Fanconi's syndrome.

Algorithm 1.4

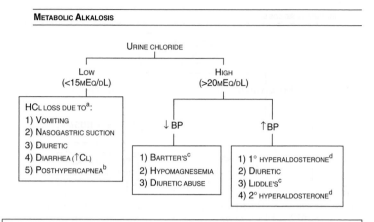

METABOLIC ALKALOSIS

URINE CHLORIDE

LOW (<15mEq/dL)

HIGH (>20mEq/dL)

HCL LOSS DUE TO[a]:
1) VOMITING
2) NASOGASTRIC SUCTION
3) DIURETIC
4) DIARRHEA ($\uparrow$CL)
5) POSTHYPERCAPNEA[b]

↓ BP
1) BARTTER'S[c]
2) HYPOMAGNESEMIA
3) DIURETIC ABUSE

↑BP
1) 1° HYPERALDOSTERONE[d]
2) DIURETIC
3) LIDDLE'S[c]
4) 2° HYPERALDOSTERONE[d]

[a] These conditions are all known as "contraction alkaloses," or "chloride-responsive alkaloses." The contraction in extracellular volume creates a hypochloremic state. The kidney resorbs extra bicarbonate from the tubules due to the loss of chloride anion (tubules need a different anion to maintain electrical neutrality). Administration of chloride anion in the form of normal saline will correct the alkalosis.

[b] Patients who are hypercapnic undergo renal compensation, with resorption of extra bicard from the tubules to offset the respiratory acidosis. When the hypercapnia is corrected (e.g., via intubation) the kidneys must adjust and resorb less bicard. Until they adjust, the patient will have a posthypercapnic metabolic alkalosis.

[c] See Appendix B for Bartter's & Liddle's.

[d] 1° hyperaldosteronism is known as Conn's syndrome. See Endocrinology, Section III.D. 1.2° hyperaldosteronism can be caused by renal artery stenosis (see Nephrology, Section V), Cushing's syndrome (see Endocrine, Section III.B), congestive heart failure, and hepatic cirrhosis.

Algorithm 1.5

RESPIRATORY ACID-BASE DIFFERENTIAL

RESPIRATORY ALKALOSIS	RESPIRATORY ACIDOSIS
• CNS LESION	• MORPHINE/SEDATIVES
• PREGNANCY	• STROKE IN BULBAR AREA OF BRAIN STEM
• HIGH ALTITUDE	• ONDINE'S CURSE (CENTRAL SLEEP APNEA)
• SEPSIS/INFECTION	• COPD (EMPHYSEMA, ASTHMA, BRONCHITIS)
• SALICYLATE TOXICITY	• ADULT RESPIRATORY DISTRESS SYNDROME
• LIVER FAILURE	• CHEST WALL DISEASE (POLIO, KYPHOSCOLIOSIS, MYASTHENIA GRAVIS, MUSCULAR DYSTROPHY)
• ANXIETY (HYPERVENTILATION)	• OBESITY
• PAIN/FEAR (HYPERVENTILATION)	• HYPOPHOSPHATEMIA (DIAPHRAGM REQUIRES LOTS OF ATP DUE TO HIGH ENERGY DEMAND)
• CONGESTIVE HEART FAILURE	• SUCCINYLCHOLINE (PARALYSIS FOR INTUBATION)
• PULMONARY EMBOLUS	• PLEURAL EFFUSION
• PNEUMONIA	• PNEUMOTHORAX
• HYPERTHYROIDISM	
• COMPENSATION FOR A 1° ACIDOSIS	

Check for the presence of a mixed disorder by comparing the change in CO_2 and HCO_3 from normal (normal CO_2 = 40, normal HCO_3 = 24).

Acute respiratory acidosis: HCO_3^- increases by 1 for every 10 the CO_2 increases.
Acute respiratory alkalosis: HCO_3^- decreases by 2 for every 10 the CO_2 decreases.
Chronic respiratory acidosis: HCO_3^- increases by 3.5 for every 10 the CO_2 increases.
Chronic respiratory alkalosis: HCO_3^- decreases by 5 for every 10 the CO_2 decreases.

It's easy to remember the compensations by organizing them in the following table.

	ACIDOSIS	ALKALOSIS
Acute	1	2
Chronic	3–4 (3.5)	5

Change in HCO_3^- per 10 change in CO_2.
Just remember = 1 : 2 : 3–4 : 5!

Algorithm 1.6

EVALUATION OF HYPONATREMIA

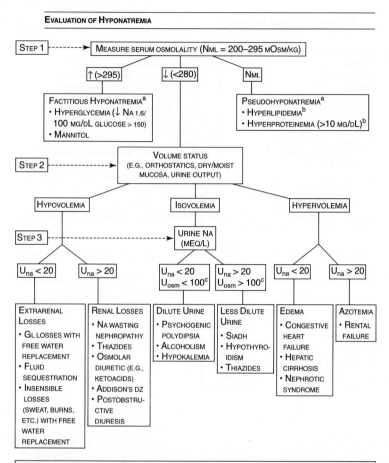

[a] Pseudohyponatremia is a lab artifact due to serum volume occupation by lipid or protein, resulting in an apparent decrease in the amount of Na per given volume of serum. Factitious hyponatremia is a true decrease in serum Na concentration (but normal total body Na) caused by glucose or mannitol osmotically drawing water into the serum.

[b] These disorders are characterized by ≥ 10mOsm/kg gap between the calculated & and the measued serumosmolarity. Serum osmolarity is calculated by $(2*Na) + (BUN/2.8) + (glucose/18)$. The gap is due to the presence of solutes detected by the lab but not accounted for in the osmolality calculation.

[c] U_{osm} = urine osmolality.

Algorithm 1.7

EVALUATION OF HYPERNATREMIA

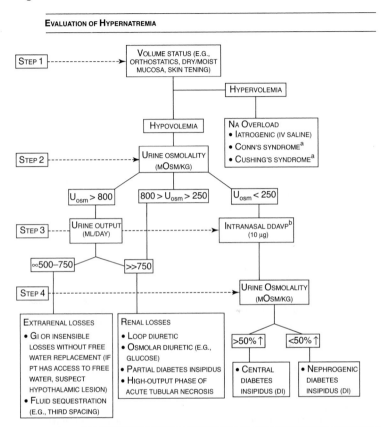

^a See Endocrinology, Section III.B.1 and III.D.1 for Cushing's syndrome and Conn's syndrome.
^b DDAVP = long-acting antidiuretic hormone analogue. Patients with central DI respond by successfully increasing the concentration of their urine by 50%. Patients with nephrogenic DI are unable to concentrate their urine in the presence of DDAVP. Patients with DI tend to be only mildly hypernatremic.

Algorithm 1.8

EVALUATION OF HYPOKALEMIA

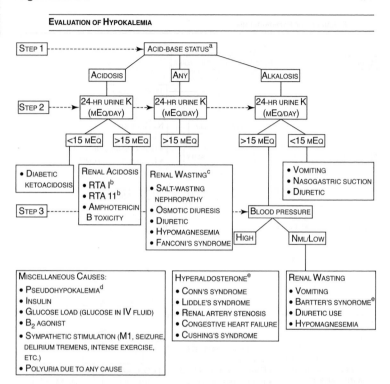

^{a} Metabolic acidosis or alkalosis. Please see Acid-Base algorithms to determine acid-base status.

^{b} RTA = Renal Tubular Acidosis. See Nephrology, Section III.F for a full description.

^{c} Salt wasting nephropathies are tubulointerstitial disorders (e.g., pyelonephritis, renal medullary dz, acute tubular necrosis & allergic interstitial nephritis). For Fanconi's syndrome, see Nephrology, Section III.F.2.

^{d} Pseudohypokalemia is seen in conditions with very high white blood cell counts (e.g., leukernia). The while cells take up potassium while they are sitting in the blood draw tube, creating spurious results.

^{e} See Endocrinology, Sections III.B & D for Cushing's & Conn's syndromes, IV.C for congenital adrenal hyperplasia, Nephrology, Section V for renal artery stenosis, and Appendix B for Liddle's & Bartter's syndromes.

Algorithm 1.9

EVALUATION OF HYPERKALEMIA

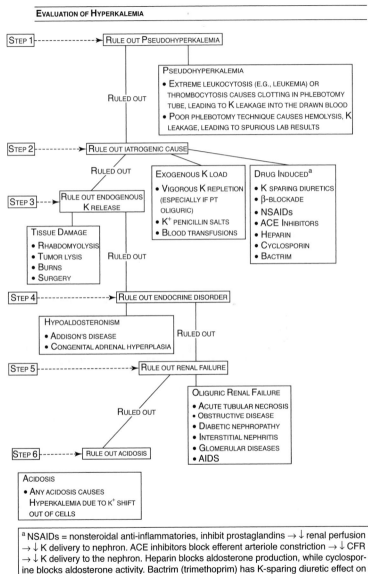

STEP 1 ----------> RULE OUT PSEUDOHYPERKALEMIA

PSEUDOHYPERKALEMIA
- EXTREME LEUKOCYTOSIS (E.G., LEUKEMIA) OR THROMBOCYTOSIS CAUSES CLOTTING IN PHLEBOTOMY TUBE, LEADING TO K LEAKAGE INTO THE DRAWN BLOOD
- POOR PHLEBOTOMY TECHNIQUE CAUSES HEMOLYSIS, K LEAKAGE, LEADING TO SPURIOUS LAB RESULTS

RULED OUT

STEP 2 ----------> RULE OUT IATROGENIC CAUSE

RULED OUT

EXOGENOUS K LOAD
- VIGOROUS K REPLETION (ESPECIALLY IF PT OLIGURIC)
- K^+ PENICILLIN SALTS
- BLOOD TRANSFUSIONS

DRUG INDUCED[a]
- K SPARING DIURETICS
- β-BLOCKADE
- NSAIDs
- ACE INHIBITORS
- HEPARIN
- CYCLOSPORIN
- BACTRIM

STEP 3 ----------> RULE OUT ENDOGENOUS K RELEASE

TISSUE DAMAGE
- RHABDOMYOLYSIS
- TUMOR LYSIS
- BURNS
- SURGERY

RULED OUT

STEP 4 ----------> RULE OUT ENDOCRINE DISORDER

HYPOALDOSTERONISM
- ADDISON'S DISEASE
- CONGENITAL ADRENAL HYPERPLASIA

RULED OUT

STEP 5 ----------> RULE OUT RENAL FAILURE

RULED OUT

OLIGURIC RENAL FAILURE
- ACUTE TUBULAR NECROSIS
- OBSTRUCTIVE DISEASE
- DIABETIC NEPHROPATHY
- INTERSTITIAL NEPHRITIS
- GLOMERULAR DISEASES
- AIDS

STEP 6 ----------> RULE OUT ACIDOSIS

ACIDOSIS
- ANY ACIDOSIS CAUSES HYPERKALEMIA DUE TO K^+ SHIFT OUT OF CELLS

[a] NSAIDs = nonsteroidal anti-inflammatories, inhibit prostaglandins → ↓ renal perfusion → ↓ K delivery to nephron. ACE inhibitors block efferent arteriole constriction → ↓ CFR → ↓ K delivery to the nephron. Heparin blocks aldosterone production, while cyclosporine blocks aldosterone activity. Bactrim (trimethoprim) has K-sparing diuretic effect on tubules.

2. SURGERY

I. Fluid and Electrolytes

A. **Physiology** (Figure 2.1)

1. 50% to 70% of lean body weight is water; most of it is in skeletal muscle
2. Total body water (TBW) is divided into extracellular (one third) and intracellular (two thirds) compartments
3. Extracellular water
   a. Comprises 20% of lean body weight
   b. 25% intravascular and 75% extravascular (interstitial)
4. Intracellular water comprises 40% of lean body weight

B. **Fluid Management**

1. **3 for 1 Rule**
   a. By 1 to 2 hr after a 1-L infusion of isotonic saline or lactated Ringer's, only 300 ml remains in the intravascular compartment
   b. **Thus, three to four times the vascular deficit should be administered** if isotonic crystalloid solutions are used for resuscitation
2. Colloid solutions (containing high-molecular-weight molecules; e.g., albumin, hetastarch, and dextrans) stay in the intravascular space longer
3. Colloids are more expensive than crystalloids and may be most useful in the edematous pt where, for instance, 100 ml of 1% albumin solution will be able to draw approximately 400 ml from the extravascular compartment, thus decreasing edema

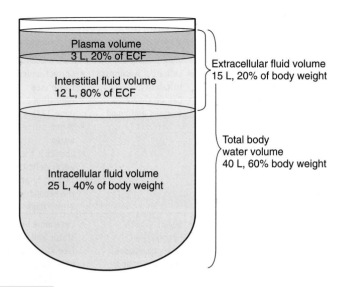

FIGURE 2.1

Distribution of fluid within the body. (From Premkumar K. *The massage connection anatomy and physiology.* Baltimore: Lippincott Williams & Wilkins, 2004.)

C. **Hydration of Surgical Pts**

1. Pts are commonly NPO (nothing by mouth) and require IV fluid hydration

2. An uncomplicated pt without oral intake loses ≥1 L of fluid per day from sweat, urine, feces, and respiration

3. Adequate fluid hydration is indicated by **urine output ≥0.5 cc/kg/hr (for typical pt ≥30 cc/hr)** and by measuring daily weight changes

4. Electrolytes should be replaced as necessary

   a. Salivary and colon secretions are high in potassium (K^+)

   b. Stomach, ileum, and bile secretions are high in Cl^-

   c. Salivary, ileum, pancreas, and bile secretions are high in HCO_3^-

D. **Common Electrolyte Disorders** (Table 2.1)

Text continues on page 140

Table 2.1 Common Electrolyte Disorders

Disorder	DDx	Si/Sx	Tx
↑ Na$^+$	• Fluid loss • Steroid use • Hypertonic fluids	• Lethargy, weakness, irritability • Can be severe → seizures and coma	• Correct underlying cause (see Algorithm 1.7, page 133) • ½ nml saline or water • Correct ½ the water deficit in first 24 hr and the second ½ over 2 to 3 days
↓ Na$^+$	• Copious bladder irrigation status post transurethral resection of the prostate (TURP) • High-output ileostomy • Hyperglycemia • Adrenal insufficiency	• Severe (<115 mmol/L) → seizures, nausea, vomiting, stupor, or coma	• Determine volume status and cause (see Algorithm 1.6, page 132) • For eu- or hypervolemic, water restrict • Correct hyperglycemia • Refractory dz → hypertonic saline
↑ K$^+$	• Acidosis • ↓ Insulin • Leukocytosis • Burns • Crush injury	• Neuromuscular and cardiac sequelae (heart block, ventricular fibrillation, asystole) • EKG → peaked T waves, flattened P waves, wide QRS, eventually a sinusoidal pattern	• Stabilize cardiac membranes with IV calcium gluconate • Glucose and insulin infusion • Albuterol and loop diuretics • Binding resins (Kayexalate) and dialysis longer term • Reverse cause (see Algorithm 1.9, page 135)

Table 2.1 *Continued*

Disorder	DDx	Si/Sx	Tx
↓ K⁺	• Diarrhea, nasogastric suction, vomiting • Diuretics, metabolic alkalosis • Cushing's, burns, β-agonists, ↓ Mg²¹	• Ectopy, T-wave depression, prominent U waves • Also ventricular tachycardia and ↑ sensitivity to digoxin	• See Table 1.41 • Reverse cause (see Algorithm 1.8, page 134)
↑ Ca²⁺	• Malignancy (number one cause in inpatients) • Disorders involving bone, parathyroid, or kidneys • Acute pancreatitis	• Altered mental status, muscle weakness, ileus, constipation, nausea, vomiting • Nephrolithiasis • QT-interval shortening	• Hydration and loop diuretics • Bisphosphonates • Calcitonin
↓ Ca²⁺	• Blood transfusion • Parathyroid resection • ↓ Mg⁺⁺ • Renal failure	• Chvostek's and Trousseau's signs • Paresthesias, tetany, seizures, weakness, mental status changes • QT interval prolonged	• Calcium gluconate • Vitamin D supplement
↑ Mg²⁺	• Overzealous Mg²⁺ supplements in patients with renal failure	• Lethargy, weakness, ↓ deep tendon reflexes • Paralysis, ↓ BP and heart rate (HR) • Prolonged PR and QT intervals	• Calcium gluconate • Nml saline infusion with a loop diuretic • Dialysis
↓ Mg²⁺	• Diarrhea, malabsorption • Vomiting • Aggressive diuresis, alcoholism, chemoTx	• T wave and QRS widening, PR and QT intervals prolonged	• MgSO₄

(continued)

Table 2.1 *Continued*

Disorder	DDx	Si/Sx	Tx
↑ **Phos**	• Usually iatrogenic • Rhabdomyolysis • Hypoparathyroid • Hypocalcemia • Villous adenoma	• Can cause soft-tissue calcification • Heart block	• ↓ dietary phosphorus • Aluminum hydroxide • Hydration and acetazolamide • Dialysis
↓ **Phos**	• Excessive IV glucose • Hyperpara-thyroidism • Osmotic diuresis • Refeeding syndrome	• Diffuse weakness and flaccid paralysis (all because of ↓ adenosine triphosphate (ATP) production)	• Potassium phosphate or sodium phosphate

Note: Refeeding syndrome caused by a large glucose load too soon after prolonged NPO status; see ↓ in Mg^{2+}, K^+, and Phos.

II. Blood Product Replacement

A. Nml Hemostasis

1. Coagulation involves endothelium, platelets, and coagulation factors
2. Endothelial damage allows platelets to bind to subendothelium, inducing platelet release of adenosine diphosphate (ADP), 5-HT, and platelet-derived growth factor (PDGF), which promote platelet aggregation
3. Initial thrombus stabilized by fibrin laid down by coagulation factors

4. Coagulation Cascades
   a. Two coagulation pathways share factors I, II, V, and X
   b. Extrinsic pathway
      (1) Tissue thromboplastin (tissue factor) activates factor VII, which then activates factor X
      (2) Measured in vitro by prothrombin time (PT)
   c. Intrinsic pathway
      (1) Factor XII → XI → IX → VIII, activated factor VIII causes activation of the common factor X
      (2) Measured in vitro by partial thromboplastin time (PTT)
   d. Factor I = fibrin, which cross-links platelets to provide the tensile strength needed to stabilize the thrombus
5. Vitamin K is fat soluble, derived from leafy vegetables and colonic flora
   a. Cofactors for γ-carboxylation of factors II, VII, IX, and X and the anticoagulation factors proteins C and S enables them to interact with Ca^{2+}
   b. Deficiency caused by malabsorption, prolonged parenteral feeding, prolonged oral antibiotics, or ingestion of oral anticoagulants
   c. First sign is prolonged PT, because of the short half-life of factor VII

B. **Preoperative Evaluation of Bleeding Disorders**
1. Si/Sx = Hx or FHx of ↑ bleeding following minor cuts, dental procedures, menses, or past surgeries, ecchymoses, or sequelae of liver dz
2. Ask about nonsteroidal anti-inflammatory drugs (NSAID) or herbal medicine intake the wk of surgery
3. Bleeding Time
   a. Evaluates platelet function
   b. ↑ bleeding time indicates quantitative or qualitative platelet dz
   c. Also ↑ in von Willebrand's dz and vasculitis
4. Thrombin Time (TT)
   a. Measures the time to clot after the addition of thrombin, which is responsible for conversion of fibrinogen to fibrin
   b. ↑ TT may be due to ↑ fibrin, dysfibrinogenemia, disseminated intravascular coagulation (DIC), or heparin
5. **Routine preoperative lab screening is not warranted without Si/Sx suggestive of underlying disorder**

SURGERY

C. **Transfusions**

1. Packed Red Blood Cells (pRBCs)

 a. Type and screen = pt's RBCs tested for A, B, and Rh antigens and donor's serum screened for antibodies to common RBC antigens

 b. Cross-match = pt's serum checked for preformed antibodies against the donor's RBCs

 c. In trauma situations, type O negative blood is given while additional units are being typed and crossed (O positive blood can be given to male pts and postmenopausal women if no O negative is available)

 d. **1 unit pRBCs should ↑ hemoglobin by 1 g/dL and ↑ hematocrit 3%**

 e. Complications

 (1) Acute rejection

 (a) Because of preformed antibodies against the donor RBCs

 (b) Si/Sx = anxiety, flushing, tachycardia, renal failure, shock

 (c) **Most common cause is clerical error**

 (d) Recheck all paperwork and repeat cross-match

 (e) Tx = stop transfusion, IV fluids to maintain urine output

 (2) Infectious diseases

 (a) Hepatitis C virus (HCV) is by far the most common cause of hepatitis in pts who received prior transfusions, although risk of new HCV infxn now is lower with blood bank screening

 (b) Current risks (Table 2.2)

Table 2.2 Risk of Viral Infection from Blood Transfusions

Disease	Estimated Risk*
Hepatitis B	1 case per 220,000 units transfused
Hepatitis C	1 case per 230,000 units transfused
HIV	1 per 1.2 million units transfused

*Mean estimates from Jackson BR, Busch MP, Stramer SL, et al. The cost-effectiveness of NAT for HIV, HCV, and HBV in whole blood donations. *Transfusion* 2003;43:721–729.

2. Platelet Transfusions
   a. Pts do not bleed significantly until platelets <50,000/μL, so transfusion should be given only to maintain this level
   b. If pt is anticipated to experience severe blood loss intraoperatively or the pt is actively bleeding, transfuse to maintain even higher
   c. Most common complication is alloimmunization
      (1) Platelet counts fail to rise despite continued transfusion
      (2) Caused by induction of antibodies against the donor's major histocompatibility complex (MHC) type
      (3) Single-donor, human leukocyte antigen (HLA)-matched platelets may overcome problem
3. Plasma Component Transfusion
   a. Plasma products do not require cross-matching, but donor and recipient should be ABO compatible
   b. Fresh-frozen plasma (FFP)
      (1) Contains all the coagulation factors
      (2) Used to correct all clotting factor deficiencies
   c. Cryoprecipitate is rich in factor VIII, fibrinogen, and fibronectin

III. Perioperative Care

A. Preoperative Care

1. All pts require detailed H&P
2. Laboratory Tests
   a. CBC for pts undergoing procedure that may incur large blood loss
   b. Electrolytes, blood urea nitrogen (BUN), and creatinine in pts >60 yr or who have illnesses (e.g., diarrhea, liver, and renal dz) or take medications (e.g., diuretics) that predispose them to electrolyte disorders
   c. Urinalysis (UA) in pts with urologic Sx or those having urologic procedures
   d. PT and PTT in pts with bleeding diathesis or liver disease or who are undergoing neurosurgery or cardiac surgery
   e. Liver function tests (LFTs) in pts with liver disease
   f. CXR in pts with ↑ risk of pulmonary complications (e.g., obesity or thoracic procedures) and those with pre-existing pulmonary problems
   g. EKG in men >40, women >50, or young pts with pre-existing cardiac dz

SURGERY

B. **Perioperative Review of Systems**
1. Neurologic—Cerebrovascular Disease
   a. Strokes usually occur postoperatively and are caused by hypotension or emboli from atrial fibrillation
   b. Pts with a recent history of strokes should have their surgical procedure delayed 6 wk
   c. Anticoagulation should stop 2 wk prior to surgery, if possible
2. Cardiovascular
   a. Most postoperative complications are cardiac related
   b. Goldman cardiac risk index stratifies the operative risk of noncardiac surgery pts and helps in the decision of pursuing further Dx testing
   c. See Table 2.3
3. Pulmonary
   a. Pulmonary complications rarely occur in healthy pts
   b. Chronic obstructive pulmonary disease (COPD) is the most important and significant risk factor to consider
   c. Obesity, abd, and intrathoracic procedures predispose pts to pulmonary complications in the postoperative period
   d. Smoking Hx, independent of COPD, is also an important risk factor

Table 2.3 Goldman Cardiac Risk Index

Condition	Points	Concern
S$_3$ gallop, jugular venous distention (JVD)	11	Congestive heart failure
MI within 6 mo	10	Cardiac injury
Abnormal EKG rhythm	7	Diseased cardiac conduction
>5 premature ventricular contractions /min	7	Cardiac excitability/arrhythmia
Age >70	5	↑ comorbidity
General poor health	3	↑ morbidity
Aortic stenosis	3	Left ventricular outflow obstruction
Peritoneal/thoracic/ aortic surgery	3	Major surgery
Emergency	3	Emergency surgery

26 points warrants life-saving procedures only, because of ↓ risk of cardiac-related death.

4. Renal
   a. Postoperative acute renal failure → ≥50% mortality despite hemodialysis
   b. Chronic renal failure is a significant risk factor not only because of the ↑ risk of developing acute failure but because of the associated metabolic disturbances and underlying medical conditions
   c. Azotemia, sepsis, intraoperative hypotension, nephrotoxic drugs, and radiocontrast agents are risk factors for postoperative renal failure
   d. Preventive measures include expanding the intravascular volume with IV fluids and use of diuretics after administration of radiocontrast dye

5. Infxn/Immunity
   a. Infxn risk depends upon pt characteristics and surgery
   b. Advanced age, diabetes, immunosuppression, obesity, pre-existing infxn, and pre-existing illness all ↑ risk
   c. Surgical risk factors include GI surgery, prosthetic implantation, preoperative wound contamination, and duration of the operation
   d. Prophylaxis
      (1) To prevent surgical wound infxns, antibiotics should be administered before the skin incision is made—stop prophylactic antibiotics within 24 hrs postoperatively
      (2) Appropriate choice of the antibiotics depends on the procedure
      (3) Give all pts with prosthetic heart valves antibiotic prophylaxis to prevent bacterial endocarditis

6. Hematologic
   a. Deep venous thrombosis (DVT) prevented by early ambulation and mechanical compression stockings
   b. Subcutaneous heparin may be substituted for compression stockings
   c. Pulmonary embolus should always be considered as a cause of postoperative acute-onset dyspnea

7. Endocrinology
   a. Adrenal insufficiency
      (1) Surgery creates stress for the body; normally the body reacts to stress by secreting more corticosteroids

(2) Response may be diminished in pts taking corticos-teroids for ≥1 wk preoperatively and pts with primary adrenal insufficiency

(3) Hence, for these pts, steroid replacement is needed, and **hydrocortisone is given before, during, and after surgery to approximate the response of the nml adrenal gland.** If these measures are not taken, then adrenal crisis may occur.

(4) Adrenal crisis

(a) Life-threatening complication of adrenal insufficiency

(b) **Si/Sx = unexplained hypotension and tachycardia despite fluid and vasopressor administration**

(c) Tx = corticosteroids dramatically improve BP

C. Fever

1. Intraoperative Fever

   a. DDx = transfusion reaction, malignant hyperthermia, or prior infxn

   b. Malignant hyperthermia

      (1) Triggered by several anesthetic agents; e.g., halothane, isoflurane, and succinylcholine

      (2) Tx = dantrolene, cooling measures, ICU monitoring

2. Postoperative Fever

   a. **Mnemonic for causes: the 5Ws**

      (1) **W**ind (lungs)

      (2) **W**ater (urinary tract)

      (3) **W**ound

      (4) **W**alking (DVT)

      (5) **W**onder drug (drug reaction)

   b. Immediate postoperative fever includes atelectasis, *Streptococcus* and *Clostridium* wound infxns, and aspiration pneumonia

   c. 1 to 2 days postoperatively look for indwelling vascular line infxn, aspiration pneumonia, and infectious pneumonia

   d. Tx = encourage early postoperative ambulation, incentive spirometry use postoperatively, treat infxns with appropriate antibiotics

IV. Trauma

A. **General**

1. Trauma is the major cause of death in those <40 yrs
2. Management broken into 1° and 2° surveys

B. **Primary Survey = ABCDE**

1. **A** = **A**irway
   a. All pts immobilized due to ↑ risk of spinal injury
   b. Maintain airway with jaw thrust or mandible/tongue traction, protecting cervical spine
   c. If pt is likely to vomit, position them in a slightly lateral and head-down position to prevent aspiration
   d. If airway cannot be established, a large-bore (14-gauge) needle can be inserted into the cricothyroid membrane
   e. Do not perform tracheotomy in the field or ambulance
   f. Unconscious pts need endotracheal (ET) tube (Glasgow Coma Scale <8 intubate)

2. **B** = **B**reathing
   a. Assess chest expansion, breath sounds, respiratory rate, rib fractures, subQ emphysema, and penetrating wounds
   b. Life-threatening injuries to the lungs or thoracic cavity are
      (1) Tension pneumothorax
         (a) Causes contralateral mediastinal shift, distended neck veins (↑ central venous pressure [CVP]), hypotension, absent breath sounds, and hyperresonance to percussion on the affected side
         (b) Tx = immediate chest tube or 14-gauge needle puncture of affected side
      (2) Open pneumothorax → Tx = immediate closure of the wound with dressings and placement of a chest tube
      (3) Flail chest
         (a) Caused by multiple rib fractures that form a free-floating segment of chest wall that moves paradoxically to the rest of the chest wall, resulting in an inability to generate sufficient inspiratory or expiratory pressure to drive ventilation
         (b) Tx = intubation with mechanical ventilation
      (4) Massive hemothorax
         (a) Injury to the great vessels with subsequent hemorrhage into the thoracic cavity
         (b) Tx = chest tube, surgical control of the bleeding site

SURGERY

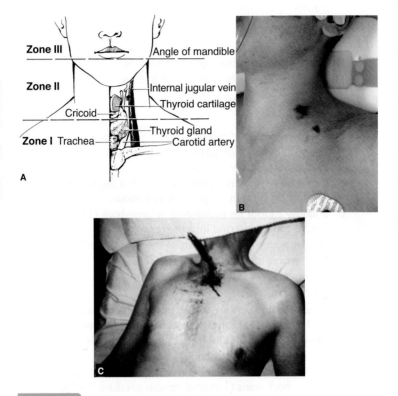

FIGURE 2.2

(A) Anterior view of the neck. Significant structures and the zones of the neck are illustrated. (From Harwood-Nuss A, Wolfson AB, Londen CD, et al., eds. *The clinical practice of emergency medicine,* 3rd Ed. Philadelphia: Lippincott Williams & Wilkins, 2001, with permission.) (B) Gunshot wound in Zone 1 of neck. (Courtesy of Mark Silverberg, MD.) (C) Stab wound in Zone 1 of neck. (Courtesy of Lewis J. Kaplan, MD.) (B,C from Greenberg MI, Hendrickson RG, Silverberg M, et al. *Greenberg's text-atlas of emergency medicine.* Philadelphia: Lippincott Williams & Wilkins, 2004, with permission.)

    c. Neck injuries can be life threatening (Figure 2.2)
      (1) Neck trauma: three zones
        (a) Zone I: clavicle to cricoid cartilage. Structures at greatest risk in this zone are the great vessels, aortic arch, trachea, esophagus, lung apices, cervical spine, spinal cord, and cervical nerve roots
        (b) Zone II: cricoid cartilage to the angle of the mandible. Important structures in this region include the carotid

and vertebral arteries, jugular veins, pharynx, larynx, trachea, esophagus, cervical spine, and spinal cord

   (c) Zone III: angle of the mandible to the base of the skull. Salivary and parotid glands, esophagus, trachea, cervical spine, carotid arteries, jugular veins, and major cranial nerves

(2) Assessment: four-vessel angiography is routinely used to evaluate stable pts sustaining penetrating wounds to Zones I and III that pierce the platysma

(3) Tx

   (a) Zone II injuries are routinely explored especially if platysma is pierced or if pt is unstable

   (b) Never send an unstable pt to a radiographic suite

   (c) If surgical exposure and access to bleeding vessels proves impractical, such as in Zone III, then therapeutic embolization or occlusion of damaged vessels may be warranted

d. Esophageal injury: Gastrografin swallow or direct visualization

e. Thoracic surgery consult

   (1) Follow Advanced Trauma Life Support (ATLS) guidelines for pt stabilization and surgical exploration.

3. **C** = **C**irculation

   a. Two large-bore IVs placed in upper extremities (if possible)

   b. For severe shock, place a central venous line

   c. O-negative blood on standby for any suspected significant hemorrhage

4. **D** = **D**isability

   a. Neurologic disability assessed by history, careful neurologic examination (Glasgow coma scale), laboratory tests (blood alcohol level, blood cultures, blood glucose, ammonia, electrolytes, and urinalysis [UA]), and skull x-rays

   b. Loss of consciousness

      (1) DDx = **AEIOU TIPS** = **A**lcohol, **E**pilepsy, **E**nvironment (temp), **I**nsulin($+/-$), **O**verdose, **U**remia (electrolytes), **T**rauma, **I**nfection, **P**sychogenic, **S**troke

      (2) Tx = Coma cocktail = dextrose, thiamine, naloxone, and O_2

   c. ↑ Intracranial pressure (ICP) → HTN, bradycardia, and bradypnea = Cushing's triad

   d. Tx = ventilation to keep $PaCO_2$ at 30–40 mm Hg, controlling fever, administration of osmotic diuretics (mannitol), corticosteroids, and even bony decompression (burr hole)

5. **E** = Exposure
   a. Remove all clothes without moving pt (cut off if necessary)
   b. Examine all skin surfaces and back for possible exit wounds
   c. Ensure pt not at risk for hypothermia (small children)

C. **Secondary Survey**
   1. Identify all injuries, examine all body orifices
   2. Periorbital and mastoid hematomas ("raccoon eyes" and Battle's sign), hemotympanum, and cerebrospinal fluid (CSF) otorrhea/rhinorrhea → basilar skull fractures
   3. Glasgow coma scale should be performed (Table 2.4)
   4. Deaths from abd trauma usually result from sepsis because of hollow viscus perforation or hemorrhage if major vessels are penetrated
   5. Dx
      a. If pt stable, diagnostic peritoneal lavage, abd Utz, or CT scan
      b. If pt unstable, surgical laparotomy
      c. If blood noted at urethra, perform retrograde urethrogram before placement of a bladder catheter; hematuria suggests significant retroperitoneal injury and requires CT scan for evaluation; take pt to OR for surgical exploration if unstable

Table 2.4 Glasgow Coma Scale

Finding		Finding	
Eye Opening	Points	Motor Response	Points
Spontaneous	4	To command	6
To voice	3	Localizes	5
To stimulation (pain)	2	Withdraws	4
No response	1	Abnormal flexion	3
Verbal Response		Extension	2
Oriented	5	No response	1
Confused	4		
Incoherent	3		
Incomprehensible	2		
No response	1		

Glasgow coma scale score <8 indicates severe neurologic injury; intubation must be performed to secure airway.

Table 2.5 Differential Diagnosis of Shock

Type	Cardiac Output	Pulmonary Capillary Wedge Pressure	Peripheral Vascular Resistance
Hypovolemic	↓	↓	↑
Cardiogenic	↓	↑	↑
Septic	↑	↓	↓

    d. Check for compartment syndrome of extremities; Si/Sx = tense, pale, paralyzed, paresthetic, and painful extremity; Tx = fasciotomy

  6. Tx = Surgical Hemostasis

D. **Shock**

  1. DDx (Table 2.5)

  2. Correction of defect (Table 2.6)

  3. Shock in trauma can also be neurogenic or hypovolemic

  4. Neurogenic because of blood pooling in splenic bed and muscle from loss of autonomic innervation

  5. Tx = usually self-limiting; can be managed by placing pt in supine or Trendelenburg position

Table 2.6 Correction of Defect in Shock

Type	Defect	First-Line Treatment
Hypovolemic	↓ Preload	Two large-bore IVs, crystalloid or colloid infusions (see Section I. Fluids and Electrolytes), replace blood losses with the **3 for 1** rule = give 3 L of fluid per liter of blood loss
Cardiogenic	Myocardial failure	Pressors—dobutamine first line, can add dopamine and/or norepinephrine, supplemental oxygen
Septic	↓ Peripheral vascular resistance	Norepinephrine to vasoconstrict peripheral arterioles, prevent vascular progression to multiple organ dysfunction syndrome (MODS), give resistance IV antibiotics as indicated, supplemental oxygen

V. Burns

A. Partial Thickness

1. 1° and 2° burns are limited to epidermis and superficial dermis
2. Si/Sx = skin is red, blistered, edematous, skin underneath blister is pink or white in appearance, very painful
3. Infxn may convert to full-thickness burns

B. Full Thickness

1. 3° and 4° burns affect all layers of skin and subcutaneous tissues
2. Si/Sx = skin initially is painless, dry, white, charred, cracked, insensate
3. 4° burns also involve muscle and bone
4. All full-thickness burns require surgical treatment
5. Percentage of body surface area (BSA) affected (Figure 2.3 and Table 2.7)
6. Tx = Resuscitation, Monitor Fluid Status, Remove Eschars
   a. Consider any facial burns or burning of nasal hairs as a potential candidate for acute respiratory distress syndrome (ARDS) and airway compromise
   b. Fluid resuscitation
      (1) Parkland formula = % BSA × weight (kg) × 4, formula used to calculate volume of crystalloid needed
      (2) Give half of fluid in first 8 hr; remainder given over next 16 hr
   c. CXR to rule out inhalation injury
   d. Labs → PT/PTT, CBC, type and cross, arterial blood gas (ABGs), electrolytes, UA
   e. Irrigate and débride wound, IV and topical antibiotics (silver sulfadiazine, mafenide, Polysporin), tetanus prophylaxis, and stress ulcer prophylaxis
   f. Transfer to burn center if pt is very young or old, burns >20% BSA, full-thickness burns >5% BSA, coexisting chemical or electrical injury, facial burns, or pre-existing medical problems
   g. Make pt NPO until bowel function returns; pt will have extremely ↑ protein and caloric requirements with vitamin supplementation
   h. Excision of eschar to level of bleeding capillaries and split-thickness skin grafts
   i. **Marjolin's ulcer = squamous cell carcinoma arising in an ulcer or burn**
   j. **Curling's ulcer = acute duodenal ulcer seen in burn patients**

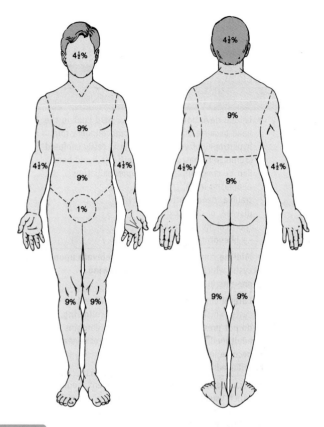

FIGURE 2.3

Rule of nines for calculating body surface area. (From Nettina SM. *The Lippincott manual of nursing practice*, 7th Ed. Philadelphia: Lippincott Williams & Wilkins, 2001.)

Table 2.7 Body Surface Area in Burns

Palm of hand	1%	Upper extremities*	9%
Head and neck*	9%	Lower extremities*	18%
Anterior trunk*	18%	Genital area*	1%
Posterior trunk*	18%		

*In adults.

VI. Neck Mass Differential (Table 2.8)

Table 2.8 Neck Mass Differential Diagnosis

Disease	Characteristics	Dx Findings	Tx
Congenital			
Torticollis	• Lateral deviation of head because of hypertrophy of unilateral sternocleidomastoid • Can be congenital, neoplasm, infxn, trauma, degenerative disease, or drug toxicity (particularly D_2 blockers → phenothiazines)	Rock hard knot in the sternocleidomastoid that is easily confused with the hyoid bone upon palpation	Muscle relaxants and/or surgical repair
Thyroglossal duct cyst	• **Midline** congenital cysts, which usually presents in childhood	**Cysts elevate upon swallowing**	Surgical removal
Branchial cleft cyst	• **Lateral** congenital cysts, which usually do not present until adulthood, when they become infected or inflamed	**Do not elevate upon swallowing,** aspirate contains cholesterol crystals	Surgical excision
Cystic hygroma	• Occluded lymphatics, which usually present within first 2 yrs of life • **Lateral or midline**	Translucent, benign mass painless, soft and compressible	Surgical excision
Dermoid cyst	• **Lateral or midline** • Solid mass composed of an overgrowth of epithelium	**No elevation with swallowing**	Surgical excision
Carotid body tumor → paraganglioma	• Palpable mass at bifurcation of common carotid artery • Not a vascular tumor, but originate from neural crest cells in the carotid body within the carotid sheath • Rule of 10: 10% malignant, 10% familial, 10% secrete catecholamines	**Pressure on tumor can cause brady-cardia and dizziness, will move in horizontal direction but not in vertical direction**	Surgical excision with prior emobolization of feeding vessels

Table 2.8 *Continued*

Disease	Characteristics	Dx Findings	Tx
Acquired-Inflammatory			
Cervical lymphadenitis	• Bilateral lymphadenopathy is usually viral, caused by Epstein Barr virus, cytomegalovirus, or HIV • Unilateral is usually bacterial, caused by *S. aureus,* group A and B Strep Other Causes • Cat scratch fever (*Bartonella henselae*), transmitted via scratch of young cats • Scrofula because of tuberculosis • *Actinomyces israelii* → sinuses drain pus containing "sulfur granules" • Kawasaki's syndrome • Lymphoma	Fine-needle aspirate and culture	Per cause: Viral → supportive; bacteria → antibiotics; Kawasaki's → IVIG; Lymphoma → chemotherapy
Thyroid			
Goiter	• Enlargement of thyroid gland • Usually 2° to ↓ iodine intake, inflammation or use of goitrogens	Fine-needle aspirate, thyroid-stimulating hormone, levels	Treat underlying condition
Malignancy	• See Internal Medicine, section V.F.	Fine-needle aspirate	Surgical excision, followed by radioactive iodine as indicated

VII. Surgical Abdomen (Figures 2.4, 2.5, and 2.6)

A. **Right Upper Quadrant (RUQ)** (Table 2.9A)

B. **Right Lower Quadrant (RLQ)** (Table 2.9B)

C. **Left Upper Quadrant (LUQ)** (Table 2.9C)

D. **Left Lower Quadrant (LLQ)** (Table 2.9D)

E. **Midline** (Table 2.9E)

F. **Tx**

    1. Generally all above surgical conditions will require **NPO, nasogastric (NG) tube, IV fluids, and cardiac monitoring**

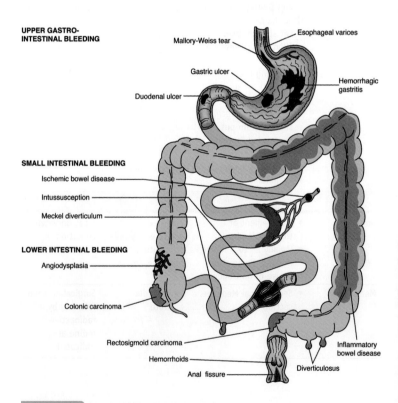

FIGURE 2.4

Common causes of GI bleeding. (Image from Rubin E, Farber JL. *Pathology*, 3rd Ed. Philadelphia: Lippincott Williams & Wilkins, 1999.)

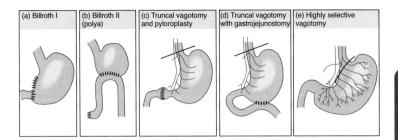

FIGURE 2.5

Operations for peptic ulceration. **(A)** Partial gastrectomy with Billroth I anastomosis. The ulcer and the ulcer-bearing portion of the stomach are resected. **(B)** Partial gastrectomy with creation of a duodenal loop (Billroth II, Polya). **(C)** Truncal vagotomy and pyloroplasty. The main nerves are divided to eliminate nervous stimulation of the stomach, reducing the acid secretory capacity, and gastric emptying is maintained with pyloroplasty. **(D)** Truncal vagotomy with gastrojejunostomy. The main nerves are divided and gastric emptying maintained with gastrojejunostomy. **(E)** Highly selective vagotomy. Innervation of the acid-producing area of the stomach is interrupted, leaving the nerve supply to the antrum and pylorus intact. This does not affect gastric emptying, so a drainage procedure is not required. (Adapted from Axford JS. *Medicine.* Oxford: Blackwell Science, 1996, with permission.)

2. IV antibiotics as needed
3. Surgery for hemostasis and life-threatening conditions, consult appropriate surgical service (obstetric, pediatric surgery, etc.) as indicated

VIII. Esophagus

A. Hiatal Hernia

1. Majority of pts with reflux have hiatal hernia (80%)
2. Si/Sx = gastroesophageal reflux disease (GERD) and chest pain
3. Dx = barium swallow to identify anatomic variations
4. Two Types of Hiatal Hernias
   a. Type I
      (1) Sliding hiatal hernia, more common than the type II hernia
      (2) Consists of movement of the gastroesophageal junction and stomach up into the mediastinum
      (3) Tx = antacids as per GERD

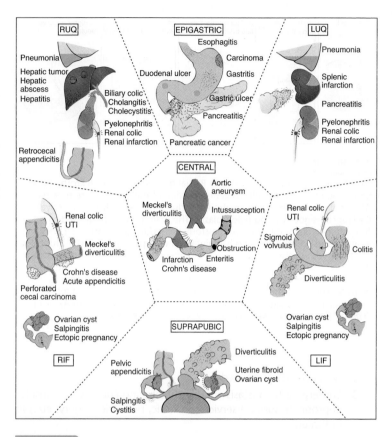

FIGURE 2.6 Acute abd pain.

  b. Type II
    (1) Herniation of the stomach fundus through the diaphragm parallel to the esophagus
    (2) Tx = mandatory surgical repair due to ↑ risk of strangulation
B. **Achalasia**
  1. Most common motility disorder; affects 70% of pts with scleroderma
  2. Loss of esophageal motility and failure of lower esophageal sphincter (LES) relaxation; may be caused by ganglionic degeneration or Chagas' disease; results in the dilatation of the proximal esophagus

Text continues on page 162

Table 2.9A Right Upper Quadrant Differential Diagnosis

Disease	Characteristics
Biliary colic	• Si/Sx = constant right upper quadrant (RUQ) to epigastric pain • Utz → gallstones but no gallbladder wall thickening or pericholecystic fluid
Cholecystitis	• Si/Sx = fever, RUQ tenderness, **Murphy's sign** (inspiratory arrest upon deep palpation of RUQ) • Labs → moderate to severe leukocytosis, ↑ liver function tests (LFT), ↑ bilirubin • Utz → gallstones, **pericholecystic fluid**, thickened gallbladder wall
Choledocholithiasis	• Si/Sx = RUQ pain worse with fatty meals, jaundice • Utz → common bile duct dilatation • Labs → ↑ LFTs, ↑ bilirubin
Pneumonia*	• Si/Sx = pleuritic chest pain and fever • CXR → infiltrate, labs → leukocytosis
Fitz-Hugh-Curtis syndrome*	• Syndrome of perihepatitis caused by ascending *Chlamydia* or *N. gonorrhoeae* salpingitis • Si/Sx = RUQ pain, fever, Hx or Si/Sx of salpingitis • Labs → leukocytosis but nml bilirubin and LFTs • Utz → nml gallbladder and biliary tree but fluid around the liver and gallbladder
Cholangitis	• Life threatening • Si/S ◊ **Charcot's triad** = fever, jaundice, and RUQ pain ◊ **Reynolds' pentad**: add hypotension and mental status change • Labs → leukocytosis, blood Cx → enteric organisms, ↑ LFTs, ↑ bilirubin • Utz and CT → biliary duct dilatation from obstructing gallstones • Dx with ERCP or percutaneous transhepatic cholangiography (PTC)
Hepatitis*	• Si/Sx = RUQ pain/tenderness, jaundice, fever • Labs → ↑ LFTs, ↑ bilirubin, leukocytosis, ⊕ hepatitis virus serologies • Utz rules out other causes of RUQ pain

*Medical treatment indicated unless patient absolutely requires surgery for cure.

SURGERY

Table 2.9B	Right Lower Quadrant Differential Diagnosis
Disease	**Characteristics**
Appendicitis	• Si/Sx = right lower quadrant (RLQ) pain/tenderness originally diffuse and then migrating to **McBurney's point** (⅓ the distance from the anterior superior iliac spine to the umbilicus), fever, diarrhea • Perform rectal exam to rule out retroperitoneal appendicitis • Labs → leukocytosis, fecalith on plain film or abd CT • Decision to take to OR based mostly on clinical picture
*Yersinia enterocolitis**	• Si/Sx = fever, diarrhea, severe RLQ pain make it hard to distinguish from appendicitis • Labs → fecal culture
Ectopic pregnancy	• Si/Sx = crampy to constant lower abd pain, vaginal bleeding, tender adnexal mass, menstrual irregularity • Labs → anemia, ↑ human chorionic gonadotropin (hCG), culdocentesis reveals blood
Salpingitis/ Tubo-ovarian abscess (TOA)	• Si/Sx = lower abd/pelvic pain (constant to crampy, sharp to dull), purulent vaginal discharge, cervical motion tenderness, adnexal mass • Wet mount → white blood cells (WBC), endocervical Cx ⊕ for *N. gonorrhoeae* or *Chlamydia* • Utz → TOA, CT scan can help rule out appendicitis
Meckel's diverticulum	• **1-10-100 rule: 1%–2% prevalence, 1–10 cm in length, 50–100 cm proximal to ileocecal valve, or rule of 2s: 2% of the population, 2% are symptomatic (usually before age 2), remnants are roughly 2 in, found 2 ft from ileocecal valve and found 2× as common in males** • Si/Sx = GI bleed (melena, hematochezia), small bowel obstruction (intussusception, Littre's hernia), Meckel's diverticulitis (similar presentation to appendicitis) • Nuclear medicine gastric scan to detect gastric mucosa present in 50% of Meckel's diverticula or tagged red blood cell (RBC) scan to detect bleeding source
Ovarian torsion	• Si/Sx = acute onset, sharp unilateral lower abd/pelvic pain, pain may be intermittent because of incomplete torsion, pain related to change in position, nausea and fever present, tender adnexal mass • Utz and laparoscopy confirm Dx
Intussusception	• Most common in infants 5–10 mo • SiSx = infant crying with pulling legs up to abdomen, dark, red stool (**currant jelly**), vomiting, shock • Barium or air contrast enema → diagnostic "coiled spring" sign

*Medical treatment indicated unless patient absolutely requires surgery for cure.

Table 2.9C Left Upper Quadrant Differential Diagnosis

Disease	Characteristics
Peptic ulcer*	• Si/Sx = epigastric pain relieved by food or antacids • Perforated ulcers present with sudden upper abd pain, shoulder pain, GI bleed • Labs → endoscopy or upper GI series
Myocardial infarction*	• Si/Sx = chest pain, dyspnea, diaphoresis, nausea • Labs → EKG, troponins, creatine kinase–MB
Splenic rupture	• Si/Sx = tachycardia, broken ribs, Hx of trauma, hypotension • **Kehr's sign** = left upper quadrant pain and referred left shoulder pain • Labs → leukocytosis • X-ray → fractured ribs, medially displaced gastric bubble • CT scan of abdomen preferred method of Dx

*Medical treatment indicated unless patient absolutely requires surgery for cure.

Table 2.9D Left Lower Quadrant Differential Diagnosis

Disease	Characteristics
Diverticulitis*	• Si/Sx = left lower quadrant (LLQ) pain and mass, fever, urinary urgency • Labs → leukocytosis • CT scan and Utz → thickened bowel wall, abscess—do not use contrast enema
Sigmoid volvulus	• Si/Sx = elderly, chronically constipated patient, abd pain, distention, obstipation • X-ray → **inverted U**, contrast enema → **bird's beak deformity**
Pyelonephritis*	• Si/Sx = high fever, rigors, costovertebral angle tenderness, Hx of UTI • Labs → pyuria, ≈ urine culture
Ovarian torsion	• See RLQ (Table 2.9B)
Ectopic pregnancy	• See RLQ (Table 2.9B)
Salpingitis	• See RLQ (Table 2.9B)

*Medical treatment indicated unless patient absolutely requires surgery for cure.

SURGERY

Table 2.9E Midline Differential Diagnosis

Disease	Characteristics
Pancreatitis	• Si/Sx = severe epigastric pain radiating to the back, nausea/vomiting, signs of hypovolemia because of "third spacing," ↓ bowel sounds • In hemorrhagic pancreatitis, there are ecchymotic appearing skin findings in the flank (**Grey Turner's sign**) or periumbilical area **(Cullen's sign)** • Labs → leukocytosis, ↑ serum and urine amylase, ↑ lipase • X-ray → dilated small bowel or transverse colon adjacent to the pancreas, called **"sentinel loop"** • CT → phlegmon, pseudocyst, necrosis, abscess
Pancreatic pseudocyst	• Si/Sx = sequelae of pancreatitis, if pancreatitis Sx do not improve, check for pseudocyst; may cause fever or shock in infected or hemorrhagic cases • CT and Utz → fluid-filled cystic mass
Abd aortic aneurysm (AAA)	• Si/Sx = usually aSx, rupture presents with back or abd pain and shozzck, compression on duodenum or ureters can cause obstructive Sx, palpable pulsatile periumbilical mass • X-ray (cross-table lateral films), Utz, CT, aortography reveal aneurysm
Gastroesophageal rflux disease[a]	• Si/Sx = position-dependent (supine worse) substernal or epigastric burning pain, regurgitation, dysphagia, hoarse voice • Dx by barium swallow, manometric or pH testing, esophagoscopy
Myocardial infarction*	• See LUQ (Table 2.9C)
Peptic ulcer*	• See LUQ (Table 2.9C)
Gastroenteritis*	• Si/Sx = diarrhea, vomiting, abd pain, fever, malaise, headache • Labs → stool studies not usually indicated except in severe cases

*Medical treatment indicated unless patient absolutely requires surgery for cure.

3. Si/Sx = dysphagia of both solids and liquids, weight loss, and repulsion of undigested foodstuffs that may produce a foul odor

4. May ↑ risk of esophageal CA because stasis promotes development of Barrett's esophagus

5. Dx
   a. Barium swallow → dilatation of the proximal esophagus with subsequent narrowing of the distal esophagus; studies may also reveal esophageal diverticula
   b. Manometry → ↑ LES pressure and diffuse esophageal spasm
6. Tx
   a. Endoscopic dilation of LES with balloon cures 80% of pts
   b. Alternative is a myotomy with a modified fundoplication
   c. Surgical Tx may be used for palliation in pts with scleroderma, who may experience dysphagia or severe reflux

C. **Esophageal Diverticula (Zenker's Diverticulum)**
   1. Proximal diverticula are usually Zenker's
   2. Pulsion diverticula involving only the mucosa, located between the thyropharyngeal and cricopharyngeus muscle fibers (condition associated with muscle dysfunction/spasms)
   3. Si/Sx = dysphagia, regurgitation of solid foods, choking, left-sided neck mass, and bad breath
   4. Dx = clinically + barium swallow
   5. Tx = myotomy of cricopharyngeus muscle and removal of diverticulum

D. **Esophageal Tumors**
   1. Squamous Cell CA
      a. Most common esophageal CA, alcohol and tobacco synergistically ↑ risk of development
      b. Most commonly seen in men in the sixth decade of life
   2. AdenoCA
      a. Seen in pts with chronic reflux → Barrett's esophagus = squamous to columnar metaplasia
      b. 10% of pts with Barrett's esophagus will develop adenoCA
   3. Si/Sx for both = **dysphagia,** weight loss, hoarseness, tracheoesophageal fistula, recurrent aspiration, and possibly symptoms of metastatic disease
   4. Dx = barium study demonstrates **classic apple-core lesion;** Dx confirmed with endoscopy with biopsy, CT of abdomen and chest is also performed to determine extent of spread
   5. Tx = esophagectomy with gastric pull-up or colonic interposition with or without chemotherapy/radiation
   6. Px poor unless resected prior to spread (very rare); however, palliation should be attempted to restore effective swallowing

IX. Gastric Tumors

A. Benign tumors comprise <10% of all gastric tumors; most commonly polyps and leiomyoma

B. Stomach CA most common after 50 yr, ↑ incidence in men

C. Linked to blood group A (suggesting genetic predisposition), immunosuppression, and environmental factors

D. Nitrosamines, excess salt intake, low fiber intake, *H. pylori*, achlorhydria, chronic gastritis are all risk factors

E. Almost always adenocarcinoma; usually involves antrum, rarely fundus; aggressive spread to nodes/liver

F. Rarer Gastric Tumors

  1. Lymphoma

    a. Causes 4% of gastric CA, better Px than adenoCA

    b. Associated with *H. pylori* infxn

  2. Linitis Plastica

    a. Infiltrating, diffuse adenoCA, invariably fatal within months

    b. **This is the deadliest form of gastric CA**

G. Several classic physical findings in metastatic gastric CA

  1. **Virchow's node = large rock-hard supraclavicular node**

  2. **Krukenberg tumor = mucinous, signet-ring cells that metastasize from gastric CA to bilateral ovaries, so palpate for ovarian masses in women**

  3. **Sister Mary Joseph sign = metastasis to umbilicus, feel for hard nodule there, associated with poor Px**

  4. **Blumer's shelf = palpable nodule superiorly on rectal exam, caused by metastasis of GI CA**

H. Si/Sx for all = weight loss, anemia, anorexia, GI upset

I. Dx = biopsy

J. Tx = mostly palliative; combination surgery and chemotherapy when tolerated

K. Px = approximately 5% survival at 5 yr

X. Hernia (Table 2.10)

A. **Inguinal Hernias (Figure 2.7)**

  1. Most common hernia; more common in men

  2. Direct type = viscera protrudes directly through abd wall at Hesselbach's triangle (inferior epigastric artery, rectus sheath, and inguinal ligament), medial to inferior epigastric artery

Table 2.10 Hernia Definitions

Combined (pantaloon)	Concurrent direct and indirect hernias
Sliding	Part of the hernia sac wall is formed by a visceral organ
Richter's	Part of the bowel is trapped in the hernia sac
Littre's	Meckel's diverticulum contained inside hernia
Reducible	Able to replace herniated tissue to its usual anatomic location
Incarcerated	Hernias that are not reducible
Strangulated	Incarcerated hernia with vascular compromise → ischemia
Incisional	Herniation through surgical incision, commonly 2° to wound infxn

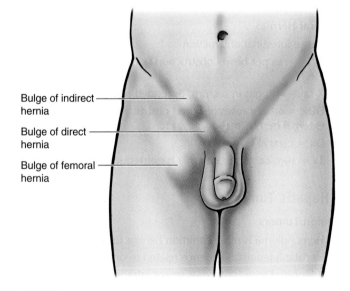

Bulge of indirect hernia

Bulge of direct hernia

Bulge of femoral hernia

FIGURE 2.7

Inguinal and femoral hernias. (From Moore KL, Dalley AF. *Clinical oriented anatomy*, 4th Ed. Baltimore: Lippincott Williams & Wilkins, 1999.)

3. Indirect type is more common (two thirds are indirect), pass lateral to inferior epigastric artery into spermatic cord covered by cremasteric muscle

4. Si/Sx = intermittent groin mass with bowel sounds that appear during Valsalva maneuvers

5. DDx = femoral hernias, which protrude below the inguinal ligament

6. Dx = physical exam some unable to completely differentiate until surgery

7. Tx = surgical repair with mesh placement

B. **Femoral Hernias (Figure 2.7)**

1. More common in women

2. Si/Sx = bulge above or below the inguinal ligament, ↑ risk of incarceration

3. Dx = clinical and/or surgical

4. Tx = surgical repair should not be delayed

C. **Visceral Hernias**

1. Cause intestinal obstruction

2. Si/Sx = as per bowel obstruction (e.g., obstipation, abd pain, etc.)

3. X-ray → no gas in rectum, distended bowel, air–fluid levels

4. DDx = other causes of bowel obstruction such as adhesions, external hernia, malignancy, etc.

5. Dx = clinical or surgical

6. Tx = surgical repair if hernia is not reducible

XI. Hepatic Tumors

A. **Benign Tumors**

1. Hemangioma is most common benign tumor of the liver

2. Hepatic adenoma incidence related to oral contraceptives

3. Adenomas may rupture → severe intraperitoneal bleed

4. Dx = Utz, CT scan

5. Tx = surgery only indicated if danger of rupture, pt symptomatic, or large amount of liver involved

B. **Malignant Tumors**

1. Metastases are the most common malignant hepatic tumors

2. Hepatocellular CA is the most common 1° hepatic malignancy
   a. Note also called "hepatoma," incorrectly implying benign tumor (historical misnomer)
   b. Most common malignancy in the world, endemic in Southeast Asia and sub-Saharan Africa because of vertical transmission of hepatitis B virus (HBV)
   c. Associated with cirrhosis, HBV and HCV infxn, alcoholism, hemochromatosis, Wilson's disease
   d. Si/Sx = weight loss, jaundice, weakness, dull and constant RUQ or epigastric pain, hepatomegaly; palpable mass or bloody ascites may also be present
   e. Labs → ↑ bilirubin, ⊕ HBV or HCV serologies, **very high α-fetoprotein (AFP) level**
   f. Dx = Utz or CT scan
   g. Tx = surgical resection and its variations offer the greatest survival rates
3. Hemangiosarcoma
   a. Associated with toxic exposure to polyvinyl chloride, Thorotrast, and arsenic
   b. Dx = Utz or CT scan
   c. Tx = surgical resection, may be curative if liver function is nml; in presence of cirrhosis, usually not effective

XII. Gallbladder

A. **Cholelithiasis = Gallstones**
   1. Higher incidence in women, multiple pregnancies, obesity (**the four Fs = female, forty, fertile, fat**)
   2. 10% of U.S. population has gallstones; complications of the disorder are what necessitate intervention
   3. Pts ≤20 yr with gallstones should undergo workup for congenital spherocytosis or hemoglobinopathy
   4. Si/Sx = aSx by definition
   5. Dx = Utz, often incidental finding that does not require therapy
   6. Tx
      a. aSx pts with gallstones do not require cholecystectomy unless there is ↑ risk for developing CA
      b. Pts with a porcelain gallbladder (calcified gallbladder walls) and those of Native American descent with gallstones are at ↑ risk of developing gallbladder CA and should receive a cholecystectomy

B. **Biliary Colic**

1. Because of gallstone impaction in cystic or common bile duct (CBD)

2. **The vast majority of people who have aSx gallstones WILL NEVER progress to biliary colic** (2% to 3% progress per year; lifelong risk = 20%)

3. Sx = sharp colicky pain made worse by eating, particularly fats

4. May have multiple episodes that resolve, but eventually this condition leads to further complications, so surgical resection of the gallbladder is required

5. Dx = Utz,; endoscopic retrograde cholangiopancreatography (ERCP)

6. Tx = cholecystectomy to prevent future complications

C. **Cholecystitis**

1. Cholecystitis is due to 2° infxn of obstructed gallbladder

   a. The EEEK! bugs: *Escherichia coli, Enterobacter, Enterococcus, Klebsiella* spp.

   b. Si/Sx = sudden onset, severe, steady pain in RUQ/ epigastrium; muscle guarding/rebound; ⊕ **Murphy's sign** (RUQ palpation during inspiration causes sharp pain and sudden cessation of inspiration)

   c. Labs → leukocytosis (may be >20,000 in emphysematous cholecystitis = presence of gas in gallbladder wall), ↑ aspartate aminotransferase/alanine aminotransferase (AST/ALT), ↑ bilirubin

   d. Dx = Utz → gallstones, pericholecystic fluid and thickened gallbladder wall; if results equivocal can confirm with radionuclide cholescintigraphy (e.g., hepatobiliary iminodi-acetic acid [HIDA] scan)—CT scan usually is not the test of choice to diagnose cholecystitis

   e. Tx

      (1) NPO, IV hydration, and antibiotics to cover Gram-negative rods and anaerobes

      (2) Demerol better for pain as morphine causes spasm of the sphincter of Oddi

      (3) Surgical resection if unresponsive or worsening

D. **Choledocholithiasis**

1. Passage of stone through the cystic duct, can obstruct CBD

2. Si/Sx = obstructive jaundice, ↑ conjugated bilirubin, hypercho-lesterolemia, ↑ alkaline phosphatase

3. Dx = Utz → CBD >9-mm diameter (Utz first line for Dx)

4. **Passage of stone to CBD can cause acute pancreatitis if the ampulla of Vater is obstructed by the stone**

5. Tx = laparoscopic cholecystectomy

E. **Ascending Cholangitis**

1. Results from 2° bacterial infxn of obstructed CBD, facilitated by obstructed bile flow

2. Obstruction usually because of choledocholithiasis but can be 2° to strictures, foreign bodies (e.g., surgical clips from prior abd surgery), and parasites

3. **Charcot's triad = jaundice, RUQ pain, fever (85% sensitive for cholangitis)—for Reynolds' pentad add altered mental status and hypotension**

4. Dx = Utz or CT → CBD dilation; definitive Dx requires ERCP or percutaneous transhepatic cholangiography (PTC)

5. This is a life-threatening emergency!

6. Tx

   a. NPO, IV hydration, and antibiotics to cover Gram-negative rods and anaerobes

   b. ERCP or PTC to decompress the biliary tree and remove obstructing stones

F. **CA**

1. Very rare, usually occurs in seventh decade of life

2. More commonly seen in females; gallstones are risk factors for developing CA

3. Most common 1° tumor of gallbladder is adenoCA

4. Frequently seen in Far East, associated with *Clonorchis sinensis* (liver fluke) infestation

5. When the tumor occurs at the confluence of the hepatic ducts forming the common duct, the tumor is called "**Klatskin's tumor**"

6. **Courvoisier's law** = gallbladder enlarges when CBD is obstructed by pancreatic CA but not enlarged when CBD is obstructed by stone

7. Courvoisier's sign is a palpable gallbladder

8. Si/Sx = as for biliary colic but persistent

9. Dx = Utz or CT to show tumor, but preoperative Dx of gallbladder CA is often incorrect

10. Tx = palliative stenting of bile ducts; can consider surgical resection for palliation only

11. Px = terminal, almost all pts die within 1 yr of Dx

XIII. Exocrine Pancreas

A. **Acute Pancreatitis**

1. Pancreatic enzymes autodigest pancreas → hemorrhagic fat necrosis, calcium deposition, and sometimes formation of pseudocysts (cysts not lined with ductal epithelium)

2. Most common causes in US = gallstones and alcohol

3. Other causes include infxn, trauma, radiation, drug (thiazides, azidothymidine [AZT], protease inhibitors), hyperlipidemia, hypercalcemia, vascular events, tumors, scorpion sting

4. Si/Sx = severe abd pain, prostration (fetal position opens up retroperitoneal space and allows more room for swollen pancreas), hypotension (because of retroperitoneal fluid sequestration), tachycardia, fever, ↑ serum amylase (90% sensitive)/ lipase, hyperglycemia, hypocalcemia

5. Dx = clinically and/or abd CT, **classic x-ray finding = sentinel loop or colon cutoff sign** (loop of distended bowel adjacent to pancreas)

6. **Classic physical findings = Grey Turner's sign (discoloration of flank) and Cullen's sign (periumbilical discoloration)**

7. Tx is aimed at decreasing stress to pancreas
   a. NPO until symptoms/amylase subside; total parenteral nutrition (TPN) if NPO for >7–10 days
   b. Demerol to control pain
   c. IV fluid resuscitation
   d. Alcohol withdrawal prophylaxis
   e. May require ICU admission if severe

8. Complications = abscess, pseudocysts, duodenal obstruction, shock lung, and acute renal failure

9. Repeated bouts of pancreatitis cause chronic pancreatitis, resulting in fibrosis and atrophy of the organ with early exocrine and later endocrine insufficiency

10. Px of acute pancreatitis determined by **Ranson's criteria** (Table 2.11)

B. **Pancreatic Pseudocyst**

1. Collection of fluid in pancreas surrounded by a fibrous capsule, no communication with fibrous ducts

2. **Suspect anytime a pt is readmitted with pancreatitis for complaints within several weeks of being discharged after a bout of pancreatitis**

Table 2.11 Ranson's Criteria

On Admission	Within 24 to 48 Hrs
Age >55, WBCs >16,000/mL, aspartate aminotransferase >250 IU/dL, lactate dehydrogenase >350, blood glucose >200, base deficit >4 mEq/L	↓ hematocrit >10%, blood urea nitrogen rise >5 mg/dL, serum calcium <8 mg/dL, arterial pO_2 <60 mmHg, fluid sequestration >6 L

- 0–2 of these → minimal mortality
- 3–5 → 10%–20% mortality
- >5 → ≥50% mortality

3. 2° to pancreatitis or trauma, as in steering wheel injury

4. Dx = Abd Utz/CT (Figure 2.8A)

5. Tx = percutaneous surgical drainage or pancreaticogastrostomy (creation of surgical fistula to drain cyst into the stomach), but small cysts will resorb on their own

6. New cysts contain blood, necrotic debris, leukocytes; old cysts contain straw-colored fluid

7. Can become infected with purulent contents, causing peritonitis after rupture

C. **Pancreatic CA**

1. Epidemiology = 90% are adenoCA, with 60% of these arising in the head of pancreas

2. More common in African Americans, cigarette smokers, and males; linked to chronic pancreatitis and diabetes mellitus

3. Si/Sx = jaundice, weight loss, abd pain; **classic sign is Trousseau's syndrome = migratory thrombophlebitis, which occurs in 10% of pts**

4. Frequently invades duodenum, ampulla of Vater, and CBD; can also cause biliary obstruction

5. Dx = Labs: ↑ bilirubin, ↑ alkaline phosphatase, ↑ CA 19-9 (not diagnostic), **CT scan** (Figure 2.8B)

6. Tx = Whipple's procedure, resection of pancreas, part of small bowel, stomach, gallbladder

7. Site of CA and extent of disease at time of Dx determines Px: usually very poor; 5-yr survival rate after palliative resection is 5%

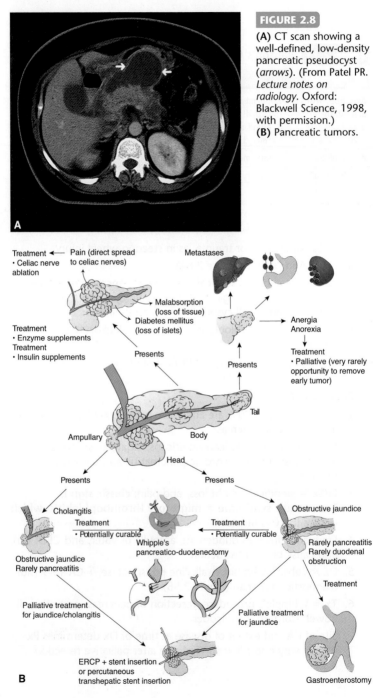

FIGURE 2.8

(A) CT scan showing a well-defined, low-density pancreatic pseudocyst (*arrows*). (From Patel PR. *Lecture notes on radiology*. Oxford: Blackwell Science, 1998, with permission.) (B) Pancreatic tumors.

Treatment
• Celiac nerve ablation

Pain (direct spread to celiac nerves)

Metastases

Malabsorption (loss of tissue)
Diabetes mellitus (loss of islets)

Anergia
Anorexia

Treatment
• Enzyme supplements
Treatment
• Insulin supplements

Treatment
• Palliative (very rarely opportunity to remove early tumor)

Presents

Presents

Tail

Ampullary

Body

Head

Presents

Presents

Cholangitis

Treatment
• Potentially curable

Treatment
• Potentially curable

Obstructive jaundice

Whipple's pancreatico-duodenectomy

Obstructive jaundice
Rarely pancreatitis

Rarely pancreatitis
Rarely duodenal obstruction

Treatment

Palliative treatment for jaundice/cholangitis

Palliative treatment for jaundice

ERCP + stent insertion or percutaneous transhepatic stent insertion

Gastroenterostomy

B

D. **Endocrine Pancreatic Neoplasm**

1. Insulinoma because hyperplasia of insulin-producing β-cells
2. Hyperglucagonemia = α–cell tumor → hyperglycemia and exfoliative dermatitis
3. Somatostatinoma = delta cell tumor → produces somatostatin, develop diabetes mellitus
4. VIPoma = secretes vasoactive intestinal peptide (VIP), prolonged watery diarrhea with severe electrolyte imbalances
5. Zollinger-Ellison syndrome
   a. Dx = clinically, elevated serum levels of insulin, glucagon, or gastrin
   b. Tx = surgical resection of the tumor

XIV. Small Intestine

A. **Small Bowel Obstruction (SBO)**

1. Most common surgical condition of the small bowel
2. Causes = peritoneal adhesions from prior surgery, hernias, and neoplasms in order of occurrence in the adult population
3. Other causes include Crohn's disease, Meckel's diverticulum, radiation enteritis, gallstone ileus, hypokalemia, narcotics, anticholinergics, acute pancreatitis, gastroenteritis, and cholecystitis
4. Si/Sx = crampy abd pain, nausea, vomiting, lack of flatus, abd tenderness, abd distention, and hyperactive, high-pitched bowel sounds
5. DDx = paralytic ileus (similar Si/Sx)
6. Dx = abd series → distended loops of small bowel proximal to the obstruction, upright film → air–fluid levels or free air beneath the diaphragm (if accompanied by bowel perforation) on a posterior/anterior (PA) chest film (Figure 2.9)
7. Tx
   a. Conservative Tx = IV fluids, NG tube decompression, and Foley catheter; partial obstructions may be successfully treated with conservative therapy
   b. Surgical candidates receive antibiotics to include both anaerobic and Gram-negative coverage
   c. Objective of surgery is to remove obstruction and resect nonviable bowel

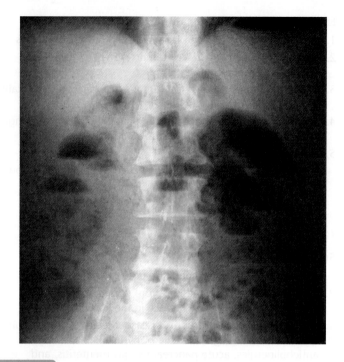

FIGURE 2.9

"Stepladder" pattern of air-fluid levels on upright view in patient with small bowel obstruction. (From Harwood-Nuss A, Wolfson AB, Linden CH, et al. *The clinical practice of emergency medicine*, 3rd Ed. Philadelphia: Lippincott Williams & Wilkins, 2001.)

B. **Small-Bowel Neoplasms**

1. Leiomyoma is most common benign tumor of the small bowel
2. Si/Sx = pain, anemia, weight loss, nausea, and vomiting; common complication is obstruction that is caused primarily by leiomyomas
3. Carcinoid tumors (small bowel is the second most common location, appendix is first) → cutaneous flushing, diarrhea, and respiratory distress
4. Malignant neoplasms in order of decreasing incidence: **adenoCA, carcinoid, lymphoma, and sarcomas**
5. Dx = biopsy, not necessarily reliable
6. Tx = surgical resection of primary tumor along with lymph nodes and liver metastases, if possible

XV. Colon

A. **Colonic Polyps: neoplastic, hamartoma, inflammatory, hyperplastic**

1. Neoplastic Polyps

   a. Most commonly adenomas and can be classified as tubular adenoma (smallest malignant potential), tubulovillous adenoma, or villous adenoma (greatest malignant potential)

   b. Mean age of pts with polyps is 55; incidence ↑ with age

   c. 50% of polyps occur in the sigmoid or rectum

   d. Si/Sx = intermittent rectal **bleeding** is most common presenting complaint

   e. Dx = colonoscopy, sigmoidoscopy, always consider family Hx

   f. Tx

      (1) Colonoscopic polypectomy or laparotomy

      (2) If invasive adenoCA is found, a colectomy is not mandatory if gross and microscopic margins are clear, if tissue is well differentiated without lymphatic or venous drainage, and polyp stalk does not invade

2. Hyperplastic Polyps

   a. Common in distal colon; comprise 90% of all polyps

   b. Most commonly benign, but can be associated with malignancy in hyperplastic polyposis syndrome

   c. Patients with multiple or large hyperplastic polyps are at ↑ risk for malignancy

3. Familial Polyposis Syndromes

   a. Familial adenomatous polyposis (FAP) has autosomal dominant inheritance of APC gene; abundant polyps throughout the colon and rectum beginning at puberty

   b. Gardner's syndrome consists of polyposis, desmoid tumors, osteomas of mandible or skull, and sebaceous cysts

   c. Turcot's syndrome is polyposis with medulloblastoma or glioma

   d. Dx = family Hx, colonoscopy; presence of congenital hypertrophy of retinal pigment epithelium predicts FAP with 97% sensitivity

   e. Tx = colectomy and upper GI endoscopy to rule out gastroduodenal lesions—a favored operation is an abd colectomy, mucosal proctectomy, and ileoanal anastomosis

4. Peutz-Jeghers Syndrome (Figure 2.10)
   a. Si/Sx = autosomal dominant inheritance, nonneoplastic hamartomatous polyps in stomach, small intestine, and colon, skin, and mucous membrane hyperpigmentation, **particularly freckles on lips**
   b. ↑ **Risk of developing CA in other tissues** (e.g., breast, pancreas)
   c. Dx = clinical and family Hx
   d. Tx = careful, regular monitoring for malignancy
5. Juvenile Polyposis Syndromes
   a. Examples include juvenile polyposis coli, generalized juvenile GI polyposis, and Cronkhite-Canada syndrome
   b. Si/Sx = hamartomatous polyps and thus carry ↓ malignant potential, similar to Peutz-Jeghers; pts with familial juvenile polyposis carry ↑ risk for GI CA
   c. Dx = clinical and family Hx
   d. Tx = polypectomy is generally reserved for symptomatic polyps

B. **Diverticular Disease**
   1. General Characteristics
      a. Approximately 50% of people have diverticula, ↑ incidence between fifth and eighth decade of life in Western countries, but **only 10% to 20% cause Sx**
      b. True diverticula = herniations involving the full bowel wall thickness
      c. True diverticula are rare, often found in cecum and ascending colon
      d. False diverticula = only mucosal herniations through muscular wall
      e. False diverticula are common, >90% found in sigmoid colon
      f. It is believed that ↑ intraluminal pressure (perhaps promoted by ↓ fiber diet) causes herniation
   2. Diverticulosis
      a. Presence of multiple false (acquired) diverticula
      b. Si/Sx = 80% are aSx and are found incidentally; can cause recurrent abd pain in LLQ and changes in bowel habits; 5% to 10% of pts present with lower GI hemorrhage that can be massive
      c. Dx = colonoscopy or barium enema to reveal herniations

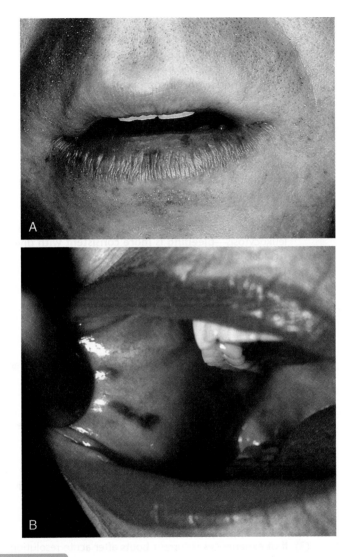

FIGURE 2.10

Peutz-Jeghers syndrome. **(A)** Pigmented macules on the lips that cross the vermilion border. (Courtesy of Jeffrey P. Callen, MD.) **(B)** Buccal and perioral pigment spots are characteristic of this syndrome. (From Yamada T, Alpers DH, Kaplowitz N, et al., eds. *Atlas of gastroenterology*, 3rd Ed. Philadelphia: Lippincott Williams & Wilkins, 2003, with permission.)

    d. Tx

      (1) aSx pts should ↑ fiber content of diet, ↓ fatty food intake, and avoid foods that exacerbate diverticular obstruction (e.g., seeds)

      (2) Surgical therapy for uncomplicated diverticulosis is **rare**

      (3) See Section E for management of GI hemorrhage

3. Diverticulitis

    a. Diverticular infxn and macroperforation resulting in inflammation

    b. Inflammation may be limited to the bowel, extend to pericolic tissues, form an abscess, or result in peritonitis

    c. Si/Sx

      (1) LLQ pain, diarrhea or constipation, fever, anorexia, and leukocytosis—**bleeding is more consistent with diverticulosis, not diverticulitis**

      (2) **Life-threatening complications from diverticulitis include large perforations, abscess or fistula formation, and obstruction**

      (3) Most common fistula associated with diverticular dz is colovesicular (presenting with recurrent UTIs)

    d. Dx

      (1) CT scan may demonstrate edema of the bowel wall and the presence/location of formed abscesses

      (2) Barium enema and colonoscopy are generally contraindicated for the acute pt, but if the pt's Sx point to obstruction or to presence of a fistula, a contrast enema is warranted

    e. Tx

      (1) Majority of pts respond to conservative Tx with IV hydration, antibiotics with coverage for Gram-negative rods and anaerobes, and NPO orders

      (2) Abscess requires CT- or Utz-guided percutaneous drainage

      (3) If pt experiences recurrent bouts after acute resolution, a sigmoid colectomy is usually considered on an elective basis

      (4) Perforation or obstruction → resection of affected bowel and construction of a temporary diverting colostomy and a Hartman pouch—reanastomosis performed 2 to 3 months postoperatively

C. **GI Hemorrhage**

1. **Bright-red blood per rectum** (BRBPR) usually points to bleeding in the **distal small bowel or colon,** although a proximal bleeding site must be considered

2. Massive lower GI hemorrhage usually is caused by diverticular disease, angiodysplasia, ulcerative colitis, ischemic colitis, or solitary ulcer (Figure 2.11)

3. Chronic rectal bleed usually is because of hemorrhoids, fissures, CA, or polyps

4. Dx

   a. Digital rectal exam (DRE) and visualization with an anoscope and sigmoidoscope to locate and Tx obvious bleeding site

   b. Endoscopy to evaluate for an upper GI bleed

   c. Angiography if pt continues to bleed despite rule out upper GI source

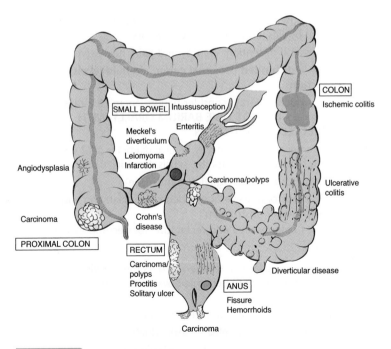

FIGURE 2.11 Lower GI bleeding.

    d. If bleeding is minimal/stopped or angiography is indeterminate and the pt is stable, the bowel should be prepped and colonoscopy performed

    e. Tagged RBC scan or barium enema if colonoscopy is non-Dx

5. Tx

    a. IV fluids and transfusions as needed to maintain hemodynamic stability

    b. Surgery is rarely required and should be considered only if bleeding persists (>90% of bleeding ceases spontaneously) despite intervention

D. Large Intestine Obstruction

1. Accounts for 15% of obstructions—most common site is sigmoid colon

2. Three most common causes are **adenoCA, scarring 2° to diverticulitis, and volvulus—consider adhesions if pt had previous abd surgery**

3. Other causes are fecal impaction, inflammatory disorders, foreign bodies, and other benign tumors

4. Si/Sx = abd distention, crampy abd pain, nausea/vomiting

5. **X-ray → distended proximal colon, air–fluid levels, no gas in rectum**

6. Dx = clinical + x-ray, consider barium enema if x-rays are equivocal—**DO NOT GIVE BARIUM ORALLY WITH SUSPECTED OBSTRUCTION**

7. Tx = emergency laparotomy if cecal diameter >12 cm or for severe tenderness, peritonitis, sepsis, free air

8. Pseudo-Obstruction **(Ogilvie's Syndrome)**

    a. Presence of massive right-sided colon dilatation with no evidence of obstruction

    b. Tx = colonoscopy and rectal tube for decompression

E. Volvulus

1. Rotation of the large intestine along its mesenteric axis— twisting can promote ischemic bowel, gangrene, and subsequent perforation

2. Most common site is **sigmoid** (70%) followed by **cecum** (30%)

3. **Commonly occurs in elderly individuals**

4. Si/Sx = obstructive symptoms, including distention, tympany, rushes, and high-pitched bowel sounds

5. Dx = clinical, confirmed by radiographic studies
   a. X-ray → dilated loops of bowel with loss of haustra with **a kidney bean appearance**
   b. Barium enema → a narrowing mimicking a **"bird's beak"** or **"ace of spades"** picture, with point of beak pointing to site of bowel rotation
6. Tx
   a. Sigmoidoscopy or colonoscopy for decompression
   b. If not successful, laparotomy with a two-stage resection and anastomosis is necessary
   c. Cecal volvulus is treated with cecopexy (attachment of mobile cecum to peritoneal membrane) or right hemicolectomy

F. **Colon CA**
   1. Epidemiology
      a. Second leading cause of CA deaths
      b. Genetic influences include tumor suppressor and proto-oncogenes
      c. Lynch syndromes I and II or hereditary nonpolyposis colorectal CA (HNPCC)
         (1) **Lynch syndrome I** is an autosomal dominant predisposition to colorectal CA with right-sided predominance (70% proximal to the splenic flexure)
         (2) **Lynch syndrome II** shows all of the features of Lynch syndrome I and also causes extracolonic CA, particularly endometrial CA, CA of the ovary, small bowel, stomach, and pancreas, and transitional cell CA of the ureter and renal pelvis
   2. Screening
      a. Age >50 yr without risk factors (strong family Hx, ulcerative colitis, etc.) → yearly stool occult blood tests, flexible sigmoidoscopy q3–5 yr or colonoscopy q10yr or barium enema q5–10 yr
      b. Colonoscopy/barium enema if polyps found
      c. Pts with risk factors require more frequent and full colonoscopies
   3. Dx
      a. Endoscopy or barium enema—biopsy not essential
      b. Obtain preoperative carcinoembryonic antigen (CEA) to follow disease; these levels will be elevated before any physical evidence of disease

4. Surgical = resection and regional lymph node dissection
5. Adjuvant Tx for metastatic dz = 5-fluorouracil (5-FU) ⊕ leucovorin or levamisole → 30% improvement in survival
6. Follow-Up
   a. Hx, physical, and CEA level q3mo for 3 yr, then follow-up every 6 mo for 2 yr
   b. Colonoscopy at 6 mo, 12 mo, and yearly for 5 yr
   c. CT and MRI for suspected recurrences

XVI. Rectum and Anus (Figure 2.11)

A. Hemorrhoids

1. Varicosity in the lower rectum or anus caused by congestion in the veins of the hemorrhoidal plexus
2. Si/Sx = anal mass, bleeding, itching, discomfort
3. Presence or absence of pain depends on the location of the hemorrhoid: internal hemorrhoid is generally not painful, whereas an external hemorrhoid can be extremely painful
4. **Thrombosed External Hemorrhoid**
   a. Not a true hemorrhoid, but subcutaneous external hemorrhoidal veins of the anal canal
   b. It is classically **painful,** tense, bluish elevation beneath the skin or anoderm
5. Hemorrhoids are classified by degrees
   a. 1° = no prolapse
   b. 2° = prolapse with defecation, but returns on its own
   c. 3° = prolapse with defecation or straining, require manual reduction
   d. 4° = not capable of being reduced
6. Dx = H&P inspection of the perianal area, digital rectal examination (DRE), anoscopy, and sigmoidoscopy
7. Tx = conservative therapy consists of a high-fiber diet, Sitz baths, stool-bulking agents, stool softeners, cortisone cream, astringent medicated pads
8. Definitive Tx = sclerotherapy, cryosurgery, rubber band ligation, and surgical hemorrhoidectomy

B. Fistula-in-Ano

1. Communication between the rectum to the perianal skin, usually 2° to anal crypt infxn

2. Infxn in the crypt forms abscess then ruptures and a fistulous tract is formed; can be seen in Crohn's disease

3. Si/Sx = intermittent or constant discharge, may exude pus, incontinence

4. Dx = physical exam

5. Tx = fistulotomy

6. Factors that predispose to maintenance of fistula patency = **FRIEND** = **F**oreign body, **R**adiation, **I**nfection, **E**pithelialization, **N**eoplasm, **D**istal obstruction

C. **Anal Fissure**

1. Epithelium in the anal canal denuded 2° to passage of irritating diarrhea and a tightening of the anal canal related to nervous tension

2. Si/Sx = **classic** presentation, a severely painful bowel movement associated with bright red bleeding

3. Dx = anoscopy

4. Tx = stool softeners, dietary modifications, and bulking agents, Botox type A, or nitroglycerin ointment

5. Surgical Tx = lateral internal sphincterotomy if pain is unbearable and fissure persists

D. **Rectal CA**

1. More common in males

2. Si/Sx = **rectal bleeding,** obstruction, altered bowel habits, and tenesmus

3. Dx = colonoscopy, sigmoidoscopy, biopsy, barium enema

4. Tx = sphincter-saving surgery, adjuvant Tx for rectal CA with positive nodal metastasis or transmural involvement includes radiation therapy and 5-fluorouracil (5-FU) chemotherapy

E. **Anal CA**

1. Most commonly squamous cell CA, others include transitional cell, adenoCA, melanoma, and mucoepidermal

2. Risk factors include fistulas, abscess, infxns, and Crohn's disease

3. Si/Sx = **anal bleeding,** pain, and mucus evacuation

4. Dx = biopsy

5. Tx = chemotherapy and radiation

XVII. Breast

A. **Mastalgia**

1. Cyclical or noncyclical breast pain NOT because of lumps

2. Tx = danazol, works by inducing amenorrhea (side effects are hirsutism and weight gain)

3. Pain worse with respiration may be due to Tietze syndrome (costochondritis)

4. Mondor's disease = thoracoepigastric vein phlebitis → skin retraction along vein course

B. **Gynecomastia**

1. Enlargement of male breast (unilateral or bilateral)

2. Lobules not found in male breast as in the female breast

3. Occurs as result of an imbalance in estrogen and androgen hormones usually occurring during puberty but can occur in old age

4. Can also be seen in hyperestrogen states, such as liver cirrhosis or drug use that inhibits liver breakdown of estrogen; e.g., alcohol, marijuana, heroin, and psychoactive drugs

5. Medication induces from cimetidine, spironolactone, antipsychotics, isoniazid, and digitalis

6. Seen in Klinefelter's syndrome and pts with a testicular neoplasm

C. **CA Risks**

1. Risk ↑ by

   a. Number one factor is gender (1% of breast CA occur in men)

   b. Age (number one factor in women)

   c. Young first menarche (<11 yr)

   d. Old at first pregnancy (>30 yr)

   e. Late menopause (>50 yr)

   f. FHx

      (1) 95% of CA are not familial

      (2) ↑ incidence in pt having a first-degree relative with history of breast CA

      (3) Autosomal dominant (not 100% penetrance) conditions with ↑ risk: BRCA-1, BRCA-2, Li-Fraumeni syndrome, Cowden's disease, and Peutz-Jeghers

   g. Prior breast CA in opposite breast

2. Risk NOT ↑ by caffeine, sexual orientation
3. Risk NOT ↑ by fibroadenoma or fibrocystic disease
4. CA occurs most frequently in upper outer quadrant (tail of Spencer)

D. **Breast Tumors**

1. **Fibroadenoma (FA)** (Figure 2.12)

a. Most common tumor in teens and young women (peak in 20s)

Algorithm 2.1

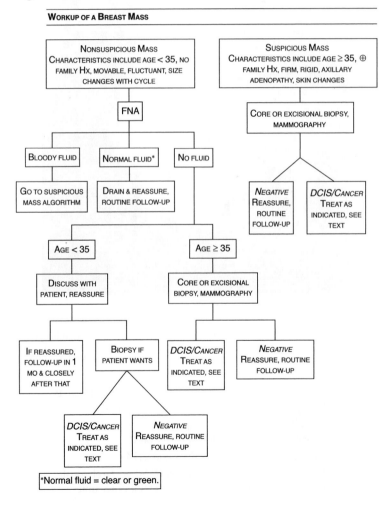

WORKUP OF A BREAST MASS

NONSUSPICIOUS MASS CHARACTERISTICS INCLUDE AGE < 35, NO FAMILY HX, MOVABLE, FLUCTUANT, SIZE CHANGES WITH CYCLE

SUSPICIOUS MASS CHARACTERISTICS INCLUDE AGE ≥ 35, ⊕ FAMILY HX, FIRM, RIGID, AXILLARY ADENOPATHY, SKIN CHANGES

FNA

CORE OR EXCISIONAL BIOPSY, MAMMOGRAPHY

BLOODY FLUID

NORMAL FLUID*

NO FLUID

NEGATIVE REASSURE, ROUTINE FOLLOW-UP

DCIS/CANCER TREAT AS INDICATED, SEE TEXT

GO TO SUSPICIOUS MASS ALGORITHM

DRAIN & REASSURE, ROUTINE FOLLOW-UP

AGE < 35

AGE ≥ 35

DISCUSS WITH PATIENT, REASSURE

CORE OR EXCISIONAL BIOPSY, MAMMOGRAPHY

IF REASSURED, FOLLOW-UP IN 1 MO & CLOSELY AFTER THAT

BIOPSY IF PATIENT WANTS

DCIS/CANCER TREAT AS INDICATED, SEE TEXT

NEGATIVE REASSURE, ROUTINE FOLLOW-UP

DCIS/CANCER TREAT AS INDICATED, SEE TEXT

NEGATIVE REASSURE, ROUTINE FOLLOW-UP

*Normal fluid = clear or green.

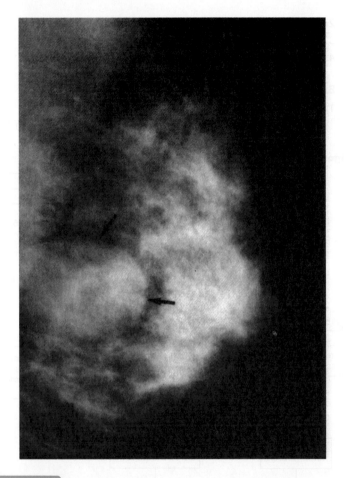

FIGURE 2.12

Fibroadenoma. Mammogram. A dominant mass (*arrows*) with smooth borders is the same density as nml breast tissue in a young woman. (Image from Rubin E, Farber JL. *Pathology*, 3rd Ed. Philadelphia: Lippincott Williams & Wilkins, 1999.)

    b. Histology = myxoid stroma and curvilinear, slit ducts

    c. FAs grow rapidly, no ↑ risk for developing CA

    d. Tx NOT required, often will resorb within several weeks; reevaluation after 1 month is standard

2. **Fibrocystic Disease** (Figure 2.13 and 2.14)

    a. Most common tumor in pts 35 to 50 yr, rarely post-menopausal, arise in terminal ductal lobular unit

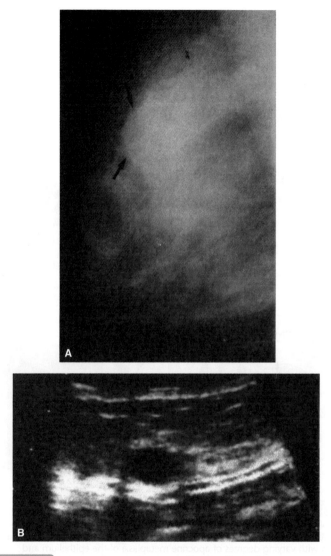

FIGURE 2.13

Fibrocystic breast disease. **(A)** Mammogram showing oval, very well-defined mass without calcifications (*arrows*). **(B)** The mass was shown to be cystic on Utz. (Both images from Rubin E, Farber JL. *Pathology*, 3rd Ed. Philadelphia: Lippincott Williams & Wilkins, 1999.)

Terminal duct lobular unit

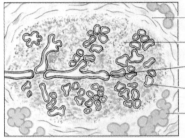

Interlobular stroma

Intralobular stroma

Intralobular duct

Terminal duct or acinus

Fat

A Nonproliferative fibrocystic change

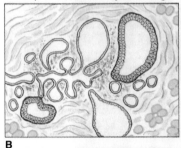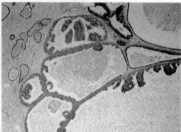

B

Proliferative fibrocystic change

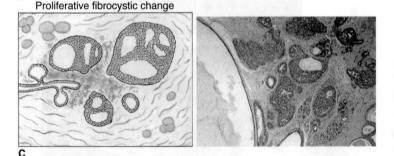

C

Histology of fibrocystic change. **(A)** Nml terminal lobular unit. **(B)** Nonproliferative fibrocystic change. This lesion combines cystic dilation of the terminal ducts with varying degrees of apocrine metaplasia of the epithelium and ↑ fibrous stroma. **(C)** Proliferative fibrocystic change. Terminal duct dilation and intraductal epithelial hyperplasia are present. (From Rubin E, Gorstein F, Rubin R, et al. *Rubin's pathology: clinicopathologic foundations of medicine,* 4th Ed. Baltimore: Lippincott Williams & Wilkins, 2005, with permission.)

    b. Pts c/o multiple bilateral small lumps tender during menstrual cycle

    c. Cysts can arise overnight, of no clinical significance

    d. Not associated with ↑ risk for CA unless biopsy specimen reveals epithelial (ductal or lobular) hyperplasia with atypia

    e. Dx/Tx = fine-needle aspiration (FNA), drainage of fluid—if aspirated fluid is bloody, send for cytology to rule out cystic malignancy

3. **Fibrous Pseudo-Lump**

    a. Parenchymal atrophy in premenopausal breast

    b. Multiple nodules will be present

4. **Intraductal Papilloma**

    a. Often presents with serous/**bloody nipple discharge (guaiac-positive)**

    b. Will be solitary growth in perimenopause but can have multiple nodules if younger

    c. **Solitary papillomas do not ↑ CA risk, but multiple papillomas DO**

5. **Intraductal Hyperplasia**

    a. Dx by biopsy, >2 cell layers in ductal epithelium, either with or without atypia

    b. If atypia is present, ↑ risk for CA later developing in EITHER breast

    c. It is NOT premalignant, it is a MARKER for future malignancy, which will not be in the same place

6. **Ductal CA in Situ (DCIS) (Figure 2.15)**

    a. Usually nonpalpable, seen as irregularly shaped ductal calcifications on mammography

    b. Unless comedonecrosis is present, not be visibly detectable

    c. Comedonecrosis common in *her2/neu* + (*c-erbB-2*+) disease

    d. This is a true premalignancy; will lead to invasive ductal CA

    e. Histology = haphazard cells along papillae (in contrast to hyperplasia, which is orderly), punched-out areas in ducts with "Roman bridge" pattern because of cells infiltrating open spaces

    f. Tx = excision of mass, ensure clean margins on excision (if not excise again with wider margins), and add postoperative radiation to reduce rate of recurrence

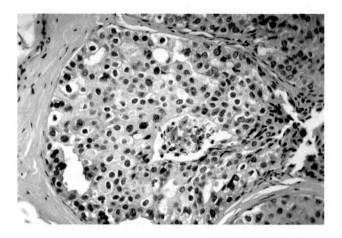

FIGURE 2.15
Ductal CA in situ, comedo-type. The terminal ducts are distended by CA in situ (intraductal CA). The centers of the tumor masses are necrotic and display dystrophic calcification. (From Rubin E, Gorstein F, Rubin R, et al. *Rubin's pathology: clinicopathologic foundations of medicine,* 4th Ed. Baltimore: Lippincott Williams & Wilkins, 2005, with permission.)

7. **Lobular Carcinoma in Situ (LCIS)**
   a. Cannot be detected clinically or by gross examination; mammography is also a poor tool for diagnosing this disease
   b. It is NOT precancerous like DCIS is, but it IS a marker for future invasive ductal CA risk
   c. Histology shows mucinous cells almost always present; "sawtooth" and clover-leaf configurations occur in the ducts

8. **Invasive Ductal CA (IDC)** (Figure 2.16)
   a. Most common breast CA, occurs commonly in mid 30s to late 50s, forms solid tumors
   b. Tumor size is the most important Px factor; node involvement is also an important Px factor
   c. Moderately differentiated IDC comes from cribriform or papillary intraductal originators
   d. Poorly differentiated IDC comes from intraductal comedo originator
   e. Forms solid tumor; many subtypes of this tumor exist (e.g., mucinous, medullary)

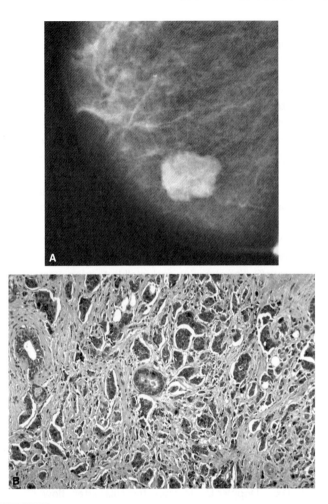

FIGURE 2.16

(A) Mammogram of breast CA (note the irregular shape and borders of the growth). (Reprinted with permission from Mitchell GW. *The female breast and its disorders*, 1st Ed. Baltimore: Williams & Wilkins, 1990.) **(B)** Ductal CA. Invasive ductal CA. Irregular cords and nests of tumor cells, derived from the same cells that compose the intraductal component **(A)**, invade the stroma. Many of the cells form ductlike structures. (Image from Rubin E, Farber JL. *Pathology*, 3rd Ed. Philadelphia: Lippincott Williams & Wilkins, 1999.)

9. **Invasive Lobular CA**
    a. Only 3% to 5% of invasive CA is lobular, present at age 45 to 56 yr, vague appearance on mammogram
    b. Pts have ↑ frequency of bilateral CA
    c. **Exhibits single file growth pattern within a fibrous stroma** (Figure 2.17)

10. **Paget's Breast Disease (NOT BONE DISEASE!)**
    a. Presents with dermatitis/macular rash over nipple or areola
    b. Underlying ductal CA almost always present

11. **Inflammatory CA**
    a. Breast has classic Sx of inflammation: redness, pain, and heat
    b. Rapidly progressive breast CA, almost always widely metastatic at presentation
    c. Px poor

E. **Mammography**
    1. Highly effective screening tool in all but young women
    2. **Dense breast tissue found in young women interferes with the test's sensitivity and specificity**
    3. All women over 50 should have yearly mammograms (proven to ↓ mortality in these pts)

XVIII. Urology

A. **Scrotal Emergencies**
    1. Testicular Torsion
        a. Usually peripubertal pt
        b. Si/Sx = acute onset testicular pain and edema, nausea and vomiting, tender, swollen testicle with transverse lie, **absent cremasteric reflex on affected side**
        c. Dx = Doppler Utz to assess testicular artery flow
        d. Tx = emergent surgical decompression, with excision of testicle if it infarcts
    2. Epididymitis
        a. Si/Sx = unilateral testicular pain, dysuria, occasional urethral discharge, fever, leukocytosis in severe cases, painful and swollen epididymis
        b. Dx = history and physical, labs → UA can be negative or show pyuria, urine Cx should be obtained, swab for *Neisseria gonorrhoeae* and *Chlamydia*
        c. Tx = antibiotics and NSAIDs

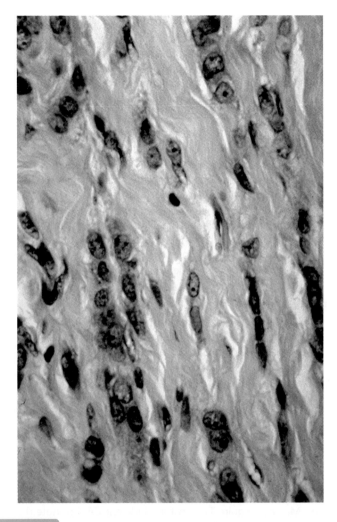

FIGURE 2.17

Invasive lobular CA. In contrast to invasive ductal CA, the cells of lobular CA tend to form single strands that invade between collagen fibers in a single pattern. The tumor cells are similar to those seen in lobular CA in situ. (From Rubin E, Gorstein F, Rubin R, et al. *Rubin's pathology: clinicopathologic foundations of medicine,* 4th Ed. Baltimore: Lippincott Williams & Wilkins, 2005, with permission.)

3. Appendix Testis Torsion of Testicular Appendage
    a. Si/Sx = similar to testicular torsion, severe tenderness over superior pole of testicle, **"blue dot" sign** of ischemic appendage, nml position and lie, **cremasteric reflex present**, testicle and epididymis not tender
    b. Dx = Utz, perfusion confirmed with nuclear medicine scan
    c. Tx = supportive, should resolve in 2 wk
4. Fournier's Gangrene
    a. Necrotizing fasciitis of the genital area
    b. Si/Sx = acute pruritus, rapidly progressing edema, erythema, tenderness, fever, chills, malaise, necrosis of skin and subcutaneous tissues, crepitus caused by gas-forming organisms
    c. Dx = history of diabetes mellitus, or immunocompromise, physical exam, labs → leukocytosis, positive blood and wound cultures (polymicrobial), x-ray → subcutaneous gas
    d. Tx emergently with wide surgical débridement and antibiotics

B. **Prostate CA**
1. Si/Sx = advanced dz causes obstructive Sx, UTI, urinary retention; pts may also present with Sx due to metastases (bone pain, weight loss, and anemia), rock-hard nodule in prostate
2. Dx = labs → anemia, azotemia, elevated serum acid phosphatase and prostate-specific antigen (PSA)—note that use of these tests for screening is controversial because of relatively low sensitivity and specificity
3. Transrectal Utz, CT scan, MRI, plain films for metastatic workup, biopsy to confirm Dx
4. Bone scan helpful to detect bony metastases (Figure 2.18)
5. Tx
    a. May not require Tx, most are indolent CA, but note that some are very aggressive and may warrant Tx depending on pt's wishes
    b. Modalities include finasteride, local irradiation, nerve sparing, or radical prostatectomy—risks of surgery include impotence and incontinence
    c. Aggressiveness of Tx depends on extent of disease and pt's age

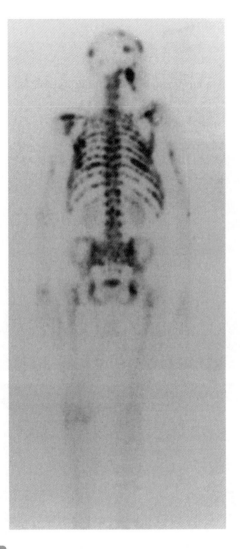

SURGERY

FIGURE 2.18

Bone scan showing multiple metastases secondary to prostatic CA. (From Crushieri A, Hennessy TPJ, Greenhalgh RM, et al. *Clinical surgery*. Oxford: Blackwell Science, 1996, with permission.)

XIX. Orthopedics

A. **Wrist Injuries**

1. Fractures

   a. Distal radius fracture (**Colles'**) occurs after fall on outstretched hand (Figure 2.19)

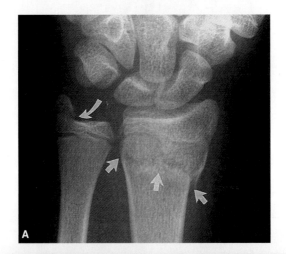

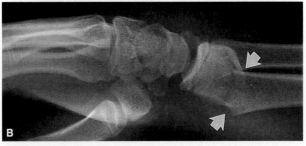

(A) Extraarticular (Colles) distal radial fracture (*arrow*) in frontal projection associated with a fracture of the base of the ulnar styloid (*curved arrow*, A). (From Harris JH Jr, Harris WH. *The radiology of emergency medicine*, 3rd Ed. Philadelphia: Lippincott-Raven, 2000, with permission.) **(B)** Extra-articular (Colles) distal radial fracture (*arrow*) in lateral projection associated with a fracture of the base of the ulnar styloid (*curved arrow*, A). (From Harris JH Jr, Harris WH. *The radiology of emergency medicine*, 3rd Ed. Philadelphia: Lippincott-Raven, 2000, with permission.)

b. Ulnar fracture occurs after direct blow; commonly seen in hockey, lacrosse, or martial arts

c. Dx = x-rays, H&P

d. Tx for both = cast immobilization for 2 to 4 wk followed by bracing

e. Scaphoid fracture

   (1) Usually 2° to falls; commonly misdiagnosed as a "wrist sprain"

   (2) Dx = clinical (pain in anatomic **snuffbox**), x-rays to confirm, bone scan or MRI for athletes who require early definitive Dx (Figure 2.20)

   (3) Tx = thumb splint for 10 wk (↑ risk of avascular necrosis)

2. Carpal Tunnel Syndrome

a. Si/Sx = pain and paresthesias in fingers worse at night

b. Dx = **Tinel's sign** (pathognomonic) = tapping median nerve on palmar aspect of wrist producing "shooting"

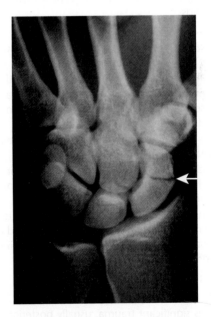

FIGURE 2.20

Scaphoid fracture. (From Bucholz RW, Heckman JD. *Rockwood & Green's fractures in adults*, 5th Ed. Philadelphia: Lippincott Williams & Wilkins, 2001.)

sensation to fingers and **Phalen's test** = wrist flexion to 60° for 30 to 60 sec reproduces pt's Sx

   c. Tx = avoid causative activities, splint wrist in slight extension, consider steroid injection into carpal canal; surgery for refractory dz

   d. Px = may require up to 1 yr before Sx resolve even after surgery

B. **Shoulder Injuries**

   1. Rotator Cuff Injury (Impingement Syndrome)

      a. Typically develops over time in pts >45 yr

      b. Si/Sx = pain/tenderness at deltoid and over anterior humeral head, difficulty lying on shoulder, ↓ internal rotation, crepitation, **Neer's sign** (pain elicited with forcible forward elevation of arm), lidocaine injection into subacromial space alleviates pain

      c. Dx = clinical, confirm with MRI

      d. Tx = NSAIDs and stretching; consider steroid injection for refractory dz, arthroscopic surgery for severe dz refractory to steroids

   2. Shoulder Dislocation

      a. Subluxation = symptomatic translation of humeral head relative to glenoid articular surface

      b. Dislocation = complete displacement out of the glenoid fossa

      c. Anterior instability (approximately 95% of cases) usually because of subcoracoid dislocation is the most common form of shoulder dislocation (Figure 2.21)

      d. Si/Sx = pain, joint immobility, arm "goes dead" with overhead motion

      e. Dx = clinical, assess axillary nerve function in neurologic exam, look for signs of rotator cuff injury, confirm with x-rays if necessary

      f. Tx = initial reduction of dislocation by various traction–countertraction techniques, 2- to 6-wk period of immobilization (longer for younger pts), intense rehabilitation; rarely is surgery required

C. **Hip and Thigh Injuries**

   1. Dislocations

      a. Requires significant trauma, usually posterior, occur in children

      b. Sciatic nerve injury may be present—do a careful neurologic exam

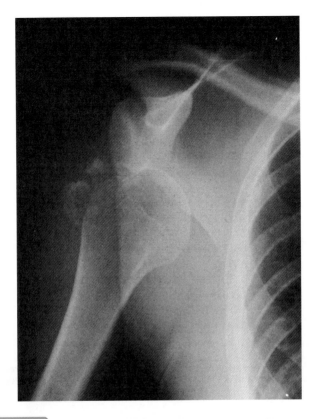

FIGURE 2.21

Anterior dislocation with a fracture of the greater tuberosity. (From Bucholz RW, Heckman JD. *Rockwood & Green's fractures in adults*, 5th Ed. Philadelphia: Lippincott Williams & Wilkins, 2001.)

c. Dx = x-rays, consider CT scan to assess any associated fractures
d. Tx
  (1) **Orthopedic emergency requiring reduction under sedation (open reduction may be required)**
  (2) Light traction for ≥5 days is strongly recommended
  (3) No weight-bearing for 3-wk minimum, followed by 3 to 4 wk of light weight-bearing activities
  (4) Follow-up imaging studies required every 3 to 6 mo for 2 yr
e. Major complication is avascular necrosis of femoral head

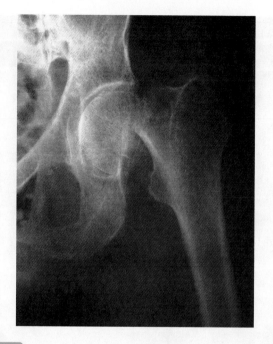

FIGURE 2.22
Femoral neck fracture. (From Bucholz RW, Heckman JD. *Rockwood & Green's fractures in adults*, 5th Ed. Philadelphia: Lippincott Williams & Wilkins, 2001.)

    2. Femoral Neck Fracture (Figure 2.22)
      a. Like hip dislocation, requires significant force
      b. Si/Sx = severe hip and groin pain worse with movement; leg may be externally rotated
      c. Dx = radiograph is definitive diagnosis
      d. Tx = operative reduction with internal fixation
  D. **Knee Injuries** (Table 2.12; Figure 2.23)

XX. Neurosurgery

A. **Head Injury**
    1. Intracranial Hemorrhage (Table 2.13; Figures 2.24 and 2.25)
    2. General Treatment
      a. Establish ABCs, intubate and ventilate unconscious pts

Table 2.12   Knee Injuries

Injury	Characteristics	Tx
Anterior cruciate ligament tear (ACL)	• Si/Sx = **presents with a "pop" in the knee**, pt may also complain of **knee instability or giving way** • **Lachman test** and/or anterior drawer finds pathologic anterior tibial translation and can Dx without imaging • MRI is most helpful to determine full extent of injury	Conservative or arthroscopic repair of tear
Posterior cruciate ligament tear (PCL)	• Tear seen during falls on flexed knee and dashboard injuries in motor vehicle accidents (MVAs) • X-rays to rule out associated injury or fracture • MRI useful to determine full extent of injury	Conservative or arthroscopic repair of tear
Collateral ligament tear	• **Medial collateral is the most commonly injured knee ligament** (lateral collateral is least commonly injured) • Seen after direct blow to lateral knee • **Commonly pt also injures ACL or PCL** • X-rays to rule out associated injury or fracture • MRI useful to determine full extent of injury	Hinge brace
Meniscus tear	• Acute trauma or more commonly due to degeneration seen with aging • Medial menisci injured three times more often, male > female • Dx = **McMurray test** = pt supine with hips flexed 90° and knee fully flexed, maneuver foot into abduction–adduction and external–internal rotation while palpating joint line for a click • MRI is standard diagnostic test (Figure 2.23)	Rest (fails >50% of time), consider arthroscopy

SURGERY

b. Maintain cervical spine precautions

c. ↑ ICP → mannitol, hyperventilate, steroids, and/or ventricular shunt

B. **Temporal Bone Fractures**

1. Transverse fractures 20% of fractures facial nerve injury and loss of hearing more likely

2. Logitudinal fractures 80% of fractures

3. Dx by fine cut CT of temporal bone and audiogram

Text continues on page 205

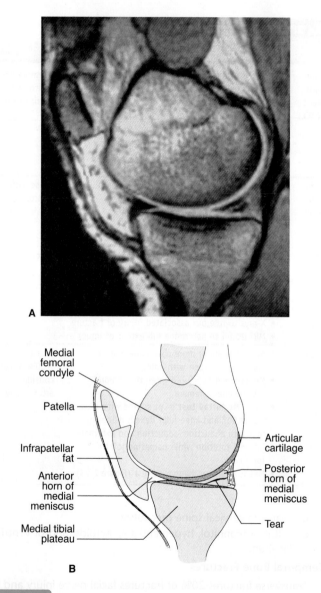

FIGURE 2.23

Tear of medial meniscus. **(A)** Sagittal MRI through the medial part of the knee joint showing a tear in the posterior horn of the medial meniscus. **(B)** The anterior horn appears nml. (Adapted from Armstrong P, Wastie M. *Diagnosticimaging*, 4th Ed. Oxford: Blackwell Science, 1998, with permission.)

Table 2.13   Intracranial Hemorrhage

Type	Bleeding Site	Characteristics	Treatment
Epidural (Figure 2.24)	Middle meningeal artery	• **Dx = CT → biconcave disk not crossing sutures** • This is a medical emergency!	Evacuate hematoma via burr holes
Subdural (Figure 2.24)	Cortical bridging veins	• Causes = trauma, coagulopathy, common in elderly • Sx may start 1–2 wks after trauma • **Dx = CT → crescentic pattern extends across suture lines** • Px worse than epidural due to ↑ risk of concurrent brain injury	Evacuate hematoma via burr holes
Subarachnoid (Figure 2.25)	Circle of Willis, often at middle cerebral artery (MCA) branch	• Causes = arteriovenous malformation, berry aneurysm, trauma • Berry aneurysms → severe sudden headache, **CN III palsy**	Berry aneurysm = surgical excision or fill with metal coil
		• Cerebrospinal fluid (CSF) xanthochromia (also seen any time CSF protein >150 mg/dL or serum bilirubin >6 mg/dL) • Dx berry aneurysm with cerebral angiogram	Nimodipine to prevent vasospasm and resultant 2° infarcts
Parenchymal	Basal ganglia, internal capsule, thalamus	• Causes = hypertension, trauma, arteriovenous malformation, coagulopathy • CT/MRI → focal edema, hypodensity	↑ ICP → mannitol, hyperventilate, steroids and/or ventricular shunt

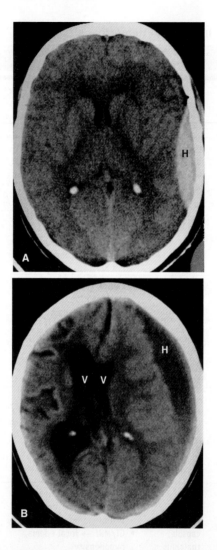

FIGURE 2.24

Extracerebral hematoma. **(A)** CT scan showing a high-density lentiform area typical of an acute epidural hematoma (*H*). **(B)** CT scan in another pt taken 1 mo after injury showing a subdural hematoma (*H*) as a low-density area. Note the substantial ventricular displacement. *V*, ventricle. (From Berg D. *Advanced clinical skills and physical diagnosis.* Oxford: Blackwell Science, 1999; Armstrong P, Wastie M. *Diagnostic imaging,* 4th Ed. Oxford: Blackwell Science, 1998, with permission.)

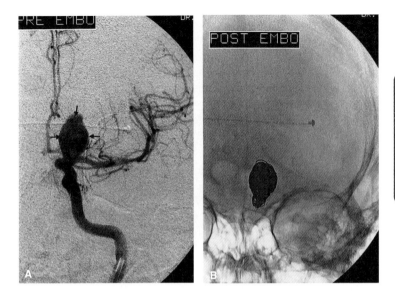

FIGURE 2.25

Aneurysm occlusion. **(A)** Carotid angiogram showing a large aneurysm (*arrows*) arising at the termination of the internal carotid artery. **(B)** Plain film after embolization of the aneurysm that is occluded with metal coils. (From Armstrong P, Wastie M. *Diagnostic imaging,* 4th Ed. Oxford: Blackwell Science, 1998, with permission.)

4. IV antibiotics and ear drops if CSF leak noted
5. Facial nerve decompression may be needed if facial nerve affected

C. **Basilar Skull Fractures**
   1. **Present with four classic physical findings: "raccoon's eyes" and Battle's sign, hemotympanum, CSF rhinorrhea, and otorrhea**
   2. "Raccoon's eyes" are dark circles (bruising) about the eyes, signifying orbital fractures (Figure 2.26)
   3. Battle's sign is ecchymoses over the mastoid process, indicating a fracture there
   4. Dx = clinical + CT
   5. Tx = supportive

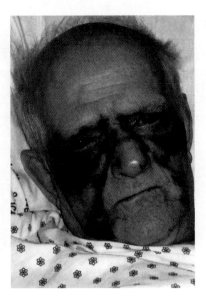

FIGURE 2.26

Raccoon eyes in basilar skull fracture.

D. **Tumors**

1. Si/Sx

   a. Headache awakening pt at night or is worse in morning after waking

   b. ↑ ICP → nausea/vomiting, **bradycardia with hypertension, Cheyne-Stokes respirations (Cushing's triad),** and papilledema

   c. ⊕ Focal deficits, frequently of CN III → fixed, dilated pupil

2. DDx (Table 2.14)

3. Dx

   a. Bx → definitive Dx

   b. Clinical suspicion + CT/MRI can diagnose lymphoma, prolactinoma, meningioma

   c. Demographics important for retinoblastoma

4. Tx = excision for all 1° tumors except prolactinoma and lymphoma

   a. First-line Tx for prolactinoma = bromocriptine (D_2 agonist inhibits prolactin secretion); second line = surgery

Table 2.14	CNS Malignancy
Type	**Characteristics**
Metastatic	Small circular lesion, often multiple, at gray–white junction—**most common CNS neoplasm: 1° =** lung, breast, melanoma, renal cell, colon, thyroid
Glioblastoma multiforme	Large, irregular, ring enhancing due to central infarction (outgrows blood supply)—**most common 1° CNS neoplasm**
Meningioma	Second most common 1° CNS neoplasm, slow growing and benign
Retinoblastoma	Occurs in children, 60% sporadic, 40% familial (often bilateral)
Medulloblastoma	Found in cerebellum in floor of fourth ventricle, common in children
Craniopharyngioma	Compresses optic chiasm (visual loss) and hypothalamus
Prolactinoma	Most common pituitary tumor; Sx = **bilateral gynecomastia, amenorrhea, galactorrhea, impotence, bitemporal hemianopsia**
Lymphoma	Most common CNS tumor in AIDS pts (100× ↑ incidence), **MRI ring-enhancing lesion difficult to distinguish from toxoplasmosis**
Schwannoma	Usually affects CN VIII (acoustic neuroma) → tinnitus, deafness, ↑ ICP

SURGERY

   b. Tx for lymphoma is radiation therapy, poor Px
   c. Tx for metastases is generally radiation therapy and support
E. **Hydrocephalus**
   1. Definition = ↑ CSF → enlarged ventricles
   2. Si/Sx = ↑ ICP, ↓ cognition, headache, focal findings; in children separation of cranial bones leads to grossly enlarged calvaria
   3. **Dx made by finding dilated ventricles on CT/MRI** (Figure 2.27)
   4. Lumbar puncture opening pressure and CT appearance are crucial to determine type of hydrocephalus
   5. Nml ICP is always communicating
      a. Hydrocephalus ex vacuo
         (1) Ventricle dilation after neuron loss (e.g., stroke, CNS dz)
         (2) Sx due to neuron loss, not ventricular dilation in this case
         (3) Tx = none indicated

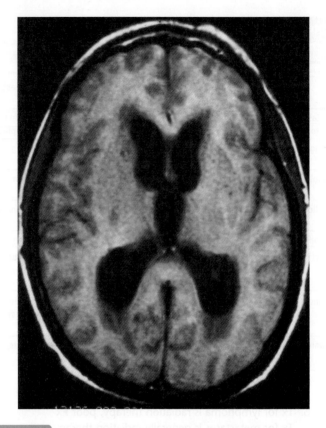

CT scan showing hydrocephalus. (From Cuschieri A, Thomas PJ, Henness RM, et al. *Clinical surgery.* Oxford: Blackwell Science, 1996, with permission.)

b. Nml pressure hydrocephalus
   (1) **Si/Sx = classic triad: bladder incontinence, dementia, ataxia ("wet, wacky, wobbly")**
   (2) Causes: 50% idiopathic, also meningitis, cerebral hemorrhage, trauma, atherosclerosis
   (3) Because of ↓ CSF resorption across arachnoid villi
   (4) Dx = clinically, or radionucleotide CSF studies
   (5) Tx = diuretic therapy, repeated spinal taps, consider shunt placement

6. ↑ ICP can be communicating or noncommunicating
   a. Pseudotumor cerebri
      (1) Communicating spontaneous ↑ ICP
      (2) **Commonly seen in obese, young females;** can be idiopathic; massive quantities of vitamin A can cause it
      (3) **CT → no ventricle dilation (may even be shrunken)**
      (4) Tx = symptomatic (acetazolamide or surgical lumboperitoneal shunt); dz is typically self-limiting
   b. Noncommunicating
      (1) Because of block between ventricles and subarachnoid space → CSF outflow obstruction at fourth ventricle, foramina of Luschka/Magendie/Munro/Magnum
      (2) Causes = congenital (e.g., Arnold-Chiari syndrome), tumor effacing outflow path, or scarring 2° meningitis or subarachnoid hemorrhage
      (3) Dx = CT
      (4) Tx = treat underlying cause if possible

XXI. Vascular Diseases

A. **Aneurysms**
   1. Abnormal dilation of an artery to **more than twice** its nml diameter
   2. Most common cause is atherosclerosis
   3. Common sites include abd aorta aneurysms (AAAs) and peripheral vessels including femoral and popliteal arteries
   4. True aneurysms involve all three layers of the vessel wall— caused by atherosclerosis and congenital defects such as Marfan's syndrome
   5. False aneurysms are "pulsatile hematomas" covered only by a thickened fibrous capsule (adventitia)—usually caused by traumatic disruption of the vessel wall or at an anastomotic site
   6. Si/Sx = mostly aSx; however, pts can present with rupture, thrombosis, and embolization; some pts complain of referred back pain and/or epigastric discomfort
   7. Rupture of AAA
      a. **Ruptured AAA is a surgical emergency,** and pt may present with **classic** abd pain, pulsatile abd mass, and hypotension
      b. The rate of rupture for a 5-cm diameter AAA is 6% per yr; rate for 6-cm diameter AAA is 10% per yr

      c. Pt's risk for rupture is ↑ by large diameter (Laplace's law), recent expansion, hypertension, and COPD; as a result, regular follow-up and control of hypertension are critical

8. Dx
   a. Palpation of a pulsatile mass in the abdomen on physical exam, confirmed with abd Utz or CT (Figures 2.28 and 2.29)
   b. CT is the best modality to determine the size of the aneurysm in a stable pt
   c. Plain film of the abdomen may demonstrate a calcified wall
   d. Aortogram most definitive Dx, also reveals size and extent

9. Tx
   a. BP control and ↓ risk factors, or surgical intervention
   b. Surgical intervention usually involves placement of a synthetic graft within the dilated wall of the AAA; surgery is recommended for **aneurysms >5 cm** in diameter in a good surgical candidate

10. Complications
    a. Myocardial infarction (MI), renal failure (because of proximity of renal vasculature off of aorta), colonic ischemia (AAAs usually involve the inferior mesenteric artery [IMA])
    b. Be aware of formation of **aortoduodenal fistula** in pts who have had a synthetic graft placed for AAA disease and present with GI bleeding

11. **Peripheral aneurysms**
    a. Most commonly in the popliteal artery
    b. 50% of popliteal aneurysms are bilateral, and 33% of pts with a popliteal aneurysm have an AAA
    c. Si/Sx = rupture is rare, and pts usually present with thrombosis, embolization, or claudication
    d. Tx = surgical if pt is symptomatic

B. **Aortic Dissection**
1. Intimal tear through which blood can flow, creating a plane between the intima and remainder of vessel wall
2. Usually confined to thoracic aorta (e.g., syphilis)
3. These planes can progress proximally and distally to disrupt blood supply to intestines, spinal cord, kidneys, and even the coronary vessels
4. In general, type A affects ascending aorta only; type B can affect both ascending and descending aorta

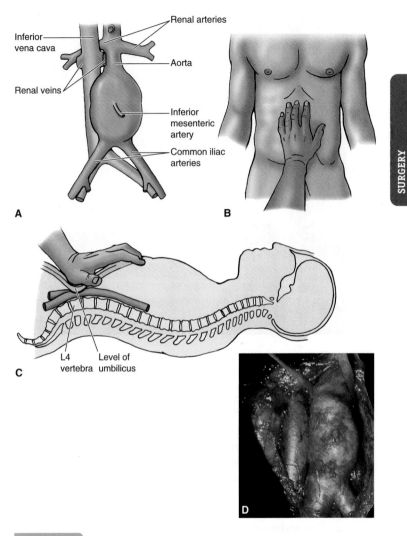

FIGURE 2.28

Pulsations of the aorta and AAA. (From Moore KL, Dalley AF II. *Clinical oriented anatomy*, 4th Ed. Baltimore: Lippincott Williams & Wilkins, 1999.)

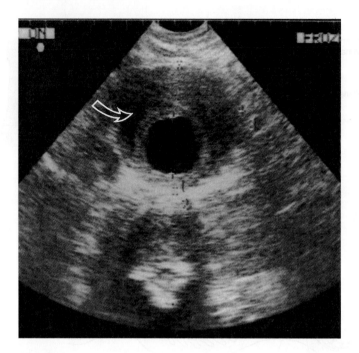

FIGURE 2.29

Abd aortic aneurysm. This is a transverse image of a large AAA with mural thrombus (*arrow*). The spine is well outlined posteriorly. (From Harwood-Nuss A, Wolfson AB, Linden CH, et al. *The clinical practice of emergency medicine*, 3rd Ed. Philadelphia: Lippincott Williams & Wilkins, 2001.)

5. Si/Sx = **classic severe tearing (ripping) chest pain in hypertensive pts that radiates toward the back**

6. Dx = clinical, confirm with CT or aortogram, but if pt unstable take immediately to OR

7. Tx
   a. Descending aortic dissection is usually medical (e.g., control of HTN) unless life-threatening complications arise
   b. In contrast, ascending dissection → immediate surgical intervention with graft placement

C. **Peripheral Vascular Disease (PVD)**

1. Caused by atherosclerotic dz in the lower extremities

2. Si/Sx = intermittent claudication, rest pain, ulceration, gangrene, reduced femoral, popliteal, and pedal pulses, dependent

rubor, muscular atrophy, trophic changes, and skin blanching on foot elevation

3. Dry gangrene is the result of a chronic ischemic state and necrosis of tissue without signs of active infxn (Figure 2.30)

4. Wet gangrene is the superimposition of cellulitis and active infxn to necrotic tissue

5. Leriche's Syndrome
   a. Aortoiliac disease → claudication in hip and gluteal muscles, impotence
   b. 5% have limb loss at 5 yr with rest pain (represents more severe ischemia); if not treated almost 50% of pts will need amputation 2° to gangrene

6. Dx
   a. Complete H&P, important to assess risk factors for atherosclerosis and limitations of lifestyle from PVD
   b. Noninvasive testing includes but is not limited to measurement of the ankle–brachial index (ABI) and duplex examination
      (1) ABI is the ratio of BP in the ankle to the BP in the arm
      (2) Pts without disease have ABIs >1.0 given the higher absolute pressure in the ankle

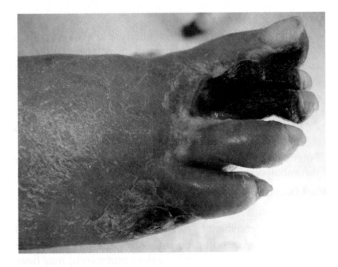

FIGURE 2.30
Dry gangrene of the toes. Image provided by Stedman's.

(3) Pts with severe occlusive disease (e.g., rest pain) generally have indices <0.4; pts with claudication generally have indices <0.7

(4) Exercise ABI most useful diagnostically; ABI may drop with exercise in a pt with PVD

(5) Duplex (Utz) examination combines Utz and Doppler instruments, can provide information regarding blood flow velocity (related to stenosis), and display blood flow as a waveform: **nml waveform is triphasic, moderate occlusive disease waveform is biphasic, and severe disease waveform is monophasic**

(6) Preoperative angiograms are classically done to confirm Dx and establish distal vessel runoff, or "road-map," vessels for the surgeon

7. Tx

a. Lifestyle modifications include smoking cessation and increasing moderate exercise

b. Pharmacotherapy is pentoxifylline

c. Minimally invasive therapy includes percutaneous balloon angioplasty (PTA) and/or atherectomy—best results for isolated lesions of high-grade stenosis in the iliac and superior femoral arteries (SFA) vessels

d. Treatment of iliac disease now involves PTA plus the placement of endoluminal stents

e. Indications for surgical intervention are severe **rest pain, tissue necrosis, nonhealing infxn, and intractable claudication**

f. Surgical treatment includes local endarterectomy with or without patch angioplasty and bypass procedures

g. Results are better with autologous vein grafts; common operation for aortoiliac disease is the aortobifemoral bypass graft, whereas disease of the SFA is commonly treated with a femoral–popliteal bypass graft

8. Potential complication = **thrombosis**, must be addressed with thrombolytic agents, balloon thrombectomy, or graft revision

D. **Vessel Disease**

1. Varicose Veins

a. Dilated, prominent tortuous superficial veins in the lower limbs

b. Commonly seen in pregnancy (progesterone causes dilation of veins) and prolonged standing professions; may have an inherited predisposition

   c. Si/Sx = may be aSx or cause itching; may have dull aching and heaviness in legs, especially at day's end

   d. Dx = clinically

   e. Tx = support hose, elevate limbs, avoid prolonged standing; sclerotherapy or surgical ablation may be indicated

2. Venous Ulcers

   a. 2° to venous hypertension, DVT, or varicose veins; usually located on the medial ankle and calf

   b. Si/Sx = **painless ulcers,** large and shallow, contain bleeding granulation tissue (Figure 2.31)

   c. Phlegmasia alba dolens (milk leg)

      (1) Venous thrombosis usually occurring in postpartum women

      (2) Si/Sx = cool, pale, swollen leg with impalpable pulses

      (3) Tx = heparin and elevation

   d. Phlegmasia cerulea dolens (venous gangrene)

      (1) Venous thrombosis with complete obstruction of arterial inflow

      (2) Si/Sx = sudden intense pain, massive edema, and cyanosis

      (3) Tx = heparin, elevation, venous thrombectomy if unresolved

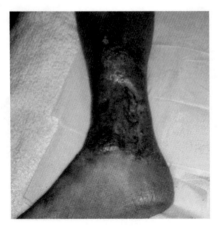

FIGURE 2.31

Venous stasis ulcer of the leg. (From Nettina SM. *The Lippincott manual of nursing practice*, 7th Ed. Philadelphia: Lippincott Williams & Wilkins, 2001.)

     e. Dx = clinical, Doppler studies of extremities

     f. Tx = reduction of swelling by elevation, compression stockings, and Unna's boots (zinc oxide paste impregnated bandage); skin grafting is rarely indicated

  3. Arterial Ulcers

     a. 2° to occlusive arterial disease

     b. Si/Sx = **painful in contrast to venous ulcers**, usually found on lower leg and lateral ankle, particularly on dorsum of the foot, toes, and heel, absent pulses, pallor, claudication, and may have "blue toes" (Figure 2.32)

     c. Dx = clinical, workup of PVD

     d. Tx = conservative management or bypass surgery

E. **Carotid Vascular Disease**

  1. Atherosclerotic plaques in carotid arteries (most commonly at carotid bifurcation)

  2. DDx of carotid insufficiency = trauma, anatomic kinking, fibromuscular dysplasia, and Takayasu's arteritis

  3. Si/Sx = carotid bruit, transient ischemic attacks (TIAs; neurologic changes that reverse in <24 hr), amaurosis fugax (transient monocular blindness), reversible ischemic neurologic

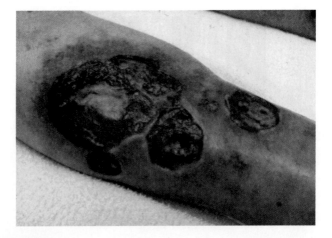

FIGURE 2.32

Arterial ulcer of the leg. (From Nettina SM. *The Lippincott manual of nursing practice*, 7th Ed. Philadelphia: Lippincott Williams & Wilkins, 2001.)

deficits (lasting up to 3 days with no permanent changes), and cerebrovascular accidents (CVAs) that result in permanent neurologic changes

4. Dx = angiography; however, duplex scanning is noninvasive, can determine location and percent stenosis, and assess plaque characteristics (e.g., soft versus calcified)

5. Tx = modification of risk factors important, anticoagulation and use of antiplatelet agents (aspirin, dipyridamole) intended to prevent thrombosis

6. Surgical therapy is carotid endarterectomy; pts usually placed on postoperative aspirin therapy

7. **Surgical Indications**

   a. **Symptomatic pt**

      (1) Carotid stenosis >70%

      (2) Multiple TIAs (risk of stroke 10% per year)

      (3) Pts who have experienced a CVA and have lesion amenable to surgery (stroke recurrence as high as 50% without surgery)

   b. In an **aSx pt** endarterectomy is controversial, but stenosis >75% is an accepted indication (AHA Consensus Statement, *Stroke* 1995;26:188–201)

8. Mortality rate of operation is very low (1%), and risk of stroke after carotid endarterectomy is reduced to 0.5% to 2%

F. **Subclavian Steal Syndrome**

1. Caused by occlusive lesion in subclavian artery or innominate artery, causing ↓ blood flow distal to the obstruction

2. This results in the "stealing" of blood from vertebral artery via retrograde flow

3. Si/Sx = arm claudication, syncope, vertigo, nausea, confusion, and supraclavicular bruits

4. Dx = angiogram, Doppler, MRI

5. Tx = **carotid–subclavian bypass**

G. **Renovascular Hypertension**

1. Caused by renal artery stenosis and subsequent activation of the renin–angiotensin pathway

2. Commonly because of atherosclerotic lesions

3. Can also be 2° to fibromuscular dysplasia, subintimal dissections, and hypoplasia of renal artery

4. Si/Sx = most pts are aSx; some present with headache, abd bruits, or cardiac, cerebrovascular, or renal dysfunction related to hypertension; sudden onset of hypertension is more consistent with a dysplastic process when compared with the slower evolving atherosclerosis

5. Surgically correctable HTN = **renal artery stenosis (most common),** pheochromocytoma, unilateral renal parenchymal disease, Cushing's syndrome, primary hyperaldosteronism, hyperthyroidism, hyperparathyroidism, coarctation of the aorta, CA, and ↑ ICP

6. Dx = definitive Dx obtained by **angiography (string of beads appearance);** others include IV pyelogram (IVP), renal scans, and renal/vein renin ratios

7. Tx = BP control and consider balloon catheter dilation of stenosis—results better with fibromuscular dysplasia versus atherosclerotic lesions; surgical correction involves endarterectomy, bypass, or resection

H. **Mesenteric Ischemia**

1. **Chronic Intestinal Ischemia**

   a. 2° to atherosclerotic lesions of at least two of the three major vessels supplying the bowel

   b. Si/Sx = **weight loss, postprandial pain, and abd bruit**

   c. Dx = definitive diagnosis is made with aortogram

   d. Tx = surgical intervention (endarterectomy, bypass from aorta to involved graft) is **indicated** in absence of malignancy (particularly pancreatic CA must be ruled out)

2. **Acute Intestinal Ischemia**

   a. Acute thrombosis of a mesenteric vessel secondary to atherosclerotic changes or emboli from the heart

   b. Si/Sx = rapid onset of pain that is out of proportion to exam, vomiting, diarrhea, and history of heart condition predisposing to emboli formation (e.g., atrial fibrillation)

   c. Dx = angiogram should be performed immediately to confirm or rule out diagnosis

   d. Tx = embolectomy/thrombectomy, resection of necrotic bowel, and bypass

3. OBSTETRICS AND GYNECOLOGY

I. Obstetrics

A. Terminology

1. Gravidity—total number of pregnancies
2. Parity—number of pregnancies carried to viability—can also express parity as four numbers: term pregnancies, preterm, abortions, and living children (TPAL)
3. Term delivery—delivery of infant after 37 wk of gestation
4. Premature delivery—delivery of infant weighing between 500 and 2,500 grams and delivery between 20 and 37 wk

B. Prenatal Care

1. The First Visit
   a. Pregnancy Dx
      (1) Si/Sx = amenorrhea, ↑ urinary frequency, breast engorgement and tenderness, nausea, fatigue, **bluish discoloration of vagina due to vascular congestion (Chadwick's sign), and softening of cervix (Hegar's sign)**
      (2) Pregnancy test
         (a) Detects human chorionic gonadotropin (hCG) or its β subunit
         (b) Rapidly dividing fertilized egg produces hCG even before implantation occurs
         (c) Commercial kits detect pregnancy 12–15 days after conception
         (d) Home tests have low false-positive rate but high false-negative rate
      (3) Utz
         (a) Gestational sac identified at 5 wk, fetal image detected by 6–7 wk, cardiac activity first noted at 8 wk
         (b) In first trimester, Utz is most accurate method to determine gestational age

    b. Obstetrical Hx
       (1) Duration of previous gestations and mode of delivery
          (e.g., nml spontaneous vaginal delivery versus cesarean
          [C]-section versus vacuum assisted)
       (2) Duration of labor, maternal, postpartum and neonatal
          complications, newborn weight, newborn sex
    c. Menstrual Hx including last menstrual period (LMP), regu-
       larity of cycles, age at menarche
    d. Contraceptive Hx (important for risk assessment, oral con-
       traceptive pills [OCPs] have been associated with birth
       defects)
    e. Medical Hx
       (1) Medicines; consider potential teratogens (Tables 3.1
          and 3.2)
       (2) FHx, social Hx including tobacco, ethanol, drug use,
          type of work, exposure to animals
       (3) Diabetes and HTN
    f. Estimated date of confinement (EDC)
       (1) **Nägele's rule = LMP + 7 days − 3 mo + 1 yr**; e.g., if
          LMP began 05/20/2007, delivery due 02/27/2008
       (2) This calculation depends on regular 28-day cycles (only
          20%–25% of women), adjustments must be made for
          longer or shorter cycles
    g. Complete physical exam with pelvic examination including
       Papanicolaou (Pap) smear, cultures for *Neisseria gonorrhea*
       and *Chlamydia,* and estimation of uterine size

Table 3.1 Teratogens

Drug	Birth Defect
Lithium	Ebstein's anomaly (single-chambered right side of heart)
Carbamazepine, valproate	Neural tube defects
Retinoic acid	CNS defects, craniofacial defects, cardiovascular effects
Angiotensin-converting enzyme inhibitor	Renal failure in neonates, renal tubule dysgenesis, ↓ skull ossification
Oral hypoglycemic	Neonatal hypoglycemia
Warfarin (Coumadin)	Skeletal and CNS defects
NSAIDs	Constriction of ductus arteriosis, necrotizing enterocolitis

Table 3.2	US Food and Drug Administration Drug Categories
Category	**Description**
A	Medication has not shown ↑ risk for birth defects in human studies.
B	Animal studies have not demonstrated a risk, and there are no adequate studies in humans, OR animal studies have shown a risk, but the risk has not been seen in humans.
C	Animal studies have shown adverse effects, but no studies are available in humans, OR studies in humans and animals are not available.
D	Medications are associated with birth defects in humans; however, potential benefits in rare cases may outweigh their known risks.
X	Medications are contraindicated (should not be used) in human pregnancy because of known fetal abnormalities that have been demonstrated in both human and animal studies.

   h. Labs include CBC, blood type with Rh status, urinalysis with culture, RPR test for syphilis, rubella titer, tuberculosis (TB) skin testing, can offer HIV antibody test

   i. If pt is not already immune to rubella, do NOT vaccinate, as the vaccine is live virus

   j. Genetic testing as indicated by Hx (e.g., hemoglobin electrophoresis in African American pt to determine sickle cell anemia likelihood)

   k. Recommend 25- to 35-lb weight gain during pregnancy

   l. Consider folate, iron, and multivitamin supplements

2. First-Trimester Visits

   a. Visit every 4 wk

   b. Assess weight gain/loss, BP, pedal edema, fundal height, urine dip for glucosuria and proteinuria (**trace glucosuria is nml because of ↑ glomerular filtration rate (GFR), but anything more than trace protein should be evaluated**)

   c. Estimation of gestational age by uterine size (Table 3.3)

     (1) Nml uterus is $3 \times 4 \times 7$ cm

     (2) Gravid uterus begins to enlarge and soften by 5–6 wk

   d. All pregnant women, regardless of age, should undergo first-trimester screening for Down's syndrome

     (1) Screen with combination of Utz and blood tests

     (2) Utz test is for nuchal translucency (NT), which measures the thickness at the back of the neck of the fetus

Table 3.3 Height of Uterus by Gestational Week

12 Wk	16 Wk	20 Wk	20–36 Wk
At pubic symphysis	Midway from symphysis to umbilicus	At umbilicus	Height (cm) correlates with weeks of gestation[a]

[a]If uterine size (cm) > gestational age (wk) by >3 wk, consider multiple gestations, molar pregnancy, or MOST COMMONLY inaccurate dating.

    (3) Blood tests include the standard triple-marker screen, including alpha fetoprotein (AFP), βhCG, and estriol
        (a) AFP is ↓ in Down's syndrome, and ↑ in multiple gestational pregnancies and neural tube defects
        (b) Estriol is also ↓ in Down's syndrome
        (c) βHCG is ↑ in Down's syndrome
        (d) The triple-marker test detects ~70% of cases of Down's syndrome, with a ~5% false positive rate
    (4) Newer test, inhibin, is also ↑ in Down's syndrome, and adding it to the triple-marker test ↑ detection of Down's syndrome to 80% (Obstetrics & Gynecology 2005 106:260–67)
    (5) Adding the PAPP-A blood test ↑ detection to >85% (NEJM 2005 353:2001–2011)
3. Second-Trimester Visits
  a. Continue every 4 wk
  b. After 12 wk, use Doppler Utz to evaluate fetal heartbeat at each visit
  c. At 17–19 wk (quickening) and beyond, document fetal movement
  d. Amniocentesis for higher risk mothers >35 years old or if Hx indicates (e.g., recurrent miscarriages, previous child with chromosomal or single gene defect, abnormal triple marker or quadruple marker screening test)
  e. Glucose screening at 24 wk (1-hr Glucola)
  f. Repeat hematocrit at 25–28 wk
4. Third-Trimester Visits
  a. Every 4 wk until wk 32, every 2 wk from wk 32–36, every wk until delivery
  b. Inquire about preterm labor (PTL) Sx: **vaginal bleeding, contractions, rupture of membranes (ROM)**

     c. Inquire about pregnancy-induced hypertension (PIH) (discussed further in Section I.D.3)

     d. Screen for *Streptococcus agalactiae* (**group B *Streptococcus* [GBS]**) at 35–37 wk

     e. RhoGAM at 28–30 wk if indicated (discussed further in Section E.5.h)

C. Physiologic Changes in Pregnancy

  1. Hematologic

     a. Pregnancy is a **hypercoagulable** state

       (1) ↑ Clotting factor levels

       (2) Venous stasis due to uterine pressure on lower-extremity great veins

     b. Anemia of pregnancy

       (1) Plasma volume ↑ approximately 50% from wk 6 to wk 30–34

       (2) Red cell mass ↑ later and to a smaller degree, causing a relative anemia of approximately 15% due to dilution

     c. Slight leukocytosis due to granulocyte demargination

     d. Platelets ↓ slightly but remain within nml limits

  2. Cardiac

     a. Cardiac output ↑ 50% (↑ in both heart rate and stroke volume)

     b. Because of ↑ flow, ↑ S_2 split with inspiration, distended neck veins, systolic ejection murmur, and S_3 gallop are nml findings

     c. **Diastolic murmurs are not nml findings in pregnancy**

     d. ↓ Peripheral vascular resistance due to progesterone-mediated smooth muscle relaxation

     e. BP ↓ during first 24 wk of pregnancy with gradual return to nonpregnant levels by term

  3. Pulmonary

     a. Nasal stuffiness and ↑ nasal secretions due to mucosal hyperemia

     b. 4-cm elevation of diaphragm due to expanding uterus

     c. Tidal volume and minute ventilation ↑ 30%–40% (progesterone mediated)

     d. Functional residual capacity and residual volume ↓ 20%

     e. Hyperventilation →↑ PO_2, ↓ PCO_2—this allows the fetal PCO_2 to remain near 40 and still be able to give off CO_2 to maternal blood (sets up a CO_2 concentration gradient across maternal–fetal circulation and PO_2 gradient allowing maternal to fetal O_2 transfer)

f. Respiratory rate, vital capacity, and inspiratory reserve do not change, total lung capacity ↓ approximately 5%

4. GI
   a. ↓ GI motility due to progesterone
   b. ↓ Esophageal sphincter tone → gastric reflux also due to progesterone
   c. ↑ Alkaline phosphatase
   d. Hemorrhoids due to constipation and ↑ venous pressure due to enlarging uterus compressing inferior vena cava

5. Renal
   a. ↓ Bladder tone due to progesterone predisposes pregnant women to urinary stasis and urinary tract infxns (UTIs)/pyelonephritis
   b. GFR ↑ 50%
      (1) ↑ GFR → glucose excretion occurs in nearly all pregnant women
      (2) Thus urine dipsticks are not useful in managing pts with diabetes
      (3) However, there should be no significant ↑ in protein loss
   c. Serum creatinine and blood urea nitrogen ↓

6. Endocrine
   a. ↓ Fasting blood glucose in mother due to fetal utilization
   b. ↑ Postprandial glucose in mother due to ↑ insulin resistance
   c. Fetus produces its own insulin starting at 9–11 wk
   d. ↑ Maternal thyroid-bonding globulin (TBG) due to ↑ estrogen, ↑ total T_3 and T_4 due to ↑ TBG
   e. Free T_3 and T_4 remain the same so pregnant women are euthyroid
   f. ↑ Cortisol and cortisol-binding globulin

7. Skin
   a. Nml skin changes in pregnancy mimic liver dz due to ↑ estrogen
   b. Can see spider angiomas, palmar erythema
   c. Hyperpigmentation occurs from ↑ estrogen and melanocyte-stimulating hormone, affects umbilicus, perineum, face (chloasma), and linea (nigra)

D. Medical Conditions in Pregnancy

  1. Gestational Diabetes Mellitus (GDM)

    a. GDM—glucose intolerance or DM first recognized during pregnancy

    b. **Number one medical complication of pregnancy, occurs in 2% of pregnancies**

    c. GDM risk factors: previous Hx of GDM, maternal age ≥30 yr, obesity, FHx of DM, previous Hx of infant weighing 4,000 g at birth, Hx of repeated spontaneous abortions or unexplained stillbirths

    d. GDM caused by placental-released hormone, human placental lactogen (HPL), which antagonizes insulin

    e. GDM worsens as pregnancy progresses because ↑ amounts of HPL are produced as placenta enlarges

    f. Maternal complications = hyperglycemia, ketoacidosis, ↑ risk of UTIs, **2-fold ↑ in PIH**, retinopathy (can occur very quickly and dramatically)

    g. Fetal complications

      (1) Macrosomia (≥4,500 g), neonatal hypoglycemia due to abrupt separation from maternal supply of glucose, hyperbilirubinemia, polycythemia, polyhydramnios (amniotic fluid volume ≥2,000 mL)

      (2) **Abruption and PTL** due to ↑ uterine size and postpartum uterine atony, **3- to 4-fold ↑ in congenital anomalies** (often cardiac and limb deformities), spontaneous abortion, and respiratory distress

    h. Dx = 1-hr Glucola screening test at 24–28 wk or at onset of prenatal care in pt with known risk factors, confirm with 3-hr glucose tolerance test

    i. Tx = strict glucose control, which significantly ↓ complications

      (1) Insulin is not required if the pt can adhere to a proper diet

      (2) **Oral hypoglycemics are contraindicated** because they cross the placenta and can result in fetal and neonatal hypoglycemia

    j. Delivery

      (1) Route of delivery determined by estimated fetal weight

      (2) If 4,500 g, consider C-section; if 5,000 g, C-section recommended

(3) Postpartum 95% of GDM pts return to nml glucose levels

(4) Glucose tolerance screening recommended 2–4 mo postpartum to pick up those few women who will remain diabetic and require Tx

2. Thromboembolic Dz

a. Incidence during pregnancy is 1%–2%, usually occurs postpartum (80%)

b. Si/Sx for superficial thrombophlebitis = swelling, tenderness, erythema, warmth (4 cardinal signs of inflammation), may be a palpable cord

c. Deep venous thrombosis (DVT) occurs postpartum due to spread of uterine infxn to ovarian veins

d. Si/Sx of DVT = persistent fever, uterine tenderness, palpable mass, but often aSx

e. Dx

(1) Doppler Utz is first line, sensitivity and specificity >90%

(2) Gold-standard is venography but this is invasive

f. Tx

(1) Superficial thrombophlebitis → leg elevation, rest, heat, NSAIDs

(2) DVT → heparin to maintain PTT 1.5–2.5 × baseline

(3) **Warfarin (Coumadin) contraindicated in pregnancy** because it crosses the placenta, is teratogenic early, and causes fetal bleeding later

g. Px

(1) 25% of untreated DVT progress to pulmonary embolism (PE)

(2) Anticoagulation ↓ progression to 5%

(3) PEs in pregnancy are treated identically to DVT

3. PIH

a. Epidemiology

(1) Develops in 5%–10% of pregnancies, 30% of multiple gestations

(2) Causes 15% of maternal deaths

(3) Risk factors = nulliparity, age >40 years, FHx of PIH, chronic HTN, chronic renal dz, diabetes, twin gestation

b. Types (Table 3.4)

c. Other Si/Sx seen in preeclampsia or eclampsia

(1) Pts have rapid weight gain (2° to edema)

(2) Peripheral lower-extremity edema is common in pregnancy; however, persistent edema unresponsive to

Table 3.4 Types of Pregnancy-Induced Hypertension

Dz	Characteristics
Preeclampsia	• HTN (>140/90 or ↑ sbp >30 mm Hg or dbp >15 mm Hg compared to previous) • New-onset proteinuria and/or edema • Generally occurring at ≥20 wk
Severe preeclampsia	• SBP >160 mm Hg or DBP >110 mm Hg • Marked proteinuria (>1g/24-hr collection or >11 on dip), oliguria, ↑ creatinine • CNS disturbances (e.g., headaches or scotomata) • Pulmonary edema or cyanosis • Epigastric or right upper quadrant pain, hepatic dysfunction
Eclampsia	• **Convulsions** in a woman with preeclampsia • 25% occur before labor, 50% during labor, and 25% in first 72 hr postpartum

DBP, diastolic blood pressure; SBP, systolic blood pressure.

rest and leg elevation or edema involving the upper extremities or face is not nml

(3) Hyperreflexia and clonus are noted

d. Tx

(1) Only cure for PIH is delivery of the baby; decision to deliver depends on severity of preeclampsia and maturity of fetus

(2) Mild pre-eclampsia + immature fetus → bed rest, preferably in left lateral decubitus position to maximize blood flow to uterus, close monitoring, tell pt to return to ER if preeclampsia worsens

(3) Severe preeclampsia/eclampsia → delivery when possible, magnesium sulfate to prevent seizure, antihypertensives to maintain BP <140/100

e. Complication of severe PIH = HELLP syndrome

(1) **HELLP** = **H**emolysis, **E**levated **L**iver enzymes, **L**ow **P**latelets

(2) Occurs in 5%–10% of women with severe preeclampsia or eclampsia, more frequently in multiparous, older pts

(3) Tx = delivery (the only cure), transfuse blood, platelets, fresh-frozen plasma as needed, IV fluids and pressors as needed to maintain BP

4. Cardiac Dz

    a. Pts with congenital heart dz have ↑ risk (1%–5%) of having a fetus with a congenital heart dz

    b. Pts with pulmonary HTN and ↑ right-sided pressures (e.g., Eisenmenger's complex) have poor Px with pregnancy

    c. Tx of preexisting cardiac dz = supportive; e.g., prevention and/or prompt correction of anemia, aggressive Tx of infxns, ↓ physical activity/strenuous work, adherence to a low-sodium diet, and proper weight gain

    d. Peripartum cardiomyopathy

        (1) Rare but severe pregnancy-associated condition

        (2) Occurs in last mo of pregnancy or first 6 mo postpartum

        (3) Risk factors = African American, multiparous, age >30 yr, twin gestation, or preeclampsia

        (4) Tx = bed rest, digoxin, diuretics, possible anticoagulation, consider post-delivery heart transplant especially in those whose cardiomegaly has not resolved 6 mo after Dx

5. Group B *Streptococcus* (GBS = *Streptococcus Agalactiae*)

    a. aSx cervical colonization occurs in up to 30% of women

    b. 50% of infants become colonized, clinical infxn in <1%

    c. Intrapartum prophylaxis with penicillin is reserved for the following situations:

        (1) PTL (<37 wk) or prolonged ROM (>18 hr) or fever in labor regardless of colonization status

        (2) Women identified as colonized with GBS through screening at 35–37 wk of gestation

        (3) Women with GBS bacteriuria or with previous infant with GBS dz

        (4) Pts with severe PCN allergies may consider clindamycin or erythromycin if no GBS resistance noted

        (5) Broader spectrum antibiotics may be needed if chorioamnionitis occurs

6. Hyperemesis Gravidarum

    a. ↑ nausea and vomiting that, unlike "morning sickness," persists past wk 16 of pregnancy

    b. Causes = ↑ hCG levels, thyroid or GI hormones

    c. Si/Sx = excessive vomiting, dehydration, hypochloremic metabolic alkalosis

    d. Dx = clinical, rule out other cause

e. Tx = fluids, electrolyte repletion, antiemetics (IV, IM, or suppositories)

f. Some pts require feeding tubes and parenteral nutrition

E. Fetal Assessment and Intrapartum Surveillance

1. Fetal Growth

   a. Measure by fundal height, if 2-cm deviation from expected fundal height during wk 18–36 → repeat measurement and/or Utz

   b. Utz is most reliable tool for assessing fetal growth

   c. In early pregnancy, measurement of gestational sac and crown–rump length correlate very well with gestational age

   d. Later in pregnancy, four measurements are done because of wide deviation in nml range: biparietal diameter of skull, abd circumference, femur length, and cerebellar diameter

2. Fetal Well-Being

   a. ≥4 fetal movements per hr generally indicate fetal well-being

   b. Nonstress test (NST)

      (1) Measures response of fetal heart rate (FHR) to movement

      (2) Nml (i.e., reactive) NST occurs when FHR ↑ by 15 bpm for 15 seconds following fetal movement

      (3) 2 such accelerations within 20 min are considered nml

      (4) Nonreactive NST → further assessment of fetal well-being

      (5) Test has a high false-positive rate (test suggests fetus is in trouble, but fetus actually is healthy), so the result must be interpreted in the context of other tests and often is repeated within 24 hr to verify results

   c. Biophysical profile

      (1) measures of fetal well-being, each rated on a scale from 0–2

         (a) Fetal breathing → ≥1 fetal breathing movement in 30 min lasting at least 30 sec

         (b) Gross body movement → ≥3 discrete movements in 30 min

         (c) Fetal tone → ≥1 episode of extension with return to flexion of fetal limbs/trunk OR opening/closing of hand

         (d) Qualitative amniotic fluid volume → ≥1 pocket of amniotic fluid at least 1 cm in two perpendicular planes

         (e) Reactive FHR → reactive NST

(2) Final score of 8–10 is nml, score of 6 is equivocal and requires further evaluation, score of ≤4 is abnormal and usually requires immediate intervention

3. Tests of Fetal Maturity

   a. Respiratory system is last fetal system to mature, so decisions regarding when to deliver a premature infant often depend on tests that assess the maturity of this system

   b. Phospholipid production (collectively known as "surfactant") remains low until 32–33 wk of gestation, but this is highly variable

   c. Lack of surfactant → neonatal respiratory distress syndrome (RDS)

   d. Phospholipids enter amniotic fluid from fetal breathing and are obtained by amniocentesis and tested for maturity

   e. Tests for fetal maturity

      (1) Lecithin/sphingomyelin (L:S) ratio

         (a) Lecithin is major phospholipid found in surfactant and ↑ as fetal lungs become mature

         (b) Sphingomyelin production remains constant throughout pregnancy

         (c) Ratio >2.0 is considered mature

      (2) Phosphatidylglycerol appears late in pregnancy; its presence generally indicates maturity

4. Intrapartum Fetal Assessment

   a. Causes of nonreassuring fetal status

      (1) Uteroplacental insufficiency

         (a) Placenta impaired or unable to provide oxygen and nutrients while removing products of metabolism and waste

         (b) Causes = placenta previa or abruption, placental edema from hydrops fetalis or Rh isoimmunization, postterm pregnancy, intrauterine growth retardation (IUGR), uterine hyperstimulation

         (c) Fetal response to hypoxia → shunting of blood to brain, heart, and adrenal glands

         (d) If unrecognized, can progress to metabolic acidosis with accumulation of lactic acid and damage to vital organs

      (2) Umbilical cord compression due to oligohydramnios, cord prolapse or knot, anomalous cord, or abnormal cord insertion

(3) Fetal anomalies include IUGR, prematurity, postterm, sepsis, congenital anomalies

b. FHR monitoring

(1) Nml FHR is 120–160 bpm

(2) Tachycardia = FHR >160 bpm for ≥10 min

    (a) Most common cause is maternal fever (which may signal chorioamnionitis)

    (b) Other causes = fetal hypoxia, immaturity, tachyarrhythmias, anemia, infxn, maternal thyrotoxicosis, or Tx with sympathomimetics

(3) Bradycardia = FHR <120 bpm for ≥10 min, caused by congenital heart block, fetal anoxia (e.g., from placental separation), and maternal Tx with β-blockers

(4) FHR variability

    (a) Reliable indicator of fetal well-being, suggesting sufficient CNS oxygenation

    (b) ↓ Variability associated with fetal hypoxia/acidosis, depressant drugs, fetal tachycardia, CNS or cardiac anomalies, prolonged uterine contractions, prematurity and fetal sleep

c. Accelerations

(1) Types and patterns of accelerations play a role in intrapartum evaluation of the fetus

(2) Accelerations

    (a) ↑ FHR of at least 15 bpm above baseline for 15–20 seconds

    (b) This pattern indicates a fetus unstressed by hypoxia or acidemia → reassuring and suggests fetal well-being

(3) Early decelerations (Figure 3.1)

    (a) ↓ FHR (not <100 bpm) that mirrors a uterine contraction (i.e., begins with onset of contraction, dips at peak of contraction, returns to baseline with end of contraction)

    (b) Results from pressure on fetal head → vagus nerve stimulated reflex response to release acetylcholine at fetal sinoatrial node

    (c) Considered physiologic and not harmful to fetus

(4) Variable decelerations (see Figure 3.1)

    (a) Do not necessarily coincide with uterine contraction

    (b) Characterized by rapid dip in FHR, often <100 bpm with rapid return to baseline

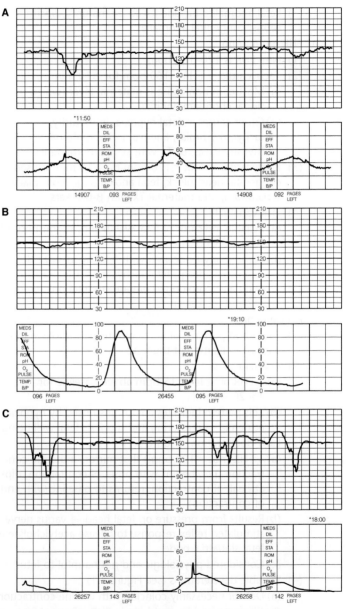

         (c) Also reflex-mediated due to umbilical cord compression

         (d) Can be corrected by shifting maternal position or amnioinfusion if membranes have ruptured and cord compression is 2° to oligohydramnios

     (5) Late decelerations (see Figure 3.1)

         (a) Begin after contraction has already started, dip after peak of contraction, returns to baseline after contraction is over

         (b) Viewed as potentially dangerous, associated with uteroplacental insufficiency

         (c) Causes include placental abruption, PIH, maternal diabetes, maternal anemia, maternal sepsis, post-term pregnancy, and hyperstimulated uterus

         (d) Repetitive late decelerations require intervention

5. Isoimmunization

   a. Development of maternal immunoglobulin (Ig)G antibodies following exposure to fetal RBC antigens

   b. Exposure commonly occurs at delivery but can occur during pregnancy

   c. In subsequent pregnancies (rarely late in the same pregnancy), these antibodies can cross the placenta → attach to fetal RBCs and hemolyze them → fetal anemia

   d. Can occur with any blood group, but most often occurs when mother is Rh-negative and fetus is Rh-positive

   e. Extent to which fetus is affected depends on amount of IgG antibodies crossing placenta and ability of fetus to replenish destroyed RBCs

   f. Worst-case scenario is hydrops fetalis

     (1) Significant transfer of antibodies across placenta → fetal anemia

     (2) Liver attempts to make new RBCs (fetal hematopoiesis occurs in liver and bone marrow) at the expense of

FIGURE 3.1

(A) Early deceleration pattern is depicted in this fetal heart rate (FHR) tracing. Note that each deceleration returns to baseline before the completion of the contraction. The remainder of the FHR tracing is reassuring. **(B)** Repetitive late decelerations in conjunction with ↓ variability. **(C)** Variable decelerations are the most common periodic change of the FHR during labor. Repetitive mild-to-moderate variable decelerations are present. Baseline is nml.

other necessary proteins → ↓ oncotic pressure → fetal ascites and edema

(3) High-output cardiac failure associated with severe anemia

g. Maternal IgG titer ≥1:16 is sufficiently high to pose risk to the fetus

h. Tx = RhoGAM

(1) Administration of antibody to the Rh antigen (Rh immune globulin = RhoGAM) within 72 hr of delivery prevents active antibody response by the mother in most cases

(2) Risk of subsequent sensitization ↓ from 15% to 2%

(3) When RhoGAM is also given at 28 wk of gestation, risk of sensitization is further reduced to 0.2%

i. RhoGAM given to Rh-negative mother if baby's father is Rh-positive or unknown

(1) At 28 wks of gestation

(2) Within 72 hr of delivery of Rh-positive infant

(3) Other times maternal–fetal blood mixing can occur

(a) At time of amniocentesis

(b) After an abortion

(c) After an ectopic pregnancy

6. Genetic Testing

a. Chromosomal abnormalities account for 50%–60% of spontaneous abortion, 5% of stillbirths, 2%–3% of couples with multiple miscarriages

b. 0.6% of all live births have a chromosomal abnormality

c. Indications for prenatal genetic testing

(1) Most common is advanced maternal age (AMA)

(a) Trisomy 21 (Down's syndrome) incidence ↑ 10-fold from age 35–45 yr, other polysomies ↑ similarly

(b) New Practice Bulletin by American College of Obstetricians and Gynecologist (ACOG) January, 2007, states that, "All pregnant women, regardless of their age, should be offered screening for Down's syndrome"

(2) Prior child with chromosome or single gene abnormality

(3) Known chromosomal abnormality such as balanced translocation or single gene disorder in parent(s)

(4) Abnormal results from screening tests, such as the triple-marker screen or quadruple-marker screen

F. Labor and Delivery
   1. Initial Presentation
      a. Labor = progressive effacement and dilation of uterine cervix resulting from contractions of uterus
      b. **Braxton Hicks contractions** (false labor) = uterine contractions without effacement and dilation of cervix
      c. 85% of pts undergo spontaneous labor and delivery between 37 and 42 wk of gestation
      d. Pts are told to come to hospital for regular contractions q5min for at least 1 hr, ROM, significant bleeding, ↓ fetal movement
      e. Initial exam upon arrival
         (1) Auscultation of fetal heart tones
         (2) Leopold maneuvers help determine fetal lie (relation of long axis of fetus with maternal long axis), determine fetal presentation (i.e., breech vs. cephalic), and position of presenting part with respect to right or left side of maternal pelvis
         (3) Vaginal examination
            (a) Check for ROM, cervical effacement, and cervical dilation (in cm)
            (b) Fetal station (level of fetal presenting part relative to ischial spines) measured from −3 (presenting part palpable at pelvic inlet) to +3 (presenting part palpable beyond pelvic outlet)
            (c) 0 station = presenting part palpable at ischial spines, significance of 0 station is that biparietal diameter (biggest diameter of fetal head) has negotiated pelvic inlet (smallest part of pelvis)
   2. Labor divided into 3 stages (Figure 3.2)
      a. Stage 1
         (1) Interval between onset of labor and full cervical dilation (10 cm)
         (2) Further subdivided into:
            (a) Latent phase = cervical effacement and early dilation
            (b) Active phase = more rapid cervical dilation occurs, usually beginning at 3–4 cm
         (3) In Stage 1, continuous monitoring of FHR, either via Doppler or internal monitoring via fetal scalp electrode

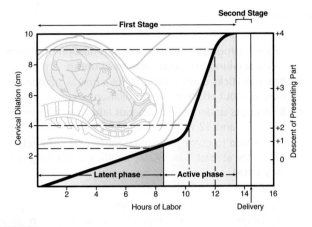

FIGURE 3.2

Schematic illustration of progress of rotation of occipitoanterior presentation in the successive stages of labor. Note relationship between changes in cervical dilation and phases of labor.

    (4) Monitoring of uterine activity by
        (a) External tocodynamometer measures frequency and duration of contractions but not intensity, OR
        (b) Intrauterine pressure catheter (IUPC) measures intensity by measuring intrauterine pressure
    (5) Analgesic (typically meperidine) and/or anesthetic (typically an epidural block that provides both continuous analgesia and anesthesia) can be given—agents usually not given until active stage of labor

  b. Stage 2 = interval between complete cervical dilation and delivery of infant
    (1) Maternal effort (i.e., pushing) accelerates delivery of fetus (↑ intra-abd pressure assists fetal descent down birth canal)
    (2) Delivery should be well controlled with protection of the perineum
    (3) If used, episiotomies usually are cut midline
    (4) After head is delivered, bulb suction of nose and mouth is performed and neck is evaluated for presence of nuchal cord
    (5) Shoulders are delivered by applying gentle downward pressure on head to deliver anterior shoulder followed by easy upward force to deliver posterior shoulder

(6) Delivery of body follows, cord is clamped and cut, and infant given to mother or placed in warmer

(7) Blood from umbilical cord sent for ABO and Rh testing as well as arterial blood gases

c. Stage 3 = interval between delivery of infant and delivery of placenta

   (1) Three signs of placenta separation

      (a) Uterus rises in abdomen signaling that placenta has separated

      (b) Gush of blood

      (c) Lengthening of umbilical cord

   (2) Excessive pulling on placenta should be avoided because of risk of uterus inversion with associated profound hemorrhage and retained placenta

   (3) Gentle traction should be applied at all times

   (4) May take up to 30 min for placenta to be expulsed

d. Stage 4 = immediate postpartum period lasting 2 hr, during which pt undergoes significant physiologic changes

   (1) Systematic evaluation of cervix, vagina, vulva, perineum, and periurethral area for lacerations

   (2) Likelihood of serious postpartum complications is greatest in first 1–2 hr postpartum

4. Abnormal Labor

a. Dystocia = difficult labor

   (1) Cause detected by evaluating the **3 Ps**

      (a) **Power**

         (i) Refers to strength, duration, and frequency of contractions

         (ii) Measured by using tocodynamometer or IUPC

         (iii) For cervical dilation to occur, ≥3 contractions in 10 min must be generated

         (iv) During active labor maternal effort comes into play as maternal exhaustion, effects of analgesia/anesthesia, or underlying dz may prolong labor

      (b) **Passenger**

         (i) Refers to estimates of fetal weight + evaluation of fetal lie, presentation, and position

         (ii) Occiput posterior presentation, face presentation, and hydrocephalus are associated with dystocia

        (c) **Passage**
- (i) Difficult to measure pelvic diameters
- (ii) Adequacy of pelvis often unknown until progress (or no progress) is made during labor
- (iii) Distended bladder, adnexal or colon masses, and uterine fibroids can all contribute to dystocia

    (2) Dystocia divided into prolongation disorders
      (a) Prolonged latent phase
- (i) Latent phase >20 hr in primigravid or >14 hr in multigravid pt is prolonged and abnormal
- (ii) Causes include ineffective uterine contractions, fetopelvic disproportion, and excess anesthesia
- (iii) Prolonged latent phase → no harm to mother or fetus

      (b) Prolonged active phase
- (i) Active phase >12 hr or rate of cervical dilation, <1.2 cm/hr in primigravid, or <1.5 cm/hr in multigravid
- (ii) Causes include excess anesthesia, ineffective contractions, fetopelvic disproportion, fetal malposition, ROM before onset of active labor
- (iii) Prolonged active phase → ↑ risk of intrauterine infxn and ↑ risk of C-section

b. Arrest disorders
- (1) 2° arrest occurs when cervical dilation during active phase ceases for ≥2 hr
- (2) Suggests either cephalopelvic disproportion or ineffective uterine contractions

c. Management of abnormal labor
- (1) Labor induction = stimulation of uterine contractions before spontaneous onset of labor
- (2) Augmentation of labor = stimulation of uterine contractions that began spontaneously but have become infrequent, weak, or both
- (3) Induction trial should occur only if cervix is prepared or "ripe"
- (4) Bishop score used to try to quantify cervical readiness for induction (Table 3.5)

d. Indications for induction = suspected fetal compromise, fetal death, PIH, premature ROM, chorioamnionitis, postdates pregnancy, maternal medical complication

Table 3.5 Bishop Score

Factor	Points			
	0	1	2	3
Dilation (cm)	Closed	1–2	3–4	≥5
Effacement (%)	0–30	40–50	60–70	≥80
Station	−30	−2, −1	0	≥+1
Position		Posterior	Mid	Anterior

Score from 9–13 is associated with highest likelihood of successful induction.
Score from 0–4 is associated with highest likelihood of failed induction.

   e. Contraindications for induction include placenta previa, active genital herpes, abnormal fetal lie, cord presentation
   f. If cervix not "ripe," prostaglandin E_2 gel can be used to attempt to ripen cervix; biggest risk is uterine hyperstimulation → uteroplacental insufficiency
   g. Another method is insertion of laminaria or rods inserted into the internal os that absorb moisture and expand, slowly dilating cervix, risks include failure to dilate, laceration, ROM, and infxn
   h. Prolonged latent phase can be managed with rest, augmentation of labor with oxytocin, and/or amniotomy that may allow for fetal head to provide greater dilating force
   i. During active phase of labor, fetal malposition and cephalopelvic disproportion must be considered and may warrant C-section versus augmentation
   j. If fetus has descended far enough, forceps or vacuum can be used; if not C-section is performed
   k. Risks of prolonged labor include infxn, exhaustion, lacerations, uterine atony with hemorrhage
   l. Breech presentation occurs in 2%–4% of pregnancies and risk ↑ in cases of multiple gestations, polyhydramnios, hydrocephaly, anencephaly, and uterine anomalies (see Figure 3.3)
5. Postpartum Hemorrhage
   a. Defined as blood loss >500 mL associated with delivery
   b. Causes = uterine atony (most common), lacerations, retained placenta
   c. **Uterine atony**

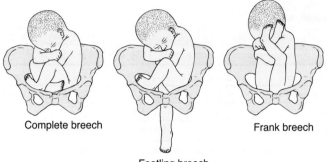

Complete breech

Frank breech

Footling breech

FIGURE 3.3

Different breech presentations.

(1) Normally uterus quickly contracts following delivery of placenta, muscle contraction compresses down on spiral arteries and prevents excessive bleeding

(2) If contraction does not occur → postpartum hemorrhage

(3) Risk factors for uterine atony = multiple gestations, hydramnios, multiparity, macrosomia, previous Hx of postpartum hemorrhage, fibroids, magnesium sulfate, general anesthesia, prolonged labor, amnionitis

(4) Dx based on clinical exam of soft, "boggy" uterus

(5) Tx

(a) Start with uterine massage to stimulate contractions

(b) IV fluids and transfusions as needed, cervix and vagina visualized for lacerations

(c) Medical Tx = oxytocin, methylergonovine maleate (Methergine; potent uterotonic always given IM; if given IV can cause severe HTN), or prostaglandins → uterine contractions

(d) If these measures are unsuccessful, surgical interventions are used and include ligation of uterine arteries, ligation of internal iliac arteries, selective arterial embolization, or hysterectomy as last resort

d. Retained placenta

(1) Occurs when separation of placenta from uterine wall or expulsion of placenta is incomplete

(2) Risk factors include previous C-section, fibroids, and prior uterine curettage

       (3) Placental tissue that abnormally implants into uterus can result in retention

       (4) Placenta accreta: placental villi abnormally adhere to superficial lining of uterine wall

       (5) Placenta increta: placental villi penetrate into uterine muscle layer

       (6) Placenta percreta: placental villi completely invade uterine muscle layer

   e. Disseminated intravascular coagulation (DIC)

       (1) Rare cause of postpartum hemorrhage

       (2) Severe preeclampsia, amniotic fluid embolism, and placental abruption are associated with DIC

       (3) Tx aimed at correcting coagulopathy

G. Postpartum Care

  1. Lactation and Breast-Feeding

    a. Engorgement occurs approximately 3 days postpartum

    b. Three causes of tender, enlarged breasts postpartum are engorgement, mastitis, and plugged duct

    c. Treat engorgement with continued breast-feeding, mastitis with antibiotics (nursing can be continued), and plugged duct with warm packs

    d. Advantages of breast-feeding = ↑ bonding between mother and child, convenience, ↓ cost, protection against infxn and allergies

    e. Breast milk provides all vitamins except vitamin K

  2. Contraception

    a. Contraception should be discussed with all pts prior to discharge

    b. Approximately 15% of women are fertile 6 wk postpartum

    c. OCPs are not contraindicated in breast-feeding women, postpartum tubal ligation should be discussed as well

  3. Postpartum Immunizations

    a. Rubella nonimmune women should be immunized (they can continue to breast-feed)

    b. Rh-negative woman who has given birth to an Rh-positive baby should receive RhoGAM

  4. Postpartum Depression

    a. Recurrence rate for pts with previous postpartum depression is 25%

b. Postpartum depression ranges from the "blues," which affects 50% of women and typically occurs day 2–3 and resolves in 1–2 wk, to postpartum depression, which affects 10% of women, to suicidal ideation, which occurs more rarely

c. Especially worrisome is a mother who has estranged herself from her newborn or has become indifferent

d. Tx depends on severity of Sx and may range from simple telephone contact to psychotherapy and medication to inpt hospitalization

5. Postpartum Uterine Infexn

a. Incidence of infxn ranges from 10%–50% depending on population, mode of delivery (C-section > vaginal delivery), and risk factors

b. Risk factors = maternal obesity, immunosuppression, chronic dz, vaginal infxn, amnionitis, prolonged labor, prolonged ROM, multiple pelvic examinations during labor, internal fetal monitoring or IUPC, C-section

c. **Most common infxn post C-section is metritis** (uterine infxn)

d. Si/Sx = fever on first or second postpartum day, uterine tenderness, ↓ bowel sounds, leukocytosis (difficult to interpret because of nml leukocytosis in puerperium)

e. DDx = same as postsurgical, see Surgery III.C.2.a

f. Metritis usually polymicrobial with aerobic and anaerobic organisms present

g. Dx = clinical

h. Tx = first-generation cephalosporin, broaden antibiotics if no response within 48–72 hr

i. Prophylactic antibiotic Tx (one-time dose) at time of C-section delivery significantly reduces incidence of postpartum infxn

H. Obstetrical Complications

1. Abortion

a. Termination of a pregnancy before viability, usually at ≤20 wk, occurs spontaneously in 15% of all pregnancies

b. Risk factors = ↑ parity, AMA, ↑ paternal age, conception within 3 mo of a live birth

c. Single pregnancy loss does not significantly ↑ risk of future loss

d. Chromosomal abnormalities cause 50% of early spontaneous abortions, mostly trisomies (the longer a pregnancy goes before undergoing spontaneous abortion, the less likely the fetus is chromosomally abnormal)

    e. Other causes = endocrine dz (e.g., thyroid), structural abnormalities (e.g., fibroids, incompetent cervix), infxn [e.g., *Listeria*; *Mycoplasma*; *Toxoplasma*; Rubella, Cytomegalovirus, Herpes Simplex Virus, and Syphilis (ToRCHs)], chronic dz (e.g., DM, systemic lupus erythematosus, renal or cardiac dz), environmental factors (e.g., toxins, radiation, smoking, alcohol)

    f. Vaginal bleeding in first half of any pregnancy is presumed to be a threatened abortion unless another Dx, such as ectopic pregnancy, cervical polyps, cervicitis, or molar pregnancy, can be made

    g. Types (Table 3.6)

2. Ectopic Pregnancy

    a. Implantation outside of uterine cavity

    b. ↑ Incidence recently because of ↑ in pelvic inflammatory dz (PID), second leading cause of maternal mortality

    c. Risk factors = previous ectopic pregnancy, previous Hx of salpingitis (scarring and adhesions impede transport of ovum down tube), age ≥35 yr, >3 prior pregnancies, sterilization failure

    d. Si/Sx = abd/pelvic pain, referred shoulder pain from hemoperitoneal irritation of diaphragm, amenorrhea, vaginal bleeding, cervical motion or adnexal tenderness, nausea, vomiting, orthostatic changes

    e. DDx = surgical abdomen, abortion, salpingitis, endometriosis, ruptured ovarian cyst, ovarian torsion

    f. Ectopic pregnancy should be suspected in any reproductive-age woman who presents with abd/pelvic pain, irregular bleeding, and amenorrhea—lag in Tx is a significant cause of mortality

    g. Dx

        (1) ⊕ Pregnancy test with Utz to determine intrauterine versus extrauterine pregnancy

        (2) Very low progesterone level strongly suggests nonviable pregnancy that may be located outside the uterine cavity; higher levels suggest viable pregnancy

    h. Tx

        (1) Surgical removal now commonly done via laparoscopy with maximum preservation of reproductive organs

        (2) Methotrexate can be used early, especially if pregnancy is <3.5 cm in diameter, with no cardiac activity on Utz

        (3) Regardless of technique used, post-Tx serial β-hCG levels must be followed to ensure proper falloff in level

Table 3.6 Types of Abortions

Threatened	• Si/Sx = vaginal bleeding in first 20 wk of pregnancy without passage of tissue or ROM, with cervix closed • Occurs in 25% of pregnancies (half go on to spontaneously abort) • ↑ Risk preterm labor and delivery, low birth weight, perinatal mortality • Dx = Utz to confirm early pregnancy is intact • If no cardiac activity by 9 wk → consider D&C procedure • hCG levels are used to identify viable pregnancies at various stages of development
Inevitable	• Si/Sx = threatened abortion with dilated cervical os and/or ROM, usually accompanied by cramping with expulsion of products of conception (POC) • Pregnancy loss is unavoidable • Tx = surgical evacuation of uterine contents and RhoGAM if mother is Rh-negative
Completed	• Si/Sx = documented pregnancy that spontaneously aborts all POCs • POCs should be grossly examined and submitted to pathology to confirm fetal tissue and/or placental villi, if none is observed must rule out ectopic pregnancy • Pts may require curettage because of ↑ likelihood that abortion was incomplete (suspected if b-hCG levels plateau or fail to decline to zero) • RhoGAM given to Rh-negative women
Incomplete	• Si/Sx = cramping, bleeding, passage of tissue, with dilated cervix and visible tissue in vagina or endocervical canal • Curettage usually needed to remove remaining POCs and control bleeding • Rh-negative pts are given RhoGAM • Hemodynamic stabilization may be required if bleeding is very heavy
Missed	• Failure to expel POC • Si/Sx = lack of uterine growth, lack of fetal heart tones, and cessation of pregnancy Sx • Evacuation of uterus required after confirmation of fetal death, suction curettage recommended for first-trimester pregnancy, dilation and evacuation (D&E) recommended for second-trimester pregnancies • DIC is serious but rare complication • Rh-negative pts receive RhoGAM
Recurrent	• Si/Sx = ≥2 consecutive or total of 3 spontaneous abortions • If early, often due to chromosomal abnormalities → karyotyping for both parents to determine if they carry a chromosomal abnormality • Examine mother for uterine abnormalities • Incompetent cervix is suspected by Hx of painless dilation of cervix with delivery of nml fetus between 18–32 wk of gestation • Tx = surgical cerclage procedures to suture cervix closed until labor or rupture of membranes occurs

(4) Rh-negative women should receive RhoGAM to avoid Rh sensitization

3. Third-Trimester Bleeding
   a. Occurs in approximately 5% of all pregnancies
   b. Half of these are due to placenta previa or placental abruption, others due to vaginal/vulvar lacerations, cervical polyps, cervicitis, cervical CA
   c. In many cases, no cause of bleeding is found
   d. Comparison of placenta previa and placental abruption (Table 3.7)

Table 3.7	Comparison of Placenta Previa and Placental Abruption	
	Placenta Previa	**Placental Abruption**
Abnormality	Placenta implanted over internal cervical os (completely or partially)	Premature separation (complete or partial) of normally implanted placenta from decidua
Epidemiology	↑ Risk grand multiparas and prior C-section	↑ risk preeclampsia, previous Hx of abruption, rupture of membranes in a pt with hydramnios, cocaine use, cigarette smoking, and trauma
Time of onset	20–30 wk	Any time after 20 wk
Si/Sx	Sudden, **painless** bleeding	**Painful** bleeding, can be heavy and painful, and frequent uterine contractions
Dx	Utz → placenta abnormal location	Clinical, based on presentation of painful vaginal bleeding, frequent contractions, and fetal distress. **Utz not useful**
Tx	Hemodynamic support, expectant management, deliver by C-section when fetus mature enough	Hemodynamic support, urgent C-section or vaginal induction if pt is stable and fetus is not in distress
Complications	Associated with two-fold ↑ in congenital malformations so evaluation for fetal anomalies should be undertaken at Dx	↑ Risk of fetal hypoxia/death, DIC may occur as a result of intravascular and retroplacental coagulation

4. Preterm Labor (PTL)

a. Regular uterine contractions at ≤10-min intervals, lasting ≥30 seconds, between 20 and 36 wk of gestation, accompanied by cervical effacement, dilation, and/or descent of fetus into the pelvis

b. Major cause of preterm birth → significant perinatal morbidity and mortality

c. Risk factors = premature rupture of membranes (PROM), infxn (UTI, vaginal, amniotic), dehydration, incompetent cervix, smoking, fibroids, placenta previa, placental abruption, many cases are idiopathic

d. Si/Sx = cramps, dull low-back pain, abd/pelvic pressure, vaginal discharge (mucous, water, or bloody), and contractions (often painless)

e. Dx = external fetal monitoring to quantify frequency and duration of contractions, vaginal exam → extent of cervical dilation/effacement

f. Utz to confirm gestational age, amniotic fluid volume (helps to determine if ROM has occurred), fetal presentation, and placental location

g. Tx focused on delaying delivery if possible until fetus is mature

(1) 50% of pts have spontaneous resolution of preterm uterine contractions

(2) IV hydration important because dehydration causes uterine irritability

(3) Empiric antibiotic Tx is given for suspected chorioamnionitis or vaginal infxn

(4) Tocolytic regimens

(a) Magnesium sulfate, β_2 agonists such as terbutaline and ritodrine, Ca^{2+} blockers such as nifedipine or indomethacin may be instituted, although they have never been shown to substantially prolong delivery for more than several days

(b) Contraindications to tocolysis = advanced labor (cervical dilation >3 cm), mature fetus, chorioamnionitis, significant vaginal bleeding, anomalous fetus, acute fetal distress, severe preeclampsia or eclampsia

(5) From 24–34 wk, steroids such as betamethasone are generally used to enhance pulmonary maturity

(6) Management of infants at 34–37 wk is individualized; survival rates for infants born at 34 wk is within 1% of the survival rate for infants born at ≥37 wk; assessment

of fetal lung maturity may help decide who to deliver between 34–37 wk

   h. Common complications include death, RDS and subsequent bronchopulmonary dysplasia, sepsis, intraventricular hemorrhage, necrotizing enterocolitis, developmental delays, and seizures

5. PROM

   a. Rupture of chorioamnionic membrane before onset of labor, occurs in 10%–15% of all pregnancies

   b. Labor usually follows PROM; 90% of pts and 50% of preterm pts go into labor within 24 hr after rupture

   c. Biggest risk is labor and delivery of preterm infant with associated morbidities/mortality, second biggest complication is infxn (chorioamnionitis)

   d. PROM at ≤26 wk of gestation is associated with pulmonary hypoplasia

   e. Dx = vaginal exam with testing of nonbloody fluid from the vagina

     (1) Nitrazine test: uses pH to distinguish alkaline amniotic fluid (pH >7.0) with more acidic urine and vaginal secretions. (*Note:* false-positive result seen with semen, cervical mucus, *Trichomonas* infxn, blood, unusually basic urine.)

     (2) Fern test: amniotic fluid placed on slide that is allowed to dry in room (up to 30 min); branching fern leaf pattern that results when the slide is completely dry is caused by sodium chloride precipitates from amniotic fluid

     (3) Utz confirms Dx by noting oligohydramnios, labor is less likely to occur if sufficient fluid remains

   f. Tx

     (1) If intrauterine infxn is suspected, empiric broad-spectrum antibiotics are started

     (2) Otherwise treat as for PTL above

6. Multiple Gestations

   a. 1 in 90 incidence in the US; incidence slightly higher in black women, slightly lower in white women.

   b. **Dizygotic twins occur when two separate ova are fertilized by two separate sperm, incidence ↑ with ↑ age and parity**

   c. Monozygotic twins represent division of the fertilized ovum at various times after conception

    d. Multiple gestations are considered high-risk pregnancies because of the disproportionate ↑ in perinatal morbidity and mortality as compared with a singleton gestation

        (1) **Spontaneous abortions and congenital anomalies occur more frequently in multiple pregnancies as compared with singleton pregnancies**

        (2) Maternal complications = anemia, hydramnios, eclampsia, PTL, postpartum uterine atony and hemorrhage, ↑ risk for C-section

        (3) Fetal complications: congenital anomalies, spontaneous abortion, IUGR, prematurity, PROM, umbilical cord prolapse, placental abruption, placenta previa, and malpresentation

    e. Average duration of gestation ↓ with ↑ number of fetuses (twins deliver at 37 wk, triplets deliver at 33 wk, quadruplets deliver at 29 wk)

    f. Twin–twin transfusion syndrome

        (1) Occurs in 10% of twins sharing a chorionic membrane

        (2) Occurs when blood flow is interrupted by a vascular anastomoses such that one twin becomes the donor twin and can have impaired growth, anemia, hypovolemia, and the other twin (recipient twin) can develop hypervolemia, HTN, polycythemia, and congestive heart failure as a result of ↑ blood flow from one twin to the other

    g. Dx of twins usually suspected when uterine size exceeds calculated gestational age and can be confirmed with Utz

    h. DDx = incorrect dates, fibroids, polyhydramnios, and molar pregnancy

    i. Delivery method largely depends on presentation of twins; usually if first fetus is in vertex presentation, vaginal delivery is attempted; if not, C-section is often performed

    j. Important to watch for uterine atony and postpartum hemorrhage because overdistended uterus may not clamp down normally

    k. ↑ Incidence of multiple gestations also seen in females taking fertility meds

II. Gynecology

A. Benign Gynecology

    1. Menstrual Cycle (Figure 3.4)

        a. Due to hypothalamic pulses of gonadotropin-releasing hormone (GnRH), pituitary release of follicle-stimulating hor-

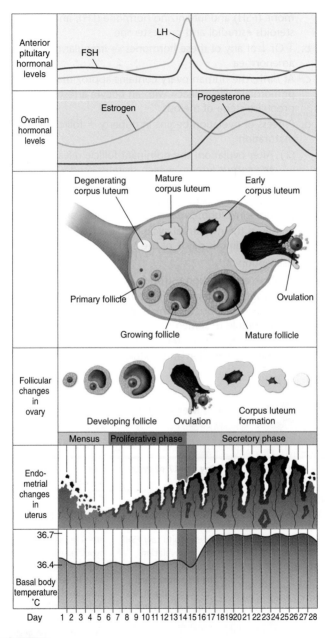

OBSTETRICS AND GYNECOLOGY

FIGURE 3.4

Nml menstrual cycle. (From Premkumar K. *The massage connection anatomy and physiology.* Baltimore: Lippincott Williams & Wilkins, 2004.)

mone (FSH) and luteinizing hormone (LH), and ovarian sex steroids estradiol and progesterone

b. ↑ Or ↓ of any of these hormones → irregular menses or amenorrhea

c. At birth, the human ovary contains approximately 1 million primordial follicles, each with an oocyte arrested in the prophase stage of meiosis

d. Process of ovulation begins in puberty = follicular maturation

   (1) After ovulation, the dominant follicle released becomes the corpus luteum, which secretes progesterone to prepare the endometrium for possible implantation

   (2) If the ovum is not fertilized, the corpus luteum undergoes involution, menstruation begins, and cycle repeats

e. Phases of the menstrual cycle (Table 3.8). First day of menstrual bleeding is day 1 of the cycle

2. Contraception

a. OCPs = combination estrogen and progestin

   (1) Progestin is major contraceptive by suppressing LH and thus ovulation, also thickens cervical mucus so it is less favorable to semen

   (2) Estrogen participates by suppressing FSH, thereby preventing selection and maturation of a dominant follicle

Table 3.8 Phases of the Menstrual Cycle (see Figure 3.4)

Follicular Phase (Proliferative Phase)	Ovulatory Phase	Luteal Phase (Secretory Phase)
Day 1–13 of cycle:	Day 13–17 of cycle:	Day 15 to first day of menses:
Estradiol-induced negative feedback on FSH and ⊕ feedback on LH in anterior pituitary leads to LH surge on days 11–13	Dominant follicle secretion of estradiol → ⊕ feedback to anterior pituitary FSH and LH, ovulation occurs 30–36 hr after the LH surge, small FSH surge also occurs at time of LH surge	Marked by change from estradiol to progesterone predominance, corpus luteal progesterone acts on hypothalamus, causing negative feedback on FSH and LH, resulting in ↓ to basal levels prior to next cycle, if fertilization and implantation do not occur → rapid ↓ in progesterone

    (3) Estrogen and progesterone together inhibit implantation by thinning endometrial lining, also resulting in light or missed menses

    (4) Monophasic pills deliver a constant dose of estrogen and progestin

    (5) Phasic OCPs alter this ratio (usually by varying the dose of progestin) that slightly ↓ the total dose of hormone per mo but also has slightly ↑ rate of breakthrough bleeding between periods

    (6) Pts usually resume fertility once OCPs are discontinued; **however, 3% may have prolonged postpill amenorrhea**

    (7) Risks and benefits (Table 3.9)

    (8) Absolute contraindications to use of OCPs = pregnancy, DVT or thromboembolic dz, endometrial CA, cerebrovascular or coronary artery dz, breast CA, cigarette smoking in women >35 yr old, hepatic dz/neoplasm, abnormal vaginal bleeding, hyperlipidemia

    (9) Alternatives to standard OCPs (Table 3.10)

3. Pap Smear

    a. Current ACOG recommendations are to begin screening 3 yrs after first intercourse or at age 21, which ever comes first.

    b. Pts with 1 sexual partner, 3 consecutive nml Pap smears, and onset of sexual activity after age 25 can be screened less frequently

Table 3.9	Risks and Benefits of Oral Contraceptives
Advantages	**Disadvantages**
• Highly reliable, failure rate <1% (failure usually related to missing pills)	• Require daily compliance
	• Does not protect against sexually transmitted dz
• Protect against endometrial and ovarian CA	• 10%–30% have breakthrough bleeding
• ↓ Incidence of pelvic infxns and ectopic pregnancies	• Side effects:
	◊ Estrogen → bloating, weight gain, breast tenderness, nausea, headaches
• Menses are more predictable, lighter, less painful	◊ Progestin → depression, acne, HTN*[a]

[a]Try lower-dose progesterone pill if HTN does not resolve. Discontinue OCPs—pts with pre-existing HTN can try OCPs if they are ≤35 yr and under good medical control.

Table 3.10 Alternatives to Oral Contraceptives

Method	Indication	Advantage	Disadvantage
Progestin-only pills ("mini-pills")	• **Lactating women**	• Can start immediately postpartum • No impact on milk production or on the baby	• ↑ Failure rate than OCP (ovulation continues in 40%) • Requires strict compliance—low dose of progesterone requires that pill be taken at same time each day
Drospirenone and ethinyl estradiol	• Contraception for 1 mo	• Drospirenone is a synthetic progestin, has antimineralocorticoid activity that diminishes salt retention versus standard progestins • One pill once per mo	• Risk of hyperkalemia
Depo-Provera (medroxy-progesterone)	• Contraception for ≥1 yr • Noncompliance with daily OCPs • Breast-feeding	• **IM injection** maintained for 14 wk	• Irregular vaginal bleed[a] • 50% pts infertile for 10 mo after last injection • Risk of abortion[b]
Norplant	• Long-term contraception	• Subcutaneous implants provide **contraception for 5 yr** • Prompt fertility following D&C	• 30% of break through pregnancies are ectopic
Patch	• Contraception for 1 mo	• Patch worn on skin like band-aid; slowly releases estrogen/progestin • Wear for 3 wks, then take off for 1 wk • 99% effective	• Does not protect against STDs • Less effective (92%) for women ≥198 pounds
Intrauterine device	• For those at low risk for STDs	• Inserted into endometrial cavity, left in place for several years	• Contraindicated in cervical or vaginal infxn, Hx of PID or infertility • Spontaneous expulsion, menstrual pain, ↑ rate of ectopic pregnancy, septic abortion and pelvic infxns

Table 3.10   *Continued*

Method	Indication	Advantage	Disadvantage
Vaginal Contraceptive Ring	• Contraception for 1 mo	• Flexible ring inserted into vagina, releases estrogen/progestin locally • Wear for 3 wks, take out for 1 wk	• If ring is expelled and stays out for ≥3 hours, must use another birth control method until new ring is in place for 7 days
Postcoital	• Emergency contraception	• **Progestin/estrogen taken within 72 hr of intercourse,** repeat in 12 hr • Allows for early termination of unwanted pregnancy	• Follow pt to ensure withdrawal bleeding occurs within 5 days • Nausea

[a]Oral estrogen or NSAIDs can ↓ bleeding, bleeding ↓ with each use, 50% pts are amenorrheic in 1 yr.
[b]Injection given within first 5 days of menses (ensuring pt not pregnant).
STD, sexually transmitted dz.

   c. Reliability depends on presence/absence of cervical inflammation, adequacy of specimen, and prompt fixation of specimen to avoid artifact

   d. If Pap → mild- or low-grade atypia → repeat Pap—atypia may spontaneously regress

   e. Recurrent mild atypia or high-grade atypia → more intensive evaluation

      (1) Colposcopy

         (a) Allows for magnification of cervix so that subtle areas of dysplastic change can be visualized, optimizing selection of Bx sites

         (b) Cervix washed with acetic acid solution, white areas, abnormally vascularized areas, and punctate lesions are selected for Bx

      (2) Endocervical curettage (ECC) → sample of endocervix obtained at same time of colposcopy so that dz further up in endocervical canal may be detected

      (3) Cone Bx

         (a) Cone-shaped specimen encompassing squamocolumnar junction and any lesions on ectocervix removed from cervix by knife, laser, or wire loop

      (b) Allows for more complete ascertainment of extent of dz, in many cases is therapeutic as well as diagnostic

      (c) Indications = ⊕ ECC, unsatisfactory colposcopy = entire squamocolumnar junction not visualized, and discrepancy between Pap and colposcopy Bx

   f. Tx = excision of premalignant or malignant lesions—if CA, see Section VIII for appropriate adjunctive modalities

4. Human Papilloma Virus (HPV) Vaccine

   a. Vaccination protects against HPV 16 and 18, which cause 70% of cervical CA, and 6 and 11, which cause 90% of genital warts

   b. Vaccination appears to be 100% effective at preventing genital warts and precancerous lesions of cervix, vulva, and vagina caused by the targeted HPV serotypes

   c. Vaccination is less effective once the virus is already contracted, so must vaccinate prior to contracting HPV

   d. Official recommendation is vaccinate all 11–12 year-old girls (can be given to girls as young as 9) and also recommended for 13–26 year-old girls/women who have not yet received or completed the vaccine series

5. Vaginitis

   a. 50% of cases due to *Gardnerella* ("bacterial vaginosis"), 25% due to *Trichomonas*, 25% due to *Candida* (↑ frequency in diabetics, women who are pregnant or have HIV)

   b. Most common presenting Sx in vaginitis is discharge

   c. Rule out noninfectious causes, including chemical or allergic sources

   d. Dx by pelvic examination with microscopic examination of discharge

   e. DDx of vaginitis (Table 3.11)

6. Endometriosis

   a. Affects 1%–2% of women (up to 50% in infertile women), peak age = 20s–30s

   b. Endometrial tissue in extrauterine locations, most commonly ovaries (60%) but can be anywhere in the peritoneum and rarely extraperitoneal

   c. Adenomyosis = endometrial implants within the uterine wall

   d. Endometrioma = endometriosis involving an ovary with implants large enough to be considered a tumor, filled with chocolate-appearing fluid (old blood) that gives them their name of "chocolate cysts"

Table 3.11 Differential Diagnosis of Vaginitis (Figure 3.5)

	Candida	Trichomonas	Gardnerella
Vaginal pH	4–5	>6	>5
Odor	None	Rancid	"Fishy" on KOH prep
Discharge	Cheesy white	Green, frothy	Variable
Si/Sx	Itchy, burning erythema	Severe itching	Variable to none
Microscopy	Pseudohyphae, more pronounced on 10% KOH prep (Figure 3.6)	Motile organisms with flagellae (Figure 3.6)	Clue cells (large epithelial cells covered with dozens of small dots) (Figure 3.6)
Tx	Fluconazole	Metronidazole—treat partner also	Metronidazole

e. Si/Sx = **the 3 Ds** = **dysmenorrhea, dyspareunia, dyschezia** (painful defecation), pelvic pain, infertility, uterosacral nodularity palpable on rectovaginal exam, severity of Sx often do not correlate with extent of dz

f. Dx requires direct visualization via laparoscopy or laparotomy with histologic confirmation

g. Tx

(1) Start with NSAIDs, can add combined estrogen and progestin pills, allowing maintenance without withdrawal bleeding and dysmenorrhea

(2) Can use progestin-only pills, drawback is breakthrough bleeding

(3) GnRH agonists inhibit ovarian function → hypoestrogen state

(4) Danazol inhibits LH and FSH midcycle surges, side effects include hypoestrogenic and androgenic (hirsutism, acne) states

(5) Conservative surgery involves excision, cauterization, or ablation of endometrial implants with preservation of ovaries and uterus

(6) Recurrence after cessation of medical Tx is common, definitive Tx requires hysterectomy, ⊕ oophorectomy (total abd hysterectomy with bilateral salpingo-

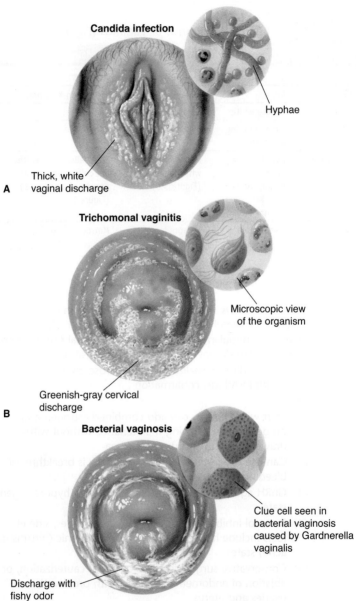

Candida infection

Hyphae

Thick, white vaginal discharge

A

Trichomonal vaginitis

Microscopic view of the organism

Greenish-gray cervical discharge

B

Bacterial vaginosis

Clue cell seen in bacterial vaginosis caused by Gardnerella vaginalis

Discharge with fishy odor

C

FIGURE 3.5

Vaginitis. **(A)** *Candida* vaginitis. **(B)** *Trichomonas* vaginitis. **(C)** Bacterial vaginosis. All assets provided by Anatomical Chart Co.

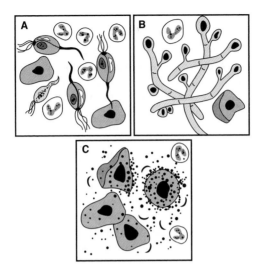

FIGURE 3.6

Microscopic preparations of samples from vaginal swabs in pts with vaginitis.
(A) Appearance of *Trichomonas vaginalis* with flagellae. **(B)** *Candida* pseudohy-
phae and hyphae. **(C)** "Clue cells" of bacterial vaginosis. (From Beckmann
CRB, Ling FW, Laube DW, et al. *Obstetrics and gynecology*, 4th Ed. Baltimore:
Lippincott Williams & Wilkins, 2002.)

oophorectomy [TAH/BSO]), lysis of adhesions, and removal of endometrial implants

(7) Pts can take estrogen replacement Tx following definitive surgery, risk of reactivation of endometriosis is very
small compared to risk of prolonged estrogen deficiency

B. Reproductive Endocrinology and Infertility

1. Amenorrhea

a. Definitions

(1) Amenorrhea = absence of menstruation

(2) 1° amenorrhea = woman who has never menstruated

(3) 2° amenorrhea = menstrual-age woman who has not
menstruated in 6 mo

b. Causes of amenorrhea

(1) **Pregnancy = most common cause**, thus every evaluation should begin with an exclusion of pregnancy before any further workup

      (2) Asherman's syndrome

         (a) Scarring of the uterine cavity after a dilatation and curettage (D&C) procedure

         (b) **Most common anatomic cause of 2° amenorrhea**

      (3) Hypothalamic deficiency due to weight loss, excessive exercise (e.g., marathon runner), obesity, drug-induced (e.g., marijuana, tranquilizers), malignancy (prolactinoma, craniopharyngioma), psychogenic (chronic anxiety, anorexia)

      (4) Pituitary dysfunction results from either ↓ hypothalamic pulsatile release of GnRH or ↓ pituitary release of FSH or LH

      (5) Ovarian dysfunction

         (a) Ovarian follicles are either exhausted or resistant to stimulation by FSH and LH

         (b) Si/Sx = those of estrogen deficiency = hot flashes, mood swings, vaginal dryness, dyspareunia, sleep disturbances, skin thinning

         (c) **Note that estrogen deficiency 2° to hypothalamic–pituitary failure does not cause hot flashes, whereas ovarian failure does**

         (d) Causes = inherited (e.g., Turner's syndrome), premature natural menopause, autoimmune ovarian failure (Blizzard's syndrome), alkylating chemotherapies

      (6) Genital outflow tract alteration, usually the result of congenital abnormalities (e.g., imperforate hymen or agenesis of uterus/vagina)

   c. Tx

      (1) Hypothalamic → reversal of underlying cause and induction of ovulation with gonadotropins

      (2) Tumors → excision or bromocriptine for prolactinoma

      (3) Genital tract obstruction → surgery if possible

      (4) Ovarian dysfunction → exogenous estrogen replacement

2. Dysfunctional Uterine Bleeding

   a. Irregular menstruation without anatomic lesions of the uterus

   b. **Usually due to chronic estrogen stimulation** (vs. amenorrhea, an estrogen deficient state), more rarely to genital outflow tract obstruction

   c. Abnormal bleeding = bleeding at intervals <21 days or >36 days, lasting >7 days, or blood loss > 80 mL

    d. Menorrhagia (excessive bleeding) usually due to anovulation

    e. Dx

        (1) Rule out anatomic causes of bleeding, including uterine fibroids, cervical or vaginal lesions or infxn, cervical and endometrial CA

        (2) Evaluate stress, exercise, weight changes, systemic dz such as thyroid, renal, or hepatic dz and coagulopathies, and pregnancy

    f. Tx

        (1) Convert proliferative endometrium into secretory endometrium by administration of a progestational agent for 10 days

        (2) Alternative is to give OCPs that suppress the endometrium and establish regular, predictable cycles

        (3) NSAIDs ⊕ iron used in pts who want to preserve fertility

        (4) **Postmenopausal bleeding is CA until proven otherwise**

3. Hirsutism and Virilization (Table 3.12)

    a. Hirsutism = excess body hair, usually associated with acne, most commonly due to polycystic ovarian dz or adrenal hyperplasia

    b. Virilization = masculinization of a woman, associated with marked ↑ testosterone, clitoromegaly, temporal balding, voice deepening, breast involution, limb–shoulder girdle remodeling

4. Menopause

    a. Defined as the cessation of menses, **average age in US is 51 yr**

    b. Suspect when menstrual cycles are not regular and predictable and when cycles are not associated with any premenstrual Sx

    c. Si/Sx = rapid onset hot flashes and sweating with resolution in 3 min, mood changes, sleep disturbances, vaginal dryness/atrophy, dyspareunia (painful intercourse), and osteoporosis

    d. Dx = irregular menstrual cycles, hot flashes, and ↑ FSH level (>30 mIU/mL)

    e. Depending on clinical scenario, other labs should be conducted to exclude other Dx that can cause amenorrhea, such as thyroid dz, hyperprolactinemia, pregnancy

Table 3.12 Differential Diagnosis of Hirsutism and Virilization

Dz	Characteristics	Tx
Polycystic ovarian dz	• **#1 cause of androgen excess and hirsutism** • Etiology likely related to LH overproduction • Si/Sx = oligomenorrhea or amenorrhea, anovulation, infertility, hirsutism, acne • Labs →↑ **LH/FSH**, ↑ **testosterone**	• Break feedback cycle with OCPs → ↓ LH production • Weight loss may allow ovulation, sparing fertility • Refractory pts may require clomiphene to ovulate
Sertoli-Leydig cell tumor	• Ovarian tumors secreting testosterone, usually in women age 20–40 yr • Si/Sx = **rapid onset** of hirsutism, acne, amenorrhea, virilization • Labs →↓ **LH/FSH**, ↑↑↑ **testosterone**	• Removal of involved ovary (tumors usually unilateral) • 10-yr survival = 90%–95%
Congenital adrenal hyperplasia	• Usually due to 21-α-hydroxylase defect • Autosomal recessive, variable penetrance • When severe → virilized newborn, milder forms can present at puberty or later • Labs →↑ **LH/FSH**, ↑ **DHEA***	• Glucocorticoids to suppress adrenal androgen production

*DHEA, dehydroepiandrosterone.

   f. Tx

     (1) **First line is estrogen hormone replacement Tx (HRT)**

     (2) HRT can consist of via continuous estrogen with cyclic progestin to allow controlled withdrawal bleeding or daily administration of both estrogen and progestin, which does not cause withdrawal bleeding

     (3) HRT now is known to ↑ the risk of cardiovascular events (stroke and myocardial infarction) and may ↑ the risk of breast CA

     (4) Raloxifene

       (a) Second-generation tamoxifen-like drug = mixed estrogen agonist/antagonist, Food and Drug

Administration (FDA) approved to prevent
osteoporosis

(b) Raloxifene shown to act like estrogen in bones (good),
↓ serum low-density lipoprotein (good), but does not
stimulate endometrial growth (good) (unlike tamoxifen and estrogen alone), also ↓ the risk of breast CA

(5) **Calcium supplements are not a substitute for estrogen replacement**

5. Infertility
   a. Defined as failure to conceive after 1 yr of unprotected sex
   b. Affects 10%–15% of reproductive-age couples in the US
   c. Causes = abnormal spermatogenesis (40%), anovulation
      (30%), anatomic defects of the female reproductive tract
      (20%), unknown (10%)
   d. Dx
      (1) **Start workup with male partner not only because it
          is the most common cause,** but because the workup is
          simpler, noninvasive, and more cost-effective than infer-
          tility workup of the female
      (2) **Nml semen excludes male cause in >90% of couples**
      (3) Workup of female partner should include measurement
          of basal body temperature, which is an excellent screen-
          ing test for ovulation
          (a) Temperature drops at time of menses, then rises
              2 days after LH surge at the time of progesterone rise
          (b) Ovulation probably occurs 1 day before first temper-
              ature elevation and temperature remains elevated for
              13–14 days
          (c) Temperature elevation >16 days suggests pregnancy
      (4) Anovulation
          (a) Hx of regular menses with premenstrual Sx (breast
              fullness, ↓ vaginal secretions, abd bloating, mood
              changes) strongly suggests ovulation
          (b) Sx such as irregular menses, amenorrhea episodes,
              hirsutism, acne, galactorrhea, suggest anovulation
          (c) FSH measured at day 2–3 is best predictor of fertility
              potential in women, FSH >25 IU/L correlates with
              poor Px
          (d) Dx confirm with basal body temperature, serum
              progesterone (↑ postovulation, >10 ng/mL →
              ovulation), endometrial Bx

(5) Anatomic disorder

    (a) **Most commonly results from an acquired disorder, especially acute salpingitis 2° to *Neisseria gonorrhoeae* and *Chlamydia trachomatis***

    (b) Endometriosis, scarring, adhesions from pelvic inflammation or previous surgeries, tumors, and trauma can disrupt nml reproductive tract anatomy

    (c) Less commonly, a congenital anomaly such as septate uterus or reduplication of the uterus, cervix, or vagina is responsible

    (d) **Dx with hysterosalpingogram**

e. Tx

    (1) Anovulation → restore ovulation with use of ovulation-inducing drugs

        (a) First line = clomiphene, an estrogen antagonist that relieves negative feedback on FSH, allowing follicle development

        (b) Anovulatory women who bleed in response to progesterone are candidates for clomiphene, as are women with irregular menses or midluteal progesterone levels <10 ng/mL

        (c) 40% get pregnant, 8%–10% ↑ rate of multiple births, mostly twins

        (d) If no response, FSH can be given directly → pregnancy rates of 60%–80%, multiple births occur at ↑ rate of 20%

    (2) Anatomic abnormalities → surgical lysis of pelvic adhesions

    (3) If endosalpinx is not intact and transport of ovum is not possible, an assisted fertilization technique, such as in vitro fertilization, may be used with 15%–25% success

C. Urogynecology

    1. Pelvic Relaxation and Urinary Incontinence

        a. ↑ Incidence with age, birth trauma, obesity, chronic cough

        b. Si/Sx = prolapse of urethra (urethrocele), uterus, bladder (cystocele), or rectum (rectocele), pelvic pressure and pain, dyspareunia, bowel and bladder dysfunction, and urinary incontinence

        c. Types of urinary incontinence (Figure 3.7)

            (1) Stress incontinence = bladder pressure exceeds urethral pressure briefly at times of strain or stress, such as coughing or laughing

TYPES

STRESS
Pelvic floor injury

URGE
Detrusor instability

NEUROPATHIC
Head injury
Spinal injury
Peripheral nerve injury

ANATOMICAL
Vesicovaginal fistula

FEATURES

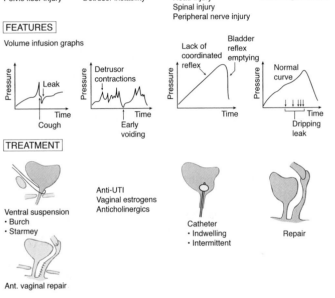

TREATMENT

Ventral suspension
• Burch
• Starmey

Ant. vaginal repair

Anti-UTI
Vaginal estrogens
Anticholinergics

Catheter
• Indwelling
• Intermittent

Repair

FIGURE 3.7

Urinary incontinence.

    (2) Urge incontinence and overflow incontinence result from neuropathic bladder resulting in loss of control of bladder function, resulting in involuntary bladder contraction (urge) or bladder atony (overflow)

d. Dx = urodynamic testing, assess for underlying medical conditions such as diabetes, neurologic dz, genitourinary surgery, pelvic irradiation, trauma, and medications that may account for Sx

e. Tx = correct underlying cause

    (1) Kegel exercises to tone pelvic floor

    (2) Insertion of pessary devices to add structural support

      (3) Useful drugs = anticholinergics, oxybutynin/tolterodine tartrate, β-agonists

      (4) Surgical repair aimed at restoring structures to original anatomic position

D. Gynecology Oncology

  1. Endometrial CA

    a. Most commonly adenoCA, with approximately 40,000 new cases per year

    b. "Estrogen-dependent" CA

      (1) Estrogen source can be glandular from the ovary

      (2) Extraglandular from peripheral conversion of androstenedione to estrone or from a granulosa cell tumor

      (3) Exogenous from oral estrogen, cutaneous patches, vaginal creams, and tamoxifen (reduces risk of breast CA by 50% but associated with $3\times \uparrow$ incidence of endometrial CA)

    c. Risk factors

      (1) Unopposed postmenopausal estrogen replacement Tx

      (2) Menopause after age 52 yr

      (3) Obesity, nulliparity, feminizing ovarian tumors (e.g., ovarian granulosa cell tumors), chronic anovulation, polycystic ovarian syndrome, postmenopausal (75% of pts), diabetes

    d. Si/Sx = abnormal uterine bleeding, especially post-menopausal—any woman >35 yr with abnormal uterine bleeding should have a sample of endometrium taken for histologic evaluation

    e. DDx = endometrial hyperplasia

      (1) Abnormal proliferation of both glandular and stromal elements, can be simple or complex

      (2) Atypical hyperplasia

        (a) Significant numbers of glandular elements that exhibit cytologic atypia and disordered maturation

        (b) Analogous to CA in situ (CIS) → 20%–30% risk for malignancy

    f. Dx

      (1) Pap smear is NOT reliable in Dx of endometrial CA; however, if atypical glandular cells of undetermined significance (AGCUS) are found on the smear, then endometrial evaluation is mandatory

      (2) Bimanual exam for masses, nodularity, induration, and immobility

      (3) Endometrial Bx by ECC, D&C, hysteroscopy with directed Bx

g. Tx

    (1) Simple or complex hyperplasia → progesterone to reverse hyperplastic process promoted by estrogen (e.g., Provera for 10 days)

    (2) Atypical hyperplasia → hysterectomy because of likelihood that it will become invasive endometrial CA

    (3) Endometrial CA

      (a) TAH/BSO, lymph node dissection

      (b) Adjuvant Tx may include external-beam radiation

      (c) Tx for recurrence is high-dose progestins (e.g., Depo-Provera)

h. Px

    (1) **Most important prognostic factor is histologic grade**

    (2) G1 is highly differentiated, G2 is moderately differentiated, G3 is predominantly solid or entirely undifferentiated CA

    (3) **Depth of myometrial invasion is second most important Px factor**

    (4) Pt with G1 tumor that does not invade the myometrium has a 95% 5-yr survival, pt with G3 tumor with deep myometrial invasion has 5-yr survival rate closer to 20%

2. Uterine Leiomyomas = Fibroids

  a. Benign tumors, growth related to estrogen production, usually most rapid growth occurs perimenopausally

  b. Most common indication for hysterectomy (30% of cases)

  c. Si/Sx = bleeding (usually menorrhagia or ↑ amount and duration of flow), pelvic pressure, pelvic pain often manifested as dysmenorrhea

  d. Dx = Utz, confirm with tissue sample by either D&C or Bx (especially in postmenopausal pts)

  e. Tx

    (1) If Sx are mild → reassurance and observation

    (2) Medical Tx → estrogen inhibitors such as GnRH agonists shrink uterus, resulting in a simpler surgical procedure or can be used as a temporizing measure until natural menopause occurs

(3) Surgery → myomectomy indicated in young pts who want to preserve fertility (risk of intraoperative and post-operative hemorrhage ↑ compared to hysterectomy); hysterectomy is considered definitive Tx but should be reserved for symptomatic women who have completed childbearing

3. Leiomyosarcoma
   a. Rare malignancy accounting for only 3% of CA involving uterine corpus
   b. ↑ Suspicion for postmenopausal uterine enlargement
   c. Si/Sx suggestive of sarcoma = postmenopausal bleeding, pelvic pain, and ↑ vaginal discharge
   d. Tx = hysterectomy with intraoperative lymph node Bx
   e. Surgical staging same as that for endometrial adenoCA
   f. Survival rate is much lower than that for endometrial CA, only 50% of pts survive 5 yr
   g. Adjunctive therapies are of minimal benefit

4. Cervical CA
   a. Annual Pap is most important screening tool available to detect dz
   b. Risk factors = early sexual intercourse, multiple sexual partners, HPV infxn (especially types 16, 18), cigarette smoking, early childbearing, and immunocompromised pts
   c. Average age at Dx = 50 yr but can occur much earlier
   d. 85% are of squamous cell origin, 15% are adenocCA arising from endocervical glands
   e. Si/Sx = postcoital bleeding, but there is no classic presentation for cervical CA
   f. Dx = Pap screening, any visible cervical lesion should be Bx
   g. Tx
      (1) Local dz → hysterectomy + lymph node dissection—ovaries may remain → survival >70% at 5 yr
      (2) Extensive or metastatic dz → pelvic irradiation → survival <40% at 5 yr
   h. Prevention—see HPV vaccine, section II.A.4

5. Ovarian Neoplasms (Table 3.13)

6. Vulvar and Vaginal CA
   a. Vulvar intraepithelial neoplasia (VIN)
      (1) VIN I and II = mild and moderate dysplasia, ↑ risk progressing to advanced stages and then CA

Table 3.13 Ovarian Neoplasms

Neoplasm	Characteristics	Tx
Benign cysts	• Functional growth resulting from failure of nml follicle to rupture • Si/Sx = pelvic pain or pressure, rupture of cyst → acute severe pain and hemorrhage mimicking acute abdomen • Confirm cyst with Utz	• Typically self-limiting • Rupture may require laparotomy to stop bleeding
Benign Tumors: more common than malignant, but risk of malignancy ↑ with age		
Epithelial cell	• Serous cystadenoma most common type, almost always benign unless bilateral → ↑ risk of malignancy • Other types = mucinous, endometrioid, Brenner tumors, all rarely malignant • Dx = clinical, can see on CT/MRI	• Surgical excision
Germ cell	• Teratoma is most common (also called "dermoid cyst") • Very rarely malignant, contain differentiated tissue from all three embryologic germ layers • Si/Sx = unilateral cystic, mobile, nontender adnexal mass, often aSx • Dx confirmed with Utz	• Excision to prevent ovarian torsion or rupture
Stromal cell	• Functional tumors secreting hormones • Granulosa tumor makes estrogens → gynecomastia, loss of body hair, etc. • Sertoli-Leydig cells make androgens, virilize females	• Excision
Malignant Tumors		

- Usually occur in women >50 yr
- Risk factors = low parity, ↓ fertility, delayed childbearing—**OCP use is a protective factor**
- Ovarian is the most lethal gynecologic CA due to lack of early detection → ↑ rate of metastasis (60% at Dx)
- Dz typically are aSx until extensive metastasis has occurred
- Can follow dz with CA-125 marker, not specific enough for screening
- Yearly pelvic exams remain most effective screening tool

(continued)

OBSTETRICS AND GYNECOLOGY

Table 3.13 *Continued*

Malignant Tumors

- Si/Sx = vague abd/pelvic complaints; e.g., distention, early satiety, constipation, pelvic pain, urinary frequency; shortness of breath due to pleural effusion may be only presenting Sx
- Tx = debulking surgery with chemotherapy and radiotherapy

Epithelial cell	• Cause 90% of all ovarian malignancies • Serous cystadenoCA is most common, often originate from benign precursors • Others = endometrioma and mucinous cystadenoCA	• Excision
Germ cell	• Most common ovarian CA in women <20 yr • Can produce hCG or AFP, useful as tumor markers • Subtypes = dysgerminoma, which is very radiosensitive, and immature teratoma	• Radiation first-line • Chemotherapy second-line • 5-yr survival >80% for both
Stromal cell	• Granulosa cell makes estrogen, can result in 2° endometriosis or endometrial CA • Sertoli-Leydig tumor makes androgens	• Total hysterectomy with oophorectomy

  (2) VIN III = CIS
  (3) Si/Sx = pruritus, irritation, presence of raised lesion
  (4) Dx = Bx for definitive Dx
  (5) DDx includes Paget's dz, malignant melanoma
  (6) Tx = excision, local for VIN I and II and wide for VIN III
b. Vulvar CA
  (1) 90% are squamous
  (2) Usually presents postmenopausally
  (3) Si/Sx = pruritus, with or without presence of ulcerative lesion
  (4) Tx = excision
  (5) 5-yr survival rate is 70%–90% depending on nodal status; if deep pelvic nodes are involved, survival is a dismal 20%
c. Vaginal CIS and CA are very rare
  (1) 70% of pts with vaginal CIS have either previous or co-existent genital tract neoplasm

   (2) Tx = radiation, surgery reserved for women with extensive dz

7. Gestational Trophoblastic Neoplasia (GTN) = Hydatidiform Mole or Molar Pregnancy
   a. Rare variation of pregnancy in which a neoplasm is derived from abnormal placental tissue (trophoblastic) proliferation
   b. Usually a benign dz called a "molar pregnancy"
      (1) A complete mole (90%) has no fetus and is 46 XX
      (2) An incomplete mole has a fetus and molar degeneration, and is 69 XXY
   c. Persistent or malignant dz develops in 20% of pts (mostly in complete moles)
   d. Si/Sx = exaggerated pregnancy Sx, with missing fetal heart tones and enlarged uterus (size > dates), painless bleeding commonly occurs in early second trimester
   e. Pts can present with PIH
   f. Dx = Utz and ↑↑↑ hCG levels
   g. Tx = removal of uterine contents by D&C and suction curettage
   h. Non-metastatic persistent GTN is treated with methotrexate
   i. Follow-up = check that hCG levels are appropriately dropping
   j. Contraception is recommended during first yr of follow-up

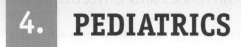

4. PEDIATRICS

I. Development

A. **Developmental Milestones (see Table 4.1)**

B. **Puberty (see Table 4.2)**

II. Infections

A. **ToRCHS (see Table 4.3)**

B. **Infant Botulism**

1. Acute, flaccid paralysis caused by *Clostridium botulinum* neurotoxin that irreversibly blocks acetylcholine release from peripheral neurons

2. Dz acquired via **ingestion of spores in honey** or via inhalation of spores

3. 95% cases in infants age 3 wk to 6 mo, peak 2–4 mo

4. Si/Sx = constipation, lethargy, poor feeding, weak cry, ↓ spontaneous movement, hypotonia, drooling, ↓ gag and suck reflexes, as dz progresses → **loss of head control and respiratory arrest**

5. Dx = clinical, **based on acute onset of flaccid descending paralysis with clear sensorium, without fever or paresthesias,** can confirm by demonstrating botulinum toxin in serum or toxin/organism in feces

6. Tx = intubate, supportive care, no antibiotics or antitoxin needed in infants

C. **Exanthems (see Table 4.4)**

D. **Vaccinations (see Figure 4.1)**

III. Respiratory Disorders

A. **Otitis Media (OM)**

1. Defined as inflammation of middle ear space

    a. Dx = fever, erythema of tympanic membrane (TM), bulging of the pars flaccida portion of the TM, opacity of the TM, otalgia

Table 4.1 Developmental Milestones

Age	Gross Motor	Fine Motor	Language	Social/Cognition
Newborn	Head side to side, **Moro (startle) and grasp reflex**			
2 mo	Holds head up	Swipes at object	Coos	Social smile
4 mo	Rolls front to back	**Grasps object**	Orients to voice	Laughs
6 mo	Rolls back to front, **sits upright**	Transfers object	Babbles	**Stranger anxiety, sleeps all night**
9 mo	Crawl, pull to stand	**Pincer grasp,** eats with fingers	**Mama-dada (non-specific)**	Waves bye-bye, responds to name
12 mo	**Stands**	**Mature pincer**	**Mama-dada (specific)**	Picture book
15 mo	**Walks**	Uses cup	4–6 words	**Temper tantrum**
18 mo	Throws ball, walks upstairs	Uses spoon for solids	Names common objects	**Toilet training may begin**
24 mo	Runs, up/down stairs	Uses spoons for semisolids	**2-word sentence)** (2 words at 2 yr	Follows 2-step command
36 mo	Rides tricycle	Eats neatly with utensils	**3-word sentence** (3 word at 3 yr)	Knows first and last names

Table 4.2 Tanner Stages

Boys	Girls
Testicular enlargement at 11.5 yr*	Breast buds at 10.5 yr*
↑ in genital size	Pubic hair
Pubic hair	Linear growth spurt at 12 yr
Peak growth spurt at 13.5 yr*	Menarche at 12.5 yr*

*Yrs represent population averages.

Table 4.3	The ToRCHS
Dz	**Characteristics**
Toxoplasmosis	• Acquired in mothers via ingestion of poorly cooked meat or through contact with cat feces • Carriers common (10%–30%) in population, only causes neonatal dz if acquired during pregnancy (1%) • One third of women who acquire during pregnancy transmit infxn to fetus and one third of fetuses are clinically affected • Sequelae = intracerebral calcifications, hydrocephalus, chorioretinitis, microcephaly, severe mental retardation, epilepsy, intrauterine growth retardation (IUGR), hepatosplenomegaly • Screening is useless because acquisition prior to birth is common and clinically irrelevant • Pregnant women should be told to avoid undercooked meat, wash hands after handling cat, do not change litter box • If fetal infxn established → Utz to determine major anomalies and provide counseling regarding termination if indicated
Rubella	• First-trimester maternal rubella infxn → 80% chance of fetal transmission • Second trimester → 50% chance of transmission to fetus; third trimester → 5% • Si/Sx of fetus = IUGR, cataracts, glaucoma, chorioretinitis, patent ductus arteriosus, pulmonary stenosis, atrial or ventricular septal defect, myocarditis, microcephaly, **hearing loss, "blueberry muffin rash,"** mental retardation • Dx confirmed with IgM rubella antibody in neonate's serum or viral culture • Tx = prevention by universal immunization of all children against rubella, there is no effective therapy for active infxn
Cytomegalovirus (CMV)	• Number one congenital infxn, affecting 1% of births • Transmitted through bodily fluids/secretions, infxn often aSx • 1° seroconversion during pregnancy →↑ risk of severely affected infant, but congenital infxn can occur if mother reinfected during pregnancy • Approximately 1% risk of transplacental transmission of infxn, approximately 10% of infected infants manifest congenital defects of varying severity • Congenital defects = microcephaly, intracranial calcifications, severe mental retardation, chorioretinitis, IUGR • 10%–15% of aSx but exposed infants develop later neurologic sequelae

Table 4.3 *Continued*

Dz	Characteristics
Herpes simplex virus	• **C-section delivery for pregnant women with active herpes** • Vaginal → 50% chance that the baby will acquire the infxn and is associated with significant morbidity and mortality • Si/Sx = vesicles, seizures, respiratory distress, can cause pneumonia, meningitis, encephalitis → impaired neurologic development after resolution • Tx = acyclovir (↓ mortality)
Syphilis	• Transmission from infected mother to infant during pregnancy nearly 100%, **occurs after the first trimester in the vast majority of cases** • Fetal/perinatal deaths in 40% of affected infants • Early manifestations in first 2 yr, later manifestations in next 2 decades • Si/Sx of early dz = jaundice, ↑ liver function tests, hepatosplenomegaly, hemolytic anemia, rash followed by desquamation of hands and feet, wartlike lesions of mucous membranes, **blood-tinged nasal secretions (snuffles), diffuse osteochondritis, saddle nose (2° to syphilitic rhinitis)** • Si/Sx of late dz = **Hutchinson teeth** (notching of permanent upper 2 incisors), mulberry molars (both at 6 yr), bone thickening (frontal bossing), **anterior bowing of tibia (saber shins)** • Dx = Rapid plasma regain/Venereal Dz Research Laboratory (RPR/VDRL) and fluorescence treponemal antigen (FTA) serologies in mother with clinical findings in infant • Tx 5 procaine penicillin G for 10–14 days

b. Effusions can also be seen as meniscus of fluid behind the TM indicative of poor pressure equalization by Eustachian tubes

c. OM with effusion common in young children because of their Eustachian tubes being smaller and more horizontal, making drainage and pressure equalization more difficult

d. Pathogens = *S. pneumoniae, Hemophilus influenzae, Moraxella catarrhalis*

e. Also commonly caused by viral pathogens

f. Tx = amoxicillin or azithromycin (first line), augmented penicillins or TMP-SMX (second line)

Text continues on page 277

Table 4.4 Viral Exanthems

Dz/Virus	Si/Sx
Measles (Rubeola)/ Paramyxovirus	• Erythematous maculopapular rash, **erupts 5 days after onset of prodromal Sx, begins on head and spreads to body, lasting 4–5 days,** resolving from head downward • **Koplik spots (white spots on buccal mucosa) are pathognomonic** but leave before rash starts so often not found when pt presents • **Dx = fever and Hx of the 3 Cs: cough, coryza, conjunctivitis**
Rubella (German measles)/ Togavirus	• **Suboccipital lymphadenopathy** (very few dzs do this) • Maculopapular rash begins on face then generalizes • Rash lasts 5 days, fever may accompany rash on first day only • May find reddish spots of various sizes on soft palate
Hand, foot, and mouth dz/Coxsackie A virus	• Vesicular rash on hands and feet with ulcerations in mouth • Rash clears in approximately 1 wk • Contagious by contact
Roseola infantum (Exanthem subitum)/ HHV-6	• **Abrupt high fever persisting for 1–5 days even though child has no physical Sx to account for fever and does not feel ill** • When fever drops, macular or maculopapular rash appears on trunk and then spreads peripherally over entire body, lasts 24 hr
Erythema infectiosum (fifth dz)/ Parvovirus B19	• **Classic sign = "slapped cheeks,"** erythema of the cheeks • Subsequently an erythematous maculopapular rash spreads from arms to trunk and legs forming a reticular pattern • **Dz is dangerous in sickle cell pts (and other anemias) because of tendency of parvovirus B19 to cause aplastic crises** **Beware of exposure to pregnant mothers because of high risk of fetal complications**
Varicella (chicken pox) Varicella zoster virus (VZV)	• Highly contagious, crops of pruritic "teardrop" vesicles that break and crust over, start on face or trunk (centripetal) and spread to extremities • New lesions appear for 3–5 days and typically take 3 days to crust over, so rash persists for approximately 1 wk • **Lesions are contagious until they crust over** • Zoster (shingles) = reactivation of old varicella infxn, painful skin eruptions are seen along the distribution of dermatomes that correspond to the affected dorsal root ganglia

Dx = clinical for all; Tx = supportive for all.
HHV-6, human herpes virus 6.

Recommended Immunization Schedule for Persons Aged 0–6 Years—UNITED STATES • 2008

For those who fall behind or start late, see the catch-up schedule

Vaccine ▼ Age ▶	Birth	1 month	2 months	4 months	6 months	12 months	15 months	18 months	19–23 months	2–3 years	4–6 years
Hepatitis B [1]	HepB	HepB		see footnote 1		HepB					
Rotavirus [2]			Rota	Rota	Rota						
Diphtheria, Tetanus, Pertussis [3]			DTaP	DTaP	DTaP		DTaP				DTaP
Haemophilus influenzae type b [4]			Hib	Hib	Hib [4]	Hib					
Pneumococcal [5]			PCV	PCV	PCV	PCV				PPV	
Inactivated Poliovirus			IPV	IPV		IPV					IPV
Influenza [6]						Influenza (Yearly)					
Measles, Mumps, Rubella [7]						MMR					MMR
Varicella [8]						Varicella					Varicella
Hepatitis A [9]						HepA (2 doses)				HepA Series	
Meningococcal [10]											MCV4

Range of recommended ages

Certain high-risk groups

This schedule indicates the recommended ages for routine administration of currently licensed childhood vaccines, as of December 1, 2007, for children aged 0 through 6 years. Additional information is available at www.cdc.gov/vaccines/recs/schedules. Any dose not administered at the recommended age should be administered at any subsequent visit, when indicated and feasible. Additional vaccines may be licensed and recommended during the year. Licensed combination vaccines may be used whenever any components of the combination are indicated and other components of the vaccine are not contraindicated and if approved by the Food and Drug Administration for that dose of the series. Providers should consult the respective Advisory Committee on Immunization Practices statement for detailed recommendations, including for **high-risk conditions**: http://www.cdc.gov/vaccines/pubs/ACIP-list.htm. Clinically significant adverse events that follow immunization should be reported to the Vaccine Adverse Event Reporting System (VAERS). Guidance about how to obtain and complete a VAERS form is available at www.vaers.hhs.gov or by telephone, 800-822-7967.

FIGURE 4.1

Immunization schedules. (Courtesy of www.cdc.gov/vaccines/recs/schedules.) (continued)

PEDIATRICS

Recommended Immunization Schedule for Persons Aged 7–18 Years—UNITED STATES • 2008

For those who fall behind or start late, see the green bars and the catch-up schedule

Vaccine ▼ Age ▶	7–10 years	11–12 years	13–18 years
Diphtheria, Tetanus, Pertussis[1]	see footnote 1	Tdap	Tdap
Human Papillomavirus[2]	see footnote 2	HPV (3 doses)	HPV Series
Meningococcal[3]	MCV4	MCV4	MCV4
Pneumococcal[4]		PPV	
Influenza[5]		Influenza (Yearly)	
Hepatitis A[6]		HepA Series	
Hepatitis B[7]		HepB Series	
Inactivated Poliovirus[8]		IPV Series	
Measles, Mumps, Rubella[9]		MMR Series	
Varicella[10]		Varicella Series	

Legend:
- Range of recommended ages
- Catch-up immunization
- Certain high-risk groups

This schedule indicates the recommended ages for routine administration of currently licensed childhood vaccines, as of December 1, 2007, for children aged 7–18 years. Additional information is available at www.cdc.gov/vaccines/recs/schedules. Any dose not administered at the recommended age should be administered at any subsequent visit, when indicated and feasible. Additional vaccines may be licensed and recommended during the year. Licensed combination vaccines may be used whenever any components of the combination are indicated and other components of the vaccine are not contraindicated and if approved by the Food and Drug Administration for that dose of the series. Providers should consult the respective Advisory Committee on Immunization Practices statement for detailed recommendations, including for **high risk conditions:** http://www.cdc.gov/vaccines/pubs/ACIP-list.htm. Clinically significant adverse events that follow immunization should be reported to the Vaccine Adverse Event Reporting System (VAERS). Guidance about how to obtain and complete a VAERS form is available at www.vaers.hhs.gov or by telephone, **800-822-7967.**

FIGURE 4.1 *(continued)*

g. If chronic effusions or repeated infxns are present, surgical placement of pressure equalization (tubes may be indicated)

h. Note: Adults with unilateral serous effusion need to have a nasopharyngeal mass ruled out

i. Complication of OM and mastoiditis

(1) Intracranial-subdural abscess, epidural abscess, temporal lobe abscess, lateral sinus thrombosis, meningitis

(2) Extracranial-facial paralysis, labrynthitis, and subperiosteal abscess

(3) Subperiosteal abscess

(a) Bezold's abscess = infxn penetrates tip of mastoid and pus travels along sternocleidomastoid muscle and forms an abscess in posterior triangle of neck

(b) Postauricular abscess = most common subperiosteal abscess, occurs posterior to auricle, displacing ear

(4) Ear, nose, and throat (ENT) consult for surgical drainage and IV antibiotics

2. Bullous Myringitis

a. Associated with *Mycoplasma* infxn

b. Presents with large blebs on tympanic membrane

c. Tx = erythromycin

3. Unilateral Serous OM

a. Presents in adults, caused by nasopharyngeal masses obstructing the Eustachian tube

b. Dx = MRI of head, endoscopic visualization, and bx

B. **Bronchiolitis**

1. Commonly seen in children age <2 yr, peak incidence at 6 mo

2. **>50% because of respiratory syncytial virus (RSV);** others include parainfluenzae and adenovirus

3. Si/Sx = mild rhinorrhea and fever progress to cough, wheezing with crackles, tachypnea, nasal flaring, $\downarrow$ appetite

4. Dx by culture or antigen detection of nasopharyngeal secretions

5. Tx = bronchodilators, oxygen (O_2) as needed

C. **Upper Respiratory Dz (see Table 4.5; Figures 4.2 and 4.3A,B)**

D. **Pneumonia**

1. Common etiologies vary with age

a. Newborns get *Streptococcus agalactiae* (group B *Streptococcus*), Gram-negative rod, *Chlamydia trachomatis*

Table 4.5 Pediatric Upper Respiratory Disorders

Dz	Cause	Si/Sx	Labs	Tx
Croup (Laryngotracheo-bronchitis)	Para-influenza, influenza, RSV, *Mycoplasma*	**Presents in fall and winter, 3 mo–3 yr old, barking cough, inspiratory stridor, Sx worse at night,** hoarse voice, preceded by URI	**Neck x-ray → "steeple sign" (Figure 4.2)**	O₂, cool mist, racemic epinephrine (Epi) and steroids if severe, ribavirin may be used for immuno-compromised
Pertussis	*Bordetella pertussis*	**Pertussis presents with 3 stages:** 1) Catarrhal stage = 1–2 wk of cough, rhinorrhea, wheezing; 2) Paroxysmal stage = 2–4 wk of paroxysmal cough with **"whoops";** 3) convales-cent stage = 1–2 wk of persistent chronic cough. Can also cause chronic cough in adults	DFA or serology, culture on Bordet-Gengou medium	Macrolide to shorten infectious period, does not affect duration of Sx, otherwise supportive

Table 4.5 *Continued*

Dz	Cause	Si/Sx	Labs	Tx
Epiglottitis	*H. influenzae* type B	**Medical emergency! Fulminant inspiratory stridor, drooling, sits leaning forward (Figure 4.3A),** dysphagia, "hot potato" voice—very rare now in era of vaccination	**"Thumb print" sign on lateral neck film (Figure 4.3B),** cherry-red epiglottitis on endoscopy	**Examine pt in OR,** intubate as needed, ceftriaxone
Bacterial tracheitis	*Staphylococcus* and *Streptococcus.* spp.	Inspiratory stridor, high fever, toxic appearing	Leukocytosis	Vancomycin or ceftriaxone
Foreign-body aspiration		**Usually presents after age 6 mo** (need to grasp object to inhale it) with **inspiratory stridor** (chronic), wheeze, ↓ breath sounds, dysphagia, unresolved pneumonia	CXR → hyper-inflation on affected side (see Figure 4.4)	Endoscopic or surgical removal

URI, upper respiratory infxn.

PEDIATRICS

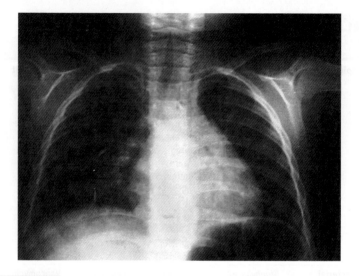

FIGURE 4.2

The "steeple sign" in the soft tissue of the neck on x-ray in a child with croup. (From Harwood-Nuss A, Wolfson AB, Linden CH, et al. *The clinical practice of emergency medicine,* 3rd Ed. Philadelphia: Lippincott Williams & Wilkins, 2001.)

    b. Infants get *S. pneumoniae, H. influenzae, Chlamydia, Staphylococcus aureus, Listeria monocytogenes,* and viral

    c. Preschoolers get RSV, other viruses, and *Mycoplasma*

    d. Adolescents get *S. pneumoniae, Mycoplasma,* and *Chlamydia*

2. Si/Sx = cough (productive in older children), fevers, nausea/vomiting, diarrhea, tachypnea, grunting, retractions, crackles

3. *Chlamydia* causes classic "staccato cough" and conjunctivitis, pts afebrile

4. RSV causes wet cough, often with audible wheezes

5. *Staphylococcus* infxns may be associated with skin lesions

6. Dx = rapid antigen detection or culture of secretions, CXR → infiltrates

7. Tx = infants get hospitalized, bronchodilators and O_2 for RSV, erythromycin for atypical dz (e.g., *Chlamydia, Mycoplasma*), cefuroxime for bacteria

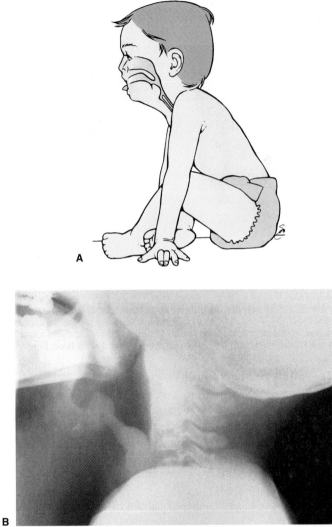

FIGURE 4.3

(A) Classic posture of a child with epiglottitis, sitting forward on hands, mouth open, tongue out, head forward and tilted up in a sniffing position in an effort to relieve the acute airway obstruction. (From Nettina SM. *The Lippincott manual of nursing practice,* 7th Ed. Lippincott Williams & Wilkins, 2001.) **(B)** Epiglottitis on lateral neck x-ray. Note the classic "thumb print" sign below the jaw. (From Harwood-Nuss A, Wolfson AB, Linden CH, et al. *The clinical practice of emergency medicine,* 3rd Ed. Philadelphia: Lippincott Williams & Wilkins, 2001.)

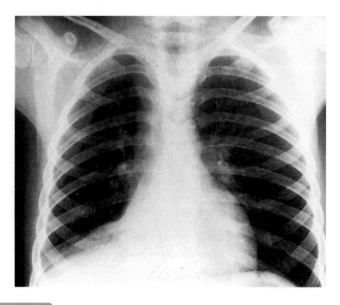

FIGURE 4.4

CXR film of a child admitted with fever and cough who failed to respond to Tx. At bronchoscopy, a toy-car steering wheel was found in the right intermediate bronchus. The radiography shows collapse of the right middle and lower lobes with loss of definition of the right hemidiaphragm and right heart border.

E. **Epiglottitis (Supraglottitis)** (Figure 4.4)
   1. Presents in children, caused by *H. influenzae* type B (HiB). Examine airway in operating room to prevent bronchospasm and airway obstruction
   2. Rare now because of efficacy of HiB vaccine
   3. Presents with acute airway obstruction, sudden airway emergency, inspiratory stridor, drooling, high fever, dysphagia, no cough, neck pain
   4. Rarely seen in adults, usually caused by *S. pneumoniae* or *S. aureus*
   5. Classic x-ray finding is "**thumb sign**" on lateral neck film
   6. Tx = immediate airway intubation, stabilize airway and observe, IV antibiotics

F. **Stridor** (see Figure 4.5)
   1. Laudible high-pitched noisy breathing caused by air turbulence
   2. Inspiratory stridor—supraglottis affected

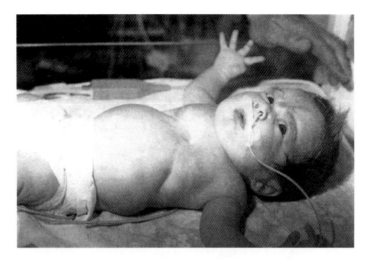

FIGURE 4.5

Baby with severe upper airway obstruction.

3. Biphasic stridor (inspiratory/expiratory)—glottic or subglottic narrowing
4. Most common pediatric noninfectious cause—laryngomalacia (see Figure 4.6)
5. Most common pediatric infectious cause is viral croup
6. Other causes—subglottic hemangioma, polyps, foreign body, vascular rings. Vocal cord paralysis (see Figure 4.7)
7. Tx = stabilize airway. Humidified O_2, steroids, and nebulized racemic epinephrine as needed
8. ENT consult, x-ray, lateral neck and chest x-ray, and airway fluoroscopy, to evaluate airway if stable
9. Immediate stabilization of airway if unstable, direct laryngoscopy and bronchoscopy to further evaluate airway once pt stabilized

G. **Adenoiditis** (see Figure 4.8)
   1. Commonly seen in young children
   2. Si/Sx = frequent OM episodes, snoring at night, constant mouth breathers, constant nasal congestion, and hypernasal voice
   3. Pts develop adenoid facies from always having mouth open
   4. Tx = surgical removal of adenoids

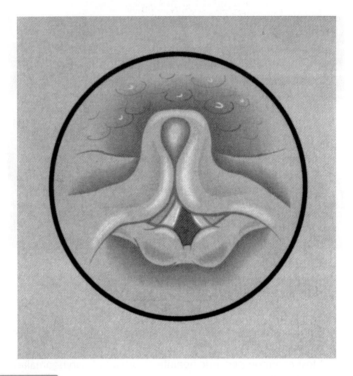

FIGURE 4.6

Laryngomalacia.

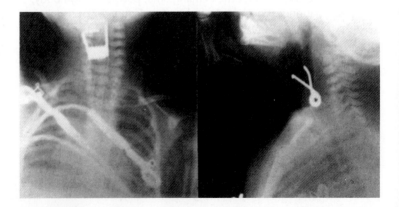

FIGURE 4.7

An unexpected foreign body in a 6-wk-old baby, causing stridor.

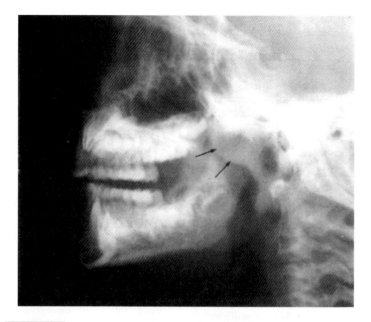

FIGURE 4.8

A lateral soft-tissue x-ray showing adenoid enlargement.

IV. Musculoskeletal

A. Limp

1. Painful limp usually is acute onset, may be associated with fever and irritability, toddlers may refuse to walk

2. DDx painful limp (see Table 4.6; Figure 4.9)

3. Painless limp usually has insidious onset, may be because of weakness or deformity of limb 2° to developmental hip dysplasia, cerebral palsy, or leg-length discrepancy

B. Collagen Vascular Dz

1. Juvenile Rheumatoid Arthritis

   a. Chronic inflammation of ≥1 joints in pt ≤16 yr old

   b. Most common in children age 1–4 yr; females > males

   c. Three categories = systemic, pauciarticular, polyarticular (see Table 4.7)

   d. Dx = Sx persists for 3 consecutive mo with exclusion of other causes of acute/chronic arthritis or collagen vascular dz

Table 4.6 Pediatric Painful Limp

Dz	Characteristics	Tx
Septic arthritis	• Number one **cause of painful limp in 1–3-yr-old** • Usually monoarticular hip, knee, or ankle • Causes = *S. aureus* **(most common)**, *H. influenzae*, *Neisseria gonorrhoeae* • Si/Sx = **acute-onset pain**, arthritis, fever, ↓ range of motion, child may lie still and refuse to walk or crawl, ↑ **WBC**, ↑ **ESR** • X-ray → joint space widening • Dx = joint aspiration → **WBC ≥10,000 with neutrophil predominance,** low glucose	Tx = drainage, antibiotics appropriate to Gram stain or cultures
Toxic synovitis	• Most common in boys 5–10 yr old, may precede viral URI • Si/Sx = **insidious onset pain**, low-grade fever, **WBC and ESR nml** • **Typically no tenderness, warmth, or joint swelling** • X-ray → usually nml • Dx → technetium scan → ↑ **uptake of epiphysis**	Rest and analgesics synovitis for 3–5 days
Aseptic avascular necrosis	• Legg-Calvé-Perthes dz = head of femur, Osgood-Schlatter = tibial tubercle, Köhler's bone dz = navicular bone • Legg-Calvé-Perthes → usually 4–9 yr old (boys/girls = 5:1), bilateral in 10%–20% of cases, ↑ incidence with delayed growth and ↓ birth weight • Si/Sx = **afebrile, insidious-onset hip pain, inner thigh, or knee,** ↑ pain with movement, ↓ with rest, antalgic gait, **nml WBC and ESR** • X-ray → **femoral head sclerosis** ↑ width of femoral neck (see Figure 4.9) • Dx → technetium scan → ↓ **uptake in epiphysis**	↓ Weight bearing on affected side over long time

Table 4.6 *Continued*

Dz	Characteristics	Tx
Slipped capital femoral epiphysis	• Often in **obese male adolescents** (8–17 yr old), 20%–30% bilateral • 80% → slow, progressive, 20% → acute, associated with trauma • Si/Sx → **dull, aching pain** in hip or knee, ↑ pain with activity • X-ray → lateral movement of femur shaft in relation to femoral head, looks like **"ice-cream scoop falling off cone"** • Dx = clinical	Surgical pinning
Osteomyelitis	• Neonates → *S. aureus* (50%), *S. agalactiae, Escherichia coli* • Children → *Staphylococcus, Streptococcus, Salmonella* (sickle cell) • Si/Sx young infants → fever may be only symptom • Si/Sx older children → fever, malaise, ↓ extremity movement, edema • X-ray lags changes by 3–4 wk • Dx → neutrophilic leukocytosis, ↑ ESR (50%), blood cultures, bone scan (90% sensitive), **MRI is the gold standard**	Antibiotics for 4–6 wk

    e. Tx = nonsteroidal anti-inflammatory drugs (NSAIDs), low-dose methotrexate, prednisone only in acute febrile onset

2. Kawasaki's Dz (Mucocutaneous Lymph Node Syndrome)

    a. Large- and medium-vessel vasculitis in children, usually under <5 yr, predilection for Japanese children

    b. Dx = fever >104°F (40°C) for >5 days, unresponsive to antibiotics, ⊕ 4 of 5 of the following criteria **(mnemonic: CRASH):**

        (1) **C**onjunctivitis

        (2) **R**ash, primarily truncal

        (3) **A**neurysms of coronary arteries

        (4) **S**trawberry tongue, crusting of lips, fissuring of mouth, and oropharyngeal erythema

        (5) **H**ands and feet show induration, erythema of palms and soles, desquamation of fingers and toes

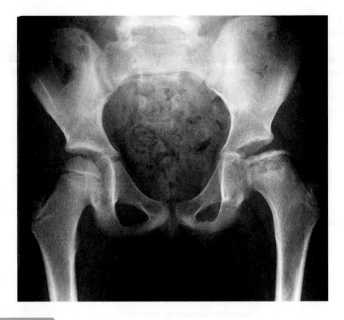

FIGURE 4.9

X-ray film of the hips of a 5-yr-old child with Legg-Calvé-Perthes dz. Note the ↑ density, flattening, and fragmentation of the left capital femoral epiphysis.

    c. Complications = cardiac involvement; 10%–40% of untreated cases show evidence of coronary vasculitis (dilation/aneurysm) within first weeks of illness

    d. Tx = IVIG to prevent coronary vasculitis, **high-dose aspirin—prednisone is contraindicated and will exacerbate the dz!**

    e. Px

       (1) Response to IVIG and aspirin is rapid, two thirds of pts afebrile within 24 hr

       (2) Evaluate pts 1 wk after discharge, repeat echocardiography 3–6 wk after onset of fever; if baseline and repeat echo do not detect any coronary abnormalities, further imaging is unnecessary

  3. Henoch-Schönlein Purpura

    a. Immunoglobulin IgA small-vessel vasculitis, related to IgA nephropathy (Berger's dz)

Table 4.7	Types of Juvenile Rheumatoid Arthritis
Systemic Still's dz (10%–20%)	• High, **spiking fevers** with return to nml daily, generalized lymphadenopathy • **Rash of small, pale pink macules with central pallor on trunk and proximal extremities with possible involvement of palms and soles** • **Rash classically appears with fever and wanes as fever goes away** • Joint involvement may not occur for wks to mo after fever • One third have disabling chronic arthritis
Pauciarticular (40%–60%)	• Involves ≤4 joints, large joints primarily affected (knees, ankles, elbows, asymmetric) • Other Si/Sx = fever, malaise, anemia, lymphadenopathy, **chronic joint dz is unusual** • Divided into 2 types ◊ Type 1 (most common) → girls <4 yr old, ↑ risk for chronic iridocyclitis, 90% antinuclear antibody (ANA)+ ◊ Type 2 → boys >8 yr old, ANA2, 75% HLA-B271, ↑ risk of ankylosing spondylitis or Reiter's later in life
Polyarticular	• ≥5 joints involved, small and large, insidious onset, fever, lethargy, anemia • Two types depending on whether or not rheumatoid factor is present • Rheumatoid factor ⊕ → 80% girls late onset, more severe, rheumatoid nodules present, 75% ANA+ • Rheumatoid factor 2 → occurs any time during childhood, mild, rarely associated with rheumatoid nodules, 25% ANA+

b. Si/Sx = **pathognomonic palpable purpura** on legs and buttocks (in children), abd pain, may cause intussusception

c. Tx = self-limited, rarely progresses to glomerulonephritis

C. **Histiocytosis X**

1. Proliferation of histiocytic cells resembling Langerhans' skin cells

2. Three Common Variants

a. Letterer-Siwe dz

(1) Acute, aggressive, disseminated variant, usually fatal in infants

(2) Si/Sx = hepatosplenomegaly, lymphadenopathy, pancytopenia, lung involvement, recurrent infxns

  b. Hand-Schüller-Christian
   (1) Chronic progressive variant, presents prior to age 5 yr
   (2) **Classic triad = skull lesions, diabetes insipidus, exophthalmus**
  c. Eosinophilic granuloma
   (1) Extraskeletal involvement generally limited to lung
   (2) Has the best Px, rarely fatal, sometimes spontaneously regresses

V. Metabolic

A. Congenital Hypothyroidism

1. Because of 2° agenesis of thyroid or defect in enzymes
2. **T_4 during first 2 yr of life is crucial for nml brain development**
3. Birth Hx → nml Apgar score, prolonged jaundice ($\neq$ indirect bilirubin)
4. Si/Sx = presents at age 6–12 wk with poor feeding, lethargy, **hypotonia, coarse facial features, large protruding tongue**, hoarse cry, constipation, developmental delay
5. Dx = $\downarrow T_4$, ↑ thyroid-stimulating hormone
6. Tx = levothyroxine replacement
7. **If Dx delayed beyond 6 wk, child will be mentally retarded**
8. Newborn screening is mandatory by law

B. Newborn Jaundice

1. Physiologic jaundice is clinically benign, occurs 24–48 hr after birth
 a. Characterized by unconjugated hyperbilirubinemia
 b. 50% of neonates have jaundice during first wk of life
 c. Results from ↑ bilirubin production and relative deficiency in glucuronyl transferase in the immature liver
 d. Requires no Tx
2. **Jaundice present AT birth is ALWAYS pathologic**
3. Unconjugated Hyperbilirubinemia
 a. Caused by hemolytic anemia or congenital deficiency of glucuronyl transferase (e.g., Crigler-Najjar and Gilbert's syndromes)
 b. Hemolytic anemia can be congenital or acquired
  (1) Congenital because of spherocytosis, glucose-6-phosphate dehydrogenase (G6PD), pyruvate kinase deficiency

(2) Acquired because of ABO/Rh isoimmunization, infxn, drugs, twin–twin transfusion, chronic fetal hypoxia, delayed cord clamping, maternal diabetes

4. Conjugated Hyperbilirubinemia (see Table 4.8)
   a. Infectious causes = sepsis, the ToRCH group, syphilis, *L. monocytogenes*, hepatitis
   b. Metabolic causes = galactosemia, a_1-antitrypsin deficiency
   c. Congenital causes = extrahepatic biliary atresia, Dubin-Johnson and Rotor syndromes

5. Tx = phototherapy with blue light (not ultraviolet (UV) light, which can harm skin and retina) to break down bilirubin pigments and Tx underlying cause

6. Tx urgently to prevent mental retardation 2° to kernicterus (bilirubin precipitation in basal ganglia)

C. Reye Syndrome

1. Acute encephalopathy and fatty degeneration of the liver associated with **use of salicylates in children with varicella or influenza-like illness**

2. Most cases in children age 4–12 yr old

3. Si/Sx = biphasic course with prodromal fever → aSx interval → abrupt onset vomiting, delirium, stupor, hepatomegaly with abnormal liver function tests, may rapidly progress to seizures, coma, and death

4. Dx = clinical $\oplus \uparrow\uparrow$ liver enzymes, nml cerebrospinal fluid (CSF)

5. Tx = control of ↑ intracranial pressure because of cerebral edema (major cause of death) with mannitol, fluid restriction,

Table 4.8	Differential Diagnosis of Neonatal Jaundice by Time of Onset
Within 24 hr of birth	• Hemolysis (ABO/Rh isoimmunization, hereditary spherocytosis) • Sepsis
Within 48 hr of birth	• Hemolysis • Infxn • Physiologic
After 48 hr	• Infxn • Hemolysis • Breast milk (liver not mature to handle lipids of breast milk) • Congenital malformation (biliary atresia) • Hepatitis

PEDIATRICS

give glucose because glycogen stores are commonly depleted

6. Px = ↑ chance to progress into coma if ≥3-fold ↑ in serum ammonia level, ↓ prothrombin not responsive to vitamin K

7. Recovery rapid in mild dz, severe dz may → neuropsychological defects

D. Febrile Seizures

1. Usually occurs between age 3 mo and 5 yr, associated with fever without evidence of CNS infxn or other defined cause

2. Most common convulsive order in young children, rarely develops into epilepsy

3. Risk = very high fever (≥102°F [39°C]) and FHx; seizure occurs during rise in temperature, not at the peak of temperature

4. Si/Sx = commonly tonic–clonic seizure with most lasting <10 min with a drowsy postictal period

5. Note: If seizure lasts >15 min, most likely because of infxn or toxic process and careful workup should follow

6. Dx = clinical, routine lab tests should be performed only to evaluate fever source, EEG not indicated unless febrile seizure is atypical (complex febrile seizure)

7. Consider lumbar puncture to rule out meningitis

8. Tx = careful evaluation for source of fever, control of fever with antipyretics, parental counseling, and reassurance to ↓ anxiety

9. Px = 33%–50% of children experience recurrence of seizure

VI. Genetic and Congenital Disorders

A. Failure to Thrive (FTT)

1. Failure of children to grow and develop at an appropriate rate

2. Because of inadequate calorie intake or inadequate calorie absorption

3. Can be idiopathic or because of gastroesophageal reflux, urinary tract infxns, cardiac dz, cystic fibrosis, hypothyroidism, congenital syndromes, lead poisoning, malignancy

4. Additional factors include poverty, family discord, neonatal problems, maternal depression

5. Dx requires three criteria

   a. Child <2 yr old with weight <3rd to 5th percentile for age on >1 occasion

b. Child <2 yr old whose weight is <80% of ideal weight for age

c. Child <2 yr old whose weight crosses 2 major percentiles downward on a standardized growth chart

d. Exceptions = children of genetically short stature, small-for-gestational-age infants, preterm infants, normally lean infants, "overweight" infants whose rate of height gain ↑ while rate of weight gain ↓

6. Tx

a. Organic causes → treat underlying condition and provide sufficient caloric supplementation

b. Idiopathic → observe the parent feeding the infant and educate parents on appropriate formulas, foods, and liquids for the infant

c. In older infants and children, it is important to offer solid foods before liquids, ↓ distractions during meal times, and child should eat with others and not be force-fed

d. Monitor closely for progressive weight gain in response to adequate calorie feeding

7. Px poor in first year of life because of maximal postnatal brain growth during the first 6 mo of life—one third of children with nonorganic FTT are developmentally delayed

B. **Craniofacial Abnormalities**

1. Mildest form is bifid uvula, no clinical significance

2. Cleft Lip (Figure 4.10)

a. Can occur unilaterally or bilaterally, because of failure of fusion of maxillary prominences

b. **Unilateral cleft lip is the most common malformation of the head and neck**

c. Does not interfere with feeding

d. Tx = surgical repair

3. Cleft Palate (Figure 4.10)

a. Can be anterior or posterior (determined by position relative to incisive foramen)

b. Anterior cleft palate because of failure of palatine shelves to fuse with primary palate

c. Posterior cleft palate because of failure of palatine shelves to fuse with nasal septum

d. **Interferes with feeding, requiring a special nipple for the baby to feed**

e. Tx = surgical repair

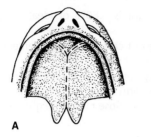
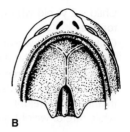
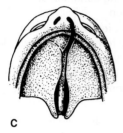
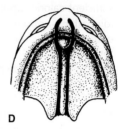
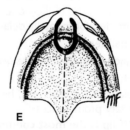

FIGURE 4.10

Different forms of cleft palate: **(A)** cleft uvula, **(B)** cleft soft and hard palate, **(C)** total unilateral cleft palate and cleft lip, **(D)** total bilateral cleft palate and cleft lip, and **(E)** bilateral cleft lip and jaw. (From Snell RS. *Clinical anatomy*, 7th Ed. Lippincott Williams & Wilkins. 2003.)

4. Macroglossia
   a. Congenitally enlarged tongue seen in Down's syndrome, gigantism, hypothyroidism
   b. Can be acquired in amyloidosis and acromegaly
   c. Different from glossitis (redness and swelling, with burning sensation) seen in vitamin B deficiencies
   d. Tx is directed at underlying cause

C. **Patau's Syndrome**
1. **Caused by trisomy 13**
2. Si/Sx → arrhinencephaly, holoprosencephaly

D. **Edward's Syndrome**
1. **Caused by trisomy 18**
2. Si/Sx → arrhinencephaly, corpus callosum agenesis, microcephaly

E. **Down's Syndrome**
1. **Invariably caused by trisomy 21, ↑ risk if maternal age >35 yr**
2. Si/Sx → cardiac septal defects, psychomotor retardation, classic Down's facies, ↑ risk of leukemia, premature Alzheimer's dz
3. Down's facies (Figure 4.11) = flattened occiput (brachycephaly), **epicanthal folds, up-slanted palpebral fissures, speckled irises (Brushfield spots)**, protruding tongue, small ears, redundant skin at posterior neck, **hypotonia, simian crease in palms (50%)**
4. Px = typically death in 30s–40s

F. **Turner's Syndrome**
1. **Number one cause of 1° amenorrhea**, because of XO genotype
2. Si/Sx = newborns have ↑ skin at dorsum of neck **(neck webbing) (Figure 4.12)**, lymphedema in hands and feet, as they develop → short stature, ptosis, **coarctation of aorta, amenorrhea but uterus is present**, juvenile external genitalia, bleeding because of GI telangiectasias, no mental retardation
3. Tx = hormone replacement to allow 2° sex characteristics to develop

G. **Fragile X Syndrome**
1. X-linked dominant trinucleotide repeat expansion disorder
2. **Number one cause of mental retardation in boys**
3. Si/Sx = long face, prominent jaw, large ears, enlarged testes (postpubertal), developmental delay, mental retardation
4. Tx = none

H. **Arnold-Chiari Malformation**
1. Congenital disorder
2. Si/Sx = caudally displaced cerebellum, elongated medulla passing into foramen magnum, flat skull base, hydrocephalus, meningomyelocele, and aqueductal stenosis
3. Px = death as neonate or toddler

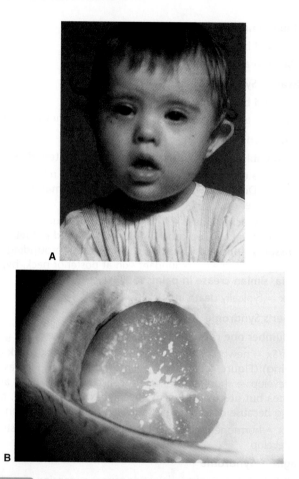

FIGURE 4.11

(A) Typical facial features of the child with Down's syndrome. (From Bickley LS, Szilagyi P. *Bates' guide to physical examination and history taking*, 8th Ed. Philadelphia: Lippincott Williams & Wilkins, 2003.) (B) Discrete flakes in the anterior and posterior cortex in a 26-yr-old man with Down's syndrome. An incomplete, cortical, star-shaped opacity is also evident. (From Tasman W, Jaeger E. *The Wills eye hospital atlas of clinical ophthalmology*, 2nd Ed. Philadelphia: Lippincott Williams & Wilkins, 2001.)

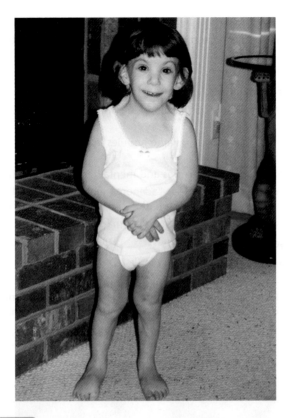

FIGURE 4.12

Neck webbing in a 3-yr-old girl with Turner's syndrome. (From Nettina SM. *The Lippincott manual of nursing practice*, 7th Ed. Lippincott Williams & Wilkins, 2001.)

I. **Neural Tube Defects**

1. Associated with ↑ α-fetoprotein levels in maternal serum

2. **Preventable by folic acid supplements during pregnancy**

3. Si/Sx = spina bifida (posterior vertebral arches do not close) and meningocele (no vertebrae cover lumbar cord)

4. Tx = prevention; neurologic deficits often remain after surgical correction

J. **Fetal Alcohol Syndrome**

1. Seen in children born to alcoholic mothers

2. Si/Sx = characterized by facial abnormalities and developmental defects (mental and growth retardation), **smooth philtrum of lip,** microcephaly, atrial septal defect (ASD)

3. Tx = prevention

K. **Tuberous Sclerosis**

1. Autosomal-dominant multinodular proliferation of multinucleated astrocytes

2. Forms small tubers = white nodules in cortex and periventricular areas

3. Characterized by seizures and mental retardation in infancy

4. Classic physical finding is "adenoma sebaceum" = small adenomas on the face in a distribution similar to acne (Figure 4.13)

5. Associated with rhabdomyosarcoma in children

L. **Congenital Pyloric Stenosis**

1. Causes projectile vomiting in first **2 wk–2 mo of life**

2. More common in boys and in first-born children

3. **Pathognomonic physical finding is palpable "olive" nodule in midepigastrium,** representing hypertrophied pyloric sphincter

4. If olive is not present, diagnosis made by Utz

5. Tx = longitudinal surgical incision in hypertrophied muscle

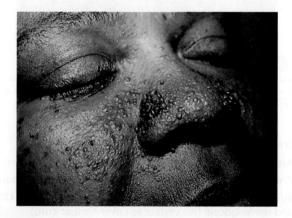

FIGURE 4.13

Tuberous sclerosis. This pt has adenoma sebaceum (angiofibromas). Note the similarity to acne lesions. (Hall J. *Sauer's manual of skin diseases,* 8th Ed. Philadelphia: Lippincott Williams & Wilkins, 2000.)

M. **Congenital Heart Dz**

1. ASD
   a. Usually aSx, often found on routine preschool physicals
   b. Predispose to congestive heart failure (CHF) in second and third decades, also predispose to stroke because of embolus bypass tract (Eisenmenger's complex)
   c. Si/Sx = loud S_1, **wide fixed-split S_2**, midsystolic ejection murmur
   d. = Echocardiography
   e. Tx = surgical patching of bypass, more important for females because of eventual ↑ cardiovascular stress of pregnancy

2. Ventricular Septal Defect (VSD)
   a. **Most common congenital heart defect**, 30% of small-to-medium defects close spontaneously by age 2 yr
   b. Si/Sx = small defects may be completely aSx throughout entire life, large defects → CHF, ↓ development/growth, frequent pulmonary infxns, holosystolic murmur over entire precordium, maximally at fourth left intercostal space
   c. Eisenmenger's complex = R → L shunt 2° to pulmonary HTN
      (1) Right ventricular (RV) hypertrophy → flow reversal through the shunt, so that an R → L shunt develops
      (2) Causes cyanosis 2° because of lack of blood flow to lung
      (3) Allows venous thrombi (e.g., deep venous thrombosis [DVT]) to bypass lung, causing systemic paradoxical embolization
   d. Dx = echocardiography
   e. Tx = complete closure for simple defects

3. Tetralogy of Fallot
   a. Four physical defects comprising the tetralogy (Figure 4.14A)
      (1) VSD
      (2) Pulmonary outflow obstruction
      (3) RV hypertrophy
      (4) Overriding aorta (aorta inlet spans both ventricles)
   b. Si/Sx = acyanotic at birth, ↑ cyanosis over first 6 mo, **"Tet spell"** = acute cyanosis and panic in child, child adopts a squatting posture to improve blood flow to lungs, **CXR shows classic boot-shaped contour** because of RV enlargement (Figure 4.14B)

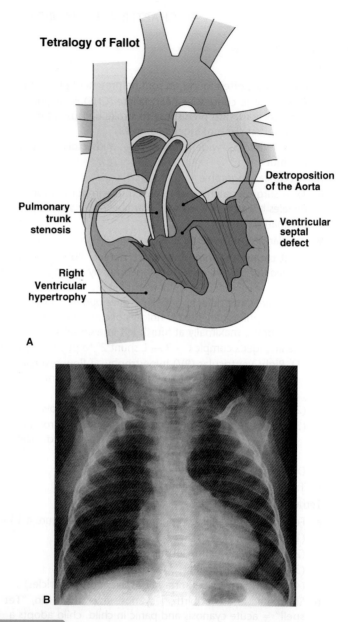

    c. Dx = echocardiography

    d. Tx = surgical repair of VSD, repair of pulmonary outflow tracts

4. Transposition of the Great Arteries

    a. Aorta comes off right ventricle, pulmonary artery off left ventricle

    b. Must have persistent arteriovenous communication or dz is incompatible with life (can be via patent ductus arteriosus [PDA] or persistent foramen ovale)

    c. Si/Sx = marked cyanosis at birth, early digital clubbing, often no murmur, **CXR → enlarged egg-shaped heart** and ↑ pulmonary vasculature

    d. Dx = echocardiography

    e. Tx = surgical switching of arterial roots to nml positions with repair of communication defect

    f. Px = invariably fatal within several mos of birth without Tx

5. Coarctation of the Aorta

    a. Congenital aortic narrowing, often aSx in young child

    b. Si/Sx = ↓ BP in legs with nml BP in arms, **continuous murmur over collateral vessels in back, classic CXR sign = rib notching**

    c. Dx confirmed with aortogram or CT

    d. Tx = surgical resection of coarctation and reanastomosis

6. PDA

    a. ↑ Incidence with premature births, predisposes pt to endocarditis and pulmonary vascular dz

    b. Si/Sx = **continuous machinery murmur heard best at second left interspace, wide pulse pressure,** hypoxia

    c. Dx = echocardiography or cardiac catheterization

    d. Tx = indomethacin (block prostaglandins, induces closure) for infants, surgical repair for older children

VII. Trauma and Intoxication

A. Child Abuse (see Figure 4.15)

1. Can be physical trauma, emotional, sexual, or neglect

2. Nutritional neglect is the most common etiology for under-weight infants

3. Most common perpetrator of sexual abuse is family member or family friends; 97% of reported offenders are males

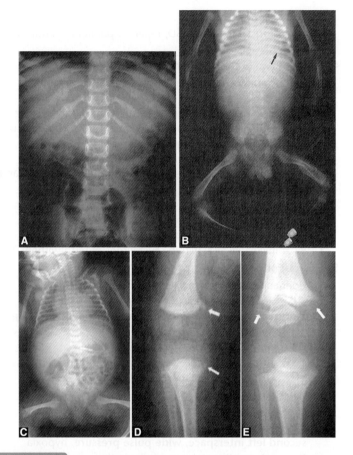

FIGURE 4.15

Skeletal survey in child abuse. **(A)** Infant with multiple old rib injuries and gastric distension. (From Reece RM, Ludwig S, eds. *Child abuse: medical diagnosis and management,* 2nd Ed. Philadelphia: Lippincott Williams & Wilkins, 2001, with permission.) **(B)** Radiograph of the trunk and extremities of a victim of child abuse showing healed misaligned fracture of the left femur and healing rib fractures (*arrow*) on the left. (From Jones NL. *Atlas of forensic pathology.* Philadelphia: Lippincott Williams & Wilkins, 1996, with permission.) **(C)** "Babygram": a single frontal radiograph of the long bones and axial skeleton may mask subtle injuries because of geometric distortion and exposure variation. **(D)** Frontal radiograph of the knee showing a characteristic metaphyseal "corner" fracture of the distal femur (*arrows*). **(E)** Another infant's knee demonstrating the typical and highly specific "bucket-handle" fracture of the distal femur (*arrows*). (A–E courtesy of Evan Geller. From Greenberg MI, Hendrickson RG, Silverberg M, et al. *Greenberg's text-atlas of emergency medicine.* Philadelphia: Lippincott Williams & Wilkins, 2004, with permission.)

4. **Physicians are required by law to report suspected child abuse or neglect (law provides protection to mandated reporters who report in good faith); clinical and lab evaluations are allowed without parental/guardian permission**

5. Epidemiology
   a. 85% of children reported to Child Protective Services (CPS) are <5 yr old, 45% are <1 yr old
   b. 10% of injuries to children <5 yr old seen in the emergency room (ER) are because of abuse, and 10% of abuse cases involve burns
   c. **High-risk children** = premature infants, children with chronic medical problems, colicky babies, those with behavioral problems, children living in poverty, children of teenage parents, single parents, or substance abusers

6. Si/Sx = injury is unexplainable or not consistent with Hx, bruises are the most common manifestation
   a. Accidental injuries seen on shins, forearms, hips
   b. Less likely to be accidental, are bilateral and symmetric, seen on buttocks, genitalia, back, back of hands, different color bruises (repeat injuries over time)
   c. Fractures highly suspicious for abuse: those because of pulling or wrenching, causing damage to the metaphysis

7. **Classic Findings**
   a. Chip fracture, where the corner of metaphysis of long bone is torn off with damage to epiphysis
   b. Periosteum spiral fracture before infant can walk
   c. Rib fractures

8. Dating fracture can be done by callus formation (callus appears in 10–12 days)

9. Burns
   a. Shape/pattern of burn may be diagnostic
   b. **Cigarette** → circular, punched out lesions of similar size, hands and feet common
   c. **Immersion** → most common in infants, affecting buttocks and perineum (hold thighs against abdomen), or with scalded line clearly demarcated on thighs or waist without splash marks
   d. Stocking-glove burn on hands or feet

10. Injury to head is the most common cause of death from physical abuse; infants can present with convulsions, apnea, ↑ intracranial

pressure, subdural hemorrhages, retinal hemorrhages (marker for acceleration/deceleration injuries), or in a coma

11. Sexual Abuse

   a. Child may talk to mother or teacher, friend, relative about situation

   b. Si/Sx = vaginal, penile, or rectal pain; erythema; discharge; bleeding; chronic dysuria; enuresis; constipation; encopresis

   c. Behaviors = sexualized activity with peers or objects, seductive behavior

12. Dx

   a. Labs → prothrombin time/partial thromboplastin time (PT/PTT) and platelets to screen for bleeding diathesis

   b. Consider bone survey in children <2 yr old, plain films or MRI for severe injuries or refusal/inability to communicate

   c. For sexual abuse, collect specimens of offender's sperm, blood, and hair; collect victim's nail clippings and clothing, obtain *Chlamydia* and *Gonorrhea* cultures from mouth, anus, and genitalia

   d. Dx is tentatively based on H&P, record all information, photograph when appropriate

13. Tx

   a. Medical, surgical, psychiatric Tx for injuries

   b. Report immediately, do not discharge before talking to CPS

   c. Admit pt if injuries are severe enough, if Dx is unclear, or if no other safe placement is available

B. **Poisonings**

   1. Accidental seen in younger children momentarily left unsupervised, usually a single agent ingested or inhaled (plants, household products, medications)

   2. Intentional seen in adolescents/adults, toxic substances for recreational purposes or overdose taken with intent to produce self-harm

   3. Epidemiology

      a. Nearly 50% of cases occur in children <6 yr old, as a result of an accidental event or as abuse

      b. 92% occur at home; 60% with nonpharmacologic agent, 40% with pharmacologic agent

      c. Ingestion occurs in 75% of cases, 8% dermal, 6% ophthalmic, 6% inhalation

Table 4.9 Pediatric Toxicology

Si/Sx	Possible Toxin
Lethargy/coma	Ethanol, sedative-hypnotics, narcotics, antihistamines, antidepressants, neuroleptic
Seizures	Theophylline, cocaine, amphetamines, antidepressants, antipsychotics, pesticides
Hypotension (with bradycardia)	Organophosphate pesticides, β-blockers
Arrhythmia	Tricyclic antidepressants, cocaine, digitalis, quinidine
Hyperthermia	Salicylates, anticholinergics

4. Hx is crucial during initial contact with pt or guardian
   a. Evaluation of severity (aSx, Sx)
   b. Age and weight
   c. Time, type, amount, and route of exposure
   d. Past medical Hx
5. Si/Sx (see Table 4.9)
6. Tx
   a. Syrup of ipecac followed by clear liquid (water) induces vomiting, should not use in children <6 mo old, those with depressed sensorium, pts with seizures, or those who ingested strong acids or bases
   b. Lavage usually unnecessary in children, may be useful with drugs that ↓ gastric motility
   c. Charcoal may be most effective and safest procedure to prevent absorption, repeat doses every 2–6 hr with cathartic for first dose; ineffective in heavy metal or volatile hydrocarbon poisoning

VIII. Adolescence

A. Epidemiology
1. Injuries
   a. 50% of all deaths in adolescents attributed to injuries
   b. Many occur under the influence of alcohol and other drugs
   c. Older adolescents more likely to be killed in motor vehicle accidents, whereas younger adolescents are at risk for drowning and fatal injuries with weapons

        d. Homicide rate is 5× higher for African American males than Caucasian males

  2. Suicide

      a. Second leading cause of adolescent death

      b. Females more likely to attempt than males but males are 5× more likely to succeed than females

      c. Pts with pre-existing psychiatric problems or those who abuse alcohol and drugs more likely to attempt suicide

  3. Substance Abuse

      a. Major cause of morbidity in adolescents

      b. Average age at first use is 12–14 yr

      c. 1 of every 2 adolescents has tried an illicit drug by high school graduation

      d. Survey of high school seniors (1994–1995) noted that 90% had experience with alcohol and ≥40% had tried marijuana

  4. Sex

      a. 61% of all male and 47% of all female high school students have had sex

      b. Health risks of early sexual activity are unwanted pregnancies and sexually transmitted dz (STDs) such as *Gonorrhea*, *Chlamydia*, and HIV

      c. 86% of all STDs occur among adolescents and young adults 15–29 yr old

      d. More than 1 million adolescent girls become pregnant yearly; 33% are <15 yr old—this is the second major cause of morbidity in adolescents

  5. Eating Disorders

      a. Anorexia nervosa occurs in 0.5% of adolescent girls and bulimia in 1%–3%

      b. Si/Sx = cardiovascular symptoms, fluid and electrolyte abnormalities, amenorrhea, ↓ bone density, anemia, parotid gland enlargement, tooth decay, constipation (hallmark of anorexia)

      c. Adolescents with anorexia lose 15% of ideal body weight and appear sick, but those with bulimia may look well nourished

      d. Anorexia nervosa is seen at 2 peak ages (14.5 yr and 18 yr), but 25% of girls with anorexia may be <13 yr old

B. Confidentiality

  1. Most issues revealed by adolescents to physicians in an interview are confidential

2. **Exceptions** include suicidal or homicidal behavior or sexual or physical abuse

3. Physicians are strongly encouraged to inform adolescents about confidentiality at the beginning of the interview to help develop a trusting relationship between adolescent and physician

C. Screening

1. Annual risk behavior screening in every adolescent is strongly recommended

2. **HEADSSS** assessment allows physicians to evaluate critical areas in each adolescent's life that may be detrimental to growth and development

   a. **H**ome environment → who does adolescent live with?; any recent changes?; quality of parental interaction (if applicable)?; has s/he ever run away from home?

   b. **E**mployment and **E**ducation → is child in school?; favorite subjects?; academic performance?; are friends in school?; any recent changes?; does child have a job?; future plans?

   c. **A**ctivities → what does child like to do in spare time?; who does child spend time with?; involved in any sports/exercise?; hobbies?; attends parties or clubs?

   d. **D**rugs → has child ever used tobacco?; alcohol?; marijuana?; other illicit drugs?; if so, when was the child's last use?; how often?; do friends or family members use drugs?; who does the child use these substances with?

   e. **S**exual activity → sexual orientation?; is child sexually active?; number of sexual partners?; does the child use condoms or other forms of contraception?; any Hx of STDs or pregnancy?

   f. **S**uicide → does the child ever feel sad, tired, or unmotivated?; has the child ever felt that life was not worth living?; any feelings of wanting to harm self?; if so, does the child have a plan?; has the child ever tried to harm self in the past?; does the child know anyone who has attempted suicide?

   g. **S**afety → does the child use a seat belt or bike helmet?; does the child enter into high-risk situations?; does the child have access to a firearm?

PEDIATRICS

5. FAMILY MEDICINE

I. Headache

A. **Si/Sx and DDx (Table 5.1)**

B. **Dx**

1. **Temporal arteritis Dx requires temporal artery Bx**
2. **Trigeminal neuralgia Dx requires head CT or MRI** to rule out sinusitis, cerebellopontine angle neoplasm, multiple sclerosis, or herpes zoster
3. **Subarachnoid hemorrhage requires** confirmation by CT scan or lumbar puncture to detect CSF xanthochromia (can be detected 6 hrs after onset of headache)
4. Suspect intracranial lesion causing headache in **pts >50 or pts with headaches immediately upon waking up**
5. **Suspect** ↑ **intracranial pressure (ICP) in pts awakened in middle of night by headache, who have projectile vomiting, or who have focal neural deficits; obtain head CT**

C. **Tx (Table 5.2)**

II. Ears, Nose, and Throat

A. **Otitis Externa**

1. **Ear pain, itchy, draining ear, pulling on pinna or pushing on tragus causes pain (Figure 5.1)**
   a. **Bacterial**
      (1) *Pseudomonas* is usual cause in swimmers, diabetics, or pts with eczema
      (2) Tx = fluoroquinolone ear drops, keep water out of ears, may need wick placed in canal to facilitate distribution of ear drops within external auditory canal and prevent closure of canal
   b. **Fungal**
      (1) Otomycosis is commonly caused by *Candida* or *Aspergillus*
      (2) Tx = acetic acid ear drops, nystatin and triamcinilone ointment to canal, water precautions

Table 5.1 Summary of Headaches

Type	Epidemiology	Characteristics
Tension	Usually after age 20 yr (rarely after age 50 yr)	• Most common headache type • **Bilateral, band-like, dull in quality** • Worse with stress; not aggravated by activity • Chronic headache associated with depression
Cluster	**Male**/female = 6:1; Mean age 30 yr	• **Unilateral**, stabbing peri/retro-orbital pain, lasting 15 min to 3 hr • Seasonal attacks occur in series (6×/day) lasting wks, followed by mo of remission • **Associated with ipsilateral lacrimation (85%), ptosis, nasal congestion, and rhinorrhea** • Often occurs within 90 min of onset of sleep
Migraine	80% have positive FHx **Female**/male = 3:1	• Classically, headache is **unilateral (60%)** with **aura (only 15%)**; pt looks for quiet place to rest • Visual aura: **scotoma** (blind spots), **teichopsia** (jagged zigzag lines), **photopsias** (shimmering lights), or **rhodopsins** (colors) • Accompanied by **nausea and photophobia** • Triggered by stress, odors, certain foods, alcohol, menstruation, or sleep deprivation
Temporal arteritis (giant cell)	**Female**/male = 2:1 Age >50 yr	• **Unilateral temporal** headache • **Associated with jaw claudication, temporal artery tenderness with palpation, ESR ≥50** • 50% also have polymyalgia rheumatica • If not treated leads to optic neuritis and **blindness** • Screen by ESR; Dx with temporal artery Bx

FAMILY MEDICINE

(continued)

Table 5.1 *Continued*

Type	Epidemiology	Characteristics
Trigeminal neuralgia	Peak age at 60 yr	• Episodic, severe pain shooting from side of mouth to ipsilateral ear, eye, or nose
Withdrawal headache		• Common cause of frequent headaches • Can be withdrawal from various drugs
Subarachnoid hemorrhage		• Head trauma is most common cause • Spontaneous: usually berry aneurysm rupture • Classically the "worst headache of my life"
Temporal mandibular joint (TMJ) disorders	Can be related to osteoarthritis or previous trauma to TMJ	• Temporomandibular disorders (TMD), medical and dental conditions affecting the TMJ, and/or the muscles of mastication • Si/Sx = chronic ear pain, headache, jaw stiffness, facial pain, pain with chewing, jaw joint pain, jaw joint noises, and grinding (Bruxism) or clenching one's teeth

   c. **Viral**

      (1) Ramsay Hunt syndrome (herpes zoster oticus) caused by reactivation of Varicella Zoster Virus (VZV) in the geniculate ganglia (CN VII)

      (2) Si/Sx = painful vesicles in external auditory meatus

      (3) Tx = acyclovir to prevent progression to meningitis and facial nerve palsy

  2. In diabetics, get CT/MRI of temporal bone to rule out osteomyelitis and malignant otitis externa, which requires surgical debridement

  3. Gradenigo Syndrome = osteomeylitis of petrous apex bone causing ipsilateral otorrhea, eye pain, abducens paralysis (CN VI), and diplopia, requiring emergency referral to Neurosurgery or Neuro-otology

Table 5.2   Treatment of Headache

Headache	Tx
Tension	• NSAIDs or acetaminophen • Prophylaxis with antidepressants or β-blockers
Cluster	• Acutely 100% O_2, sumatriptan,[a] or dihydroergotamine • Prophylaxis with verapamil, lithium, methysergide, or ergotamine
Migraine	• Acutely sumatriptan,[a] dihydroergotamine, NSAIDs, antiemetics • Prophylaxis with **β-blockers** (first line) or calcium blockers
Temporal arteritis	• Start Tx with corticosteroids as soon as suspected to avoid blindness • Never delay Tx while awaiting confirmatory Bx results
Trigeminal neuralgia	• Carbamazepine (first line) or phenytoin, clonazepam, valproic acid
Withdrawal	• NSAIDs
Subarachnoid hemorrhage	• Immediate neurosurgical evaluation and nimodipine to reduce incidence of post-rupture vasospasm and ischemia
Temporal mandibular joint disorders	• NSAIDs/relaxation techniques/stress reduction • Muscle relaxants • Dental appliance (mouth guard) • Provide muscle relaxation and support for the jaw joints (TMJ) • Refer to dental/oral surgery

[a]Sumatriptan contraindicated with known coronary dz or ergot drugs taken within 24 hr.

B. **Inner Ear Dz**
1. Tinnitus (Ringing in the Ears)
   a. Objective (heard by observer) or subjective (heard only by pt)
   b. Causes = foreign body in external canal, pulsating vascular tumors, or medications (aspirin), hearing loss
   c. Dx = obtain audiogram to assess hearing thresholds
   d. Tx underlying cause, hearing aids may help with hearing loss related tinnitus
2. Vertigo is the feeling that the surroundings are spinning when eyes are open, whereas in dizziness pt feels as if s/he, not the surroundings, is spinning (Table 5.3)

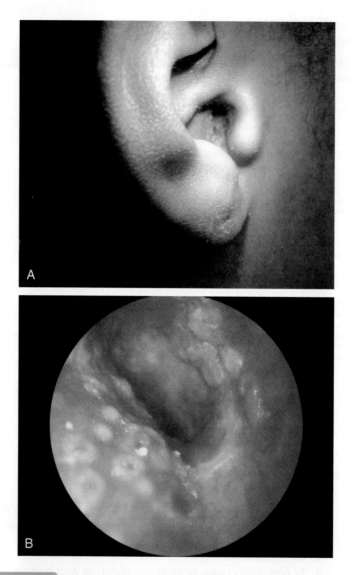

FIGURE 5.1

Otitis externa. **(A)** View of infected ear. (Courtesy of Christy Salvaggio. From Greenberg MI, Hendrickson RG, Silverberg M, et al. *Greenberg's text-atlas of emergency medicine.* Philadelphia: Lippincott Williams & Wilkins, 2004, with permission.) **(B)** External auditory canal. (From Benjamin B, Hawke M, Stammberger H. *A color atlas of otorhinolaryngology.* Philadelphia: JB Lippincott, 1995, with permission.)

Table 5.3 Causes of Vertigo

Dz	Characteristics	Tx
Benign positional vertigo	• Sudden, episodic vertigo with head movement lasting for secs	Epley maneuver
Ménière's dz	• Dilation of membranous labyrinth resulting from excess endolymph • **Classic triad = aural fullness (hearing loss), tinnitus, and episodic vertigo lasting several hours**	1) Low sodium, low caffeine diet 2) Medical (thiazide diuretics, anticholinergics, antihistamines) 3) Surgery as a last resort
Viral labyrinthitis	• Preceded by viral respiratory illness • Vertigo lasting days to weeks	Meclizine, vestibular rehab
Acoustic neuroma	• CN VIII schwannoma, commonly affects vestibular portion but can also affect cochlea • Si/Sx = vertigo, sudden deafness, tinnitus • Dx = MRI of cerebellopontine angle	Local radiation or surgical excision

C. **Hearing Loss**
  1. Sensorineural Hearing Loss
     a. 2° to sensory damage of the organ of corti in the cochlea or retrocochlear damage such as from an acoustic neuroma or other CN VIII nerve damage
     b. May be of sudden onset, but most often slowly progressive
        (1) Presbycusis—gradual loss of high frequency hearing as a person ages
        (2) Sudden hearing loss is an emergency and immediate ENT referral should be made for appropriate Dx and Tx
        (3) Bilateral hearing loss commonly associated with drugs; i.e., loop diuretics, aminoglycosides, salicylates, and cisplatin
     c. Potential causes include idiopathic, acoustic neuroma, congenital genetic, autoimmune, infxn, inheritance, trauma, or toxins affecting nerve or cochlea
     d. Alport's syndrome
        (1) Autoimmune sensorineural hearing loss, lens dislocation, hematuria

       (2) Most likely X-linked dominant inheritance

       (3) Thinning glomerular basement membrane and glomerulonephritis resulting in hematuria

    e. Congenital—refers to sensorineural hearing loss at birth, does not specify etiology

       (1) Etiologies include genetic, infectious; i.e., exposure of fetus to CMV, rubella or syphilis in utero

       (2) Tx = hearing aids, cochlear implants and steroids commonly used. ENT consult recommended

2. Conductive Hearing Loss

    a. Due to malfunction of conduction pathway such as damage or obstruction affecting middle ear or external ear

    b. Examples include otitis media, excess cerumen, otosclerosis, cholesteatoma, or perforated tympanic membrane

    c. Mixed hearing loss (sensorineural and conductive) can be seen in chronic middle ear infxn

    d. Usually correctable with surgery or appropriate Tx

    e. Pts often benefit from hearing aids

3. Diagnostic Hearing Tests

    a. Weber's test

       (1) Vibrating tuning fork (512 Hz) is placed midline on top of head

       (2) Lateralization of hearing to one ear more than the other indicates ipsilateral conductive loss or contralateral sensorineural loss

    b. Rinne's test (comparison of air conduction to bone conduction)

       (1) Vibrating tuning fork (512 Hz) placed next to ear, then when no longer heard placed against mastoid process until no longer heard

       (2) Normally air conduction should persist twice as long as bone conduction

       (3) Positive Rinne = air conduction heard longer and louder than bone conduction (this is the nml finding)

       (4) Negative Rinne = bone conduction is heard longer than air conduction, indicating a conductive hearing loss in that ear

    c. Audiogram

       (1) A graphic representation of a pt's pure-tone responses to various auditory frequency stimuli (250–8000 Hz)

(2) Should be obtained in all pts with changes in hearing or new onset tinnitus or vertigo

(3) Hearing is considered nml when hearing thresholds are less than 20 decibels

(4) Air-bone gaps (a difference between the air conduction and the bone conduction lines) exist when there is a conductive hearing loss

(5) Asymmetric hearing loss may be indicative of an acoustic neuroma and further testing is needed with auditory brain response measurements and/or MRI with gadolinium

D. **Epistaxis**

1. Most commonly involve nasal septum.

2. Blood supply of septum: anterior and posterior ethmoidal arteries, sphenopalatine artery, nasal septal branch of labial artery, greater palatine artery, all converging in anterior septum in Little's area or Kiesselbach's plexus

3. 90% of bleeds occur at Kiesselbach's plexus (anterior nasal septum)

4. Posterior bleeding more common in elderly

5. Blood supply to septum: anterior and posterior ethmoids → internal carotid artery, sphenopalatine, labial, and greater palatine → external carotid

6. **No. 1 cause of epistaxis in children is trauma (induced by exploring digits)**

7. Also precipitated by rhinitis, nasal mucosa dryness, septal deviation and bone spurs, alcohol, antiplatelet medication, bleeding diathesis, cocaine abuse, chronic HTN, and hereditary hemorrhagic telangiectasia

8. Tx

   a. Direct pressure, topical nasal vasoconstrictors; i.e., oxymetazoline, phenylephrine, silver nitrate cautery (don't cauterize same location on both sides of septum to prevent septal perforation)

   b. Consider anterior nasal packing if unable to stop

   c. Five percent origination in posterior nasal cavity requiring packing to occlude choanae—pts with posterior packing or balloon should be admitted to hospital for airway observation as they are at ↑ risk for hypoventilation and ↓ oxygen saturations

   d. Interventional radiology embolization of affected vessels

    e. Surgical ligation of internal maxillary artery, ethmoidal arteries, or affected vessels to stop bleeding

    f. Pts need to be placed on antistaphylococcal prophylaxis meds while nose is packed.

    g. Topical vasoconstrictors may be contraindicated in pts with HTN

    h. Repeat bleeding should prompt hematologic workup for bleeding diathesis; i.e., hemophilia, von Willebrand's dz, platelet function defects

E. **Sinusitis**

    1. Maxillary sinuses most commonly involved

    2. DDx **(Table 5.4)**

    3. Dx = CT scan showing inflammatory changes or bone destruction (Figure 5.2)

    4. Potential complications of sinusitis include meningitis, abscess formation, orbital infxn, osteomyelitis

Table 5.4 Sinusitis

	Organisms	Si/Sx	Tx
Acute bacterial (<4 wk)	*Streptococcus pneumoniae, Haemophilus influenzae, Moraxella catarrhalis*	**Purulent rhinorrhea**, headache, **pain on sinus palpation**, fever, **halitosis**, anosmia, **tooth pain**	Saline nasal lavage, decongestants, antibiotics (TMP-SMX or amoxicillin) can be considered
Chronic bacterial (>3 mo)	*Bacteroides, S. aureus, Pseudomonas, Streptococcus* spp.	Same as for acute but lasts longer, risk of progression to brain abscess or sphenoid sinus thrombophlebitis, loss of vision, and/or cavernous sinus thrombosis	Saline nasal lavage, nasal steroids if related to allergies; surgical correction of obstruction (e.g., septal deviation or nasal polyps); antibiotics controversial
Fungal	*Aspergillus*—**diabetics get** Mucormycosis!	Usually seen in immunocompromised pts, black nasal turbinates	Emergent antifungal Tx, emergent surgery

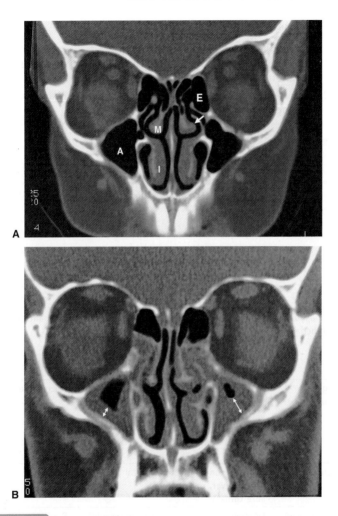

FIGURE 5.2

Coronal CT scan. **(A)** Nml sinuses. Note the excellent demonstration of the bony margins. The *arrow* points to the middle meatus into which the maxillary antrum and frontal, anterior, and middle ethmoid sinuses drain. A, maxillary antrum; E, ethmoid sinus; I, inferior turbinate; M, middle turbinate. **(B)** Sinusitis. Mucosal thickening prevents drainage of the sinuses. Both antra are almost opaque. The *arrows* indicate mucosal thickening in the antra. (From Armstrong P, Wastie ML. *Diagnostic imaging*, 4th Ed. Oxford: Blackwell Scientific, 1998, with permission.)

FAMILY MEDICINE

F. **Pharyngitis (Table 5.5)**

G. **Peritonsillar Abscess (Quinsy)**

   1. Loculation of pus in the peritonsillar space (between tonsil and superior constrictor)

   2. May be related to previous tonsillar infxn, dental caries, or allergies

Table 5.5 Pharyngitis

Dz	Si/Sx	Dx	Tx
Group A Strep throat	High fever, severe throat pain without cough, edematous tonsils with white or yellow exudate, cervical adenopathy	• H&P 50% accurate • Antigen agglutination kit for screening • Throat swab culture is gold standard	Penicillin to prevent acute rheumatic fever
Membranous (diphtheria)	High fever, dysphagia, drooling, **can cause respiratory failure** (airway occlusion)	**Pathognomonic gray membrane on tonsils extending into throat**	**STAT antitoxin**
Fungal (*Candida*)	Dysphagia, sore throat with white, cheesy patches in oropharynx (oral thrush), **seen in AIDS and small children**	Clinical or endoscopy	Fluconazole
Adenovirus	**Pharyngoconjunctival fever (fever, red eye, sore throat)**	Clinical	Supportive
Mononucleosis (Ebstein-Barr virus)	Generalized lymphadenopathy, exudative tonsillitis, palatal petechiae, splenomegaly	• ⊕ **Heterophile antibody** • **skin rash** in pts given ampicillin	Supportive. Pt should avoid contact sports to avoid splenic rupture due to splenomegaly
Herpangina (coxsackie A)	Fever, pharyngitis, body ache, tender vesicles along tonsils, uvula, and soft palate	Clinical	Supportive

3. May be caused by anaerobic bacteria, but mostly caused by same agents seen in pharyngitis and tonsillitis

4. Si/Sx = fever, drooling, odynophagia, trismus, and a muffled voice, soft palate and uvula are displaced and peritonsillar fluctuant swelling that is extremely painful to touch

5. Tx = airway stabilization, incision and drainage, antibiotic Tx, and fluids, Quinsy tonsillectomy immediately versus wait 6 wk and perform tonsillectomy

H. **Lemierre's Syndrome**

1. Thrombophleitis of internal jugular (IJ) vein

2. Usually 2° to oropharyngeal infxn with anaerobic Gram-negative rods, most commonly *Fusobacterium necrophorum*

3. Si/Sx = severe odynophagia, dysphagia, fevers, chills, rigors, neck swelling or pain, occasionally a palpable cord may be felt along IJ clot, septic emboli commonly metastasize to lungs forming cavitations and abscesses

4. Tx = antibiotics targeting *F. necrophorum* and other oral facultative anaerobes, and possible surgical drainage of abscesses or surgical ligation of clot if unresponsive to antibiotics and continued emboli

I. **Retropharyngeal Abscess**

1. An abscess formed from breakdown and necrosis of enlarged lymph nodes in retropharyngeal space

2. More common in children and usually following a severe pharyngeal infxn or longstanding upper respiratory infxn

3. Si/Sx = toxic appearing, drooling stridor, high fever, head tilted to one side, dysphagia, odynophagia. Unilateral bulging noted within oropharynx

4. Dx = CT scan with contrast, lateral neck, airway fluoroscopy

5. Tx = Stabilize airway, IV antibiotics, ENT consult and surgery if Sx don't improve or pt unstable

III. Outpatient Gastrointestinal Complaints

A. **Dyspepsia**

1. Si/Sx = upper abd pain, early satiety, postprandial abd bloating or distention, nausea, vomiting, often exacerbated by eating

2. DDx = peptic ulcer, gastroesophageal reflux dz (GERD), CA, gastroparesis, malabsorption, intestinal parasite, drugs (e.g., NSAIDs), etc.

3. Dx = clinical

4. Tx = empiric for 4 wk, if Sx not relieved → endoscopy

   a. Avoid caffeine, alcohol, cigarettes, NSAIDs; eat frequent small meals; reduce stress; maintain ideal body weight; elevate head of bed

   b. H_2 blockers and antacids, or proton pump inhibitor

   c. Empiric **antibiotics for *Helicobacter pylori* are NOT indicated for nonulcer dyspepsia**

B. **GERD**

1. Causes = obesity, relaxed lower esophageal sphincter, esophageal dysmotility, hiatal hernia

2. Si/Sx = heartburn occurring 30–60 min post-prandial and upon reclining, usually relieved by antacid self-administration, dyspepsia, postprandial burning sensation in esophagus, regurgitation of gastric contents into the mouth, cough, hoarseness, globus sensation

3. Atypical Si/Sx sometimes seen = asthma, chronic cough/laryngitis, atypical chest pain

4. Upper endoscopy → tissue damage but may be nml in 50% of cases

5. Dx = clinical, can confirm with ambulatory pH monitoring

6. Tx

   a. First line = lifestyle modifications: avoid lying down post-prandial, avoid spicy foods and foods that delay gastric emptying, reduce meal size, lose weight

   b. If medications, proton pump inhibitors are the most effective option long term with H_2 receptor antagonists useful for rapid onset and breakthrough Sx

   c. Often will require maintenance Tx since Sx return upon discontinuation

   e. For severe, refractory dz, can consider surgical fundoplication, relieves Sx in 90% of pts, may be more cost-effective in younger pts or those with severe dz

7. Sequelae

   a. **Barrett's esophagus** (Figure 5.3)

      (1) Chronic GERD → metaplasia from squamous to columnar epithelia in lower esophagus

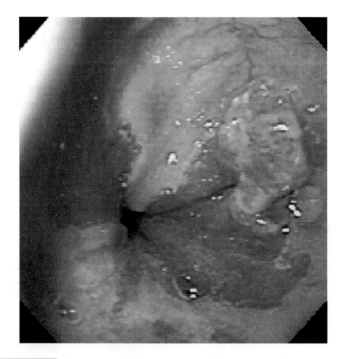

FIGURE 5.3

Barrett's esophagus with an early adenoCA identified on surveillance endoscopy. (From Yamada T, Alpers DH, Kaplowitz N, et al, eds. *Atlas of gastroenterology*, 3rd Ed. Philadelphia: Lippincott Williams & Wilkins, 2003, with permission.)

        (2) Requires close surveillance with endoscopy and aggressive Tx as 30% progress to **adenoCA**

        (3) Multiple FDA approved Tx, including radiofrequency ablation, photodynamic Tx, cryotherapy, endoscopic mucosal resection

    b. Peptic stricture

        (1) Results in gradual solid food dysphagia often with concurrent improvement of heartburn Sx

        (2) Endoscopy establishes Dx

        (3) Requires aggressive proton pump inhibitor Tx and surgical opening if unresponsive

C. Diarrhea

  1. Diarrhea = stool weight >300 g/day (nml = 100–300 g/day)

  2. Small-bowel dz → stools typically voluminous, watery, and fatty

3. Large-bowel dz → stools smaller in volume but more frequent
4. Prominent vomiting suggests viral enteritis or *Staphylococcus aureus* food poisoning
5. Malabsorption diarrhea characterized by high-fat content
   a. Lose fat-soluble vitamins, iron, calcium, and B vitamins
   b. Can cause iron deficiency, megaloblastic anemia (B_{12} loss), and hypocalcemia
6. General Tx = oral rehydration, IV fluids, and electrolytes (supportive)
7. Specific diarrheas (Table 5.6)
8. Common infectious pathogens for diarrhea (Table 5.7)

Table 5.6	Diarrheas		
Type	**Characteristics**	**Dx**	**Tx**
Infectious	• **#1 Cause of acute diarrhea** • Causes include Enterovirus spp. and **Norwalk virus (cause of cruise-ship diarrhea),** which cause noninflammatory diarrhea, bacteria that cause inflammatory diarrhea (Campylobacter #1, *E. coli* for traveler's diarrhea, *Salmonella, Shigella, Clostridium difficile* with antibiotic exposure), and parasites (*Giardia, Entamoeba, Cryptosporidium*) • Si/Sx = vomiting, pain; blood/mucus, and fevers/chills suggest invasive dz	• Stool leukocytes, Gram stain and culture, Ova and parasites (O&P) for parasitic • *C. difficile* toxin test	• Ciprofloxacin for patients with fever or those with inflammatory diarrhea or positive stool culture for a diarrheal bacterial pathogen • Metronidazole or oral vancomycin for *C. difficile*[a]

Table 5.6 *Continued*

Type	Characteristics	Dx	Tx
Osmotic	• Causes = lactose intolerance, oral Mg, sorbitol/mannitol	• ↑ Osmotic gap • Check fecal fat	• Withdraw inciting agent
Secretory	• Causes = toxins (cholera), enteric viruses, ↑ dietary fat	• Nml osmotic gap • Fasting → no change	• Supportive
Exudative	• Mucosal inflammation → plasma and serum leakage • Causes = enteritis, TB, colon CA, inflammatory bowel dz	• ↑ ESR & CRP • Radiologic imaging or colonoscopy to visualize intestine	• Varies by cause (see appropriate section of text)
Rapid transit	• Causes = laxatives, surgical excision of intestinal tissue	• Hx of surgery or laxative use	• Supportive
Encopresis	• Oozing around fecal impaction in children or sick elderly	• Hx of constipation	• Fiber-rich diet and laxatives
Celiac sprue	• Gluten allergy (wheat, barley, rye, oats contain gluten) • Si/Sx = weakness, failure to thrive, growth retardation • Classic rash = **dermatitis herpetiformis** = pruritic, red papulovesicular lesions on shoulders, elbows and knees • 10%–15% of pts develop intestinal lymphoma	**Antiendomysial, antitissue transglutaminase, and antigliadin antibodies typically positive: Dx confirmed by small-bowel Bx - pathognomonic blunting of villi**	Avoid dietary gluten
Tropical sprue	• Diarrhea probably caused by a tropical infxn	Dx = clinical	Tetracycline ⊕ folate

(continued)

Table 5.6 *Continued*

Type	Characteristics	Dx	Tx
Tropical sprue *(continued)*	• Si/Sx = glossitis, diarrhea, weight loss, steatorrhea		
Whipple's dz	• GI infxn by *Tropheryma whippelii* • Si/Sx = diarrhea, arthritis, rash, anemia	Dx = Bx → p-aminosalicylic acid (PAS) ⊕ macrophages in intestines	Penicillin or tetracycline
Lactase deficiency	• Most of world is lactase deficient as adults, losing the deficiency as they emerge from adolescence • Si/Sx = abd pain, diarrhea, flatulence after ingestion of any lactose-containing product	Dx = clinical	Avoid lactose or take exogenous lactase
Intestinal lymphangiectasia	• Seen in children, congenital or acquired dilation of intestinal lymphatics leads to marked GI protein loss • Si/Sx = diarrhea, hypoproteinemia, edema	Dx = jejunal Bx	Supportive
Pancreas dz	• Typically seen in pancreatitis and cystic fibrosis due to deficiency of pancreatic digestive enzymes • Si/Sx = foul-smelling steatorrhea, megaloblastic anemia (folate deficiency), weight loss	Hx of prior pancreatic dz	Pancrease supplementation

*aVancomycin is more effective for severe dz.
CRP, C-reactive protein.

Table 5.7 Infectious Causes of Diarrhea

	Bacterial	Viral	Parasitic
Etiology	E. coli, Shigella, Salmonella, Campylobacter jejuni, Vibrio parahaemolyticus, Vibrio cholera, Yersinia enterocolitica	Rotavirus Norwalk virus	Giardia lambia, Cryptosporidium, Entamoeba histolytica
Tx	Ciprofloxacin	Supportive	Metronidazole

IV. Urogenital Complaints

A. Urinary Tract Infxn (UTI)

1. Epidemiology
   a. 40% of females have ≥1 UTI, 8% have bacteriuria at a given time
   b. Most common in sexually active young women, elderly, posturethral catheter or instrumentation—rare in males (↑ risk with prostate dz)
   c. Caused by *Escherichia coli* (80%), *Staphylococcus saprophyticus* (15%), other Gram-negative rods
2. Si/Sx = **burning during urination,** urgency, sense of incomplete bladder emptying, hematuria, lower abd pain, nocturia
3. Systemic Sx = fever, chills, **back pain suggest pyelonephritis**
4. Dx = **Urinalysis (UA)** → **pyuria;** ⊕ bacteria on Gram stain; ⊕ culture results
5. Tx = fluoroquinolone, narrow based on cultures
6. Men cured within 7 days of Tx do not warrant further workup, but **adolescents and men with pyelonephritis or recurrent infxn require renal Utz and IV pyelogram (IVP) to rule out anatomic etiology**
7. UTI 2° to bacterial prostatitis requires 6–12 wk of antibiotics
8. aSx bacteriuria
   a. Defined as urine culture >100,000 colony-forming units (CFUs)/mL but no Sx
   b. Only Tx in (i) pregnant pts (use penicillins or nitrofurantoin), or (ii) pts with renal transplant, (iii) about to undergo genitourinary procedure, (iv) severe vesicular-ureteral reflux, or (v) struvite calculi

FAMILY MEDICINE

B. **Sexually Transmitted Dz (STDs) (Table 5.8). See Section C for AIDS.**

C. **Acquired Immunodeficiency Syndrome (AIDS)**

1. Epidemiology
   a. AIDS is a global pandemic (currently the fastest spread is in southeast Asia and central Europe)
   b. **Heterosexual transmission is the most common mode worldwide**
   c. Homosexual transmission is still the most common mode in the US, but IV drug users and their sex partners are the fastest growing population of human immunodeficiency virus (HIV) ⊕ pts

2. HIV Biology
   a. Retrovirus with the usual *gag, pol,* and *env* genes
   b. p24 is a core protein encoded by *gag* gene, can be used clinically to follow dz progression
   c. gp120 and gp41 are envelope glycoproteins that are produced on cleavage of gp160, coded by *env*
   d. Reverse transcriptase (coded by *pol*) converts viral RNA to DNA, so it can integrate into the host's DNA
   e. Cellular entry is by binding to both CD4 and an additional ligand (can be CXCR4, CCR5, others) that typically is a cytokine receptor
   f. HIV can infect CD4⊕ T cells, macrophages, thymic cells, astrocytes, dendritic cells, and others
   g. The mechanisms of T cell destruction are not well understood but probably include direct cell lysis, induction of cytotoxic T lymphocyte responses against infected CD4⊕ cells, and exhaustion of bone marrow production (suppression of production of T cells)
   h. In addition, the virus induces alterations in host cytokine patterns, rendering surviving lymphocytes ineffective

3. Dz Course
   a. In most pts, AIDS is relentlessly progressive and death occurs within 10–15 yr of HIV infxn
   b. Long-term survivors
      (1) Up to 5% of pts are "long-term survivors," meaning the dz does not progress even after 15–20 yr without Tx
      (2) This may be the result of infxn with defective virus, a potent host immune response, or genetic resistance of the host

Table 5.8 Sexually Transmitted Diseases

Dz	Characteristics	Tx
Herpes simplex virus (HSV)	• Most common cause of genital ulcers (causes 60%–70% of cases) • Si/Sx = **painful vesicular and ulcerated** lesions 1- to 3-mm diameter, onset 3–7 days after exposure • Lesions generally resolve over 7 days • 1° infxn also characterized by malaise, low-grade fever, and inguinal adenopathy in 40% of pts • Recurrent lesions are similar appearing, but milder in severity and shorter in duration, lasting approximately 2–5 days • Dx confirmed with direct fluorescent antigen (DFA) staining, Tzanck prep, serology, HSV PCR, or culture	• Tx = acyclovir, famciclovir, or valacyclovir to ↓ duration of viral shedding and shorten initial course
Pelvic inflammatory dz (PID)	• *Chlamydia trachomatis* and *Neisseria gonorrhea* are 1° pathogens, but PID is polymicrobial involving both aerobic and anaerobic bacteria • PID includes endometritis, salpingitis, tuboovarian abscess (TOA), and pelvic peritonitis • Infertility occurs in 15% of pts after 1 episode of salpingitis, ↑ to 75% after ≥3 episodes • Risk of ectopic pregnancy ↑ 7–10 times in women with Hx of salpingitis • Dx = abd, adnexal, and cervical motion tenderness and at least + of the following: ⊕ Gram stain, temp >38°C, WBC >10,000, pus on culdocentesis or laparoscopy, TOA on bimanual or Utz	• Toxic pts, ↓ immunity and noncompliant should be Tx as inpts with IV antibiotics • Can use azithromycin or fluoroquinolone + metronidazole or cephalosporin + doxycycline • Start antibiotic as soon as PID is suspected, even before culture results are available
Human Papillomavirus (HPV)	• Serotypes **6 and 11** most commonly associated with **Genital Warts** • Serotypes **16 and 18** most commonly associated with **Cervical CA**	• Topical podophyllin or trichloroacetic acid, if refractory → cryosurgery or excision

(continued)

FAMILY MEDICINE

Table 5.8 *Continued*

Dz	Characteristics	Tx
Human Papillomavirus (HPV) *(continued)*	• Incubation period varies from 6 wk to 3 mo, spread by direct skin-to-skin contact • Infxn after single contact with an infected individual results in 65% transmission rate • Si/Sx = condyloma acuminata (genital warts) = soft, fleshy growths on vulva, vagina, cervix, perineum, anus • Dx = clinical, confirmed with Bx	• If pregnant, C-section recommended to avoid vaginal lesions **Note—Gardasil**, approved by FDA, a quadrivalent vaccine indicated in girls and women 9–26 years of age for the **prevention** of cervical CA, precancerous or dysplastic lesions, and genital warts caused by HPV Types 6, 11, 16, and 18
Syphilis (*Treponema pallidum*)	• Si/Sx = **painless ulcer** with bilateral inguinal adenopathy, chancre heals in 3–9 wk • Because of lack of Sx, Dx of 1° syphilis is often missed • 4–8 wk after appearance of chancre, 2° dz → fever, lymphadenopathy, maculopapular rash affecting palms and soles, condyloma lata in intertriginous areas • Dx = serologies, VDRL/RPR for screening, FTA-ABS to confirm	• Benzathine penicillin G

(3) People with homozygous deletions of CCR5 or other viral coreceptors are highly resistant to infxn with HIV, whereas heterozygotes are less resistant

c. Although pts can have no clinical evidence of dz for many years, **HIV has no latent phase in its life cycle;** clinical silence in pts who eventually progress is the result of daily, temporarily successful host repopulation of T cells

d. Death usually is caused by opportunistic infxns or malignancies

(1) Opportunistic infxns typically onset after CD4 counts fall <200

(2) When CD4 counts are <200, all pts should be on permanent TMP-SMX prophylaxis against *Pneumocystis* pneumonia (PCP) and *Toxoplasma* encephalitis

(3) When CD4 counts are <50, all pts should receive azithromycin prophylaxis against *Mycobacterium avium-intracellulare* complex (MAC)

(4) Kaposi's sarcoma = common skin CA found in homosexual HIV pts, thought to be caused by cotransmission of human herpes virus-8 (HHV-8)

(5) Non-Hodgkin's Lymphomas, typically high grade and aggressive, are far more common in HIV pts than non-HIV pts and are also harder to treat

(6) Other dz found in AIDS pts include generalized wasting and dementia

4. Tx

  a. Highly Active Antiretroviral Tx (HAART)

(1) Generally involves combination of a minimum of three active antiviral agents—now can administer one pill once per day that has three active drugs in it

(2) Can use resistance testing to determine to which agents a pt's virus is susceptible

(3) Initiate HAART if pt has an AIDS-defining opportunistic infxn or CA, or if the pt's CD4 count is <350 per μl

(4) Give TMP-SMX prophylaxis if CD4 count is <200

(5) Give azithromycin prophylaxis if CD4 count is <75

D. **Hematuria**

1. Red/brown urine discoloration 2° to RBCs, correlates with presence of >5 RBCs/high-powered field on microanalysis

2. Can be painful or painless

  a. Painless = 1° renal dz (tumor, glomerulonephritis), tuberculosis (TB) infxn, vesicular dz (bladder tumor), prostatic dz

  b. Painful = nephrolithiasis, renal infarction, UTI

3. DDx = myoglobinuria or hemoglobinuria, where hemoglobin dipstick is ⊕ but no RBCs are seen on microanalysis

4. Dx = finding of RBCs in urinary sediment

  a. UA → WBCs (infxn) or RBC casts (glomerulonephritis)

  b. CBC → anemia (renal failure), polycythemia (renal cell CA)

    c. Urogram will show nephrolithiasis and tumors (Utz → cystic versus solid)

    d. Cystoscopy only after UA and IVP; best for lower urinary tract

  5. Tx varies by cause

E. Prostate

1. Benign Prostatic Hyperplasia (BPH)

    a. Hyperplasia of the periurethral prostate causing bladder outlet obstruction

    b. Common after age 45 (autopsy shows that 90% of men older than 70 have BPH)

    c. Does not predispose to prostate CA

    d. Si/Sx urinary frequency, urgency, nocturia, ↓ size and force of urinary stream leading to hesitancy and intermittency, sensation of incomplete emptying worsening to continuous overflow incontinence or urinary retention, rectal exam → enlarged prostate (classically a rubbery vs. firm, hard gland that may suggest prostate CA) with loss of median furrow

    e. Labs → prostate-specific antigen (PSA) elevated in up to 50% of pts, not specific, so not useful marker for BPH

    f. Dx based on symptomatic scoring system; i.e., prostate size >30 mL (determined by Utz or exam), maximum urinary flow rate (<10 mL/s), and post-void residual urine volume (>50 mL)

    g. Tx = α-blocker (e.g., terazosin), 5α-reductase inhibitor (e.g., Finasteride); avoid anticholinergics, antihistaminergics, or narcotics

    h. Refractory dz requires surgery = transurethral resection of prostate (TURP); open prostatectomy recommended for larger glands (>75 g)

2. Prostatitis

    a. Si/Sx = fever, chills, low back pain, urinary frequency and urgency, tender, possible fluctuant and swollen prostate

    b. Labs → leukocytosis, pyuria, bacteriuria

    c. Dx = clinical

    d. Tx = systemic antibiotics

3. Prostate CA

    a. Most common CA in males, second most common cause of CA death (first = lung)

    b. It is adenoCA histologically

    c. More common in African Americans, rare in Asians

    d. PSA ↑ in 90% of adenoCA pts, but not specific, **controversy over use as a screening tool**, used to follow Tx by watching for dropping PSA levels

    e. Gleeson score (pathological grading)

       (1) Add scores of two of most common patterns (scored from 1 to 5)

       (2) If only one pattern multiply by 2

       (3) Scores range from 2 to 10, higher score → worse Px

    f. Metastasis occurs via lymph or blood, commonly causes **osteoblastic** lesions in bone

    g. Tx = surgery, hormones, and/or radiation Tx

F. Impotence

   1. Affects 30 million men in US, strongly associated with age (approximately 40% among 40-yr-olds and 70% among 70-yr-olds)

   2. Causes

    a. 1° erectile dysfunction = never been able to sustain erections

       (1) Psychological (sexual guilt, fear of intimacy, depression, anxiety)

       (2) ↓ testosterone 2° to hypothalamic-pituitary-gonadal disorder

       (3) Hypothyroidism or hyperthyroidism, Cushing's syndrome, ↑ prolactin

    b. 2° erectile dysfunction = acquired, >**90% from an organic cause**

       (1) Vascular dz = atherosclerosis of penile arteries and/or venous leaks causing inadequate impedance of venous outflow

       (2) Drugs = diuretics, clonidine, CNS depressants, tricyclic antidepressants, high-dose anticholinergics, antipsychotics

       (3) Neurologic dz = stroke, temporal lobe seizures, multiple sclerosis, spinal cord injury, autonomic dysfunction 2° to diabetes, post-TURP or open prostatic surgery

   3. Dx

    a. Clinical, rule out above organic causes

    b. **Nocturnal penile tumescence** testing differentiates psychogenic from organic—nocturnal tumescence is involuntary, ⊕ in psychogenic but not in organic dz

4. Tx
   a. Cyclic GMP-specific phosphodiesterase 5 (PDE5) inhibitors
      (1) Examples include: (e.g., sildenafil = Viagra, tadalafil = Cialis, vardenafil = Levitra)
      (2) Inhibition of PDE5 → improves relaxation of smooth muscles in corpora cavernosa
      (3) Side effects = transient headache, flushing, dyspepsia, rhinitis, transient visual disturbances (blue hue) is very rare, drug may lower blood pressure → **use of nitrates is an absolute contraindication,** deaths have resulted from combo
   b. Vacuum-constriction devices use negative pressure to draw blood into penis with band placed at base of penis to retain erection
   c. Intracavernosal prostaglandin injection has mean duration of approximately 60 min; risks = penile bruising/bleeding and priapism
   d. Surgery = penile prostheses implantation; venous or arterial surgery
   e. Testosterone Tx for hypogonadism
   f. Behavioral Tx and counseling for depression and anxiety

V. Common Sports Medicine Complaints

A. Plantar Fasciitis

1. Inflamed plantar fascia band originating from the medial calcaneal tuberosity, which fans and inserts on the flexor mechanism of the toes at the metatarsal heads
2. Inflammatory condition common in runners and dancers who use repetitive, maximal plantar flexion of the ankle and dorsiflexion of the metatarsophalangeal joints
3. Si/Sx = pain in heel with first morning step (dorsiflexion), irritated and inflamed fascia is stretched causing severe pain
4. Tx = morning stretches/exercises and NSAIDs, rarely steroid injection or surgery

B. Low Back Pain

1. 80% of people experience low back pain—second most common complaint in 1° care (next to common cold)
2. **50% of cases recur within the subsequent 3 yr**
3. **Majority of cases attributed to muscle strains,** but always consider disk herniation

4. Si/Sx of disk herniation = shooting pain down leg (sciatica), pain on **straight leg raise (>90% sensitive)**, and pain on **crossed straight leg raise (>90% specific, not sensitive)**

5. Dx
   a. **Always rule out RED FLAGS** (see below) with H&P exam
   b. If no red flags detected, presume Dx is muscle strain and not serious—**no radiologic testing is warranted**
   c. Dz not remitting after 4 wk of conservative Tx should be evaluated further with repeat H&P; consider radiologic studies
   d. Red Flags (Table 5.9)

6. Tx
   a. No red flags → conservative with acetaminophen (safer) or NSAIDs, **muscle relaxants have not been shown to help;** avoid narcotics
   b. **Strict bed rest is NOT warranted** (extended rest shown to be debilitating, especially in older pts)—encourage return to nml activity, low-stress aerobic, and back exercises
   c. **90% of cases resolve within 4 wk with conservative Tx**
   d. Red flags:
      (1) Fracture → surgical consult
      (2) Tumor → urgent radiation/steroid ($\downarrow$ compression), then excise
      (3) Infxn → abscess drainage and antibiotics per pathogen
      (4) Cauda equina syndrome → emergent surgical decompression
      (5) Spinal stenosis → complete laminectomy
      (6) Radiculopathy → anti-inflammatories, nerve root decompression with laminectomy or microdiscectomy only if (i) sciatica is severe and disabling, (ii) Sx persist for 4 wk or worsening progression, and (iii) strong evidence of specific nerve root damage with MRI correlation of level of disk herniation

C. **Shoulder Dislocation**
   1. Subluxation = symptomatic translation of humeral head relative to glenoid articular surface
   2. Dislocation = complete displacement out of the glenoid
   3. Anterior instability (approximately 95% of cases) usually as a result of subcoracoid dislocation is the most common form of shoulder dislocation

Table 5.9 Low Back Pain Red Flags

Dz	Si/Sx	Diagnostic Studies
Fracture	• Hx of trauma (fall, car accident) • Minor trauma in elderly (e.g., strenuous lifting)	• Spine x-rays
Tumor	• **Pt age >50 yr** (accounts for >80% of CA cases) or <20 yr • Prior Hx of CA • **Constitutional Sx** (fever/chills, weight loss) • Pain worse when supine or at night	• Spinal MRI is gold standard, can also get CT
Infxn	• Immunosuppressed pts • Constitutional Sx • Recent bacterial infxn or IV drug abuse	• Blood cultures, spinal MRI to rule out abscess
Cauda equine syndrome	• Acute urinary retention, **saddle anesthesia**, lower-extremity weakness or paresthesias, and ↓ reflexes, ↓ anal sphincter tone	• Spinal MRI
Spinal stenosis	• Si/Sx = **pseudoclaudication** (neurogenic) with pain ↑ with walking **and standing;** relieved by sitting or leaning forward	• Spinal MRI
Radiculopathy (herniation compressing spinal nerves)[a]	• Sensory loss: (**L5** → **L**arge toe/medial foot, **S1**→ **S**mall toe/lateral foot) • Weakness: (L1–L4 → quadriceps, L5 → foot dorsiflexion, S1 → plantar flexion) • ↓ Reflexes (L4 → patellar, S1 → Achilles)	• **Clinical**—MRI may confirm clinical Dx but false-positive results are common (clinically insignificant disk herniation) (see Figure 5.4)

[a]Radiculopathy ≠ herniation; radiculopathy indicates evolving spinal nerve impingement and is a more serious Dx than simple herniation indicated by straight leg testing and sciatica.

4. Si/Sx = pain, joint immobility, arm "goes dead" with overhead motion

5. Dx = clinical, assess axillary nerve function in neurologic exam, look for signs of rotator cuff injury, confirm with x-rays if necessary

6. Tx = initial reduction of dislocation by various traction—countertraction techniques, 2- to 6-wk period of immobilization

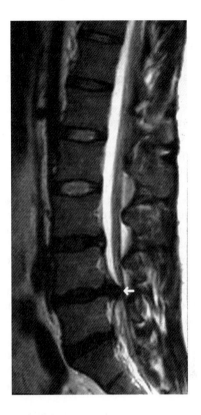

FIGURE 5.4

MRI scan showing a prolapsed disk at L4–5 with posterior deviation of the theca (*arrow*).

(longer for younger pts), intense rehabilitation; rarely is surgery required

D. **Clavicle Fracture**
   1. Occurs primarily as a result of contact sports in adults
   2. Si/Sx = pain and deformity at clavicle
   3. Dx = clinical, confirm fracture with standard AP view x-ray
   4. Must rule out subclavian artery injury by checking pulses, brachial plexus injury with neurologic examination, and pneumothorax by checking breath sounds
   5. Tx = sling until range of motion is painless (usually 2–4 wk)

E. **Elbow Injuries**

1. Epicondylitis (Tendinitis)

    a. Lateral epicondylitis **(tennis elbow)**

        (1) Usually in tennis player (>50%) or participants in racquetball, squash, fencing

        (2) Si/Sx = pain 2–5 cm distal and anterior to lateral picondyle reproduced with wrist extension while elbow is extended

    b. Medial epicondylitis **(golfer's elbow)**

        (1) Commonly in golf, racquet sports, bowling, baseball, swimming

        (2) Si/Sx = acute onset of medial elbow pain and swelling localized 1 or 2 cm area distal to medial epicondyle, pain usually reproduced with wrist flexion and pronation against resistance

    c. Tx for both = ice, rest, NSAIDs, counterforce bracing, rehabilitation

    d. Px for both varies, can become chronic condition; surgery sometimes indicated (débridement and tendon reapproximation)

2. Olecranon Fracture

    a. Usually direct blow to elbow with triceps contraction after fall on flexed upper extremity

    b. Tx = long arm cast or splint in 45- to 90-degree flexion for ≥3 wk

    c. Displaced fracture requires open reduction and internal fixation

3. Dislocation

    a. Elbow joint most commonly dislocated joint in children, second most in adults (next to shoulder)

    b. Fall onto outstretched hand with fully extended elbow (posterolateral dislocation) or direct blow to posterior elbow (anterior dislocation)

    c. May be seen in child after child's arm is jerked by hurried parent or guardian **(nursemaid's elbow)**

    d. Key is associated nerve injury (ulnar, median, radial, or anterior interosseous nerve), vascular injury (brachial artery), or other structural injury (associated coronoid process fracture common)

    e. Tx = reduce elbow by gently flexing supinated arm, long arm splint, or bivalved cast applied at 90-degree flexion

4. Olecranon Bursitis
   a. Inflammation of bursa under olecranon process
   b. Seen with direct blow to elbow by collision or fall on artificial turf
   c. Si/Sx = swollen and painful posterior elbow with restricted motion
   d. Dx = clinical, confirm with bursa aspiration to rule out septic bursitis
   e. Tx = bursa aspiration, compression dressing and pad

F. **Ankle Injuries**

1. Achilles Tendonitis
   a. 2° to overuse, commonly seen in runners, gymnasts, cyclists, and volleyball players
   b. Si/Sx = swelling or erythema along area of Achilles tendon with tenderness 2–5 cm proximal to calcaneus
   c. Evaluate for rupture = Thompson test (squeezing leg with passive plantar flexion) positive only with complete tear
   d. Tx = rest, ice, NSAIDs, taping or splinting to ↓ stress and ↑ support
   e. Rupture requires long leg cast for 4 wk, short leg walking cast for 4 wk, then heel lift for 4 wk
   f. Open repair speeds recovery and is recommended with complete tears in younger pts

2. Ankle Sprains
   a. Lateral sprain occurs when ankle is plantar-flexed (90% of sprains)
   b. Anterior drawer sign is done with foot in 10- to 15-degree plantar flexion
   c. Medial sprain is rare (10%) because ligament is stronger
   d. Dx = multiple view x-rays both free and weight-bearing
   e. Tx = **RICE** = **R**est (limit activity ± crutches), **I**ce, **C**ompression (ACE bandage), **E**levation above level of heart to ↓ swelling
   f. Severe sprains may benefit from casting, open repair rarely indicated

VI. Nutrition

A. **Nutritional Assessment**

1. Diet history: Many methods can be used to assess a pt's nutritional status, whatever method used must start with a careful history of nutritional intake

2. Labs occasionally used:
   a. Serum albumin levels: Half life 18–20 days, nml levels 3.5–5.5 g/dL, severe malnutrition <2.1 g/dL
   b. Serum pre-albumin levels: Half life 2–4 days, nml levels 15.7–29.6 mg/dL, severe malnutrition <8 mg/dL
   c. Serum transferrin levels: Half life 8–9 days, nml levels 200–400 mg/dL, severe malnutrition <100 mg/dL
   d. Serum retinal-binding protein: Half-life 12 hr, reflects very recent changes in protein and caloric intake, influenced by vitamin A intake
   e. 24 hr collection for urine urea nitrogen to assess nitrogen balance before and after starting nutritional Tx—nitrogen losses are proportional to catabolic state

3. Anthropometric Measurements
   a. Ideal body weight (IBW)
      (1) Males: Height of 5 ft, ideal weight 106 lb and add 6 lb +/− 10% (frame size) for each additional inch over 5 ft
      (2) Females: Height of 5 ft, ideal weight 100 lb and add 5 lb +/− 10% (frame size) for each additional inch over 5 ft
      (3) Percent IBW = (actual weight/IBW) × 100, severely malnourished <69%, overweight >120%, morbidly obese = 200%
   b. Body mass index (BMI)
      (1) Useful in Dx of obesity, correlated with total body fat
      (2) Nml range is 19.0–26.0, pts with a BMI between 26.1 and 29.0 are considered overweight
      (3) BMI >30 is considered obese
      (4) Formula: BMI = Weight (Kg)/ Height (m^2)
   c. Triceps skin fold
      (1) Measurements obtained using skin fold calipers on triceps of nondominant arm
      (2) Results compared with standardized tables and provide an estimate of overall subcutaneous fat stores.

4. Calculating Nutritional Requirements
   a. Caloric requirements: Harris-Benedict equation (kcal/kg/day) calculates resting metabolic rate
      (1) Men: 66 + 13.7 (weight [kg]) + 5 (height [cm]) − 6.9 (age [yr])
      (2) Women: 665 + 9.6 (weight) + 1.8 (height) − 4.7 (age)
   b. Estimated caloric requirements
      (1) Unstressed person: 25–35 kcal/kg/day
      (2) Hospitalized pt: 35–45 kcal/kg/day
      (3) Severely ill (ICU) pt: 50–70 kcal/kg/day
   c. Protein requirements
      (1) Maintenance: 1.0–1.5 g/kg/day
      (2) Repletion: 1.5–2.0 g/kg/day
      (3) Excessive loss: 2.0–2.5 g/kg/day
   d. Lipid requirements
      (1) Usually 25%–30% of total calories
      (2) Essential fatty acids are 2%–4% of those calories
5. Nutritional Supplements
   a. Enteral feeding is the preferred method of nutritional supplementation. Whenever possible feed the gut
      (1) Enteral feeding maintains gut integrity, reduces the risk of sepsis from gut bacteria
      (2) May be administered orally, per nasogastric, gastrostomy, or jejunostomy tube. All carry the risk of aspiration, but jejunostomy has the lowest
      (3) May be continuous or intermittent bolus feedings
      (4) Least expensive, most convenient
   b. Parenteral feeding
      (1) Useful when pt is on bowel rest, and gut should not or cannot be fed
      (2) Total parenteral nutrition (TPN) requires central venous access. Solutions are a hyperosmolar mixture of dextrose, amino acids, vitamins, minerals, trace elements, electrolytes, and, in some institutions, fat emulsions are also directly added to mixture
      (3) Provides pts with all the necessary daily requirements
      (4) Monitor pts carefully when starting TPN. Electrolytes, liver enzymes, white count, and fluid status. These pts are at high risk for hyperglycemia, infxn, hypophos-phatemia, hyponatremia, hepatic steatosis, and biliary dz

(5) When discontinuing TPN, you should slowly taper the person off of TPN. This will prevent hypoglycemia by allowing pts insulin levels to slowly return to nml

B. **Vitamins and Nutrition**

Nutrient	Deficiency	Excess
B₁ (thiamine)	**Dry beriberi → neuropathy** Wet beriberi → high-output cardiac failure Either → Wernicke-Korsakoff's syndrome	
B₂ (riboflavin)	**Cheilosis (mouth fissures)**	
B₃ (niacin)	Pellagra → dementia, diarrhea, dermatitis **Also seen in Hartnup's dz (dz of tryptophan metabolism)**	
B₅ (pantothenate)	**Enteritis, dermatitis**	
B₆ (pyridoxine)	**Neuropathy (frequently caused by isoniazid Tx for TB)**	
B₁₂ (cyanocobalamin)	**Pernicious anemia (lack of intrinsic factor) → neuropathy, megaloblastic anemia, glossitis**	
Biotin	**Dermatitis, enteritis (caused by ↑ consumption of raw eggs, due to the avidin in raw eggs blocking biotin absorption)**	
Chromium	**Glucose intolerance (cofactor for insulin)**	
Copper	**Leukopenia, bone demineralization**	
Folic acid	**Neural tube defects, megaloblastic anemia**	
Iodine	**Hypothyroidism, cretinism, goiter**	
Iron	**Plummer-Vinson syndrome = esophageal webs, spoon nails**	**Hemochromatosis → multiorgan failure (bronze diabetes)**
Selenium	**Myopathy (Keshan's dz, see Appendix A)**	
Vitamin A	**Metaplasia of respiratory epithelia (seen in cystic fibrosis due to failure of fat-soluble vitamin absorption), xerophthalmia, night**	**Pseudotumor cerebri (can be caused by consuming polar**

	blindness (lack of retinal in rod cells), acne, Bitot's spots, frequent respiratory infxns (respiratory epithelial defects)	bear livers), headache, nausea, vomiting, skinpeeling
Vitamin C	Scurvy: poor healing, hypertrophic bleeding gums, easy bruising, deficient osteoid mimicking rickets	
Vitamin D	Rickets in kids, osteomalacia in adults	Kidney stones, dementia, constipation, abd pain, depression
Vitamin E	Fragile RBCs, sensory and motor peripheral neuropathy	
Vitamin K	Clotting deficiency	
Zinc	Poor wound healing, ↓ taste and smell, alopecia, diarrhea, dermatitis, depression (similar to pellagra)	
Calories	Marasmus = total calorie malnutrition → pts look deceptively well but are immunosuppressed, poor wound healing, impaired growth	
Protein	Kwashiorkor = protein malnutrition → edema/ascites, immunosuppression, poor wound healing, impaired growth and development	

VII. Hoarseness

A. **Hoarseness (Dysphonia)**

1. Perceived rough quality of the voice (caused by structural or functional abnormalities)
2. Many causes:
   a. **Congenital**—laryngeal webs, clefts, cysts
   b. **Infectious**—papillomatosis, viral, bacterial and fungal laryngitis, tuberculosis
   c. **Inflammatory**—reflux laryngitis, rheumatoid arthritis
   d. **Iatrogenic**—recurrent laryngeal nerve damage occurring during neck or cardiothoracic surgery
   e. **Traumatic**—vocal fold nodules, polyps, arytenoids dislocation, laryngeal framework disruption (fracture), and postintubation
   f. **Endocrine**—hypothyroidism, hyperthyroidism

g. **Connective tissue dz**—scleroderma, sarcoidosis
h. **Neoplastic**
   (1) Benign—HPV, granuloma, laryngeal chondroma
   (2) Malignant (1°)—squamous cell CA (larynx/lung) or thyroid CA invading recurrent laryngeal nerve (RLN)
   (3) Malignant (metastasis)
i. **Neurologic**—vocal fold paralysis, multiple sclerosis, viral neuronitis, spasmodic dysphonia
j. **Senile larynx (old age)** (Hoarseness differential by Dr. Ramon Franco)

B. **Larynx (Neoplasms)**
1. Benign—most common is papilloma (HPV), chondroma, adenoma, chemodectoma (cherry red), and hemangioma
2. Malignant—squamous cell CA most common
   a. Sx = hoarseness, stridor, otalgia, dyspnea, hemoptysis, weight loss, and adenopathy
   b. Tx = Surgery, chemotherapy, or radiation

6. PSYCHIATRY

I. Introduction

A. **DSM-IV** *(Diagnostic & Statistical Manual of Mental Disorders, Fourth Ed.)* **(Table 6.1)**

1. The DSM-IV lists current US diagnostic criteria for psychiatric conditions

2. **The United States Medical Licensing Examination (USMLE) will rely on DSM-IV diagnostic criteria, with DSM-V projected to come out in 2011; USMLE will take some time to catch up to any changes**

B. **Principles of Psychiatry for the USMLE (more complex in real life)**

1. Major psychiatric Dx requires **significant impairment in the pt's life**

2. **Always rule out drug abuse** (frequent comorbidity in psychiatric dz)

3. **Combination Tx** (pharmacology and psychotherapy) **is superior** to either alone, but **pharmacologic Tx is first line for severe dz in acute setting**

4. **Criteria for hospitalization (any single criterion is acceptable)**

   a. Danger to self (suicide)

   b. Danger to others

   c. Unable to provide food, clothing, shelter (grave disability)

5. Psychiatric dz is chronic—if asked about dz course, **"cures" are rare**

6. Px depends on Sx onset, insight, and premorbid function (Table 6.2)

Table 6.1	DSM-IV Classifications
Axis	**Type of Disorder**
I	Clinical Disorders
II	Personality disorders/mental retardation
III	Medical conditions
IV	Social and environmental factors
V	Level of functioning

Table 6.2 Prognosis of Psychiatric Disorders

Px	Sx Onset	Insight[a]	Premorbid Function
Favorable	Acute	Good	High
Unfavorable	Subacute/chronic	Poor	Low

[a]Insight refers to pt who recognizes Sx are abnormalities and is distressed by them.

II. Mood Disorders

A. **Major Depressive Disorder (MDD)**
  1. Syndrome of **repeated major depressive episodes**
  2. One of the most common psychiatric disorders, with lifetime prevalence of 15%–25%, with a greater incidence in women and elderly (often overlooked)
  3. Si/Sx for depression in general
     a. Major Si/Sx = ↓ **mood** and/or **anhedonia** (inability to experience pleasure)
     b. Others = insomnia (less commonly hypersomnia), ↓ appetite/weight loss (less commonly ↑ appetite/weight gain), fatigue, ↓ concentration, guilt or feeling worthless, recurrent thoughts of death and suicide
     c. **Commonly presents with various somatic complaints and ↓ energy level rather than complaints of depression—** beware of clinical scenarios in which pts have multiple unrelated physical complaints
  4. DDx = dysthymic disorder, bipolar disorder, medical dz **(classically hypothyroidism)**, bereavement
  5. Dx requires 2 depressive episodes to continue for ≥2 wk each, separated by ≥2 mo
  6. Tx (Table 6.3)
     a. Psychotherapy = **psychodynamic** (understanding self/inner conflicts), **cognitive/behavioral** (recognizing negative thought or behavior and altering thinking/behavior accordingly), **interpersonal** (examines relation of Sx to negative/absent relationships with others)
     b. **Electroconvulsive Tx (ECT)** is effective for refractory cases, main side effect is short-term memory loss

B. **Dysthymic Disorder**
  1. Si/Sx = as per major depressive episodes but is continuous
  2. Dx = **steady Sx duration for minimum of 2 yr**—dysthymic disorder is longer but less acute than MDD

Table 6.3 Pharmacologic Therapy for Depression[a]

Drug	Examples	Side Effects
SSRIs[b]	Fluoxetine, paroxetine, sertraline, citalopram, escitalopram	Favorable profile: rare impotence
TCAs[b]	Amitriptyline, desipramine, imipramine, nortriptyline	More severe: confusion, sedation, **orthostatic hypotension, prolonged QRS duration** (think autonomic/cholinergic)
MAOIs[b]	Phenelzine, tranylcypromine	Very severe: classic syndromes • **Serotonin syndrome =** caused by **MAOI interaction with SSRIs, meperidine (Demerol), pseudoephedrine**, and others; presents with hyperthermia, muscle rigidity, altered mental status • **Hypertensive crisis =** malignant HTN when ingested with foods rich in **tyramine** (wine and cheese)
SNRIs	Duloxetine, mirtazapine	Mirtazapine associated with agranulocytosis

[a]Takes 2–6 wk for effect.
[b]SSRIs are first line; TCAs are second line; monoamine oxidase inhibitors (MAOIs) are third line; serotonin-norepinephrine reuptake inhibitors (SNRIs) are newest options.

3. If major depressive episode takes place during the 2 yr of dysthymia, then by definition the Dx is MDD rather than dysthymic disorder
4. Tx = as per MDD

C. **Bereavement**
1. **Bereavement** is a commonly asked test question!
2. Si/Sx = in an older adult whose partner has died: feeling sad, losing weight, and sleeping poorly (depression Sx)
3. Dx: key is **how much time** has elapsed since the partner died—**if Sx persist for >2 mo, Dx is MDD rather than nml bereavement**
4. Although bereavement is nml behavior, grief management may be helpful

D. **Bipolar Disorder (Manic-Depression)**

1. Seen in 1% of population, genders equally affected but **often presents in young people**, whereas **major depression is a dz of middle age (40s)**

2. Si/Sx = abrupt onset of ↑ **energy**, ↓ **need to sleep, pressured speech** (speaks quickly to the point of making no sense), ↓ attention span, **hypersexuality, spending large amounts of money**, engaging in outrageous activities (e.g., directing traffic at an intersection while naked)

3. DDx = cocaine and amphetamine use, personality disorders (see Section V.B., cluster B), schizophrenia (see Section III), hypomania

4. Dx
   a. **Manic episode causes significant disability**, whereas hypomania presents with identical Sx but no significant disability
   b. Episodes **must last ≥1 wk and should be abrupt, not continuous**, which would suggest personality disorder or schizophrenia
   c. **Bipolar I** = manic episode with or without depressive episodes (pts often have depressive episodes before experiencing mania)
   d. **Bipolar II** = depressive episodes **with hypomanic episodes** but, by definition, **the absence of manic episodes**
   e. **Rapid cycling** = 4 episodes (depressive, manic, or mixed) in 12 mo; can be precipitated by antidepressants

5. Tx
   a. Hospitalization, often involuntary because manic pts rarely see the need
   b. **Valproate** or **carbamazepine** are first line, **lithium** second line
   c. Valproate and carbamazepine cause **blood dyscrasias**
   d. Lithium blood levels must be checked because of frequent toxicity, including **tremor** and polyuria resulting from **nephrogenic diabetes insipidus**

6. Px worse than major depression, episodes more frequent with age

E. **Drug-Induced Mania**

1. Cocaine and amphetamines are major culprits

2. Si/Sx = as per mania, also tachycardia, HTN, dilated pupils, **ECG arrhythmia, or ischemia in young people is highly suggestive**

3. Dx = urine or serum toxicology screen
4. Tx = calcium channel blockers for acute autonomic Sx, drug Tx programs longer term

III. Psychosis

A. **Si/Sx**

1. **Hallucinations and delusions** are hallmark
   a. Hallucination = false sensory perception not based on real stimulus
   b. Delusion = false interpretation of external reality
   c. Can be paranoid, grandiose (thinking one possesses special powers), religious (God is talking to the pt), or ideas of reference (every event in the world somehow involves the pt)

B. **DDx (Table 6.4)**

C. **Tx**

1. Hospitalization if voices tell pts to hurt themselves or others, or if condition is disabling to the point that pts cannot care for themselves
2. Pharmacologic Tx (Table 6.5)
   a. All antipsychotics act as dopamine blockers
   b. Differences among agents relate to side-effect profile (Table 6.6)
   c. Compliance to drugs can be improved with **depot form of haloperidol,** which administers a 1-mo supply of drug in 1 IM injection
3. Psychotherapy can improve social functioning
   a. Behavioral Tx teaches social skills that allow pts to deal more comfortably with other people
   b. Family-oriented Tx teaches family members to act in more appropriate, positive fashion

D. **Px**

1. Schizophrenia is a chronic, episodic dz, recovery from each relapse typically leaves pt below former baseline function
2. Presence of negative Sx (e.g., flat affect) marks poor Px
3. High-functioning prior to psychotic break marks better Px

Table 6.4 Diagnosis of Psychotic Disorders

Dz	Characteristics
Schizophrenia	• **Presents in late teens to 20s (slightly later in women), very strong genetic predisposition** • Often accompanied by **premorbid** sign, including poor school performance, poor emotional expression, lack of friends • Positive Sx = hallucinations (**more often auditory than visual**) and delusions • Negative Sx = lack of affect, alogia (lack of speech) • Other Sx = disorganized behavior and/or speech • **Schizophrenia lasts ≥6 continuous mo** • **Schizophreniform disorder lasts 1–6 mo** • **Brief psychotic disorder lasts 1 day–1 mo,** with full recovery of baseline functioning—look for acute stressor; e.g., death of a loved one
Other psychoses	• Schizoaffective disorder = meets criteria for mood disorders and schizophrenia • Delusional disorder = **nonbizarre delusions** (they could happen; e.g., pt's spouse is unfaithful, a person is trying to kill the pt), without hallucinations, disorganized speech, or disorganized behavior
Mood disorders	• Major depression and bipolar disorder can cause delusions and, in extreme cases, hallucinations—can be difficult to differentiate from schizophrenia
Delirium	• Seen in pts with underlying illnesses, often in ICU (ICU psychosis) • **Pts are not orientated to person, place, time.** • **Severity waxes and wanes even during the course of 1 day** • Resolves with Txt of underlying dz
Drugs	• LSD and PCP → predominantly visual, taste, touch, or olfactory hallucination • Cocaine and amphetamines → paranoid delusions **and classic sensation of bugs crawling on the skin (formication)** • Anabolic steroids → bodybuilder with bad temper, acne, shrunken testicles • Corticosteroids → psychosis/mood disturbances early in course of Tx
Medical	• Metabolic, endocrine, neoplastic, and seizure dz can all cause psychosis • **Look for associated Si/Sx not explained by psychosis,** including focal neurologic findings, seizure, sensory/motor deficits, abnormal lab values

LSD, lysergic acid diethylamide; PCP, phencyclidine

Table 6.5 Antipsychotic Drugs

Drug		Adverse Effects[a]
Typical Antipsychotics[b]		
Chlorpromazine	Low potency	↑ Anticholinergic effects, ↓ movement disorders
Haloperidol	High potency	↓ Anticholinergic effects, ↑ movement disorders
Atypical Antipsychotics[b]		
Clozapine	For refractory dz	No movement disorders; 1% incidence of agranulocytosis mandates wkly CBC
Risperidone	First line	Rare movement disorders, but can occur at high doses Linked to new onset diabetes
Olanzapine, quetiapine, ziprasidone, aripiprazole	First line	No movement disorders Linked to new onset diabetes

[a]Anticholinergic effects = dry mouth, blurry vision (miosis), urinary retention, constipation.
[b]Atypical agents have much lower incidence of movement disorders.

IV. Anxiety Disorders

A. Panic Disorder

1. Si/Sx = mimic myocardial infarction (MI): chest pain, palpitations, diaphoresis, nausea, marked anxiety, escalate for 10 min, remain for approximately 30 min (rarely >1 hr)
2. Occurs in younger pts (average age 25)—good way to distinguish from MI
3. DDx = MI, drug abuse (e.g., cocaine, amphetamines), phobias (discussed further)
4. Dx is by exclusion of true medical condition and drug abuse
5. Panic attacks are unexpected, so if pt consistently describes panic Sx in a specific setting, phobia is a more likely diagnosis
6. Tx
   a. Selective serotonin reuptake inhibitors (SSRIs) and tricyclic antidepressants (TCAs) have similar efficacy, but SSRIs have fewer side effects
   b. Benzodiazepines work immediately, have ↑ risk of addiction

Table 6.6 Antipsychotic-Associated Movement Disorders

Disorder	Time Course	Characteristics
Acute dystonia	4 hr–4 days	• Sustained muscle spasm anywhere in the body but often in neck (torticollis), jaw, or back (opisthotonos) • Tx = immediate IV dphenhydramine
Parkinsonism	4 days–4 mo	• Cog-wheel rigidity, shuffling gait, resting tremor • Tx = benztropine (anticholinergic)
Tardive dyskinesia	4 mo–4 yr	• Involuntary, irregular movements of the head, tongue, lips, limbs, and trunk • Tx = immediately change medication or ↓ doses because effects often are permanent
Akathisia	Any time	• Subjective sense of discomfort → restlessness: pacing, sitting down and getting up • Tx = lower medication doses
Neuroleptic malignant syndrome	Any time	• Life-threatening muscle rigidity → fever, ↑ BP/HR, rhabdomyolysis appearing over 1–3 days • Can be easily misDx as ↑ psychotic Sx • Labs → ↑ WBC, ↑ creatine kinase, ↑ transaminases, ↑ plasma myoglobin, as well as myoglobinuria • Tx = supportive: immediately stop drug, give dantrolene (inhibits Ca release into cells), cool pt to prevent hyperpyrexia

    c. Therefore, start benzodiazepine for immediate effects, add a TCA or SSRI, taper off the benzodiazepine as the other drugs kick in

    d. Cognitive/behavioral Tx and **respiratory training** (to help pts recognize and overcome desire to hyperventilate) are helpful

B. **Agoraphobia**

    1. Sx = fear of being in situations where getting out would be very difficult should a panic attack arise

2. Theorized that pts develop agoraphobia because they have experienced enough unexpected panic attacks to know that the attacks can come at any time

3. Dx = clinical, look for evidence of social/occupational dysfunction

4. Tx (for phobias in general)

   a. β-blockers useful for prophylaxis in phobias related to performance

   b. **Exposure desensitization** = exposure to noxious stimulus in increments while undergoing concurrent relaxation Tx

C. **Obsessive–Compulsive Disorder (OCD)**

1. **Obsessions = recurrent thought; compulsions = recurrent act**

2. Sx = obsessive thought causes anxiety, and the compulsion is a way of temporarily relieving that anxiety (e.g., pt worries whether s/he locked the door; going back to see if the door is locked relieves the anxiety), but because relief is only temporary the pt performs compulsion repeatedly

3. Obsessions commonly involve **cleanliness/contamination** (washing hands), doubt, symmetry (elaborate rituals for entering doorways, arranging books, etc.), and sex

4. Dx = pt should be disturbed by their obsessions and **should recognize their absurdity** in contrast to obsessive–compulsive personality disorder, where pt sees nothing wrong with compulsion

5. Tx = SSRIs (first line) or clomipramine, psychotherapy in which the pt is literally forced to overcome the behavior

D. **Posttraumatic Stress Disorder (PTSD)**

1. Dx requires a traumatic, violent incident that effectively scars the person involved; the experiences of Vietnam vets are emblematic of this disorder

2. Sx

   a. **Pt relives the initial incident via conscious thoughts or dreams**

   b. Due to resultant subjective and physiologic distress, the pt avoids any precipitating stimuli and **hence often avoids public places and activities**

   c. Pt may suffer restricted emotional involvement/responses and may experience a detachment from others

   d. **Depression is common; look for moodiness, diminished interest in activities, and difficulties with sleeping and concentrating**

3. DDx = **Acute Stress Disorder**
   a. Dx also requires a traumatic incident, but Sx are more immediate (within 4 wk of the event) and limited in time (<4 wk)
   b. Sx are different; imagine being so traumatized that you are in a daze, where nothing seems real and you have trouble remembering what has happened (commonly seen in victims of sexual assault)

4. Tx
   a. SSRIs are first line, TCAs can be used for refractory pts
   b. **Beware of giving benzodiazepines because of high association between substance abuse and PTSD!**
   c. Psychotherapy takes two approaches
      (1) Exposure Tx: the idea is to confront one's demons by "reliving" the experience (either stepwise or abruptly)
      (2) Relaxation techniques: think of the two modalities as attacking the source versus controlling the Sx

5. Px = variable, but the predictive factors are similar to schizophrenia: abrupt Sx and strong premorbid functioning lead to better outcomes

E. **Generalized Anxiety Disorder**
   1. Sx = worry for most days for at least 6 mo, irritability, inability to concentrate, insomnia, fatigue, restlessness
   2. DDx = specific anxieties, including separation anxiety disorder, anorexia nervosa, hypochondriasis
   3. **Dx requires evidence of social dysfunction** (e.g., poor school grades, job stagnation, or marital strains) to rule out "nml" anxiety
   4. Tx = psychotherapy because of chronicity of the problem
      a. Cognitive/behavioral Tx = teaching pt to recognize his/her worrying and finding ways to respond to it through behavior and thought patterns
      b. **Biofeedback and relaxation** techniques, in particular, can help the pt deal with physical manifestations of anxiety; e.g., heart rate
      c. Pharmacotherapy includes buspirone or β-blockers (works for peripheral Sx; e.g., tachycardia, but not for worry itself)

V. Personality Disorders

A. General Characteristics

1. Sx = pervasive pattern of maladaptive behavior causing functional impairment; consistent behavior often can be traced back to childhood

2. Typically present to psychiatrists because behavior is causing significant problems for others; e.g., colleagues at work, spouse at home, **or for the medical staff in the inpt or clinic setting (typical USMLE question)**

3. **Pts usually see nothing wrong with their behavior (ego-syntonic),** contrast with pts who recognize their hallucinations as abnormal (ego-dystonic)

4. Ego Defenses

   a. Unconscious mental process that individuals resort to in order to quell inner conflicts and anxiety that are unacceptable to the ego

   b. Examples include "denial" and "projection"

5. Tx = psychotherapy, medication used for peripheral Sx (e.g., anxiety)

B. Clusters

1. **Cluster A** = paranoid, schizoid, and schizotypal personalities, often thought of as **"weird" or "eccentric"**

2. **Cluster B** = borderline, antisocial, histrionic, and narcissistic personalities, **"dramatic" and "aggressive"** personalities

3. **Cluster C** = avoidant, dependent, and obsessive–compulsive personalities, **"shy" and "nervous"** personalities

C. Specific Personality Disorders (Table 6.7)

D. Other Ego Defenses

1. Acting out: transforming unacceptable feeling into actions, often loud ones (tantrums)

2. Altruism: constructive service to others that brings pleasure and personal satisfaction (Volunteering for Medical Missions)

3. Denial: refusal to accept external reality because it is too threatening

4. Displacement: redirection of some emotion from a real source to a substitute person or object

Table 6.7 Specific Personality Disorders

Disorder	Characteristics
Paranoid (cluster A)	• Negatively misinterpret the actions, words, intentions of others • Often use **projection** as ego defense (attributing to other people impulses and thoughts that are unacceptable to their own selves) • **Do not hold fixed delusions** (delusional disorder) **or experience hallucinations** (schizophrenia)
Schizoid (cluster A)	• Socially withdrawn, introverted, little external affect • Do not form close emotional ties with others (often feel no need) • Can recognize reality
Schizotypal (cluster A)	• **Believe in concepts not considered real by the rest of society (magic, clairvoyance),** display the prototypical ego defense: **fantasy** • Not necessarily psychotic (can have brief psychotic episodes) • Like schizoids, they are often quite isolated socially • **Often related to schizophrenics (unlike other cluster A disorders)**
Antisocial (cluster B)	• Violate the rights of others, break the law (e.g., theft, substance abuse) • Can be quite seductive (particularly with the opposite sex) • **For Dx, pt must have exhibited the behavior by a certain age (15—think truancy) but must be of a certain age (at least 18—adult)** • **Popular USMLE topic; you may have to differentiate it from conduct disorder (bad behavior, but Dx of children/adolescents)**
Borderline (cluster B)	• Volatile emotional lives, swing wildly between idealizing and devaluing other people (**splitting** ego defense = people are very good or bad) • **Commonly asked on USMLE;** typical scenario is a highly disruptive hospitalized pt; on interview, he (but usually she) says some nurses are incompetent and cruel but wildly praises others (including you) • Exhibit self-destructive behavior (scratching or cutting themselves) • Ability to **disassociate;** they simply "forget" negative effects/experiences by covering them with overly exuberant, seemingly positive behavior

Table 6.7 *Continued*

Disorder	Characteristics
Histrionic (cluster B)	• Require the attention of everyone, use sexuality and physical appearance to get it, exaggerate their thoughts with dramatic but vague language • Use disassociation and **repression** (block feelings unconsciously)—don't confuse with **suppression** (feelings put aside consciously)
Narcissistic (cluster B)	• Feel entitled—strikingly so—because they are the best and everyone else is inferior, handle criticism very poorly
Dependent (cluster C)	• Can do little on their own, nor can they be alone
Avoidant (cluster C)	• Feel inadequate and are extremely sensitive to negative comments • Reluctant to try new things (e.g., make friends) for fear of embarrassment
Obsessive–compulsive (cluster C)	• Preoccupied with detail: rules, regulations, neatness • Isolation is a common ego-defense: putting up walls of self-restraint and detail orientation that keep away any sign of emotional effect

5. Humor: overt expression of ideas and feelings (especially those that are unpleasant to focus on or too terrible to talk about) that gives pleasure to others (e.g., Jokes about someone close to you just dying)
6. Identification: patterning behavior after someone else's
7. Intellectualization: explaining away the unreasonable in the form of logic
8. Introjection: identifying with some idea or object so deeply that it becomes a part of that person
9. Projection: attributing unacceptable thoughts, feelings, behaviors, and motives to others
10. Rationalization: making the unreasonable seem acceptable (e.g., upon being fired, you say you wanted to quit anyway)
11. Reaction formation: set aside unconscious feelings and express exact opposite feelings (show extra affection for someone you hate)
12. Regression: resorting to childlike behavior (often seen in the hospital)

13. Sublimation: taking instinctual drives (sex) and funneling that energy into a socially acceptable action (studying) behavior or emotion

14. Suppression: the conscious process of pushing thoughts into the preconscious; the conscious decision to delay paying attention to an emotion or need in order to cope with the present reality

VI. Somatoform and Factitious Disorders

A. Definitions

1. Somatoform disorder = **lack of conscious manipulation of somatic Sx**

2. Factitious disorder = **consciously faking** or manipulating Sx for purpose of "assuming the sick role" **but not for material gain**

3. Malingering = consciously faking Sx **for purpose of material gain**

B. Factitious Disorder

1. Pt may mimic any Sx, physical or psychological, to assume the sick role

2. **Pt is not trying to avoid work or win a compensation claim**

3. Münchhausen syndrome = factitious disorder with predominantly physical (not psychologic) Sx

4. Münchhausen by proxy = pt claims nonexistent Sx in someone else under his/her care; e.g., parents bringing in their "sick" children

5. DDx = malingering

6. **HINT: The USMLE may present a scenario involving nurses or other health care workers as the pts (often involving an episode of apparent hypoglycemia), look for evidence of factitious disorder (e.g., low C-peptide levels suggesting insulin self-injection)**

7. Dx is by exclusion of real medical condition

8. Tx is nearly impossible; when confronted, pts often become angry, deny everything, tell you how horrible you are, and move on to someone else

C. Somatoform Disorders

1. Somatization Disorder

a. Often female pts with problems starting before age 30, with history of frequent visits to the doctor for countless procedures and operations (often exploratory) and often history of abusive/failed relationships

b. Sx = somatic complaints involving different systems, particularly GI (nausea, diarrhea), neurologic (weakness), and sexual (irregular menses), with no adequate medical explanation based on exam/lab findings

c. Dx = rule out medical condition and material or psychologic gain

d. Tx = **continuity of care**

   (1) Schedule regular appointments so pt can express his/her Sx

   (2) Perform physical exam but do not order labs

   (3) As the therapeutic bond strengthens, strive to establish awareness in the pt that psychologic factors are involved and, if successful in doing so, arrange a psychiatric consult—but if done too early or aggressively, pt may be reluctant or resentful

2. Conversion Disorder

   a. Sx are neurologic, not multisystem, and are not consciously faked

   b. Sensory deficits often fail to correspond to any known pathway; e.g., a stocking-and-glove sensory deficit that begins precisely at the wrist, studies will reveal intact neurologic pathways, and pts rarely get hurt; e.g., pts who are "blind" will not be colliding into the wall

   c. Dx requires identification of a stressor that precipitated the Sx as well as exclusion of any adequate medical explanation

   d. Up to half of pts who receive this Dx may eventually be found to have non-psychiatric causes of illness; e.g., brain tumors, multiple sclerosis.

   e. Tx = supportive, Sx resolve within days (<1 mo), **do not tell pt that s/he is imagining the Sx, but suggest that psychotherapy may help with the distress**

   f. Px: the more abrupt the Sx, the more easily identified the stressor; the higher the premorbid function, the better the outcome

3. Hypochondriasis

   a. Sx = preoccupation with dz, pt does not complain of many Sx but misinterprets them as evidence of something serious

   b. Tx = regular visits to MD with every effort not to order labs or procedures, psychotherapy should be presented as a way of coping with stress, **again, do not tell pts that s/he is imagining the Sx**

4. Body Dysmorphic Disorder
    a. Sx = concern with body, **pt usually picks 1 feature, often on the face, and imagines deficits that other people do not see;** pt excessively exaggerates any slight imperfections, if present
    b. Look for a significant amount of emotional and functional impairment
    c. Tx = SSRIs may be helpful in some cases, surgery is not recommended

VII. Child and Adolescent Psychiatry

A. Developmental Theories

Developmental Theories				
AGE (YRS)	FREUD	ERICKSON	PIAGET	MAJOR THEME
0–1	**Oral**	**Trust vs. Mistrust**	**Sensorimotor**	**Stranger Anxiety**
	Everything goes in mouth	Child trusts all basic needs to be met.	Mastery of environment (0–2 yr)	Immense anxiety when separated from mother, between 6 and 9 mo
1–3	**Anal** Toilet training	**Autonomy versus Shame and Doubt**	**Preoperational** Symbolic terms (2–7 yr)	**Separation Anxiety** (18 mo–3 yr)
3–5	**Phallicoedipal**	**Initiative versus Guilt**	**Preoperational**	**Imaginary Friends**
6–11	**Latency**	**Industry versus Inferiority**	**Concrete Operations (7–11 yr)**	**Logical Thoughts**
11–10	**Genital**	**Identity versus Difusion**	**Formal Operations**	**Abstract Thoughts**
20–40		**Intimacy versus Isolation**		
40–65		**Generativity versus Stagnation**		
>65		**Ego Integrity versus Despair**		

B. Psychological Testing

Psychological Tests

INTELLIGENCE	
Wechsler Adult intelligence Scale—Revised (WAIS-R)	Tests ability to reason new situations, and assimilate, organize, and process this information. Tests cover verbal comprehension, performance at picture completion, block design, etc.
Wechsler Intelligence Scale for Children—Revised (WISC-R)	Tests children 6–16
Wechsler Preschool and Primary Scale of Intelligence (WPPSI)	Tests children 4–6
PERSONALITY	
Minnesota Multiphasic Personality Inventory (MMPI)	Most common objective personality test. Determines personality type
Rorschach	Most common projective test. Ink blot designs are interpreted, and defense mechanisms and thought disorders are evaluated
ACHIEVEMENT	
Wide-Range Achievement Test (WRAT)	Evaluates content-specific knowledge. Topics include spelling, reading, math, and science

C. Autism and Asperger's Syndrome

1. Autism is the prototypic **pervasive developmental disorder,** pervasive because the disorder encompasses so many areas of development: language, social interaction, emotional reactivity

2. The expression "living in his own world" captures this tragic disorder; the autistic child fails to develop nml interactions with others and seems to be responding to internal stimuli

3. Si/Sx
    a. Becomes evident before age 3 yr, often much earlier
    b. Baby does not seem to be concerned with the mother's presence or absence and makes no eye contact; as the baby becomes older, deficiencies in language (including repetitive phrases and made-up vocabulary) and abnormal behavior become more obvious

    c. Look for the behavioral aspects; the child often has a strange, persistent fascination with specific, seemingly mundane objects (vacuum cleaners, sprinklers) and may show stereotyped, ritualistic movements (e.g., spinning around)

    d. Autistic children have an inordinate need for constancy

  4. Think of Asperger's syndrome as autism **without** the language impairment

  5. **Contrary to older thought, poor parenting/bonding is not a cause of autism!—parents need reassurance about this**

  6. **Also, there is no medical evidence linking vaccines (Thimersol) to autism**

D. **Depression**

  1. Depression may present slightly differently depending on the age group

    a. Preschool children may be hyperactive and aggressive

    b. Adolescents show boredom, irritability, or openly antisocial behaviors

  2. Should look for the same Sx as described for adult depression: depressed mood, anhedonia, neurovegetative changes, etc.

  3. Tx

    a. Unlike adult depression, use of antidepressants is much more controversial with far fewer data supporting its effectiveness

    b. **Note:** children's mood disorders are especially sensitive to psychosocial stressors, so family Tx is a major consideration

E. **Separation Anxiety**

  1. Look for a child who seems a bit too attached to his parents or any other figures in his life; the child is worried that something will happen to these beloved figures or that some terrible event will separate them

  2. Si/Sx = sleep disturbances (nightmares, inability to fall asleep alone) and somatic Sx during times of separation (headaches, stomach upset at school)

  3. Tx = desensitizing Tx (gradually increasing the hours spent away from parents), in some cases imipramine is used

F. **Oppositional Defiant/Conduct Disorder**

  1. Differentiate the two by words and action (bark versus bite)

  2. Oppositional defiant disorder Si/Sx ("bark")

    a. Pts are argumentative, temperamental, and defiant, more so with people they know well (they may seem harmless to you)

    b. They are often friendless and perform poorly in school

3. Conduct Disorder Si/Sx ("Bite")
   a. Pts bully others, start fights, may show physical cruelty to animals, violate/destroy other people's property (setting fires), steal things, stay out past curfews, or run away
   b. Pts do not feel guilty for any of these behaviors
   c. Glimpse into the child's family life often reveals pathology in the form of substance abuse or negligence
4. Oppositional defiant disorder may lead to conduct disorder, but the two are not synonymous
5. Tx = providing a setting with strict rules and expected consequences for violations of them

G. **Attention-Deficit Hyperactivity Disorder (ADHD)**
   1. Si/Sx can be divided into the components suggested by their name
      a. Attention-deficit Sx = inability to focus on or perform tasks completely, easily distracted by random stimuli
      b. Hyperactivity Sx are more outwardly motor; child is unable to sit still, talks excessively, and can never "wait his turn" in group games
   2. Dx requires that Sx be present before age 7 yr
   3. Tx = methylphenidate, an amphetamine
      a. Parents and teachers notice improvement in the child's behavior
      b. Because of concerns about impeding the child's growth, drug holidays are often taken (e.g., no meds over weekends or vacations)
      c. Children with ADHD do better with an extremely structured environment featuring consistent rules and punishments
      d. Px is variable, some children show remissions of hyperactivity, but quite a few continue to show Sx through adolescence and adulthood; children with ADHD have a higher likelihood of developing conduct disorders or antisocial personalities

H. **Tourette's Disorder**
   1. Tics are involuntary, stereotyped, repetitive movements or vocalizations
   2. **Tourette's Dx requires both a motor tic and a vocal tic present for ≥1 yr**
   3. **Vocal tics often are obscene or socially unacceptable (coprolalia), which is a cause of extreme embarrassment to the pt**

4. Tx = haloperidol is effective but not required in mild cases

5. Psychotherapy is unhelpful in treating the tics per se but can be helpful in dealing with the emotional stress caused by the disorder

I. **Anorexia and Bulimia Nervosa**

1. Eating disorders are by no means limited to children, but because they often start in adolescence, they are mentioned here

2. Both disorders are associated with a profound disturbance in body image and its role in the person's sense of self-worth

3. Anorexia Si/Sx

   a. **By definition, anorexic pts are below their expected body weight** because they do not eat enough, often creating elaborate rituals for disposing of food in meal settings; e.g., cutting meat into tiny pieces and rearranging them constantly on the plate

   b. **Amenorrhea occurs 2° to weight loss**

4. Bulimia Si/Sx

   a. More common than anorexia, **characterized by binge eating:** consuming huge amounts of food over a short period, with a perceived lack of control

   b. May be accompanied by active purging (vomiting, laxative use)

   c. **Unlike anorexics, who by definition have ↓ body weight, bulimics often have a nml appearance**

   d. **Abrasions over the knuckles** (from jamming the fingers into the mouth to induce vomiting) and **dental erosion** suggest the Dx

5. Tx

   a. Hospitalization may be required for anorexia to restore the pt's weight to a safe level, pt often resists hospitalization

   b. Monitoring serum electrolytes is essential because of vomiting; most worrisome consequence is cardiac dysfunction—as exemplified by singer Karen Carpenter, whose battle with anorexia led to her untimely death

   c. Psychotherapy is the mainstay of Tx for both dz

6. Overall, anorexia nervosa has a relatively poor Px, with persistent preoccupations with food and weight; bulimics fare slightly better

VIII. Abuse of Drugs

A. Introduction

1. Always consider drug abuse when a pt's life seems to be disintegrating; e.g., deteriorating family relations, work performance, financial stability

2. Generally (with many exceptions), withdrawal Sx are opposite those of intoxication, dysphoria is characteristic of all of them— withdrawal is a sign of physiologic dependence

3. Individual drugs (Table 6.8)

Table 6.8   Drug Intoxications and Withdrawal

Drug	Intoxication Si/Sx	Withdrawal	Tx
Alcohol	Disinhibition, ↓ cognition Screen for alcoholism with **CAGE:** • C–feeling the need to **cut** down • A–feeling **annoyed** when asked about drinking • G–feeling **guilty** for drinking • E–need a drink in the morning **(eye-opener)**	Tremor, seizures, delirium tremens (high mortality! Prevent with benzodiazepines)	See Internal Medicine III.D.4.h
Cocaine/ amphetamine	Agitation, irritability, ↓ appetite, formication, ↑ or ↓ BP and HR, cardiac arrhythmia or infarction, stroke, seizure, nosebleeds	Hypersomnolence, dysphoria, ↑ appetite	• Benzodiazepine for seizures and for BP/HR • Ca++ channel blockers for ischemia (β blockers may worsen ischemia due to un-opposed α agonism by the cocaine)

(continued)

Table 6.8 *Continued*

Drug	Intoxication Si/Sx	Withdrawal	Tx
Heroin (opioids)	Intense, fleeting, euphoria, drowsy slurred speech, ↓ memory, pupillary constriction, ↓ respiration **Triad of ↓ consciousness, pinpoint pupils, and respiratory depression should always lead to a suspicion of opioids**	Nausea/vomiting, pupillary dilation, and insomnia	• Naloxone to reverse acute intoxication • Withdrawal Tx with long methadone taper
Benzodiazepine and barbiturates	Respiratory and cardiac depression	Agitation, anxiety, delirium	• Intoxication → control airway, charcoal to reduce absorption, flumazenil can reverse benzos acutely, but can precipitate seizures so be cautious • Withdrawal Tx → taper doses
PCP	Intense psychosis, violence, rhabdomyolysis, hyperthermia	Similar, lasts for days to weeks	• Supportive, benzos or haloperidol for psychosis
LSD	Sensation is enhanced: colors are richer, music more profound, tastes heightened	Not withdrawal, but can have long-lasting psychosis	• Supportive

LSD, lysergic acid diethylamide; PCP, phencyclidine.

IX. Miscellaneous Disorders

A. Disorders of Sexuality and Gender Identity

1. Sexual identity is based on biology; e.g., men have testes
2. Gender identity is based on self-perception; e.g., biologic male perceives himself as a male
3. **Children have a firm conception of their gender identity very early (before age 3)**
4. Sexual orientation is who the person is attracted to; **homosexuality is not a psychiatric disorder**

B. Dissociative Disorder (Multiple Personality Disorder)

1. A pt seemingly possesses different personalities that can each take control at a given time
2. The pt's Hx may give some Hx of childhood trauma; e.g., abuse
3. Tx focuses on gradual integration of these personalities
4. Main differentials are **dissociative amnesia** and **dissociative fugue**
   a. Amnesia is a syndrome of forgetting a great deal of personal information
   b. Fugue refers to the syndrome of sudden travel to another place, with inability to remember the past and confusion of present identity
   c. **Neither case involves shifting between different identities**

C. Adjustment Disorder

1. Any behavioral or emotional Sx that occur in response to stressful life events in excess of what is nml
2. Obviously has a catch-all quality to it; **this will be a frequent answer option on the USMLE**
3. **Dx requires Sx within 3 mo of the stressor** (so Sx do not have to be immediate) and **must disappear within 6 mo of the disappearance of the stressor**
4. Bereavement may seem to be a type of adjustment disorder (stressor is death), but they are separate Dx
5. Depending on the setting, adjustment disorder may appear as depression or anxiety—but remember: **axis I disorders such as major depression and generalized anxiety take precedence**

D. **Impulse-Control Disorders**
1. Pts are unable to resist the drive to perform certain actions **harmful to themselves or others**
2. Note the emotional response: these individuals **feel anxiety before the action and gratification afterward**
3. Intermittent explosive disorder
    a. Discrete episodes of aggressive behavior far in excess of any possible stressor
    b. The key term is **episodic**; antisocial personalities also commit aggressive behaviors, but their aggression is present between outbursts of such behavior
4. Kleptomania
    a. Impulse to steal
    b. The object of theft is not needed for any reason (monetary or otherwise)
    c. The kleptomaniac often feels guilty after stealing
5. Pyromania
    a. Purposeful fire-setting
    b. Often a fascination with fire itself distinguishes this from the antisocial personality/conduct disorders, where the fire-setting is purposeful; e.g., revenge, and not the failure to resist an impulse
6. Trichotillomania = hair-pulling, resulting in observable hair loss

X. Sleep

A. **Nml sleep** consists of two different types:
1. Non–rapid eye movement (NREM) has four states (Table 6.9)
2. Rapid eye movement (REM)

Table 6.9	Sleep Stages
Stages	**Characteristics**
Non-REM	Early slow-wave sleep
Stage 1	Alpha waves (awake waves disappear) and theta waves (time to sleep waves occur)
Stage 2	Sleep spindles
Stages 3 and 4	Delta-wave sleep (most difficult to awake from)
REM	Dreaming (suppressed by alcohol and drugs)

B. **Sleep Stages** (see Table 6.9)

C. **Sleep Disorders**

1. Dyssomnias: difficulties with sleep

   a. Insomnia

      (1) Unable to fall asleep or stay asleep recurrently over a 1-mo period

      (2) Can be associated with stress, anxiety, drugs, and various medical and mental conditions

      (3) Tx = sleep routine, exercise, antihistamines, short course of benzodiazepines <2 wk to prevent rebound insomnia

   b. Hypersomnia

      (1) Narcolepsy: recurrent sleep attacks, associated with REM sleep and dreaming

         (a) Pts can suddenly collapse because of loss of all muscle tone (cataplexy)

         (b) Tx = stimulants such as methylphenidate or pemoline

      (2) Sleep apnea: periods of apnea occurring during sleep

         (a) Obstructive: ↑ inspiratory effort that fails to result in ↓ airflow

            (i) Most common; pts usually are obese heavy snorers who awake after a gasp for air, pts complain of excessive daytime sleepiness; spouse complains of loud snoring

            (ii) Can lead to pulmonary HTN, associated with hypothyroidism

            (iii) Tx = weight loss, continuous positive airway pressure (CPAP) at night to maintain patent airway, surgery if no relief and severely affecting lifestyle or danger to life

         (b) Mixed obstructive/central: periods of no inspiratory effort followed by inspiratory effect that is obstructed by collapse of oropharyngeal airway

         (c) Central: rare; loss of inspiratory effort

      (3) Pickwickian syndrome (central alveolar hypoventilation)

         (a) Triad of somnolence, obesity, and erythrocytosis

         (b) Gradual onset of hypercapnia, hypoxemia, and erythrocytosis

         (c) Weight of adipose on lungs and abdomen cause chronic alveolar hypoventilation

         (d) Tx = weight loss, CPAP

2. Parasomnias
   a. Night terror
      (1) Arises during NREM sleep
      (2) Child sits up suddenly in bed with diaphoresis, tachycardia, feeling frightened
      (3) Not full awake; pts usually fall back to sleep after the episode
   b. Nightmares
      (1) Occur during REM sleep
      (2) Usually occur after an emotional event, stress, or frightening movie
      (3) Pts are fully awake and have good recall of nightmare events
      (4) Also associated with drugs
   c. Sleep walking (somnambulism)
      (1) Occurs during NREM sleep
      (2) Pts get out of bed and wander around; some pts can jump out of windows or open doors
      (3) Pts usually awaken with no memory of events

7. NEUROLOGY

I. Stroke

A. Terminology

1. Stroke = sudden, nonconvulsive focal neurologic deficit
2. Transient ischemic attack (TIA) = deficit lasting ≤24 hr (usually <1 hr) but resolves completely
3. Emboli sources = **carotid atheroma (most common),** cardiac and fat emboli, endocarditis (metastasizing CA cells)
4. Lacunar infarct = small infarct in deep white mater, strongly associated with HTN and atherosclerosis
5. Watershed infarcts occur at border of areas supplied by different arteries (e.g., middle cerebral artery, anterior cerebral artery), often following prolonged hypotension

B. Presentation

1. Si/Sx depend on location of stroke (Table 7.1)
2. Wernicke's aphasia (temporal lobe lesion) = receptive, pt speaks fluently but words do not make sense: **Wernicke's is wordy**

Table 7.1 Presentation of Stroke

Si/Sx	Artery	Region (Lobe)
Amaurosis fugax (monocular blind)	Carotid (emboli)	Ophthalmic artery
Drop attack/vertigo/ CN palsy/coma	Vertebrobasilar (emboli)	Brainstem
Aphasia	Middle cerebral	Dominant frontal or temporal[a]
Sensory neglect and apraxia[b]	Middle cerebral	Nondominant frontal or temporal[a]
Hemiplegia	Middle or anterior cerebral	Contralateral parietal
Urinary incontinence and grasp reflex	Middle or anterior cerebral	Frontal
Homonymous hemianopia	Middle or posterior cerebral	Temporal or occipital

[a]Dominant = left in 99% of right-handers and >50% of left-handers.
[b]Apraxia = pt cannot follow command even if it is understood and the pt is physically capable of it.

3. Broca's aphasia (frontal lobe lesion) = expressive, pt is unable to verbalize: **Broca's is broken**
4. Edema occurs 2–4 days postinfarct, watch for this clinically (e.g., ↓ consciousness, projectile vomiting, pupillary changes) (Figure 7.1)
5. Decorticate (cortical lesion) posturing → flexion of arms
6. Decerebrate (midbrain or lower lesion) posturing → arm extension

C. **DDx**

1. Stroke, seizure (Sz), neoplasm, encephalitis, multiple sclerosis
2. Stroke causes = 35% local atheroembolic, 30% cardiac, 15% lacunar, 10% parenchymal hemorrhage, 10% subarachnoid hemorrhage, ≤1% other (e.g., vasculitis, temporal arteritis, etc.)
3. Dx = CT for acute, MRI for subacute infarct and/or hemorrhage (see Figure 7.1)
4. Rule out Sz → EEG, loss of bowel/bladder control and tongue injury
5. Lumbar puncture to rule out encephalitis and rule in intracranial bleed

D. **Tx**

1. Tissue plasminogen activator (tPA) within 3–6 hr of onset (preferably 1 hr) for occlusive dz **only** (i.e., not for hemorrhagic stroke)
2. **Intracranial bleeding is an absolute contraindication to tPA use!**
3. Correct underlying disorder; e.g., hyperlipidemia, hypertension, diabetes, valve abnormality, coagulopathy, atrial fibrillation
4. For embolic strokes give aspirin/warfarin anticoagulation for prophylaxis
5. If carotid is 70% occluded and pt has Sx → endarterectomy

E. **Px**

1. 20%–40% mortality at 30 days (20% atheroemboli, 40% bleed)
2. <one-third of pts achieve full recovery of lifestyle
3. Atheroembolic strokes recur at 10% per yr

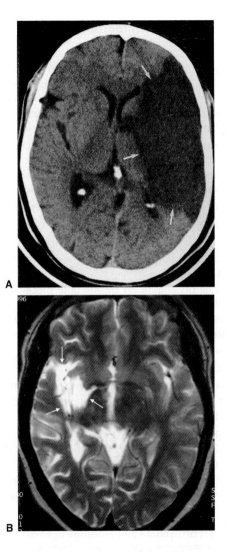

FIGURE 7.1

Cerebral infarction. **(A)** Unenhanced CT scan showing a low-density region of the left cerebral hemisphere conforming to the distribution of the middle cerebral artery (*arrows*). **(B)** MRI of another pt with a right middle cerebral artery territory infarct. The infarcted area (*arrows*) shows patchy high-signal intensity on this T2-weighted image. The *arrows* point to the anterior and posterior extents of the infarcted brain tissue. (From Armstrong P, Wastie M. *Diagnostic imaging,* 4th Ed. Oxford: Blackwell Science, 1998, with permission.)

II. Infection and Inflammation

A. Meningitis

1. 50% due to *Streptococcus pneumonia*, 25% due to *Neisseria meningitidis*; *Haemophilus influenza* rare now because of vaccination; *Listeria* seen in neonates, elderly, immunocompromised pts; group B *Streptococcus (Streptococcus agalactiae)* and *Escherichia coli* are the #1 and #2 causes of neonatal meningitis

2. Si = **Meningismus** (pt cannot touch chin to chest), ⊕ **Kernig's sign** (pt is supine with hip and knees flexed at 90 degrees, examiner cannot extend knee), ⊕ **Brudzinski's sign** (pt is supine, when examiner flexes neck, pt involuntarily flexes hip and knees)

3. Cerebrospinal fluid (CSF) differential for meningitis (Table 7.2)

4. Presentations can be acute, subacute, chronic

5. Acute
   a. Send CSF for Gram stain, bacterial cultures, herpes simplex virus (HSV) PCR
   b. Treat all pts empirically by age until specific tests return (Table 7.3)
   c. Of viral causes, only HSV (acyclovir) and HIV (AZT) can be treated—otherwise Tx is supportive
   d. Bacterial meningitis (Table 7.4)

6. Subacute/Chronic Meningitis
   a. Si/Sx = per acute but evolves over wk → mo, ± fever
   b. DDx = fungal, mycobacterial, noninfectious, other rare dzs
   c. Send CSF for fungal Cx, cytology, India Ink, TB PCR
   d. Fungal meningitis
      (1) DDx = *Cryptococcus, Coccidioides,* other rarer dz
      (2) *Cryptococcus* commonly seen in AIDS
         (a) India Ink stain will show *Cryptococcus* in CSF
         (b) Opening pressure is commonly elevated

Table 7.2 Cerebrospinal Fluid Findings in Meningitis

	Cells	Protein	Glucose
Bacterial	↑ **Neutrophils** (≥80%)	↑↑	↓↓ (≤2/3 serum)
Viral	↑ Mononuclear	± ↑	**Nml**
Subacute—Fungal and TB	↑ Mononuclear	↑↑↑↑	↓↓

Table 7.3 Empiric Therapy for Meningitis by Age

Age	Regimen	Common Etiologies
Neonates (≤1 mo)	**Ampicillin + ceftriaxone**	S. agalactiae, Listeria, E. coli
Children to teens	**Ceftriaxone + vancomycin**[a]	S. pneumonia, N. meningitidis
Adults ≤65	**Ceftriaxone + vancomycin**[a]	S. pneumonia by far most common
Adults ≥65 or with immune-compromise	**Ceftriaxone + vancomycin + ampicillin**	As for adults above, but need cover Listeria

Add acyclovir to any pt with possible HSV.
[a]Due to increasing rate of β-lactam resistance in S. pneumonia.

Table 7.4 Bacterial Meningitis

Organism	Pts	Characteristics	Tx
S. pneumoniae	**#1 cause in adults:** HIV, old age, asplenia, poor health predispose	Can progress from otitis media, sinusitis, or bacteremia	Ceftriaxone or PCN G, vancomycin if resistant to β lactams
N. meningitides	≥1 yr old or in adults in epidemics in close populations (military barracks)	**Petechiae on trunk, legs, conjunctivae—** beware of Waterhouse-Friderichsen syndrome (adrenal infarct)	Pen G; Rifampin or fluoroquinolone prophylaxis for close contacts
H. influenzae type B	Formerly #1 cause in children until vaccine	Now rare	Ceftriaxone
S. agalactiae	**#1 cause in neonates**	Acquired at birth	Ampicillin
E. coli	Common in neonates	Acquired at birth	Ceftriaxone
L. monocyto-genes	Elderly/neonates, HIV, pregnant, diabetes, steroids	Difficult CSF Gram stain/Cx, Dx → blood Cx	Ampicillin
S. aureus	Trauma/neurosurgery	Wound infxn from skin	Oxacillin/ vancomycin

NEUROLOGY

          (c) **Cryptococcal antigen in CSF invariably** ⊕

          (d) **Tx = iv amphotericin +/− 5-fluorocytosine, followed by fluconazole**

     (3) *Coccidioides*

          (a) Suspect in Arizona, California

          (b) Higher risk in African American, Hispanic, and Filipino pts

          (c) Diagnose by antibody ⊕ in serum or CSF

          (d) Tx = high dose fluconazole

  e. TB meningitis

     (1) Usually occurs in elderly by reactivation, grave Px

     (2) Dx is made by TB PCR of the CSF

     (3) Tx = **RIPE: R**ifampin, **I**NH, **P**yrazinamide, **E**thambutol

  f. Other causes = sarcoid, CA, collagen-vascular dz, drug reactions

B. **Encephalitis** Si/Sx = similar to meningitis, but focal findings are evident (Table 7.5)

C. **Abscess**

  1. Si/Sx = headache, fever, ↑ intracranial pressure (ICP), focal neurologic findings

  2. Risk factors = congenital right-to-left shunt (lung filtration bypassed), otitis, paranasal sinusitis, metastases, trauma, and immunosuppression

  3. Anaerobes and aerobes, Gram-positive cocci and Gram-negative rods can be causes

  4. Tx = antibiotics ⊕ **surgical drainage**

  5. **Brain abscesses are invariably fatal if untreated**

III. Demyelinating Diseases

A. Multiple Sclerosis (MS)

  1. Unknown etiology, but ⊕ genetic and environmental predispositions, ↑ common in pts who lived first decade of life in northern latitudes

  2. Si/Sx = relapsing asymmetric limb weakness, ↑ deep tendon reflexes (DTRs), nystagmus, tremor, scanning speech, paresthesias, optic neuritis, ⊕ Babinski sign

  3. Dx = Hx, MRI, lumbar puncture

Table 7.5 Encephalitis

Etiology	Dz	Si/Sx	Tx/Px
Toxoplasmosis	1) Transplacental congenital dz → hydrocephalus/mental retardation 2) Adults exposed via cat feces get dz if immunosuppressed—**Toxo is the #1 CNS lesion in AIDS**	**Multiple ring-enhancing lesions on MRI → focal neurologic deficits** Toxoplasmosis antibody test very sensitive	Sulfadiazine + pyrimethamine TMP-SMX prophylaxis if CD4 ≤200/μL
HSV	**#1 Cause of viral encephalitis**	**Olfactory hallucinations, bloody CSF, personality changes** EEG/MRI → temporal lobe dz	Acyclovir
Syphilis	**Meningovascular dz**	**Argyll-Robertson pupil[a]**	
	Parenchymal dz: 1) Tabes dorsalis = bilateral spinal cord demyelination 2) Dementia paralytica = cortical atrophy, neuron loss, gliosis	Pain, hypotonia, ↓ tone, ↓ DTRs ↓ proprioception, incontinence Sx = psychosis, dementia, personality change	IV penicillin
PML	Usually in AIDS, caused by JC virus	Diffuse neurologic dz	Treat the HIV
Cysticercosis	Caused by the helminth, *Taenia solium* → sz, diffuse encephalitis, edema, suspect in Hispanic pts with sz or encephalitis	Old lesions become calcified, dying lesions appear like abscesses	Albendazole + steroids

[a]Pupil accommodates but does not react to direct light.
PML, progressive multifocal leukoencephalopathy.

NEUROLOGY

4. MRI → periventricular plaques, multiple focal demyelination scattered in brain and spinal cord (**lesions disseminated in space and time**)
5. **Lumbar puncture → ↑ CSF immunoglobulins manifested as multiple oligoclonal bands on electrophoresis**
6. Tx = interferon-β or glatiramer acetate, may induce prolonged remissions in some pts
7. Px
   a. Variable types of dz, long remissions sometimes seen
   b. But can progressively decline → death in only a few years

B. **Guillain-Barré Syndrome**
1. Acute autoimmune demyelinating dz involving peripheral nerves
2. **Si/Sx = muscle weakness and paralysis ascending up from lower limbs, ↓ reflexes, can cause bilateral facial nerve palsy**
3. **Most often preceded by gastroenteritis (classically** *Campylobacter jejuni*), *Mycoplasma* or viral infxn, immunization, allergic reactions
4. Dx = Hx of antecedent stimuli (discussed earlier), CSF → **albumin-cytologic dissociation** (CSF protein ↑↑↑ without ↑ in cells seen)
5. Tx = plasmapheresis, IVIG, intubation for respiratory failure
6. Px is excellent for 80%–90% of pts, will spontaneously regress
7. Respiratory failure and death can occur in remainder

C. **Central Pontine Myelinolysis**
1. Diamond-shaped region of demyelination in basis pontis
2. **Results from rapid correction of hyponatremia, liver dz**
3. No Tx once condition has begun
4. Coma or death is common outcome

IV. Metabolic and Nutritional Disorders

A. **Carbon Monoxide Poisoning**
1. Seen in pts enclosed in burned areas or during the start of a cold winter (people are using their new gas heaters) → bilateral pallidal necrosis
2. Si/Sx = headache, nausea, vomiting, delirium, cherry-red color of lips
3. Dx = elevated carboxyhemoglobin levels
4. Tx = hyperbaric oxygen (first line) or 100% O_2

B. **Thiamine Deficiency**

1. Usually $2°$ to alcoholism
2. Beriberi peripheral neuropathy due to Wallerian degeneration
3. Wernicke's encephalopathy: **Wernicke's triad = confusion (confabulation), ophthalmoplegia, ataxia**
4. Wernicke's is related to lesions of mamillary bodies
5. Tx: give thiamine prior to glucose (e.g., thiamine should be run in IV fluid without glucose) or can exacerbate mamillary body damage

C. **B$_{12}$ Deficiency**

1. Subacute degeneration of posterior columns and lateral corticospinal tract
2. Si/Sx = weakness and $\downarrow$ vibration sense (both worse in legs), paresthesias, hyperreflexia, ataxia, personality change, dementia—**Note: neurologic deficits can occur even if no hematologic abnormalities are present!**
3. Dx is by high methylmalonic acid and homocysteine levels, which are more sensitive than B$_{12}$ levels
4. Tx = B$_{12}$ replacement (can use high-dose oral in lieu of injection provided no lack of Intrinsic Factor production exists; i.e., Pernicious Anemia)

D. **Wilson's Dz (Hepatolenticular Degeneration)**

1. Defect in copper metabolism $\rightarrow$ lesions in basal ganglia
2. Si/Sx = extrapyramidal tremors and rigidity, psychosis, manic–depression
3. **Pathognomonic $\rightarrow$ Kayser-Fleischer ring around the cornea** (Figure 7.2)
4. Dx = $\downarrow$ serum ceruloplasmin
5. Tx = penicillamine or liver transplant if drug fails

E. **Hepatic Encephalopathy**

1. Seen in cirrhosis, may result from brain toxicity $2°$ to excess ammonia and other toxins not degraded by malfunctioning liver
2. Sx = hyperreflexia, **asterixis** (flapping of extended wrists), dementia, Sz, obtundation/coma
3. Tx = lactulose, neomycin, and protein restriction to $\downarrow$ ammonia-related toxins

F. **Tay-Sachs Dz**

1. Hexosaminidase A defect $\rightarrow$ $\uparrow$ ganglioside GM$_2$

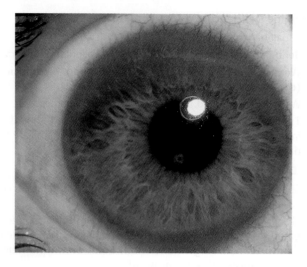

FIGURE 7.2

Kayser-Fleischer ring obscures peripheral iris details in a pt with Wilson's dz. (From Gold DH, Weingeist TA. *Color atlas of the eye in systemic disease.* Baltimore: Lippincott Williams & Wilkins, 2001.)

2. Si/Sx = **cherry-red spot on macula**, retardation, paralysis, blind
3. Dx by Bx of rectum or by enzymatic assay, no Tx

V. Seizures

A. Terminology
1. Complex Sz → loss of consciousness (LOC); simple Sz → no LOC
2. Generalized Sz = entire brain involved; partial Sz = focal area
3. Tonic Sz → prolonged contraction; clonic Sz → twitches
4. Absence = complex generalized Sz → brief LOC
5. Grand mal = complex generalized tonic–clonic Sz

B. Presentation
1. Hx of prior head trauma, stroke, other CNS dz ↑ risk for Sz
2. Si/Sx = loss of bowel/bladder control, tongue maceration, postictal confusion/lethargy, focal findings indicate epileptogenic foci
3. If pt has Hx of Sz, always check blood level of medication

Table 7.6	Seizure Therapy		
Partial	**Grand Mal**	**Absence**	**Myoclonic**
Phenytoin[a]	Valproate[a]	Ethosuximide[a]	Valproate[a]
Carbamazepine[a]	Carbamazepine	Valproate	Clonazepam
Valproate	Phenytoin	Clonazepam	

[a]First-line choice.

NEUROLOGY

C. **Tx**
   1. Tx Sz that recur or if pt has known epileptic focus (Table 7.6)
   2. Tx underlying cause: electrolyte, infxn, toxic ingestion, trauma, azotemia, stroke/bleed, delirium tremens, hypoglycemia, hypoxia
   3. **Phenytoin causes gingival hyperplasia, hirsutism**
   4. Carbamazepine causes leukopenia/aplastic anemia, hepatotoxic
   5. Valproate causes neutropenia, thrombocytopenia, hepatotoxic
   6. Stop Tx if no Sz for 2 yr and nml EEG

D. **Status Epilepticus**
   1. Continuous seizing lasting >5 min
   2. Tx = maintain and protect airway, IV benzodiazepines for immediate control, followed by phenytoin loading and phenobarbital for refractory cases
   3. **This is a medical emergency!**

VI. Degenerative Diseases

A. **Dementia versus Delirium Differential (Table 7.7)**

B. **Alzheimer's Dz (Senile Dementia of Alzheimer Type)**
   1. Most common cause of dementia—affects 5% of people age >70 yr
   2. Si/Sx = dementia, anxiety, hallucination/delusion, tremor
   3. Occurs in Down's syndrome pts at younger ages (age 30–40)
   4. Dx = clinical, with definitive Dx only possible at autopsy (neurofibrillary tangles)
   5. Tx = Cholinesterase inhibitors can slow dementia; antidepressants and antipsychotics can be used for psychosis; Memantine (Namenda), the first drug approved to treat moderate to severe stages of Alzheimer's, protects brain

Table 7.7 Dementia versus Delirium

	Dementia	Delirium
Definition	Both cause global decline in cognition, memory, personality, motor, or sensory functions	
Course	Constant, progressive	Sudden onset, waxing/waning daily
Reversible?	Usually not	Almost always
Circadian?	Constant, no daily pattern	Usually worse at night (sun-downing)
Consciousness	Nml	Altered (obtunded)
Hallucination	Usually not	Often, classically visual
Tremor	Often not	Often present (i.e., asterixis)
Causes	Alzheimer's, multiinfarct, Pick's dz, alcohol, brain infxn/tumors, malnutrition (thiamine/B$_{12}$ deficiency)	Systemic infxn/neoplasm, drugs **(particularly narcotics and benzodiazepines),** stroke, heart dz, alcoholism, uremia, electrolyte imbalance, hyper/hypoglycemia
Tx	Supportive (see below) for specifics depending on the dz	Treat underlying cause, **control Sx with haloperidol instead of sedatives**—pts are often given benzodiazepines or sedatives for agitation, but these drugs often exacerbate the delirium because they disorient pts even more

cells from damage caused by the chemical messenger glutamate

6. Px = inevitable decline in function usually over approximately 10 yrs
7. Prevention: Healthy Fit Aging, Vitamin E, Ginkgo, NSAIDS, etc.

C. **Multiinfarct Dementia**
   1. Si/Sx = acute, stepwise ↓ in neurologic function, multiple focal deficits on exam, HTN, old infarcts by CT or MRI
   2. Dx = clinical, radiographic
   3. Tx = prevent future infarcts by ↓ cardiovascular risks

D. **Pick's Dz**

1. Clinically resembles Alzheimer's, more in women, onset at younger age (50s)
2. Predominates in frontal (more personality changes seen) and temporal lobes
3. Dx = MRI → symmetric frontal or temporal atrophy, confirm by autopsy
4. Tx/Px = as per Alzheimer's

E. **Parkinson's Dz**

1. Parkinson's dz = idiopathic Parkinsonism, mid- to late-age onset
2. Parkinsonism
   a. **Syndrome of tremor, cog-wheel rigidity, bradykinesia, classic shuffling gait, mask-like facies,** ± dementia from loss of dopaminergic neurons in substantia nigra
   b. DDx = Parkinson's dz, severe depression (bradykinesia and flat affect), intoxication (e.g., manganese, synthetic heroin), phenothiazine side effects, rare neurodegenerative dz
3. Dx = clinical, rule out other causes
4. Tx
   a. Sinemet (levodopa = carbidopa) best for bradykinesia
   b. Anticholinergics (benztropine/trihexyphenidyl) for tremor
   c. Amantadine → ↑ dopamine release, effective for mild dz
   d. Surgery—Implanted deep brain electrical stimulation, or surgical pallidotomy for refractory cases
5. Px = typically progresses over yrs despite Tx

F. **Huntington's Chorea**

1. Si/Sx = progressive choreiform movements of all limbs, ataxic gait, grimacing → dementia, usually in 30s–50s (can be earlier or later)
2. Autosomal CAG triplet repeat expansion in HD gene → atrophy of striatum (especially caudate nucleus), with neuronal loss and gliosis
3. Dx = MRI → atrophy of caudate, ⊕ FHx
4. Tx/Px = supportive, death inevitable

G. **Amyotrophic Lateral Sclerosis (Lou Gehrig's Dz, Motor Neuron Dz)**

1. Si/Sx = **upper and lower motor neuron dz** → muscle weakness with fasciculations (anterior motor neurons) progressing to

denervation atrophy, hyperreflexia, spasticity, difficulty speaking/swallowing

2. Dx = clinical Hx, physical findings

3. Tx/Px = supportive, death inevitable, usually from respiratory failure

H. **Cerebral Palsy**

1. Dx = group of conditions that affect control of movement and posture. In approximately 70% of cases, cerebral palsy results from events occurring before birth that can disrupt nml development of the brain; in many cases, the cause of cerebral palsy is not known

2. Si/Sx = range from mild to severe, condition does not worsen as the child gets older

3. Types include

   a. **Spastic cerebral palsy:** most common form, individual's muscles are stiff, making movement difficult

   b. **Athetoid or dyskinetic cerebral palsy: found in** approximately 10%–20% of affected individuals, can affect the entire body, characterized by fluctuations in muscle tone, associated with uncontrolled movements

   c. **Ataxic cerebral palsy:** approximately 5%–10% of affected individuals have the ataxic form, which affects balance and coordination

4. Tx = Multidisciplinary team (pediatricians, physical medicine and rehabilitation physicians, orthopedic surgeons, physical and occupational therapists, ophthalmologists, speech/language pathologists, social workers, psychologists) working with the child and family

   a. Botox injected into spastic muscles or baclofen to ↓ spasticity

   b. Selective dorsal rhizotomy may permanently reduce spasticity by cutting some of the nerve fibers that are contributing most to spasticity

5. Px = Some pts with Tx are able to work and study, depending on severity of condition

DERMATOLOGY

I. Terminology

1. Macule = flat discoloration, <1 cm in diameter (Figure 8.1)
2. Papule = elevated skin lesion, <1 cm in diameter (Figure 8.2)
3. Plaque = elevated skin lesion, >1 cm in diameter (Figure 8.3)
4. Vesicle = small fluid-containing lesion <0.5 cm in diameter (Figure 8.4)
5. Wheal = like a vesicle but occurs transiently as in urticaria (hives) (Figure 8.5)
6. Bulla = large fluid-containing lesion, >0.5 cm in diameter (Figure 8.6)
7. Lichenification = accentuated skin markings in thick epidermis as a result of scratching (Figure 8.7)
8. Keloid = irregular raised lesion resulting from scar tissue hypertrophy (Figure 8.8)
9. Petechiae = flat, pinhead, nonblanching, red-purple lesion caused by hemorrhage into the skin: seen in any cause of thrombocytopenia
10. Purpura = larger than petechiae
11. Cyst = closed epithelium-lined cavity or sac containing liquid or semisolid material
12. Hyperkeratosis = ↑ thickness of stratum corneum (seen in chronic dermatitis)
13. Parakeratosis = hyperkeratosis with retention of nuclei in stratum corneum on histopathology and thinning of stratum granulosum (usually seen in psoriasis)
14. Acantholysis = loss of cohesion between epidermal cells (seen in pemphigus vulgaris)
15. Spongiosis = intercellular edema causing stretching and loss of desmosomal attachment, allowing formation of blisters within the epidermis (seen in acute and subacute dermatitis)

Text continues on page 390

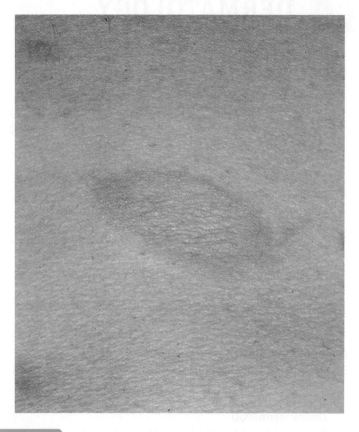

FIGURE 8.1

This erythematous macule is the typical herald patch of pityriasis rosea. (Courtesy of Dr. Steven Gammer.)

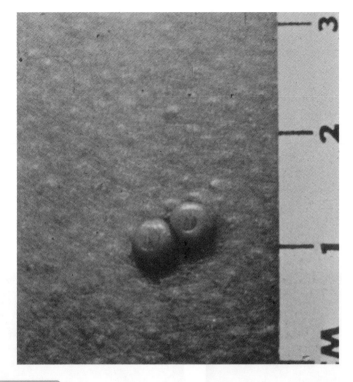

FIGURE 8.2

Papules of molluscum contagiosum. (Courtesy of Dr. Douglas Smith.)

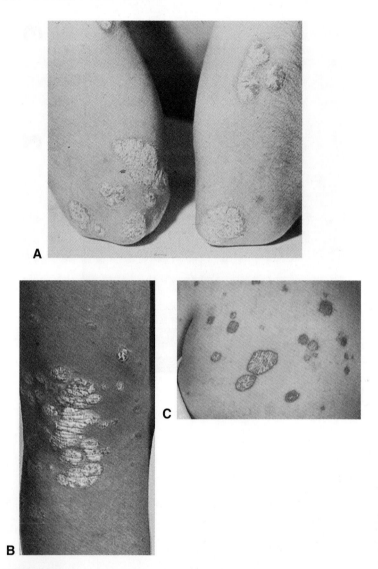

FIGURE 8.3

Erythematous plaques with silvery scales are typical of psoriasis and occur on the extensor surfaces, including the elbows **(A)** (Courtesy of Dr. Douglas Smith) and **(B)** knees (From Bickley LS. *Bate's guide to physical examination and history taking*, 8th Ed. Philadelphia: Lippincott Williams & Wilkins, 2003, with permission), but can also occur on the body **(C)**. (From Gold DH, Weingeist TA. *Color atlas of the eye in systemic disease*. Baltimore: Lippincott Williams & Wilkins, 2001.)

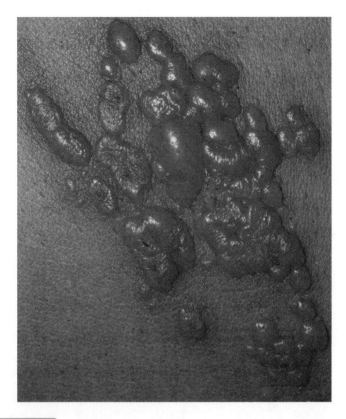

FIGURE 8.4

Vesicles of Herpes Simplex Virus (HSV) in the skin. (Courtesy of Dr. Steven Gammer.)

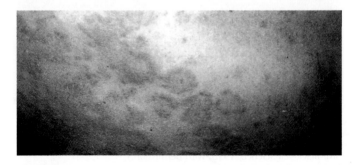

FIGURE 8.5

The ring-like wheals of urticaria. (From Axford JS. *Medicine*. Oxford: Blackwell Science, 1996, with permission.)

DERMATOLOGY

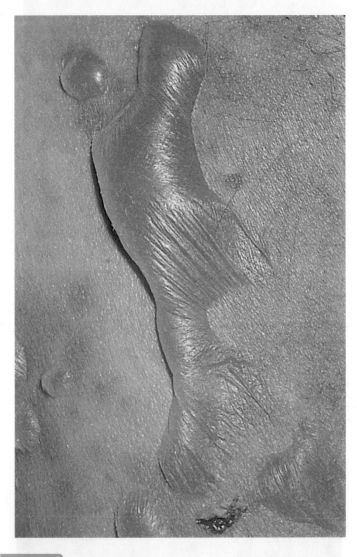

FIGURE 8.6

The large, tense bulla of bullous pemphigoid. (From Axford JS. *Medicine.* Oxford: Blackwell Science, 1996, with permission.)

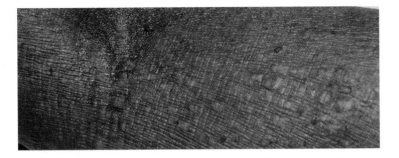

FIGURE 8.7

Lichenification caused by repeated scratching in this pt with chronic eczematous dermatitis. (Courtesy of Dr. Steven Gammer.)

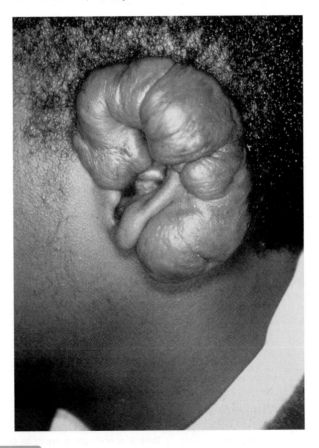

DERMATOLOGY

FIGURE 8.8

Keloid of the earlobe. (Courtesy of Dr. Douglas Smith.)

II. Topical Steroids (Table 8.1)

III. Infections

A. Acne

1. Inflammation of pilosebaceous unit caused by 2°
   Propionibacterium acnes infxn of blocked pore

2. Si/Sx = open comedones (blackheads) and closed comedones
   (whiteheads) on face, neck, chest, back, and buttocks; can become inflamed and pustular

3. Tx = topical antibiotics, Retin-A, benzoyl peroxide, systemic
   antibiotics, if acne is scarring consider isoretinoin (Accutane)

B. Impetigo

1. Superficial skin infxn of epidermis

2. Si/Sx = honey-crusted lesions or vesicles occurring most often
   in children around the nose and mouth, can be bullous or
   nonbullous (Figure 8.9)

3. Common organisms include *Staphylococcus aureus* and
   Streptococcus pyogenes

4. Tx = topical or oral antibiotics against *S. aureus* and *Strep* for
   7–10 days

C. Folliculitis

1. Si/Sx = erythematous pustules around hair follicles, commonly
   noted around beard area

Table 8.1	Use of Topical Steroids	
Potency	Drug	Use For Dz On. . .
Low	1% hydrocortisone	Face, genitals, skin folds (prevent atrophy/striae), also use in children for dz on body
Moderate	0.1% triamcinolone	Body/extremities, or ↑ dz on face, genitals, skin folds
High	Fluocinonide (Lidex)	Thick skin (palms/soles), or ↑ body dz, **do not use on face**
Very High	Diflorasone	Thick skin, or if very severe dz on body

Carrier substance: lotion = low potency; cream = mid potency; ointment = high potency.

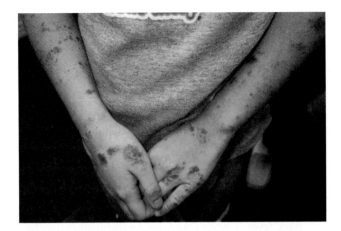

FIGURE 8.9
Crusted bullous impetigo. (Image provided by Stedman's.)

DERMATOLOGY

2. *S. aureus* most common; *Pseudomonas aeruginosa* causes "hot tub" folliculitis (organism lives in warm water), also fungi and viruses
3. Tx = local wound care, antibiotics only if severe

D. **SubQ Infxns**
   1. Cellulitis
      a. Si/Sx = spreading subQ infxn with classic signs of inflamma-tion: *rubor* (red), *calor* (hot), *dolor* (pain), and *tumor* (swelling)
      b. *Staphylococcus* and *Streptococcus* most common etiologies
      c. Tx = vancomycin, TMP-SMX, or clindamycin, narrow based on cultures
   2. Abscess
      a. Local collection of pus, often with fever, ↑ white count
      b. Tx = incision and drainage (I&D), antibiotics as above
   3. Erysipelas
      a. Cellulitis in which infxn extends to subQ tissue, leading to edema localized beneath the infxn
      b. Presents with bright red skin with peau d'orange (orange peel-like) appearance, classically on cheeks but can be elsewhere
      c. *Streptococcus* is the cause (usually Group A Strep [GAS])
      d. Treat with penicillin

4. Furuncle (Boil) and Carbuncle
   a. Furuncle = pus collection in one hair follicle, often caused by *S. aureus*
   b. Carbuncle = pus collection involving many hair follicles
   c. Tx = I&D, add antibiotics as above
5. Paronychia
   a. Infxn of skin surrounding nail margin that can extend into surrounding skin and into tendons within hand
   b. Commonly caused by *S. aureus*, also *Candida*
   c. Tx = warm compress, I&D if area is purulent, add antibiotics if severe
6. Necrotizing Fasciitis
   a. Infxn from skin layers down to fascial planes with severe pain, fever, ↑ white count, local inflammation may be deceptively absent but pt will appear very ill (i.e., "pain out of proportion to exam findings")
   b. Caused by *S. pyogenes* (GAS), *Clostridium perfringens*, and now described with community acquired Methicillin-resistant *S. aureus* (MRSA) infxn
   c. Tx = **immediate, extensive surgical débridement, add penicillin (for *Strep* and *Clostridium*) + vancomycin (for MRSA) + clindamycin (protein synthesis inhibitor, so shuts down production of toxins that mediate the tissue necrosis)**
   d. Px = ↑↑↑ mortality unless débridement is rapid and extensive

E. **Scarlet Fever**
1. *S. pyogenes* (GAS) is the cause
2. Si/Sx
   a. **"Sunburn with goose bumps"** rash, finely punctate, erythematous but blanches with pressure, initially on trunk, generalizes within hours
   b. Sandpaper rough skin, **strawberry tongue**, beefy-red pharynx, circumoral pallor
   c. **Pastia's lines = rash, most intense in creases of axillae and groin**
   d. Eventual desquamation of hands and feet as rash resolves
   e. Systemic Sx include fever, chills, delirium, sore throat, cervical adenopathy, all of which appear at same time as rash

    3. Complications include rheumatic fever and glomerulonephritis

    4. Tx = penicillin

F. **Hidradenitis Suppurativa**

    1. Si/Sx = plugged apocrine glands presenting as inflamed masses in groin/axilla, become secondarily infected

    2. Tx = surgical débridement and antibiotics

G. **Erythrasma**

    1. Si/Sx = irregular erythematous rash found along major skin folds (axilla, groin, fingers, toes, and breasts) (Figure 8.10)

    2. Commonly seen in adult diabetics, caused by *Corynebacterium* spp.

    3. Dx = Wood's lamp of skin → **coral-red fluorescence, KOH prep negative**

    4. Tx = erythromycin

DERMATOLOGY

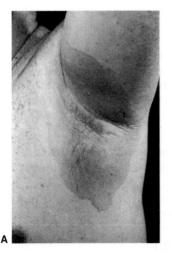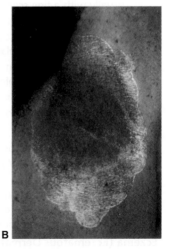

A   B

FIGURE 8.10

Erythrasma. **(A)** Nml light. **(B)** Coral-red axillary fluorescent as a result of proporphyria III, elaborated by *Corynebacterium minutissimum* under Wood's lamp. (From Axford JS. *Medicine.* Oxford: Blackwell Science, 1996, with permission.)

IV. Common Disorders

A. Psoriasis

1. Si/Sx = pink plaques with silvery-white scaling **occurring on extensor surfaces such as elbows and knees** (see Figure 8.3B), scalp (classically with involvement behind the ears), lumbosacral, glans penis, intergluteal cleft, and **fingernail pitting with onycholysis,** (Figure 8.11A), and can be associated with arthritis (Figure 8.11B)

2. Classic finding = **Auspitz sign** → removal of overlying scale causes pinpoint bleeding because of thin epidermis above dermal papillae

3. Classic finding = **Köbner's phenomenon** → psoriatic lesions appear at sites of cutaneous physical trauma (skin scratching, rubbing, or wound)

4. Psoriasis Variants

   a. Guttate psoriasis typically presents in a child or young adult, often after a streptococcal infxn, with acute eruption of small, drop-like, 1–10 mm diameter, salmon-pink papules, usually with a fine scale

   b. Pustular psoriasis is often localized to palms and soles, but can be generalized; presents with pustular lesions rather than classic psoriatic plaque (Figure 8.12)

   c. Inverse psoriasis presents with lesions in the intertriginous areas (e.g., axillae, groin, below the breasts) that are erythematous and appear like candidal infxns or tinea cruris

4. Dx = clinical, Bx is criterion standard

5. Tx

   a. Localized lesions can be treated with topical steroids

   b. PUVA (**P**soralens + **UV A** light) effective for diffuse dz, but may ↑ risk of skin CA

   c. Methotrexate, cyclosporine, or TNF antagonists (e.g., infliximab, etanercept) are options for refractory, diffuse dz, especially if arthritis coexists

B. Eczema (Eczematous Dermatitis)

1. Family of superficial, intensely pruritic, erythematous skin lesions

2. Atopic Dermatitis

   a. Si/Sx = **an "itch that rashes,"** rash 2° to scratching chronic pruritus, commonly found on the face in infancy; later in

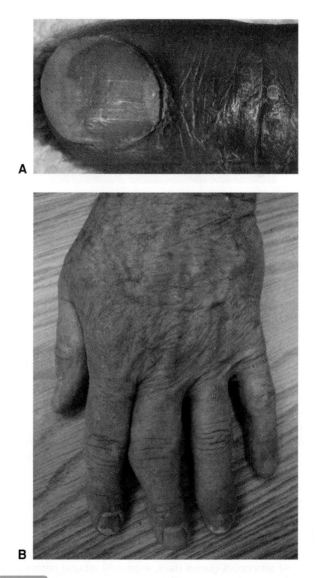

FIGURE 8.11

(A) Involvement of the hands leads to pitting of the fingernails and onycholysis (lifting of the nail off the nailbed). (Courtesy of Dr. Steven Gammer.)
(B) Psoriatic arthritis. This pt has severe psoriatic arthritis with marked deformities. (Image provided by Stedman's.)

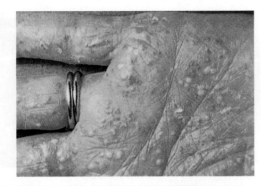

FIGURE 8.12

Pustular psoriasis.

childhood can present on the flexor surfaces such as antecubital and popliteal fossa (see Figure 8.7)
   b. Atopy
      (1) Inherited predisposition to asthma, allergies, and dermatitis
      (2) Dx is clinical
      (3) Tx = avoid irritants or triggers, keep skin moist with lotions, use steroids and antihistamines for Sx relief of itching and inflammation
3. Contact Dermatitis
   a. Si/Sx = linear pruritic rash at site of contact
   b. Caused by delayed-type hypersensitivity reaction after exposure to poison ivy, poison oak, nickel, or chemicals
   c. Dx is clinical, Hx of exposure crucial
   d. Tx = as per atopic dermatitis
4. Dishydrotic eczema causes multiple pruritic papules and vesicles on the hand and sides of fingers
5. Seborrheic Dermatitis
   a. Si/Sx = erythema, scaling, white flaking (dandruff) in areas of sebaceous glands (face, especially around nasolabial folds, scalp, groin, axilla, and external ear) (Figure 8.13)
   b. Called "cradle cap" in infants
   c. Dx = clinical and KOH prep to rule out fungal infxn
   d. Tx = selenium shampoo on face and trunk, steroids for severe dz

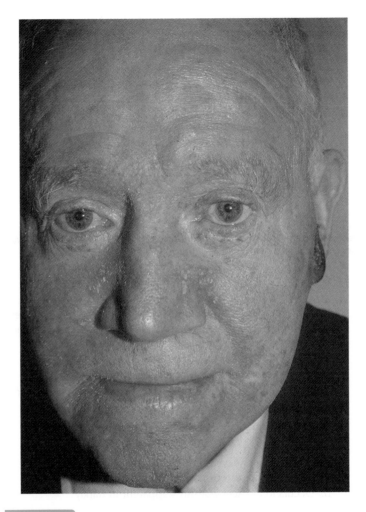

FIGURE 8.13

Seborrheic dermatitis.

C. **Urticaria (Hives)**

1. Common disorder caused by mast cell degranulation and histamine release
2. Si/Sx = transient papular wheals, intensely pruritic, surrounded by erythema, **dermographism** (write word on the skin and it remains imprinted as erythematous wheals, Figure 8.14)

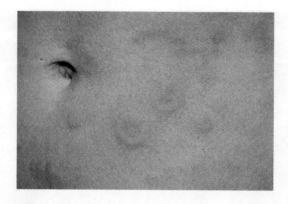

FIGURE 8.14

Urticarial wheals (acute urticaria). (From Axford JS. *Medicine*. Oxford: Blackwell Science, 1996, with permission.)

   3. Most lesions are immunoglobulin (Ig)E-mediated (type I hyper-sensitivity), but exercise, certain chemicals in sensitive pts, and inhibitors of prostaglandin synthesis (e.g., aspirin) also can cause IgE-independent reactions

   4. Dx = skin testing or aspirin or exercise challenge

   5. Tx = avoidance of triggers, antihistamines, steroids, epinephrine

   6. Can cause respiratory emergency requiring intubation

D. **Hypopigmentation**

   1. Vitiligo

      a. **Loss of melanocytes** in discrete areas of skin, appearing as sharply demarcated depigmented patches (Figure 8.15)

      b. Occurs in all races but most apparent in darkly pigmented pts

      c. Chronic condition that may be autoimmune in nature

      d. Associated with thyroid dz in 30% of pts, especially women

      e. Tx = minigrafting, total depigmentation, chronic UVA/UVB light Tx

      f. Px = some pts remit over long term, others never do

   2. Albinism

      a. **Melanocytes are present** but fail to produce pigment due to tyrosin ase deficiency

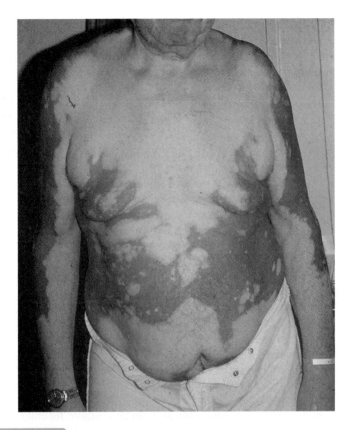

FIGURE 8.15

Extensive vitiligo. (Courtesy of Dr. Steven Gammer.)

DERMATOLOGY

    b. Si/Sx = white skin and eyelashes, nystagmus, iris translucency, ↓ visual acuity, ↓ retinal pigment, and strabismus

    c. Tx = avoid sun exposure, sunscreens

    d. Px = oculocutaneous form predisposes to skin CA

3. Pityriasis Alba

    a. Nonpathologic areas of hypopigmentation on face or upper extremities

    b. Can be 2° to prior infxn or inflammation, often regress over time

    c. Differentiated from tinea versicolor by KOH prep

E. **Hyperpigmentation**

1. Freckle (ephelis) is caused by nml melanocyte number but ↑ melanin within basal keratinocytes, darkens with sun exposure

2. Lentigo is pigmented macules caused by melanocyte hyperplasia that, unlike freckles, does not darken with sun exposure

3. Nevocellular Nevus

   a. Common mole, benign tumor derived from melanocytes

   b. Variations of nevi

      (1) Blue nevus = black-blue nodule present at birth, often mistaken for melanoma

      (2) Spitz nevus = red-pink nodule, often seen in children, confused with hemangioma or melanoma

      (3) Dysplastic nevus = atypical, irregularly pigmented lesion with ↑ risk of transformation into malignant melanoma, may be associated with an autosomal dominant inherited syndrome

   c. Dx = Bx; if Tx required, Tx is excision

4. Mongolian Spot

   a. A benign, macular blue-gray birthmark usually on the sacral area of healthy infants

   b. Often seen in newborns of Asian, African, or Native American descent

   c. Usually present at birth or appears within the first wks of life and typically disappears spontaneously within 4 yrs but can persist

   d. Lesions appear bruise-like and can be mistaken for child abuse, so good history of lesions is critical

   e. Dx = clinical, no Tx necessary

5. Melasma (Chloasma)

   a. Masklike hyperpigmentation on face seen in pregnancy

   b. Sunlight accentuates pigmentation, which typically fades postpartum

   c. Tx = minimize facial exposure to sun or use hydroquinone cream (works for any hyperpigmentation)

6. Hemangioma

   a. Group of "birthmarks," capillary hemangiomas present at birth

   b. Port-wine stains (purple-red on face or neck) (Figure 8.16)

      (1) Can be associated with Sturge-Weber syndrome (see Table 8.3)

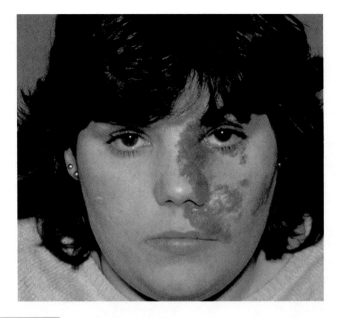

FIGURE 8.16

Port wine stain in a pt with Sturge-Weber syndrome. (From Gold DH, Weingeist TA. *Color atlas of the eye in systemic disease*. Baltimore: Lippincott Williams & Wilkins, 2001.)

      (2) Must screen for glaucoma and CNS dz (CT scan)

      (3) Tx = laser Tx, will not regress spontaneously

  c. Strawberry hemangiomas (bright-red raised lesions) are benign, most disappear on their own

  d. Cherry hemangiomas (benign small red papule); Tx with laser Tx

7. Xanthoma

  a. Yellowish papules, often accumulations of foamy histiocytes

  b. Can be idiopathic or associated with familial hyperlipidemia (Figure 8.17)

  c. If seen on eyelids they are called "xanthelasma"

  d. Tx = ↓ hyperlipidemia, surgically excise papules as needed

8. Pityriasis Rosea (Figure 8.18)

  a. Erythematous maculopapular rash with scale apparent in center

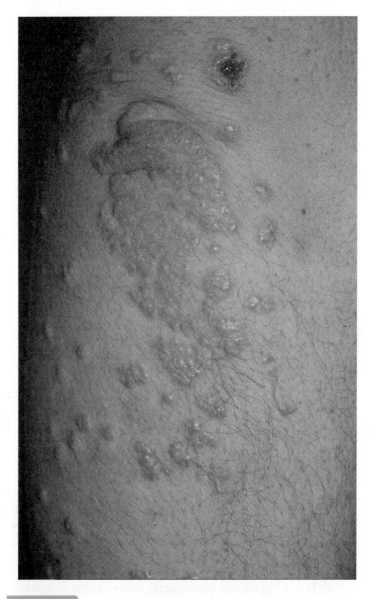

FIGURE 8.17

Multiple xanthoma (called eruptive xanthoma) in a pt with severe hypercholesterolemia. (Courtesy of Dr. Steven Gammer.)

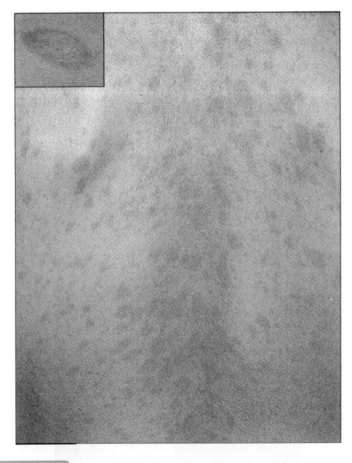

FIGURE 8.18

The herald patch (*inset*) of pityriasis rosea is typically found on the trunk and is much larger than the other papules (courtesy of Dr. Steven Gammer). Note the Christmas tree distribution of the lesions following the skin lines in a concave shape up vertically close to the spine and horizontally along the sides. (From Graham-Brown R, Burns T. *Lecture notes on dermatology*, 7th Ed. Oxford: Blackwell Science, 1996:211, with permission.)

b. Often preceded by a "herald patch" on trunk
c. **Can appear on back in a Christmas tree distribution**
d. Tx = sunlight, otherwise spontaneously remits in 6–12 wk
9. Erythema Nodosum (Figure 8.19)
a. Inflammation of subQ fat (panniculitis) and adjacent vessels
b. Characteristic lesions are **tender red nodules occurring on the lower legs** and sometimes forearms

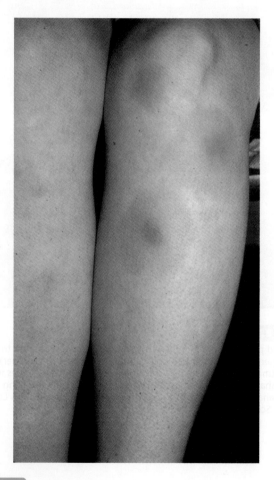

FIGURE 8.19
Erythema nodosum on the shins.

      c. Usually resolves in 6–8 wk, Tx directed at underlying cause

      d. Common causes

        (1) Infxns = *Mycoplasma, Chlamydia, Coccidioides immitis, Mycobacterium leprae,* and others

        (2) Drugs = sulfonamides and contraceptive pills

        (3) Inflammatory bowel dz, sarcoidosis, rheumatic fever

        (4) Pregnancy

10. Dermatomyositis (see Internal Medicine VI.E.3)

11. Seborrheic Keratosis (Figure 8.20)

    a. Black or brown benign plaques, appear to be stuck onto skin surface

    b. Commonly seen in elderly, runs in families

    c. Can be mistaken for melanoma

    d. The sign of Lesser-Trélat is the association of multiple eruptive seborrheic keratoses with internal malignancy, most commonly adenoCA of the GI tract

12. Acanthosis Nigricans (Figure 8.21)

    a. Black velvety plaques on flexor surfaces and intertriginous areas

    b. Seen in obesity and endocrine disorders (e.g., diabetes)

    c. Can mark underlying malignancy (e.g., GI/GU, lymphoma)

13. Bronze Diabetes = 1° Hemochromatosis

    a. Familial defect causing intestinal hyperabsorption of iron

    b. **Classic triad: ↑ skin pigmentation, cirrhosis, diabetes mellitus**

    c. Other Sx = cardiomyopathy, pituitary failure, arthropathies

    d. **Clinical pearl: hemochromatosis is the likely Dx in any pt with osteoarthritis involving the metacarpophalangeal joints**

    e. Dx = transferrin saturation (iron/total iron-binding capacity) ≥50%

    f. Tx = phlebotomy, which improves survival if started early

F. **Verrucae (Warts)**

  1. Verruca vulgaris = hand wart

  2. Verruca plana (flat wart) smaller than vulgaris, seen on hands and face

  3. Human papilloma virus (HPV) types 1–4 cause skin and plantar warts

  4. HPV-6 and HPV-11 cause anorectal and genital warts (condyloma acuminatum)

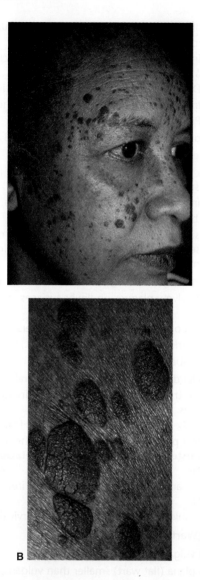

(A) The black plaques of seborrheic keratosis appear to be "stuck-on."
(B) A close-up of their velvety/warty surface. (Both images courtesy of Dr. Steven Gammer.)

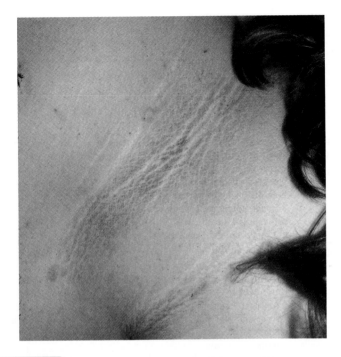

FIGURE 8.21

The fine, velvety plaque of acanthosis nigricans. (Courtesy of Dr. Steven Gammer.)

    5. HPV-16, HPV-18, HPV-31, HPV-33, HPV-35 cause cervical CA

    6. Condylomata lata are flat warts caused by *Treponema pallidum* (syphilis)

V.   Cancer (Table 8.2)

VI.   Neurocutaneous Syndromes (Phakomatoses) (Table 8.3)

VII. Blistering Disorders

A. Pemphigus Vulgaris (PG)

    1. PG is a rare autoimmune disorder, **affecting 20- to 40-yr-olds**

    2. Si/Sx = **flaccid epidermal bullae** that easily slough off leaving large denuded areas of skin (Nikolsky's sign) (Figure 8.28), ↑ risk of 2° infxn

Table 8.2 Skin Cancer

Dz	Si/Sx	Tx	Px
Basal cell CA	Most common skin CA, classic **"rodent ulcer"** seen on face, with **pearly translucent borders and fine telangiectasias**, not usually found on lips (Figure 8.22)	Excision	Excellent—almost never metastasize
Squamous cell CA	Common in elderly, appears as erythematous nodules on sun-exposed areas that eventually ulcerate and crust, **frequently preceded by actinic keratosis = rough epidermal lesions on sun-exposed** areas such as lower lip, ears and nose (Figure 8.23)	Excision, radiation	Metastasize more basal cell than but not as much as melanoma
Malignant melanoma	Seen in lightly pigmented individuals with ↑ sun exposure (Figure 8.24) — diagnose with **ABCDEs** ◊ **A**symmetry = malignant, symmetry = benign ◊ **B**order = irregular; benign = smooth ◊ **C**olor = multicolored; benign = one color ◊ **D**iameter >6 mm; benign = <6 mm ◊ **E**levation = raised above skin; benign = flat ◊ **E**nlargement = growing; benign = not growing	Excision, chemo if metastasis likely	High rate of metastasis → **#1 skin CA killer, risk of mets ↑ with depth of invasion on Bx**
Kaposi's sarcoma	Connective tissue CA caused by human herpes virus-8, appears as red-purple plaques or nodules on skin and mucosa, frequently affects lungs and GI viscera, almost exclusively seen in AIDS pts (Figure 8.25)	HIV drugs, chemo	Benign unless damages internal organs
Cutaneous T-cell lymphoma	"Mycosis fungoides," presents with erythematous patches and plaques that may ultimately ulcerate, rash can precede malignancy by yrs, a leukemic phase of dz called "Sézary syndrome"	PUVA, topical chemo, radiation	Life expectancy 7–10 yr without Tx

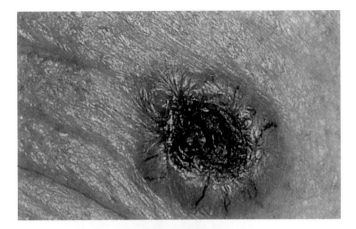

FIGURE 8.22

The rodent ulcer of basal cell CA. Note the telangiectasias as the borders. (From Axford JS. *Medicine.* Oxford: Blackwell Science, 1996, with permission.)

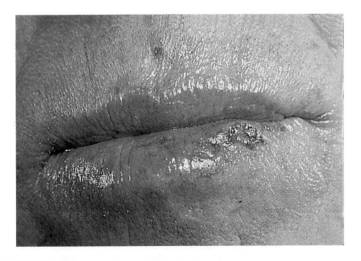

FIGURE 8.23

Squamous cell CA of the lip (early ulcer). (From Axford JS. *Medicine.* Oxford: Blackwell Science, 1996, with permission.)

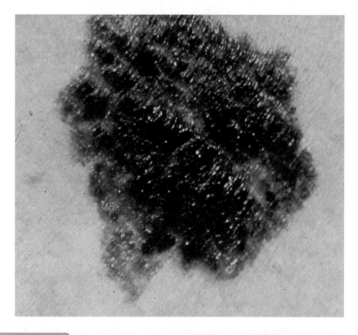

FIGURE 8.24

A melanoma with ABCDEs. The lesion is Asymmetric, with irregular Borders, is Multicolored, has a large Diameter, and is Elevated (plaque not macule). It was also Enlarging. (Courtesy of Dr. Douglas Smith.)

3. DDx = bullous pemphigoid
4. Dx = skin Bx → **immunofluorescence surrounding epidermal cells** showing "tombstone" fluorescent pattern
5. Tx = high-dose oral steroids, antibiotics for infxn
6. Px = **often fatal if not treated**

B. **Bullous Pemphigoid**

1. Common autoimmune dz affecting **mostly the elderly**
2. Resembles PG but much less severe clinically
3. Si/Sx = **hard, tense bullae** that do not rupture easily and usually heal without scarring if uninfected (Figure 8.29)
4. Dx = skin Bx → immunofluorescence as a **linear band along the basement membrane, with** ↑ **eosinophils** in dermis
5. Tx = oral steroids
6. Px = much better than PG

Text continues on page 416

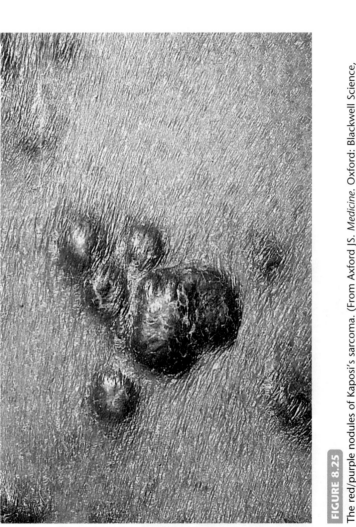

FIGURE 8.25

The red/purple nodules of Kaposi's sarcoma. (From Axford JS. *Medicine.* Oxford: Blackwell Science, 1996, with permission.)

DERMATOLOGY

Table 8.3 Neurocutaneous Syndromes (Phakomatoses)

Dz[a]	Characteristics
Tuberous sclerosis (Figure 8.26)	Ash leaf patches (hypopigmented macules), Shagreen spots (leathery cutaneous thickening), adenoma sebaceum of the face, **sz, mental retardation**
Neurofibromatosis (NF) (Figure 8.27)	Si/Sx = **café-au-lait spots**, neurofibromas, meningiomas, acoustic neuromas, Kyphoscoliosis—NF-2 causes bilateral acoustic neuromas
Sturge-Weber syndrome (see Figure 8.16)	Si/Sx = **port-wine hemangioma of face** in CN V distribution, mental retardation, sz
Von Hippel-Lindau syndrome	Si/Sx = multiple hemangiomas in various organs, ↑ frequency of renal cell CA and polycythemia (↑ erythropoietin secretion)

[a]All are autosomal dominant except Sturge-Weber, which has no genetic pattern.

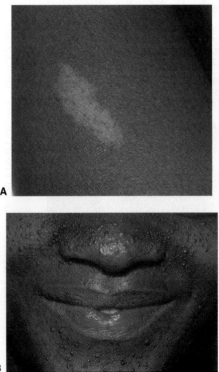

FIGURE 8.26

(A) The ash leaf patch and (B) adenoma sebaceum characteristic of tuberous sclerosis.

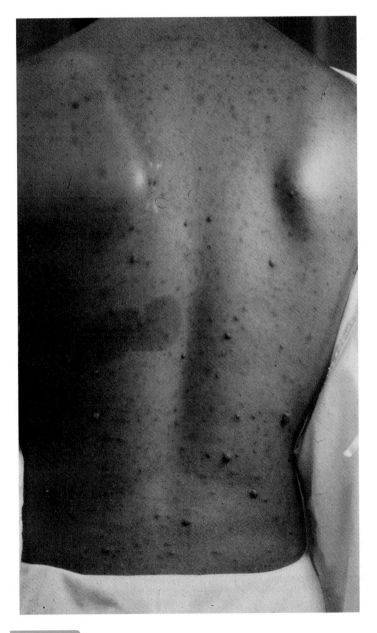

FIGURE 8.27

Several neurofibromas and a large café-au-lait spot. (Courtesy of Dr. Steven Gammer.)

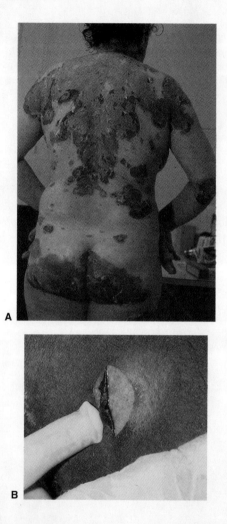

FIGURE 8.28

(A) The flaccid bullae of pemphigus vulgaris slough easily, leaving inflamed, denuded areas of skin. **(B)** Nikolsky's sign is present due to the weak attachment of the bullae to the underlying epidermis. (Courtesy of Dr. Steven Gammer.)

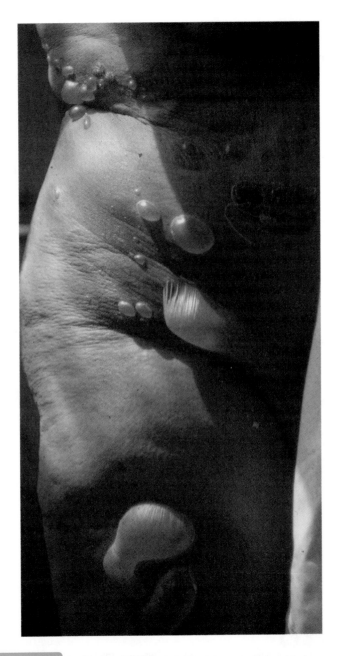

FIGURE 8.29
Multiple tense bullae of bullous pemphigold. (Courtesy of Dr. Steven Gammer.)

415

C. **Erythema Multiforme**

1. Hypersensitivity reaction to drugs, infxns, or systemic disorders such as malignancy or collagen vascular dz

2. Si/Sx = **diffuse, erythematous targetlike lesions** in many shapes (hence name "multiforme"), often accompanying a herpes eruption (Figure 8.30A)

3. **Stevens-Johnson syndrome = severe febrile form (sometimes fatal) → hemorrhagic crusting also affects lips and oral mucosa** (Figure 8.30B)

4. Dx = clinical, Hx of herpes infxn or drug exposure

5. Tx = stop offending drug, prevent eruption of herpes with acyclovir

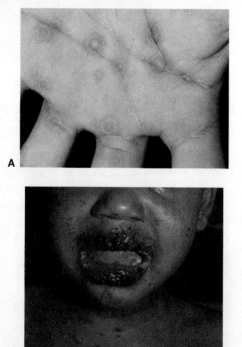

A

B

FIGURE 8.30

(A) The target-like lesions of erythema multiforme. (B) Stevens-Johnson syndrome is a more severe presentation of erythema multiforme, in which mucosal surfaces are involved as well. (Courtesy of Dr. Steven Gammer.)

D. **Porphyria Cutanea Tarda**
   1. Autosomal dominant defect in heme synthesis (50% ↓ in uroporphyrinogen decarboxylase activity in RBC and liver)
   2. Si/Sx = blisters on sun-exposed areas of face and hands, ↑ hair on temples and cheeks, **no abd pain** (differentiates from other porphyrias)
   3. Dx = Wood's lamp of urine → **urine fluoresces with distinctive orange-pink color because of** ↑ **levels of uroporphyrins**
   4. Tx = sunscreen, phlebotomy, chloroquine, no alcohol
   5. Px = remitting/relapsing, exacerbations resulting from viral hepatitis, hepatoma, alcohol abuse, estrogen, sunlight

VIII. Vector-Borne Diseases

A. **Bacillary Angiomatosis (Peliosis Hepatis)**
   1. Si/Sx = weight loss, abd pain, **rash with red or purple vascular lesions**, from papule to hemangioma size, located anywhere on skin and disseminated to any organ
   2. DDx = Kaposi's sarcoma, cherry hemangioma
   3. **Almost always seen in HIV ⊕ pts or homeless population**
   4. Caused by *Bartonella* spp., leading to dysregulated angiogenesis
   5. **Cat-scratch dz caused by *Bartonella henselae* transmitted by kitten scratches; trench fever caused by *Bartonella quintana* spread by lice**
   6. Dx = histopathology with Wharthin-Starry silver stain, visualization of organisms in lesion, blood culture, and polymerase chain reaction (PCR) can be done
   7. Tx = erythromycin

B. **Lyme Dz**
   1. Si/Sx = fever, chills, headaches, facial paralysis, lethargy, photophobia, meningitis, myocarditis, arthralgia, and myalgias
   2. **Classic rash = erythema chronicum migrans → erythematous annular plaques with a red migrating border, central clearing, and induration**
   3. Dx = PCR for *Borrelia burgdorferi* DNA, or skin Bx of migrating edge looking for causative spirochete
   4. Prevent by spraying skin and clothes with DEET or permethrin; wear long pants in woods to prevent tick bite *(Ixodes dammini, Ixodes pacificus)*

DERMATOLOGY

    5. Postexposure (i.e., after tick bite) prophylaxis with single dose doxycycline

    6. Once infected → high-dose penicillin, ceftriaxone, doxycycline or tetracycline for 2–4 wk

C. Rocky Mountain Spotted Fever

    1. Si/Sx = acute-onset fever, headache, myalgias, classic rash

    2. Rash = **erythematous maculopapular, starting on wrists and ankles then moving toward palms, soles, and trunk**

    3. Rash may lead to cutaneous necrosis because of disseminated intravascular coagulation-induced occlusion of small cutaneous vessels with thrombi

    4. Dx by Hx (exposure to outdoors or tick bite from *Dermacentor* spp.), serologies for *Rickettsia rickettsii*, skin Bx

    5. Doxycycline or chloramphenicol

IX. Parasitic Infections

A. Scabies

    1. Si/Sx = erythematous, **markedly pruritic papules and burrows located in intertriginous areas** (e.g., finger and toe webs, groin), lesions contagious (Figure 8.31)

    2. Dx = microscopic identification of *Sarcoptes scabiei* mite in skin scrapings

    3. Tx = pt and all close contacts apply Permethrin 5% cream to entire body for 8–10 hr, then repeat in 1 wk, wash all bedding in hot water the same day

    4. Lindane cream is less effective, associated with adverse effects in kids

    5. Symptomatic relief of hypersensitivity reaction to dead mites may be treated with antihistamines and topical steroids

B. Pediculosis Capitis (Head Louse)

    1. Si/Sx = can be aSx, or pruritus and erythema of scalp may be noted, common in school-age children

    2. Dx = microscope exam of hair shaft (Figure 8.32), nits may fluoresce with Wood's lamp

    3. Permethrin shampoo or gel to scalp, may need to repeat

C. Pediculosis Pubis ("Crabs")

    1. Si/Sx = very **pruritic papules in pubic area**, axilla, periumbilically in males, along eyelashes, eyebrows, and buttocks

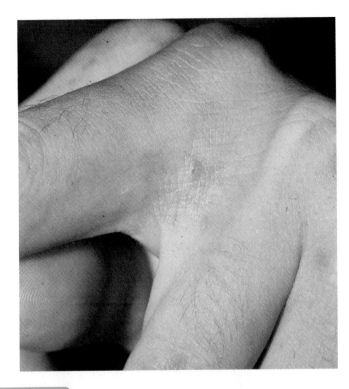

FIGURE 8.31

A papule located in the finger web is classic for scabies. (Courtesy of Dr. Steven Gammer.)

2. Dx = microscopic identification of lice, rule out other sexually transmitted dz (STDs)

3. Tx = apply Permethrin 5% shampoo for 10 min, then repeat in 1 wk

D. **Cutaneous Larva Migrans (Creeping Eruption)**

1. Si/Sx = erythematous, pruritic, **serpiginous threadlike lesion** marking burrow of migrating nematode larvae, often on back, hands, feet, buttocks (Figure 8.33)

2. Organism = hookworms: *Ancylostoma*, *Necator*, *Strongyloides*

3. Dx = Hx of unprotected skin lying in moist soil or sand, Bx of lesion, lesion moves very slowly (e.g., 1–2 cm per day)

4. Tx = ivermectin orally or thiabendazole topically

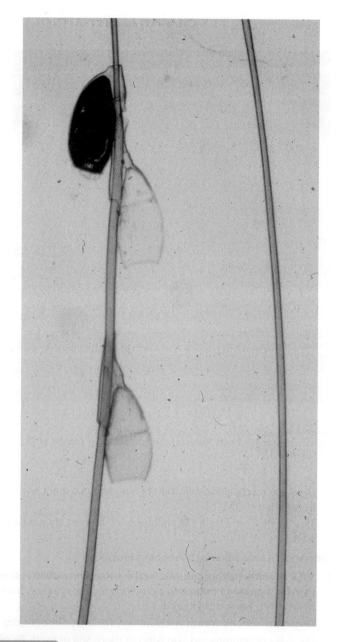

A louse and an empty casing attached to hair shaft. (Courtesy of Dr. Steven Gammer.)

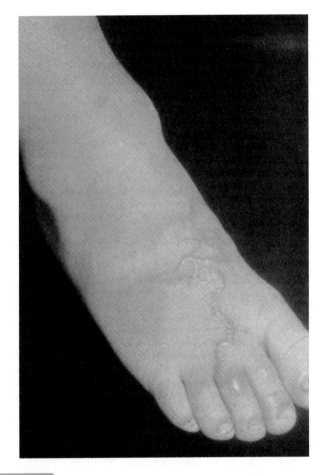

FIGURE 8.33

Cutaneous larva migrans. The skin shows a creeping eruption with the characteristic serpiginous, raised lesion. (From Sun T. *Parasitic disorders: pathology diagnosis, and management,* 2nd Ed. Baltimore: Lippincott Williams & Wilkins, 1999.)

E. Larva Currens

1. Si/Sx = rapidly moving linear, erythematous streaks in skin, moves 1–2 cm per hour

2. Caused by disseminated infxn by *Strongyloides*

3. Dx by ova and parasite exam (O&P) of stool or sputum (for hyperinfxn syndrome, in a very sick pt), or Bx

4. Tx = ivermectin

X. Fungal Cutaneous Disorders (Table 8.4)

Table 8.4 Fungal Cutaneous Disorders

Dz	Si/Sx	Dx	Tx
Tinea	• Erythematous, pruritic, scaly, well-demarcated plaques, typically annular (ring-like) with raised borders • Tinea cruris is intertriginous (typically groin) • Tinea corporis (i.e., ringworm) is on torso • Tinea capitis is on scalp, associated with hair loss and broken hair shafts • Tinea pedis is on foot (i.e., athlete's foot)	Clinical or KOH prep	Topical antifungal (oral needed for tinea capitis)
Onychomycosis	• Fingernails or toenails appear thickened, yellow, degenerating	Clinical or KOH prep	PO itraconazole or fluconazole
Tinea versicolor	• Caused by *Pityrosporum ovale* (a.k.a., *Malassezia furfur*) • Multiple sharply marginated erythematous or hyperpigmented macules on face and trunk noticed in summer because macules will not tan—in a dark-skinned individual it can appear like vitiligo, but it is distinguished by multiple, individual circular lesions	KOH prep → yeast and hyphae with classic **spaghetti and meatball appearance**	Selenium sulfide shampoo daily on affected areas for 7 days
Candida	• Erythematous scaling plaques, often in intertriginous areas (groin, breast, buttocks, web of hands)—distinguish from tinea cruris by the presence of satellite lesions beyond the edges of the main infxn (Figure 8.34A) • Oral thrush → cottage cheese-like white plaques on mucosal surface (Figure 8.34B) • Can extend to esophagus and cause dysphagia and odynophagia	KOH prep → budding yeast and pseudo-hyphae	Topical Nystatin or oral fluconazole

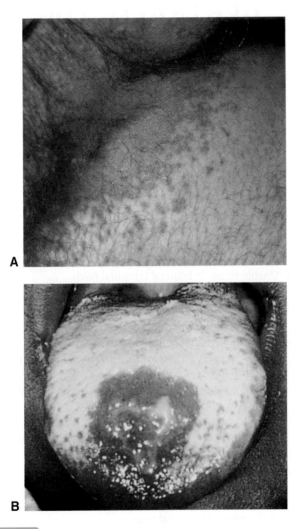

FIGURE 8.34

(A) An erythematous intertriginous infxn is usually Candida if there are "satellite lesions" beyond the edges of the main infxn. (Courtesy of Dr. Steven Gammer.) **(B)** Thrush on the tongue (From Weber J, Kelley J. *Health assessment in nursing*, 2nd Ed. Philadelphia: Lippincott Williams & Wilkins, 2003.)

9. OPHTHALMOLOGY

I. Eyes

A. Classic Syndromes or Sx

1. Amblyopia
   a. ↓ vision 2° to failure of development of the pathway between the retina and visual cortex before age 7
   b. Usually affects one eye, can be 2° to cataract, severe refractive error, or strabismus
   c. Si/Sx = esotropia (inwardly rotated "crossed eyes") or exotropia (outwardly rotated "walled eyes"), diplopia, and refractive error not correctable with lenses
   d. Tx = early correction of cause of visual acuity disturbance

2. Bitemporal Hemianopsia (Figure 9.1)
   a. Unable to see in bilateral temporal fields
   b. Usually caused by a pituitary tumor

3. Internuclear ophthalmoplegia
   a. **Classically found in multiple sclerosis**
   b. Lesion of median longitudinal fasciculus
   c. Si/Sx = inability to adduct the ipsilateral eye past midline on lateral gaze (inability to perform conjugate gaze)
   d. Caused by lack of communication between contralateral CN VI nucleus and ipsilateral CN III nucleus

4. Parinaud's Syndrome
   a. Midbrain tectum lesion → bilateral paralysis of upward gaze
   b. Commonly associated with pineal tumor

5. Marcus-Gunn Pupil
   a. Because of afferent defect of CN II, pupil will not react to direct light but will react consensually when light is directed at the nml contralateral eye
   b. **Characterized by ⊕ swinging flashlight test**
      (1) Swing penlight quickly back and forth between eyes
      (2) Denervated pupil will not constrict to direct stimulation and **instead will actually appear to dilate when light is shone in it** because it is dilating back to baseline when consensual light is removed from other eye

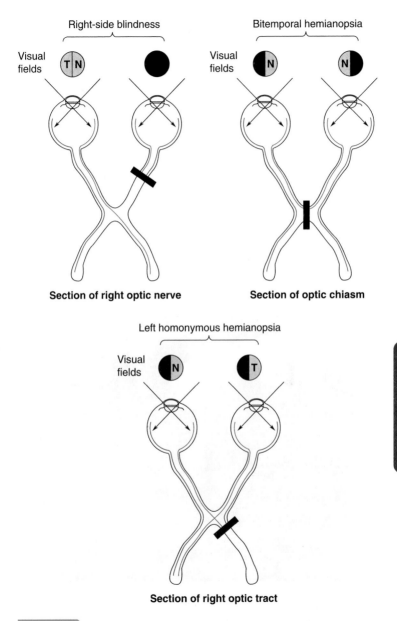

FIGURE 9.1

Visual Field Defects. (From Moore KL, Dalley AF. *Clinical oriented anatomy*, 4th Ed. Baltimore: Lippincott Williams & Wilkins, 1999.)

6. Argyll-Robertson Pupil
   a. **Pathognomonic for 3° syphilis (neurosyphilis)**
   b. Pupils constrict with accommodation but do not constrict to direct light stimulation (pupils accommodate but do not react)
7. Lens Dislocation
   a. Occurs in homocystinuria, Marfan's and Alport's syndromes
   b. Lens dislocates superiorly in Marfan's (mnemonic: **Marfan's pts are tall, their lenses dislocate upward**), inferiorly in homocystinuria, and variably in Alport's syndrome
8. Kayser-Fleischer Ring
   a. **Pathognomonic for Wilson's dz**
   b. Finding is a ring of golden pigment around the iris (see Neurology, Figure 7.2)
9. Pterygium (Figure 9.2)
   a. Fleshy growth from conjunctiva onto nasal side of cornea
   b. Associated with exposure to wind, sand, sun, and dust

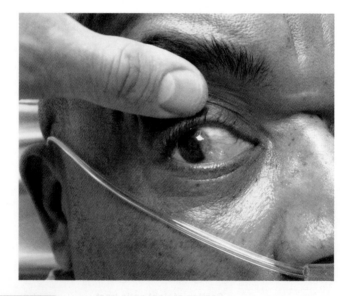

FIGURE 9.2

Right-sided pterygium. (Courtesy of Mark Silverberg, MD. From Greenberg MI, Hendrickson RG, Silverberg M, et al. *Greenberg's text-atlas of emergency medicine.* Philadelphia: Lippincott Williams & Wilkins, 2004, with permission.)

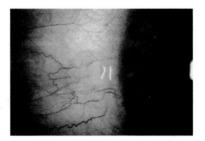

FIGURE 9.3

Clinical appearance of a pinguecula. (From James B, Chew C, Bron A. *Lecture notes on ophthalmology*, 8th Ed. Oxford: Blackwell Science, 1997, with permission.)

    c. Tx = cosmetic removal unless impairing vision; wear sunglasses and avoid dry eyes

10. Pinguecula (Figure 9.3)
    a. Benign yellowish nodules on either side of the cornea
    b. Commonly seen in pts >35
    c. Rarely grows and requires no Tx

11. Subconjunctival Hemorrhage
    a. Spontaneous onset of a painless, bright-red patch on sclera
    b. Benign, self-limited condition usually seen after overexertion

12. Retrobulbar Neuritis
    a. Caused by inflammation of the optic nerve, usually unilateral
    b. **Seen in multiple sclerosis, often is the initial sign**
    c. Si/Sx = rapid loss of vision and pain upon moving eye, spontaneously remitting within 2–8 wk, each relapse damages the nerve more until blindness eventually results
    d. Funduscopic exam is nonrevealing
    e. Tx = corticosteroids

13. Optic Neuritis
    a. Inflammation of optic nerve within the eye
    b. Causes include viral infxn, multiple sclerosis, vasculitis, methanol, meningitis, syphilis, tumor metastases
    c. Si/Sx = variable vision loss and ↓ pupillary light reflex
    d. **Funduscopic exam reveals disk hyperemia**

OPTHAMOLOGY

      e. If pt is >60 yr, Bx temporal artery to rule out temporal arteritis

      f. Tx = corticosteroids

B. **Palpebral Inflammation (Table 9.1)**

C. **Red Eye**

   1. **Assess pain, visual acuity, type of eye discharge, and pupillary abnormalities in all pts**

   2. DDx (Table 9.2)

Table 9.1	Palpebral Inflammation	
Dz	**Si/Sx**	**Tx**
Chalazion	• Inflammation of internal meibomian sebaceous gland • Presents with swelling on conjunctival surface of eyelid	None, self-limiting
Hordeolum (stye)	• Infxn of external sebaceous glands of Zeiss or Mol • Presents with tender red swelling at lid margin (Figure 9.4)	Hot compress, can add antibiotics
Blepharitis	• Inflammation of eyelids and eyelashes resulting from infxn (S. aureus) or 2° to seborrhea • Presents with red, swollen eyelid margins, with dry flakes noted on lashes • **Without Tx can extend along eyelid (cellulitis)**	Wash lid margins daily with baby shampoo, control scalp seborrhea with shampoo
Orbital cellulitis	• Marked swelling and erythema of eye, often with proptosis, ↓ vision, limited eye movement (Figure 9.5) • Distinguished from pre-septal (outside the orbit) cellulitis by change in vision and limited eye movement, which are not seen in preseptal cellulitis • **Can spread to cavernous sinus, leading to deadly thrombosis and meningitis**	Treat emergently with IV vancomycin + cefotaxime

Text continues on page 433

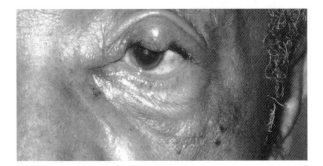

FIGURE 9.4
Stye (hordeolum).

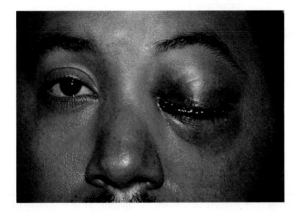

FIGURE 9.5
Orbital cellulitis presenting with massive swelling, chemosis, erythema, and poor ocular motility. (From Tasman W, Jaeger E. *The Wills eye hospital atlas of clinical ophthalmology*, 2nd Ed. Baltimore: Lippincott Williams & Wilkins, 2001.)

OPHTHALMOLOGY

Table 9.2 Red Eye

Dz	Si/Sx	Cause	Tx
Bacterial conjunctivitis	• Minimal pain, no vision changes • **Purulent** discharge • No pupillary changes • **Rarely** preauricular adenopathy (only *Neisseria gonorrhoeae*)	*S. pneumoniae, Staphylococcus* spp., *N. gonorrhoeae, Chlamydia trachomatis* (inneonates, sexually active adults)	Topical sulfacetamide or erythromycin
Viral conjunctivitis	• Minimal pain, no vision changes • **Watery** discharge • No pupillary changes • **Often preauricular adenopathy** • **Often pharyngitis** (adenovirus)	Adenovirus most common, others = HSV, varicella, EBV, influenza, echovirus, coxsackie virus	No Tx required, self-limiting dz
Allergic conjunctivitis	• No pain, vision, or pupil changes • **Marked pruritus** • **Bilateral** watery eyes	Allergy/hay fever	Antihistamine or steroid drops
Hyphema	• **Blood in anterior chamber of eye, fluid level noted** (Figure 9.6) • Pain, no vision changes • No discharge, no pupil changes	Blunt ocular trauma	Eye patch to ↓ movement
Xerophthalmia	• Minimal pain, vision blurry, no pupillary changes, no discharge • **Bitot's spots** visible on exam (desquamated, conjunctival cells) • **Keratoconjunctivitis sicca** (Sjögren's dz) **Dx by Schirmer test** (place filter paper over eyelid, if not wet in 15 min → Dx)	Sjögren's dz or vitamin A deficiency	Artificial tears, vitamin A

| Table 9.2 | *Continued* |

Dz	Si/Sx	Cause	Tx
Corneal abrasion	• **Painful, with photophobia** • No pupil changes • Watery discharge • Dx by fluorescein stain to detect areas of corneal defect	Direct trauma to eye (finger, stick, etc.)	Antibiotics, eye patch, examine daily
Keratitis	• **Pain**, photophobia, tearing • **↓ vision** • Can be caused by herpes zoster of CN V, 1st branch (Figure 9.7) • **Herpes zoster shows classic dendritic branching on fluorescein stain** (Figure 9.8) • **Pus in anterior chamber (hypopyon) is a grave sign** (Figure 9.9C)	Adenovirus, HSV, *Pseudomonas*, *S. pneumoniae*, *Staphylococcus* spp., *Moraxella* (often in contact lens wearers)	**Emergency, immediate Ophthalmology consult** Tx = topical vidarabine for herpes
Uveitis	• Inflammation of the iris, ciliary body, and/or choroid • **Pain, miosis,** photophobia • **Flare and cells** seen in aqueous humor **on slit-lamp examination** (Figure 9.9)	Seen in seronegative spondylo-arthropathy, IBD sarcoidosis, or infxn (CMV, syphilis)	Tx underlying dz
Angle-closure glaucoma	• **Severe pain** • **↓ Vision,** halos around lights • **Fixed middilated pupil** • Eyeball firm to pressure	↓ Aqueous humor outflow via canal of Schlemm—mydriatics can also cause	**Emergency,** IV mannitol and glaucoma acetazolamide, laser iridotomy for cure
Subconjunctival hemorrhage (Figure 9.8)	Spontaneous onset of painless bright red patch on sclera caused by rupture of episcleral vessel	Overexertion, valsalva, or trauma. Can also be seen in pts with uncontrolled HTN	• Self-limited • Check blood pressure

CMV, cytomegalovirus; EBV, Ebstein-Barr virus; HSV, herpes simplex virus.

OPHTHALMOLOGY

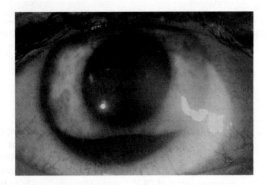

FIGURE 9.6

Hyphema. (From Moore KL, Dalley AF. *Clinical oriented anatomy*, 4th Ed. Baltimore: Lippincott Williams & Wilkins, 1999.)

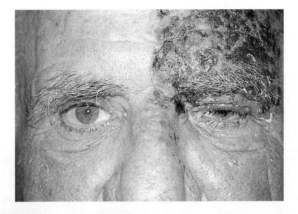

FIGURE 9.7

Herpes zoster opthalmicus. (From Tasman W, Jaeger E. *The Wills eye hospital atlas of clinical ophthalmology*, 2nd Ed. Baltimore: Lippincott Williams & Wilkins, 2001.)

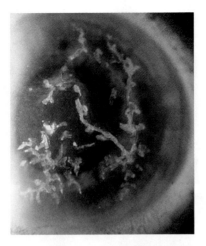

FIGURE 9.8

Classic zoster pseudo-dendrites are elevated mucous plaques with tapered ends. (From Tasman W, Jaeger EA, eds. *The Wills eye hospital atlas of clinical ophthalmology*, 2nd Ed. Philadelphia: Lippincott Williams & Wilkins, 2001, with permission.)

D. **Dacryocystitis (Tear Duct Inflammation)**

1. Infxn of lacrimal sac, usually caused by *Staphylococcus aureus*, *Streptococcus pneumoniae*, *Haemophilus influenzae*, or *Streptococcus pyogenes*

2. Si/Sx = inflammation and tenderness of nasal aspect of lower lid, purulent discharge may be noted or expressed (Figure 9.10)

3. Tx = Keflex

E. **Eye Colors**

1. **Yellow eye** (icterus) from bilirubin staining of sclera (jaundice)

2. **Yellow vision** seen in digoxin toxicity

3. **Blue sclera** classically found in osteogenesis imperfecta and Marfan's dz

4. **Opaque eye** because of cataract

   a. Opacity of lens severe enough to interfere with vision

   b. Causes = congenital, diabetes (sorbitol precipitation in lens), galactosemia (galactitol precipitation in lens), Hurler's dz (see Appendix)

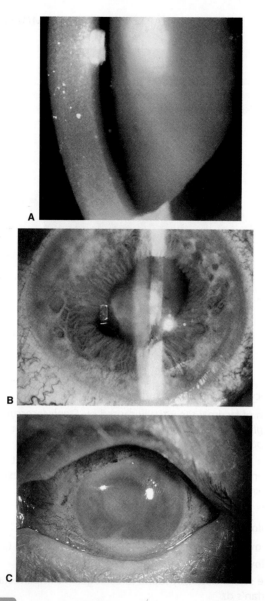

FIGURE 9.9

Signs of anterior uveitis. **(A)** Keratic precipitates on the corneal endothelium. **(B)** Posterior synechiae (adhesions between the lens and iris) give the pupil an irregular appearance. **(C)** Hypopyon, white cells have collected as a mass in the inferior anterior chamber. (From Tasman W, Jaeger E. *The Wills eye hospital atlas of clinical ophthalmology*, 2nd Ed. Baltimore: Lippincott Williams & Wilkins, 2001.)

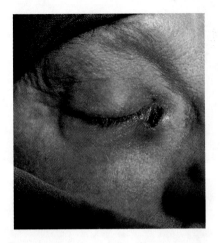

FIGURE 9.10

Dacryocystitis that, unusually, points through the skin. (From James B, Chew C, Bron A. *Lecture notes on ophthalmology*, 8th Ed. Oxford: Blackwell Science, 1997, with permission.)

F. **Retina**

1. Diabetic Retinopathy
   a. Occurs after approximately 10 yr of diabetes
      (1) Background type
          (a) Flame hemorrhages, microaneurysms, and soft exudates (cotton-wool spots) on retina (Figures 9.11A and 9.11B)
          (b) Tx is strict glucose and HTN control
      (2) Proliferative type
          (a) More advanced dz, with neovascularization easily visible around fundus (hyperemia) and hard exudates (Figure 9.11C)
          (b) Tx is photocoagulation (laser ablation of blood vessels in the retina), which slows dz progression but is not curative

2. Age-related Macular Degeneration
   a. Causes painless loss of visual acuity
   b. Dx by altered pigmentation in macula
   c. Pts often retain adequate peripheral vision
   d. Tx = antioxidants and laser Tx

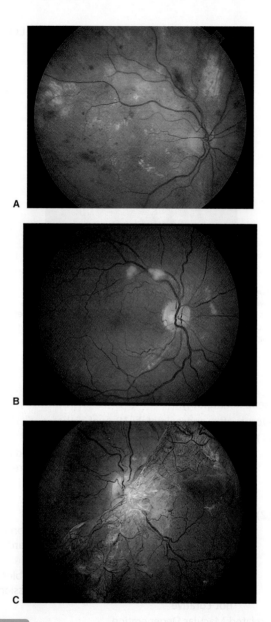

FIGURE 9.11

(A) Sign of retinal vascular dz: hemorrhage and exudate. (B) Sign of retinal vascular dz: cotton-wool spots. (C) Sign of retinal vascular dz: new vessels, here particularly florid arising at the disk. (From Tasman W, Jaeger E. *The Wills eye hospital atlas of clinical ophthalmology*, 2nd Ed. Baltimore: Lippincott Williams & Wilkins, 2001.)

3. Retinal Detachment
   a. Presents with painless, dark vitreous floaters, flashes of light (photopsias), blurry vision, eventually progressing to a curtain of blindness as detachment worsens
   b. Tx = urgent surgical reattachment
4. Retinitis Pigmentosa
   a. Slowly progressive defect in night vision (often starts in young children) with ring-shaped scotoma (blind spot) that gradually increases in size to obscure more vision
   b. Dz is hereditary with unclear transmission mode
   c. May be part of the Laurence-Moon-Biedl syndrome
   d. No Tx
5. Classic Physical Findings of Retina
   a. **Leukocoria** = absent red reflex, actually appears white, seen in retinoblastoma
   b. **Roth spots** = small hemorrhagic spots with central clearing in retina associated with endocarditis
   c. **Copper wiring, flame hemorrhages, A-V nicking** seen in subacute HTN and/or atherosclerosis
   d. Papilledema appears as disk hyperemia, blurring, and elevation, associated with ↑ intracranial pressure
   e. "Sea fan" neovascularization in sickle cell anemia
   f. Wrinkles on retina seen in retinal detachment
   g. **Cherry-red spot on macula** seen in Tay-Sachs, Niemann-Pick dz, central retinal artery occlusion
   h. Hollenhorst plaque = yellow cholesterol emboli in retinal artery
   i. Brown macule on retina = malignant melanoma (most common intraocular tumor in adults)

G. **Glaucoma**
1. Progressive optic neuropathy with characteristic visual field loss often (not always) related to ↑ intraocular pressure
2. Major cause of blindness in the aging (leading cause of blindness in African Americans)
3. Can be open or closed type
   a. Open-angle glaucoma
      (1) Causation unknown, mechanical versus vascular versus toxic (glutamate) theory
      (2) Rarely causes pain or corneal edema
      (3) Constriction of visual field in later stages

(4) Incidence ↑ with age

(5) On funduscopic examination, classic finding ↑ in size of optic cup with thinning of neural rim

(6) Tx

   (a) Medical = cholinergics, alpha-agonists, beta-blockers, carbonic anhydrase inhibitors prostaglandin analogue

   (b) Laser surgery to stretch trabecular meshwork and facilitate outflow

   (c) Surgery to facilitate alternate drainage pathway for aqueous

b. Angle-closure glaucoma

(1) Can be chronic or acute, the latter is an emergency

(2) Typically idiopathic, can be drug induced (mydriatics)

(3) Mydriatics cause the peripheral iris to move forward and occlude the aqueous fluid outflow tract

(4) Prodromal Sx = sudden pain in eye and head, halos around lights, blurry vision

(5) Acute attack causes severe throbbing pain in eye, radiating to CN V distribution, blurry vision, nausea/vomiting, fixed, mid-dilated pupil, redness

(6) This is considered an emergency because blindness can occur

(7) Tx

   (a) IV or oral acetazolamide, topical timolol, pilocarpine (stretches and pulls the iris away from the angle)

   (b) Mydriatics **not** recommended (can exacerbate condition)—laser iridotomy follows to establish alternate pathway for aqueous to flow allowing iris to bow back into position

   (c) Laser iridotomy indicated in aSx eye to prevent future occurrence of angle closure

H. **Orbital Tumors**

1. Adult

   a. Cavernous hemangioma

      (1) Most common adult tumor

      (2) Large well-circumscribed vascular tumor

   b. Metastases

      (1) Breast, lung, prostate most common

      (2) 10% of orbital tumors

      c. Lymphoid tumors
        (1) Older pts
        (2) Spectrum from benign reactive lymphoid hyperplasia to lymphoma
        (3) Orbital involvement—radiotherapy, if systemic, radiation and chemotherapy
      d. Fibrous histiocytoma—mesenchymal tumor
      e. Mucocele—cystic mass of sinuses caused by duct obstruction, frontal and ethmoid sinuses most commonly involved
      f. Fibrous dysplasia—bony tumor
      g. Schwannoma
        (1) Tumor of peripheral nerve
        (2) Seen in neurofibromatosis
  2. Pediatric
      a. Capillary hemangioma
        (1) Most common orbital tumor in children
        (2) Vascular tumor
      b. Dermoid cyst—Benign cystic mass with connective tissue and skin appendages (hair, sebaceous glands)
      c. Leukemia
        (1) Myelogenous leukemia—chloroma
        (2) Lymphocytic leukemia—can also produce orbital infiltration
      d. Rhabdomyosarcoma
        (1) Most common primary orbital malignancy in children
        (2) Px, botryoid
      e. Lymphangioma
        (1) Tumor of early childhood with large lymph channels
        (2) Often have hemorrhage
      f. Neuroblastoma
        (1) Most common metastatic tumor in children
        (2) Ecchymosis with proptosis
I. **Orbital trauma (Table 9.3)**
J. **Ophthalmic Medications (Table 9.4)**

Table 9.3 Eye Related Trauma

Dz	Si/Sx	Tx
Chemical burns	• Alkali burns most damaging. Severe pain, erythema, conjunctival injection or blanching/ necrosis complete opacification of cornea in severe cases	• Immediate irrigation of eye with nml saline and removal of particulate debris • Check vision and pH • Immediate ophthalmology consult • Complete history of events surrounding exposure and exam of eye, face, and airway
Eyelid laceration	• May be superficial or involve deeper structures such as levator muscle, tarsal plate, and orbital septem. Medial lacerations can include lacrimal system (canaliculus) • Penetrating foreign bodies must be ruled out as a cause of laceration	• Ophthalmology consult for repair of lid/lacrimal system
Foreign Body	• Pencils, glass, metal, wood, bullet • May cause corneal abrasion if hidden beneath eye lids • May be intraocular or intraorbital. CT scan is gold standard for imaging. (Never MRI: the magnet moves metallic object and may cause further damage) • Tear drop or odd shaped pupil occasionally seen with penetrating foreign bodies	• Ophthalmology consult • External examination of eyelids, orbital walls, conjunctive, visual acuity, pupils, and extraocular movements. Slit-lamp examination of cornea with fluorescein dye • Eye shield prior to transport • Stabilize any objects protruding from orbit • Give IV broad spectrum antibiotics • Give antiemetics to control nausea and vomiting and prevent ↑ intraocular pressure • Tetanus prophylaxis • Glass and some metals are inert and are well tolerated. Wood must be removed immediately to prevent endophthalmitis

Table 9.3 *Continued*

Dz	Si/Sx	Tx
Ruptured Globe (open globe injury)	• Full thickness corneal/corneoscleral/scleral otics laceration 2° to blunt or penetrating trauma	• Urgent surgical repair to close eye and IV antibi- • Orbital imaging to look for intraocular foreign bodies; BEWARE of sympathetic ophthalmia—a rare auto-immune uveitis that can affect the injured eye and then progress to uninjured eye. Tx—enucleate any irreversibly injured globes
Retinal detachment	• Commonly associated with blunt trauma to eye • Presents with painless, dark vitreous floaters, flashes of light (photopsias), and blurry vision • Progresses to a curtain of blindness in vision as detachment worsens • Retinal tear or hole visualized in periphery • Wrinkles on retina seen in retinal detachment	• Ophthalmology consult for urgent surgical reattachment
Hyphema	• Pain, blurriness blunt ocular trauma • Irregular pupil • Blood in anterior chamber of eye, fluid level noted	• Ophthalmology consult
Blowout fracture	• Thin bones of orbit "blow out" from ↑ intraorbital pressure. Most commonly orbital floor and medial wall • Enophthalmos, diplopia, and occasionally extraocular muscle entrapment, usually inferior rectus	• CT scan of orbit • Ophthalmology or • Otolaryngology consult

OPHTHALMOLOGY

(continued)

Table 9.3 *Continued*

Dz	Si/Sx	Tx
Traumatic optic neuropathy	• Caused by indirect trauma to optic nerve, direct trauma from compression by hematoma or bone fragments • Afferent papillary defect (Marcus-Gunn pupil) • Vision loss	• Ophthalmology consult • Tx controversial—observation versus IV steroids (recent large study showed no benefit of steroids or decompression)
Retrobulbar hemorrhage	• Can be seen with blunt trauma to eye and postoperatively after sinus surgery and blepharoplasty • Proptosis, resistance to retropulsion, ↑ intraocular pressure, ↓ extraocular motility, and afferent papillary defect	• Ophthalmology consult • Surgical lateral canthotomy and lateral tendon cantholysis to relieve pressure may be necessary
Ocular melanoma	• Rare tumor commonly associated with dysplastic nevus syndrome	

Table 9.4 Opthalmic Medications

Drug Class	Examples	Use	Side Effects
Anesthetics	• Proparacaine hydrochloride • Tetracaine	• ↓ corneal sensation • Inhibiting corneal blink reflex and ↓ pain • Removal of foreign bodies and examination of injured cornea	• Repeated long-term use can lead to corneal ulceration, perforation • Can cause ocular allergic reaction
Steroids (topical)	• Prednisolone • Loteprednol • Rimexolone	• Iritis	• May potentiate a herpes simplex keratitis, bacterial, or fungal infxn if misdiagnosed

Table 9.4 *Continued*

Drug Class	Examples	Use	Side Effects
Steroids (topical) *(continued)*			• Cataracts and ↑ intraocular pressure seen in long-term use of steroid eye drops (steroid induced glaucoma) • Ophthalmologist directed use only
Anticholinergics	• Short acting— Tropicamide, Cyclopentolate hydrochloride • Long acting— Scolpolamine hydrobromide, Atropine sulfate	• Mydriatic and cycloplegic agents use to fully examine retina and facilitate refraction	• Rarely nausea, vomiting, and syncope • Acute angle closure glaucoma
Adrenergics	• Phenylephrine hydrochloride	• Mydriatic only, no cycloplegic effects	• HTN and tachycardia at higher concentrations
Decongestants	• Naphazoline hydrochloride • Phenylephrine hydrochloride • Tetrahydrozaline hydrochloride	• Used to relieve red eye • Cause vasoconstriction of conjunctival vessels	• Rebound vasodilation and worsening red eye
Antibacterials	• Tobramycin • Ciprofloxacin • Sulfacetamide • Erythromycin	• Prophylactic or organism specific bacterial Tx • Under the direction of an ophthalmologist	• Allergic reactions • Tobramycin toxic to corneal epithelium
Antiviral	• Vidarabine • Trifluridine	• Herpes Simplex Virus	• Allergic reactions • Punctuate keratopathy

(continued)

Table 9.4 *Continued*

Drug Class	Examples	Use	Side Effects
NSAID	• Diclofenac • Ketorolac	• Ocular allergy	• Allergic reaction • Tachyphylaxis
Glaucoma	• Beta blockers; e.g., Timolol (nonselective), betaxolol (β-1 selecative) • Parasympathomimetics; i.e., Pilocarpine • Sympathomimetic Epinephrine (β agonist), iopidine (α agonist) • Carbonic anhydrase inhibitors (Acetazolamide)	• ↓ aqueous humor formation • ↑ outflow • ↑ outflow (β agonist), ↓ aqueous production (alpha agonist) • ↓ aqueous formation	• Systemic absorption can cause bronchospasm, bradycardia, and hypotension • Lacrimation, salivation, nausea, vomiting, and headache • HTN, headache, cardiac arrhythmias (iopidine causes allergic reaction) • Allergic reactions (sulfa base), nausea, vomiting, tingling of hands/feet. Avoid in pts with sickle cell trait or anemia, causes acidosis which ↑ sickling
Dry eye	Artificial tears	Ophthalmic lubricant	Allergic reaction to preservatives

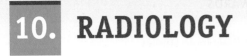

10. RADIOLOGY

I. Helpful Terms and Concepts

A. Lucent versus Sclerotic Lesions

1. On plain film, a "lucency" is a focal area of bone or tissue that has a ↓ density, usually resulting from a pathologic process

2. On x-ray, a lucent bone lesion may appear like a dark, punched-out hole in the surrounding nml bone

3. In contrast, sclerotic bone lesions appear denser than the surrounding bone, and thus on x-ray appears whiter and more intense than its surroundings

B. Hypodense versus Hyperdense

1. Tissue density on CT can be characterized by how light or dark it appears relative to surrounding nml parenchyma

2. Hypodense lesions appear darker than nml tissue, whereas hyperdense lesions are brighter

3. Air- or fluid-filled lesions, such as cysts and abscesses, are common hypodense lesions

C. Ring Enhancement

1. Ring enhancement refers to a bright intensity that can be observed surrounding many lesions on both CT and MRI

2. This usually indicates local edema around a mass lesion, and in the brain it can indicate breakdown of the blood–brain barrier

D. Radiopaque versus Radiolucent

1. The more radiopaque an object is, the brighter it appears on plain film

2. Dental fillings, bullets, and metal prostheses are very radiopaque, so they appear white on plain film

3. The more radiolucent an object is, the darker it appears on plain film

RADIOLOGY

Table 10.1	Common Radiologic Studies
Study	**Indications**
CT versus MRI	• CT → faster, less expensive, greater sensitivity for acute head trauma, better for detection of spinal cord compression • MRI → better visualization of soft tissue, allows multiplanar imaging (axial, coronal, sagittal, and oblique), no ionizing radiation
Endoscopic retrograde cholangiopancreatography (ERCP)	Pancreatitis 2° to choledocholithiasis, cholestatic jaundice
Utz[a]	Abd aortic aneurysm, gallbladder dz, renal and adrenal masses, ectopic pregnancy, kidney stones
Carotid Doppler Utz	Carotid artery stenosis, assessing flow dynamics
Intravenous pyelogram (IVP)	Genito-Urinary obstruction
Kidney, ureter, bladder (KUB) x-ray[a]	Kidney stones, solid abd masses, abd free air
Lateral decubitus chest plain film	For determination of whether a suspected pleural effusion will layer

[a]Note 80/20 rule: gallstones diagnosed 80% of the time and kidney stones 20% of the time by Utz. Kidney stones diagnosed 80% of the time and gallstones only 20% of the time by x-ray.

II. Common Radiologic Studies (Table 10.1)

III. An Approach to a Chest X-Ray (Figure 10.1)

A = Airway—is trachea midline? and **A**lignment—symmetry of clavicles

B = **B**ones—look for fractures, lytic lesions, or defects

C = **C**ardiac silhouette—normally occupies <1/2 chest width

D = **D**iaphragms—flattened (e.g., chronic obstructive pulmonary dz)?, blunted angles (effusion)?, elevated (airspace consolidation)?

E = **E**xternal soft tissues—lymph nodes (especially axilla), subQ emphysema, other lesions

F = **F**ields of the lung—opacities, nodules, vascularity, bronchial cuffing, etc.

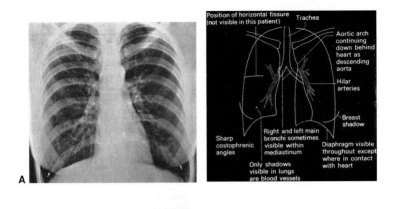

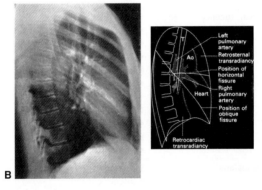

FIGURE 10.1

Nml chest. **(A)** PA view. The *arrows* point to the breast shadows of this female pt. **(B)** Lateral view. Note that the upper retrosternal area is of the same density as the retrocardiac areas and the same as over the upper thoracic vertebrae. The vertebrae are more transradiant (i.e., blacker) as the eye travels down the spine, until the diaphragm is reached. Ao, aorta; T, trachea. (From Armstrong P, Wastie M. *Diagnostic imaging*, 4th Ed. Oxford: Blackwell Science, 1998, with permission.)

IV. Common Radiologic Findings (Table 10.2)

Table 10.2 Common Radiologic Findings

Finding/Description	DDx
Multiple contrast-enhancing lesions on CT or MRI	**Neoplastic:** • Metastases (see Figure 10.2) ◊ Breast CA and bronchogenic lung CA most common ◊ Also malignant melanoma, prostate, lymphoma **Infectious:** • Bacterial abscess • Toxoplasmosis • Cysticercosis **Vascular:** • Infarct **Degenerative:** • Demyelinating dz
Nonsclerotic skull lucency	**Infectious:** • TB • Syphilis • Osteomyelitis **Neoplastic:** • Multiple myeloma • Metastases **Trauma:** • Burr hole **Endocrine:** • Hyperparathyroidism
Sclerotic bone lesions (Figure 10.3)	**Infectious:** • Osteomyelitis (presents with periosteal reaction) • Syphilis **Congenital:** • Fibrous dysplasia • Tuberous sclerosis **Neoplastic:** • Metastases—primarily prostate and breast • Lymphoma • Multiple myeloma—usually presents with multiple lesions (see Figure 1.15) • Osteosarcoma **Vascular:** • Healing fracture callus
"Bone within bone" sign	**Endocrine:** • Growth arrest and recovery • Paget's dz • Osteopetrosis **Intoxication:** Heavy metal poisoning

Table 10.2 *Continued*

Finding/Description	DDx
Inferior surface rib notching	**Vascular:** • Coarctation of the aorta—**classic finding** • Superior vena cava obstruction **Congenital:** • Chest wall A-V malformation
Ivory vertebral body Sclerotic change in single vertebra	**Neoplastic:** • Sclerotic metastases • Lymphoma **Endocrine:** • Paget's dz
Honeycomb lung Fibrotic replacement of lung parenchyma with thick-walled cysts	**Idiopathic:** • Idiopathic interstitial fibrosis • Histiocytosis X • Sarcoidosis **Congenital:** • Cystic fibrosis • Tuberous sclerosis • Neurofibromatosis **Autoimmune:** • Scleroderma • Rheumatoid arthritis **Intoxication:** • Allergic alveolitis • Asbestosis • Bleomycin • Nitrofurantoin • Cyclophosphamide
Ground glass opacities on lung CT Hazy, granular ↑ in density of lung parenchyma that usually implies an acute inflammatory process	**Inflammation:** • Interstitial pneumonia • Hypersensitivity pneumonitis • *Pneumocystic carinii* pneumonia • Alveolar proteinosis
Water-bottle-shaped heart on PA plain film	Pericardial effusions with >250 mL of fluid
Pulmonary edema Classically, severe pulmonary edema appears as **a bat's-wing shadow**	**Vascular:** • Congestive heart failure **Inflammatory:** • Adult respiratory distress syndrome • Mendelson's syndrome **Intoxication:** Smoke inhalation **Trauma:** Near drowning

RADIOLOGY

(continued)

Table 10.2 *Continued*

Finding/Description	DDx
Blunting of costophrenic angles 300–500 mL of fluid is needed before blunting of the lateral costophrenic angles becomes apparent (see Figures 10.4 and 10.5)	Pleural effusion
Kerley B lines Interlobar septa on the peripheral aspects of the lungs that become thickened by dz or fluid accumulation (see Figure 10.6)	**Vascular:** • Left ventricular failure • Lymphatic obstruction **Inflammatory:** • Sarcoidosis • Lymphangitis carcinomatosa
Multiple lung small soft tissue Densities <2 mm	**Inflammatory:** • Sarcoidosis • Miliary TB • Fungal infxn • Parasites • Extrinsic allergic alveolitis **Neoplastic:** Metastases **Endocrine:** Hemosiderosis
Lung nodules >2 cm Ghon complex—calcified granuloma classic for TB, found at lung base along hilum (see Figure 10.7)	**Neoplastic:** • Metastases • 1° lung CA • Benign hamartoma **Intoxication:** • Silicosis **Idiopathic:** • Histiocytosis X **Inflammatory:** • Sarcoidosis • TB • Wegener's • Fungal infxns • Abscess
Hilar adenopathy	**Inflammatory:** • Sarcoidosis (bilateral, eggshell calcification) • Amyloidosis **Intoxication:** • Silicosis **Neoplastic:** • Bronchogenic CA (unilateral) • Lymphoma

Table 10.2 *Continued*

Finding/Description	DDx
Cavity Annular opacity with central lucency (see Figure 10.8)	**Infectious:** • TB (apex) • Lung abscess • Fungal • Amebiasis **Neoplastic:** • Bronchogenic CA • Metastases • Lymphoma **Autoimmune:** • Rheumatoid lung dz
Unilaterally elevated diaphragm (see Figure 10.9)	**Trauma:** • Phrenic nerve palsy **Congenital:** • Pulmonary hypoplasia scoliosis **Vascular:** • Pulmonary embolism
Bilaterally elevated diaphragm	• Obesity • Pregnancy • Fibrotic lung dz
Steeple sign Narrowed area of subglottic trachea **Thumb sign**	Parainfluenza virus (croup) Epiglottitis classically caused by Haemophilus influenzae
Pneumoperitoneum Free air under the diaphragm on an upright chest film or upright abdomen **Double-wall sign on abd plain film** Appearance of the outer and inner walls of bowel is almost pathognomonic for pneumoperitoneum	**Inflammatory:** • Perforation ◊ Ulcer ◊ Diverticulitis ◊ Appendicitis ◊ Toxic megacolon ◊ Infarcted bowel Also can be: • Peritoneal dialysis • Pneumomediastinum that has tracked inferiorly • Diaphragmatic rupture
Gasless abdomen on abd plain film (see Figure 10.10)	• Obstruction • Severe ascites • Pancreatitis
Filling defects in stomach on **upper GI series**	• Gastric ulcer • Gastric CA

(continued)

RADIOLOGY

Table 10.2 *Continued*

Finding/Description	DDx
Dilated small bowel (see Figures 10.10 and 10.11)	• Mechanical obstruction ◊ Postsurgical ◊ Incarcerated hernia ◊ Intussusception • Paralytic ileus **Inflammatory:** • Celiac sprue • Scleroderma
Coffee bean sigmoid volvulus (see Figure 10.12)	• Large-bowel obstruction • Paralytic ileus
String sign on barium swallow Narrowing of the terminal ileum caused by thickening of the bowel wall	• Crohn's dz
Lead pipe sign on barium enema Smooth, narrowed colon without haustra	• Inflammatory bowel dz (see Figure 10.13)
Apple core lesion Circumferential growth in the bowel lumen	• Colon CA
Liver calcifications	**Inflammatory:** • Granuloma • Hydatid cyst **Neoplastic:** • Hepatoma
Gas in portal vein Linear lucencies that reach within 2 cm of liver capsule	**Vascular (seen in adults):** • Mesenteric infarct • Air embolism **Inflammatory (children):** • Necrotizing enterocolitis
Unilateral cystic renal mass Hypodensities with thin walls	**Inflammatory:** • Renal abscess • Hemodialysis-induced cyst • Hydatid cyst **Congenital:** • Bilateral renal cysts • Polycystic kidney dz **Neoplastic:** • Renal cell CA
String of beads on renal arteriogram Multiple dilatations alternating with strictures of both renal arteries	• Fibromuscular dysplasia

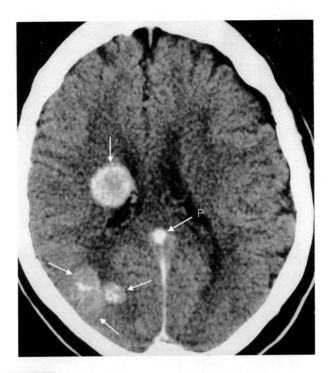

FIGURE 10.2

Metastases *(arrows)*. P, pineal. (From Armstrong P, Wastie M. *Diagnostic imaging*, 4th Ed. Oxford: Blackwell Science, 1998, with permission.)

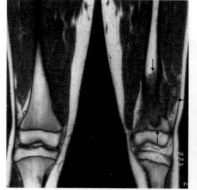
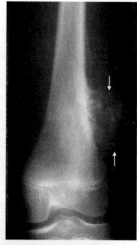
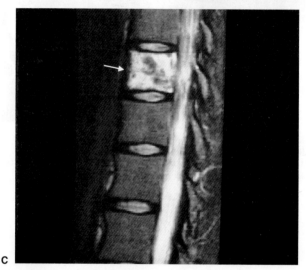

MRI of bone tumors. **(A)** T1-weighted scan of osteosarcoma in the lower shaft and metaphysis of the left femur. The extent of tumor (*arrows*) within the bone and the soft-tissue extension are both very well shown. This information is not available from the plain film. **(B)** However, the plain film provides a more specific diagnosis because the bone formation within the soft-tissue extension (*arrows*) is obvious. **(C)** T2-weighted scan of lymphoma in the T10 vertebral body (*arrow*). The very high signal of the neoplastic tissue is highly evident even though there is no deformity of shape of the vertebral body. (From Armstrong P, Wastie M. *Diagnostic imaging*, 4th Ed. Oxford: Blackwell Science, 1998, with permission.)

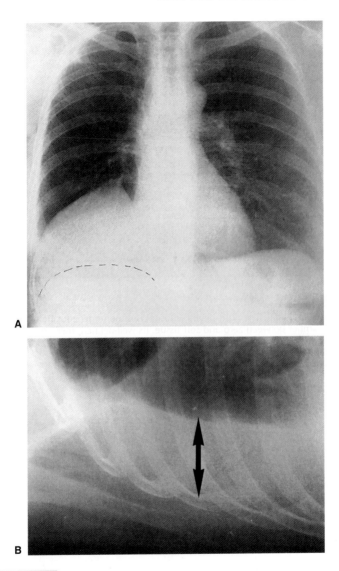

RADIOLOGY

FIGURE 10.4

Large right subpulmonary effusion (pt has had right mastectomy). Almost all the fluid is between the lung and the diaphragm. The right hemidiaphragm cannot be seen. **(A)** Estimated position is penciled in. **(B)** In the lateral decubitus view, the fluid moves to lie between the lateral chest wall and the lung edge (*arrows*). (From Armstrong P, Wastie M. *Diagnostic imaging,* 4th Ed. Oxford: Blackwell Science, 1998, with permission.)

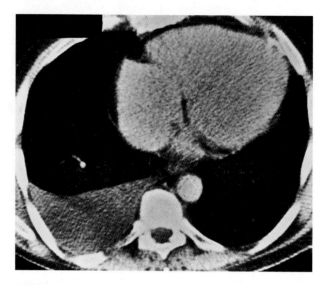

FIGURE 10.5

CT of pleural fluid. The right pleural effusion is of homogeneous density, with a CT number between zero and soft tissue. Its well-defined, meniscus-shaped border with the lung is typical. (From Armstrong P, Wastie M. *Diagnostic imaging*, 4th Ed. Oxford: Blackwell Science, 1998, with permission.)

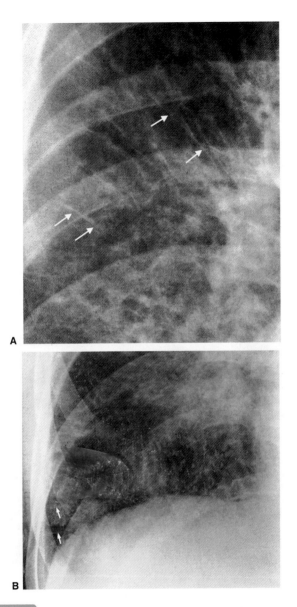

FIGURE 10.6

Septal lines. **(A)** Kerley A lines (*arrows*) in a pt with lymphangitis carcinomatosa.
(B) Kerley B lines in a pt with pulmonary edema. The septal lines (*arrows*) are
thinner than the adjacent blood vessels. The B lines are seen in the outer cm
of lung, where blood vessels are invisible or very difficult to identify. (From
Armstrong P, Wastie M. *Diagnostic imaging*, 4th Ed. Oxford: Blackwell Science,
1998, with permission.)

457

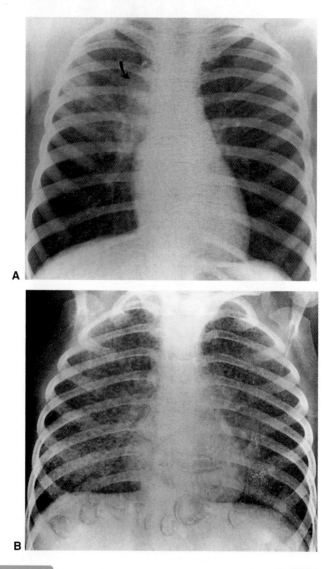

FIGURE 10.7

Tuberculosis. **(A)** 1° complex. This 7-yr-old child shows ill-defined consolidation in the right lung together with enlargement of the draining lymph nodes (*arrow*). **(B)** Miliary TB. The innumerable small nodular shadows uniformly distributed throughout the lungs in this young child are typical of miliary TB. In this instance, no 1° focus of infxn is visible. (From Armstrong P, Wastie M. *Diagnostic imaging*, 4th Ed. Oxford: Blackwell Science, 1998, with permission.)

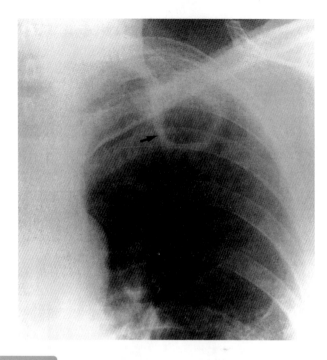

FIGURE 10.8

Fungus infxn. The cavity (*arrow*) in this pt from the southeastern U.S. was the result of North American blastomycosis. Note the similarity to TB. Other fungi; e.g., histoplasmosis, can give an identical appearance. (From Armstrong P, Wastie M. *Diagnostic imaging*, 4th Ed. Oxford: Blackwell Science, 1998, with permission.)

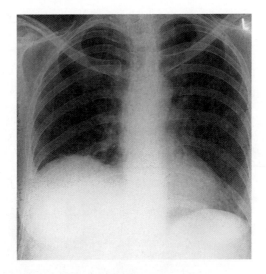

FIGURE 10.9

Elevated right diaphragm. (From Armstrong P, Wastie M. *Diagnostic imaging*, 4th Ed. Oxford: Blackwell Science, 1998, with permission.)

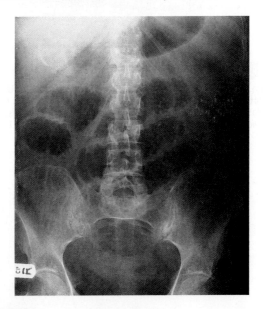

FIGURE 10.10

Small-bowel obstruction: distended small bowel and absence of gas shadows in the colon. (From Armstrong P, Wastie M. *Diagnostic imaging*, 4th Ed. Oxford: Blackwell Science, 1998, with permission.)

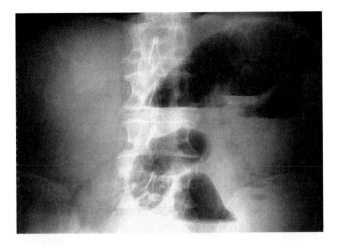

Erect film demonstrating multiple small-bowel air–fluid levels. (From Armstrong P, Wastie M. *Diagnostic imaging*, 4th Ed. Oxford: Blackwell Science, 1998, with permission.)

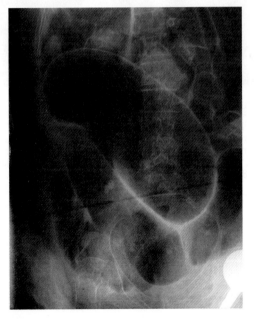

Sigmoid volvulus with a grossly distended sigmoid. (From Armstrong P, Wastie M. *Diagnostic imaging*, 4th Ed. Oxford: Blackwell Science, 1998, with permission.)

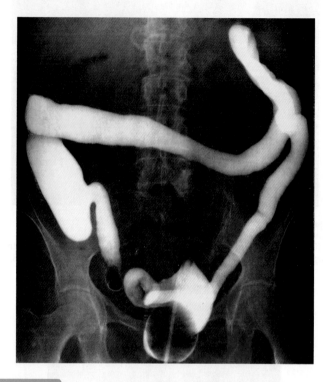

FIGURE 10.13

Ulcerative colitis. With long-standing dz, the haustra are lost and the colon becomes narrowed and shortened, coming to resemble a rigid tube. Reflux into the ileum through an incompetent ileocecal valve has occurred. (From Armstrong P, Wastie M. *Diagnostic imaging*, 4th Ed. Oxford: Blackwell Science, 1998, with permission.)

11. EMERGENCY MEDICINE

I. Toxicology

Toxin	Si/Sx	Dx	Antidote
Acetaminophen	Nausea/vomiting within 2 hr, ↑ liver enzymes, ↑ prothrombin time at 24–48 hr	Blood Level	*N*-acetylcysteine within 8–10 hr
Alkali agents	Derived from batteries, dish washer detergent, drain cleaners, ingestion causes mucosal burns → dysphagia and drooling	Clinical	Milk or water, then NPO
Anticholinergic	**Dry as a bone, mad as a hatter, blind as a bat, hot as a hare** (delirium, miosis, fever)	Clinical	Physostigmine
Arsenic	**Mees lines** (white horizontal stripes on fingernails), capillary leak, seizures	Blood level	Gastric lavage and dimercaprol
Aspirin	Tinnitus, respiratory alkalosis, **anion gap metabolic acidosis with nml S$_{Osm}$**	Blood level	Bicarbonate, dialysis
Benzodiazepine	Rapid onset of weakness, ataxia, drowsiness	Blood level	Flumazenil
β-Blockers	Bradycardia, heart block, obtundation, **hyperkalemia, hypoglycemia**	Clinical	Glucagon, IV calcium
Carbon monoxide	Dyspnea, confusion, coma, **cherry-red**	Carboxy-hemoglobin	100% O_2 or hyperbaric O_2
Cyanide	In sec to min → **almond-scented breath**, coma	Blood level	Amyl nitrite Na thiosulfate

(continued)

Toxin	Si/Sx	Dx	Antidote
Digoxin	**Change in color vision, supraventricular tachycardia with heart block,** vomiting	Blood level[a]	Antidigoxin **Fab antibodies**
Ethylene glycol	**Calcium oxalate crystals in urine, anion gap metabolic acidosis with high S_{Osm}**	Blood level	Ethanol drip, **fomepizole[a]**
Heparin	Bleeding, thrombocytopenia	Clinical	Protamine
Iron	Vomiting, bloody diarrhea, acidosis, CXR → radiopaque tablets	Blood level	Deferoxamine
Isoniazid	Confusion, peripheral neuropathy	Blood level	Pyridoxine
Lead	**Microcytic Anemia with basophilic stippling,** ataxia, retardation, peripheral neuropathy, **purple lines on gums**	Blood level	EDTA, penicillamine
Mercury	**"Erethism" = ↓ memory, insomnia, timidity, delirium (mad as a hatter)**	Blood level	Ipecac, dimercaprol
Methanol	**Anion gap Metabolic acidosis with high S_{Osm},** blindness, **optic disk hyperemia**	Blood level	Ethanol drip, bicarbonate
Opioids	CNS/respiratory depression, miosis	Blood level	Naloxone (Narcan)
Organophosphate	Incontinence, cough, wheezing, dyspnea, miosis, bradycardia, heart block, tremor	Blood level	Atropine, pralidoxime
Phenobarbital	CNS depression, hypothermia, miosis, hypotensions	Blood level	Charcoal, bicarbonate
Quinidine	Torsade de pointes (ventricular tachycardia)	Blood level[b]	IV magnesium

Toxin	Si/Sx	Dx	Antidote
Theophylline	First Sx = hematemesis, then CNS → seizures or coma, cardiac → arrhythmias, hypotension	Blood level	Ipecac, charcoal, cardiac monitor
Tricyclics	Anticholinergic Sx, QRS >100 ms, torsade de pointes	Blood level	Bicarbonate drip
Warfarin	Bleeding	↑ PT	Vitamin K

[a]See *N Engl J Med* 1999;340:832–838.
[b]Correlates in acute but not chronic toxicity.
S_{Osm}, serum osmolality.

II. Fish and Shellfish Toxins

Ciguatera

1. Most common fish-borne illness worldwide and the most common type of non-bacterial food poisoning reported in the U.S.

2. Species of fish include barracuda, grouper, snapper, and sea bass

3. The bigger the fish, the higher the concentration of ciguatoxin

4. Ciguatoxin has anticholinesterase and cholinergic properties; its toxicity is related to the competitive inhibition of calcium-regulated cell membrane sodium channels

5. Sx: Begin within 6 hr of eating a Ciguatoxic fish
    a. GI complaints: vomiting, watery diarrhea, abd cramps, lasts 24–48 hr
    b. Neurologic symptoms: paresthesia of lips and extremities, reversal of hot-cold sensation, vertigo, blurred vision, tremor, ataxia, feeling of loose painful teeth. May persist for mo and are aggravated by alcohol consumption or stress
    c. Shock: Hypotension, respiratory failure

6. Tx: prevention, supportive measures, IV Mannitol can be given for severe cases, and amitryptiline for parasthesias

Scombroid

1. A histamine like reaction associated with marine tuna, mackerel, jacks, dolphin (mahi-mahi), and bluefish

2. Scombrotoxin formed when surface bacteria Proteus and Klebsiella on the fish secrete the enzyme histidine decarboxylase and convert histidine in the fish flesh to histamine. This and other histamine-like substances act to produce the clinical effects

(continued)

Scombroid *(continued)*

3. Sx: flushing hot sensation of face and neck, pruritis, urticaria, headache, dizziness, burning sensation in mouth and throat, bronchospasm, angioedema, and hypotension can occur

4. Tx: supportive, antihistamines, cimetidine, ephinephrine, corticosteroids

Paralytic Shellfish

1. Caused by ingestion of mollusks (mussels, clams, oysters, and scallops) that have concentrated the *Saxitoxin*

2. Sx: Parasthesias of mouth and extremities, sensation of floating, ataxia, vertigo, and muscle paralysis (generalized peripheral nerve dysfunction)

3. Fatality rate of 8%–9%, with deaths occurring in 1–12 hr 2° to respiratory failure

4. *Saxitoxin* acts by inhibiting sodium channels in nerve terminals blocking nerve and muscle action potential propagation

5. Tx: supportive, no known antidote, protect airway, and consider mechanical ventilation

Neurotoxic Shellfish

1. Caused by ingestion of mollusks that have concentrated the *Brevitoxin*

2. Sx: not as bad as paralytic shellfish; parasthesis like those seen in ciguatera poisoning (hot/cold reversal), vomiting, diarrhea, no paralysis or respiratory failure. Self limited

3. Aerosolized *Brevitoxin* during a red tide at the beach can cause rhinorrhea, conjunctivitis, bronchospasm, and cough

4. *Brevitoxin* acts on the sodium channels of postganglionic cholinergic nerve fibers to inhibit transmission in skeletal muscle

5. Tx: supportive and symptomatic

Tetrodotoxin

1. Rare in US. Caused by eating Japanese puffer fish (*Fugu*), blue ringed octopus, newts, and salamanders.

2. Sxs: begin within minutes of ingestion, paresthesias of face and extremities, salivation, hyperemesis, weakness, ataxia, dysphagia, ascending paralysis, respiratory failure, hypotension, bradycardia, fixed dilated pupils

3. Tetrodotoxinis chemically related to saxitoxin, causing a similar blockade of sodium channels in nerve terminals. There are also direct effects of the toxin on the medulla, and reversible competitive blockade at the motor end plate

4. Tx: Supportive, airway and ventilatory support, anticholinesterase inhibitors; i.e., edrophonium. Px is good if pt survives first 24 hr

Source: Eastaugh J, Shepherd S. Infectious and toxic syndromes from fish and shellfish consumption: a review. *Arch Intern Med*. 1989 Aug;149(8)1735–1740.

III. Bites and Stings

Bite or Sting	Sx	Tx
Bee/Wasp	Local inflammation or anaphylactic reaction possible	Scrape out stinger if present. Wash with soap and water. **Airway**, IV fluids, O_2, Cardiac monitoring for systemic effects **Epinephrine** (1:1000) 0.3–0.5 ml SQ in adults, 0.01 ml/kg in children May be given a second time in 10–15 min **Diphenhydramine** 25–50 mg IV/IM **Methylprednisilone**: 80–120 mg IV. Prednisone taper upon stabilization
Black Widow ("red hourglass" on abdomen)	Sharp pain at site. Deep burning, aching pain along extremity. Vomiting, headache, chest tightness, and HTN. Rigid abd muscles	**Airway**, IV fluids, O_2, Cardiac monitoring for systemic effects. Antivenin can be given, skin test prior to administration. Nitrates for HTN. Wound care, tetanus prophylaxis, pain relief
Brown Recluse Spider ("brown-yellow violin" on thorax)	Pain at site, nausea, myalgias and arthralgias Fever, chills, rash, necrosis at bite site	Wound care and ice compresses Erythromycin P.O. Plastic surgery consult for significant necrosis
Snake (depends on geographical region)	Fang puncture marks, vomiting, diarrhea, restlessness, dysphagia, muscle weakness, fascicula-tions, generalized bleeding	ACLS resuscitation as needed. Type specific antivenin. Tetanus prophylaxis, monitor for compartment syndrome of affected extremity
Cats	Tender regional lymphadenopathy. Local edema, erythema, decreased range of motion (tenosynovitis). *Pasteurella* commonly involved	Copious irrigation and wound care. Augmentin P.O., IV antibiotics for immunocompromised. Tetanus prophylaxis. Close follow up

(continued)

Bite or Sting	Sx	Tx
Dogs	Local edema and erythema. *Pasteurella* also commonly involved, assess nature of bite, unprovoked worrisome for Rabies, provoked → unlikely Rabies	Copious irrigation and wound care. Tetanus prophylaxis. Rule out fractures. Augmentin P.O.
Human	Treat all knuckle injuries in a fight as a human bite. Erythema, edema, purulence, pain, fever, and chills. Aerobic and anaerobic bacteria commonly involved	Copious irrigation, tetanus prophylaxis, augmentin P.O., IV antibiotics for severe unresolving infxn or in immunocompromised. Rule out fractures. Close follow up

IV. ENT Trauma*

Dx	Si/Sx	Tx
Foreign Body	1. Ear—insect or object in ear 2. Nose—persistent unilateral nasal drainage 3. Airway—persistent pneumonia 4. Esophageal—three most common areas of narrowing and lodging of foreign bodies a. Cervical Esophagus 16 cm from dental incisors b. Cardioesophageal level 23 cm from incisors c. Gastroesophageal 40 cm from incisors	1. ENT consult for extraction. Mineral oil in ear to kill insects while you wait. Don't irrigate vegetable matter or it will swell 2. ENT consult for extraction 3. CXR PA and lateral, and pulmonary or ENT consult for bronchoscopy and extraction 4. CT scan of neck
TM perforation	• Commonly occur after a slap in the face or cotton swab in ear	• P.O. antibiotics and ear gtts • Water precautions

Dx	Si/Sx	Tx
Auricular hematoma	• Commonly seen in wrestlers with repeated trauma to ears • Ecchymotic fluctuant • If left untreated, necrosis of auricular perichondrium can occur and pts develop a cauliflower ear	1. ENT consult fluid collection 2. Incision and drainage of hematoma with drain left in place and Bolster dressing sutured in 3. P.O. antibiotics and careful follow up
Blunt laryngeal trauma	• Hoarseness, stridor, voice changes, airway obstruction, subcuta neous emphysema, and hemoptysis	• ENT consult. CXR, fiberoptic scope and CT to evaluate injury and possible fracture • Airway observation in monitored setting. May need to secure airway (tracheostomy) • Humidified oxygen and steroids. Surgery may be needed in severe trauma
Nasal Fx	• There may be external and/or internal structural deviation • Must rule out septal hematoma/septal abscess to prevent ischemic compression of perichondrium and septal cartilage necrosis leading to saddle nose deformity • Evaluate for CSF leak • Repair any superficial lacerations	1. Any nosebleed should be stopped as described in Epistaxis 2. X-rays are not very helpful. Physical exam is all you need 3. ENT consult 4. Septal hematoma/abscess must be drained with a rubber train left in place 5. Neurosurgery should be informed of potential CSF leak 6. Because of edema and severe pain most fracture (open or closed) reductions occur within 7–10 days in the OR under anesthesia if cosmesis or nasal airway is a concern 7. Antisthaphylococcus an-tibiotic prophylaxis given

(continued)

Dx	Si/Sx	Tx

Facial fracture	• LeFort fractures are the classic facial trauma fractures
	• Look for mobile palate (fractures always involve the pterygoid plates)
	  1. Types of leFort fractures
	    a. LeFort 1 = maxilla fracture
	    b. LeFort 2 = pyramidal fracture on nasofrontal suture line
	    c. LeFort 3 = total craniofacial dysjunction
		• ENT/plastics/or maxillofacial consult
		• Open versus closed reduction with fixation devices (wiring versus plating)

Mandible Fx	1. Most commonly affect the condyle, body and angle of mandible in that order 2. Multiple sites usually affected simultaneously 3. Sx: pain, malocclusion, trismus, crepitance, mucosal lacerations 4. Classified as favorable if fracture fragments pull in the direction of splinting fracture. Unfavorable if forces on fracture line pull fragments apart	1. CT and panorex views are usually diagnostic 2. Antibiotics and pain meds needed 3. Open or closed reduction of fracture is needed and can be perormed by foral surgery, plastics, or ENT

*Note: All of the above conditions should be stabilized and evaluated by an Otorhinolaryngologist.

12. ETHICS/LAW/ CLINICAL STUDIES

I. Biostatistics

A. **Table of Definitions (Table 12.1)**

B. **Study Types**

Prospective is more powerful than retrospective

Interventional is more powerful than observational

1. *Clinical trial:* **Prospective interventional trial** in which pts are randomized into an intervention group & a control group. **Randomization blunts effect of confounding factors. Blinding both clinician & pt (double-blind) further decreases bias.**

2. *Cohort study:* Population is divided by exposure status. Requires large population (cannot study rare disease). Can study multiple effects by exposure. Gives **relative risk if prospective.** Can be prospective or retrospective.

3. *Case-control study:* Pts divided into those with dz (cases) & those without dz (controls). Fewer pts are needed (good for rare disease). Can study correlation of multiple exposures. Gives **odds ratio. Always retrospective.**

Table 12.1	Biostatistics
Term	**Definition**
Sensitivity	Probability that test results will be positive in pts with disease
Specificity	Probability that test results will be negative in pts without disease
False-positive	Pt without disease who has a positive test result
False-negative	Pt with disease who has a negative test result
PPV	Positive predictive value: probability pt with positive test actually has disease
NPV	Negative predictive value: probability pt with negative test actually has no disease
Incidence	# of newly reported cases of disease divided by total population
Prevalence	# existing cases of disease divided by total population at a given time

(continued)

Table 12.1	Continued
Term	Definition
Relative risk	From cohort study (prospective)—risk of developing dz for people with known exposure compared to risk of developing dz without exposure
Odds ratio	From case-control study (retrospective)—approximates relative risk by comparing odds of developing dz in exposed pts to odds of developing dz in unexposed pts (if dz is rare, odds ratio approaches true relative risk)
Variance	Estimate of the variability of each individual data point from the mean
Std deviation	Square root of the variance
Type I error (α error)	Null hypothesis is rejected even though it is true—e.g., the study says the intervention works but it only appears to work because of random chance
Type II error (β error)	Null hypothesis is not rejected even though it is false—e.g., the study fails to detect a true effect of the intervention
Power (1 - β)	Estimate of the probability a study will be able to detect a true effect of the intervention—e.g., power of 80% means that if the intervention works, the study has an 80% chance of detecting this but a 20% chance of randomly missing it

II. Study Types

A. Prospective is more powerful than retrospective. Interventional is more powerful than observational

1. Clinical trial: **Prospective interventional trial** in which pts are randomized into an intervention group and a control group. **Randomization blunts effect of confounding factors. Blinding both clinician and pt (double-blind) further ↓ bias**

2. Cohort study: Population is divided by exposure status. Requires large population (cannot study rare dz). Can study multiple effects by exposure. Gives **relative risk if prospective.** Can be prospective or retrospective

3. Case control study: Pts divided by those with dz (cases) and those without dz (controls). Fewer pts are needed (good for rare dz). Can study correlation of multiple exposures. Gives **odds ratio. Always retrospective**

III. Calculation of Statistical Values (Table 12.2)

Sensitivity & specificity are inherent characteristics of the test—they must be given in the question. **Predictive values vary with the prevalence of the disease.** They are NOT inherent characteristics of the test; rather, they reflect an interaction of sensitivity & specificity with the frequency of the disease in the population.

Always fill the table in assuming 100 pts—it's easier to do the math this way. The prevalence of the disease (50%) tells you that 50 pts should be in the first column, because 50% of 100 pts have the disease. Therefore, 50 pts should also be in the second column (if 50 of 100 pts have the disease, 50 pts also do NOT have the disease). The sensitivity tells you that 45 of the pts in the first column should be in the top row because the test will find 90% of the 50 pts who have the disease. The specificity tells you that 40 of the pts in the second column should be in the bottom row because the test will correctly describe 80% of the 50 people who truly don't have the disease (& incorrectly claim that 20% of the 50 pts who truly don't have the disease do have the disease).

Now the disease prevalence tells you that 10 pts should be in the first column (10% of 100 pts have the disease). Therefore, 90 pts should be in the second column (if 10 of 100 pts have the disease, 90 pts do NOT have the disease). The sensitivity tells you that 9 of the pts in the first column should be in the top row because the test will find 90% of the 10 pts who have the disease. The specificity tells you that 72 of the pts in the second column should be in the bottom row because the test will correctly describe 80% of the 90 people who truly don't have the disease (& incorrectly claim that 20% of the 90 pts who don't have the disease do have the disease).

ETHICS/LAW/CLINICAL STUDIES

Table 12.2 Sample Calculation of Statistical Values

	Pt has dz	Pt does not have dz
Positive test	a = True-positive	b = False-positive
Negative test	c = False-negative	d = True-negative

PPV = a/(a + b)
NPV = d/(c + d)
Sensitivity = a/(a + c)
Specificity = d/(b + d)

Example 1:	For disease X, a theoretical screening test is **90% sensitive & 80% specific**. In Africa, where the disease has a **prevalence of 50%**, the test's **PPV = 82%** (a/[a + b] = 45/55), & the **NPV is 89%** (d/[c + d] = 40/45).

	Pt has dz	Pt does not have dz
Positive test	45	10
Negative test	5	40

Example 2:	Now study the **same test for the same disease (X)** in America, where the **prevalence of the disease is 10%**. The test characteristics remain the same: **90% sensitive & 80% specific**. The test's **PPV = 33%** (a/[a + b] = 9/27) & the **NPV = 99%** (d/[c + d] = 72/73). **The same test has drastically different predictive values depending on the disease prevalence!!!**

	Pt has dz	Pt does not have dz
Positive test	9	18
Negative test	1	72

IV. Law and Ethics (Table 12.3)

A. Legal Issues

1. Malpractice
   a. A civil wrong doing (tort), not a crime
   b. Must satisfy the four "Ds"
      (1) Dereliction: deviation from the applicable standard of care
      (2) Duty: a physician-pt relationship was established with a duty to treat
      (3) Damages: injury or measurable damages occur
      (4) Directly: injury or damages directly result from physicians actions or inactions
   c. May be required to pay compensatory damages (money) for pt's suffering

| **Table 12.3** | Ethical/Legal Terms |

Abandonment = Termination of the physician-pt relationship by the physician without reasonable notice to the pt and without the opportunity to make arrangements for appropriate continuation and follow-up care

Assault = Intentional and unauthorized act of placing another in apprehension of immediate bodily harm

Battery = Intentional and unauthorized touching of a person, directly or indirectly, without consent. A surgical procedure performed upon a person without expressed or implied consent can constitute battery unless it is done to save life in and emergency situation and consent is therefore implied

Causation = The causal connection between the act or omission of the defendant and the injury suffered by the plaintiff. The plaintiff must show causation of an injury by the defendant in order to prove negligence

Common good = (1) respect for persons; (2) social welfare; and (3) peace and security. All three of these elements dictate the common good of healthcare provision

Comparative negligence = The principle adopted by most states that reduces a plaintiff's recovery proportional to the plaintiff's degree of fault in causing the damage

Consent = Voluntary act by which one person agrees to allow another person to do something. "Expressed consent" is directly and unequivocally given, either orally or in writing. "Implied consent" is shown by signs, actions, facts, or by inaction and silence, which raise a presumption that consent has been given. It may be implied from conduct (implied-in-fact); e.g., when someone rolls up his or her sleeve and extends his or her arm for vein puncture or by the circumstance (implied-in-law); e.g., an unconscious person in an emergency situation

Damages = Money received through judicial order by a plaintiff sustaining harm, impairment, or loss to his or her person or property as the result of the accidental, intentional, or negligent act of another

Disproportionate means = Any Tx that, in the given circumstances, either offers no reasonable hope of benefit (taking into account the well-being of the whole person) or is too burdensome for the pt or others; i.e., the burdens or risks are disproportionate to or outweigh the expected benefits of the Tx

Deposition = Sworn, officially transcribed out-of-court testimony of a witness or party taken before a trial

Due care = The degree of care that a prudent and competent person engaged in the same profession would exercise under similar circumstances. A test for liability for negligence. Also called reasonable care

Duty = An obligation recognized by the law. When the pt-physician relationship exists, the pt has a right to be attended and treated by the physician according to the required standard of care and the physician has a correlative duty to provide such care

ETHICS/LAW/CLINICALS STUDIES

(continued)

Table 12.3 *Continued*

Fiduciary = Person in a position of confidence or trust who undertakes a duty to act for the benefit of another under a given set of circumstances

Futility = Efforts to achieve a result that is unreasonable or impossible. Covers Tx that: (1) will not serve any useful purpose; (2) causes needless pain and suffering; and (3) does not achieve the goal of restoring the pt to an acceptable quality of life

Good Samaritan Law = A statute, some form of which has been enacted in all 50 states and the District of Columbia, which exempts from liability a person, such as a physician passer-by, who voluntarily renders aid to an injured person but who negligently, but not unreasonably negligently, causes injury while rendering the aid

Human Dignity = Intrinsic worth that is inherent in every human being

Informed consent = Requires a physician to obtain a pt's voluntary agreement to accept Tx based upon the pt's awareness of the nature of his or her dz, the material risks and benefits of the proposed Tx, the alternative Tx and risks, or the choice of no Tx at all

Privilege = Physician-pt privilege is the right to exclude from evidence in a legal proceeding any confidential communication that a pt makes to a physician for the purpose of Dx or Tx, unless the pt consents to the disclosure

Settlement = Agreement usually involving an exchange of money for a release of the right to sue made between opposing parties in a lawsuit which resolves their legal dispute

Wrongful death = Lawsuit brought on behalf of a deceased person's survivors that alleges that death was attributable to the willful or negligent act of another

    d. Studies have shown physicians with poor communication skills and interactions with pts are most likely to be sued for malpractice

2. Informed Consent
   a. Must be obtained from pt by a physician knowledgeable in the Dx and Tx in question before any procedure
   b. Pts must be presented with their Dx, potential Tx, and the risks and benefits of each Tx
   c. A competent adult or emancipated minor must then voluntarily consent or not consent to the Tx prior to starting
   d. Considered *Battery* or *Negligence* if not obtained
   e. In an emergency, if pt is unable to consent, life-saving measures may be provided

3. Confidentiality
   a. Fosters trust in doctor-pt relationship and respects pt's privacy

    b. Can be overridden if there is a potential harm to a third party and there is no less invasive way for warning or protecting those at risk

4. *Primum Non Nocer,* Nonmaleficence
   a. "Above all, do no harm"
   b. A balance must exist in the care of pts. Risks and benefits of all interventions must be considered
   c. If a physician can't act to benefit the pt, then at least do no harm

5. Beneficence
   a. Fiduciary relationship exists between the doctor and pt
   b. Physicians are trusted to act on behalf of the well being of their pts

6. Death
   a. With the advent of cardiopulmonary life support systems, the definition of death is no longer simply a cessation of breathing or circulation
   b. Death is now also defined as complete irreversible loss of entire brain function to include cortical and brain stem function
   c. Pts must be "warm and dead" to be considered dead, there are many stories of people revived from freezing cold temperatures who were thought to be dead
   d. Persistent Vegetative State (PVS): have brain stem function but no cortical function

7. Advance Directives
   a. Allows competent pts to indicate their health-related preferences or a surrogate decision-maker prior to becoming incapacitated
   b. Living Will: Written instructions related to health-related preferences in the event the pt becomes incapacitated and is unable to communicate his or her wishes otherwise
   c. Durable Power of Attorney: A surrogate is designated to make health care decisions on behalf of the incapacitated pt
   d. Various states have limitations on Advance Directives; an attorney should be consulted if there are any questions regarding your particular state

8. Do Not Resuscitate Orders (DNR)
   a. Can only be initiated by the attending staff physician after receiving informed consent from appropriate health care decision-maker
   b. Cardiopulmonary Resuscitation (CPR) is withheld

ETHICS/LAW/CLINICALS STUDIES

c. Limited DNR orders may also be seen such as DNI (Do not Intubate) and chest compressions only

d. These should all be clearly visible to all staff so that pt's requests can be followed in an emergency

V. Doctoring

A. Introduction

1. Pt-Doctor (physician) relationship is based on trust, confidence, mutual understanding, and communication

2. Pt interviews and interactions must be conducted in a humanistic, culturally sensitive manner

3. In cooperation with other health care professionals, such as interpreters, an appreciation for racial and cultural diversity must always be conveyed

4. Nonbiased health care delivery to the pt and their family must be conveyed at all times

5. Tx plans must be realistic, mutually understood, and mutually agreed upon to achieve compliance

B. Interview

1. Introduce self to pt; assure an interpreter is present if a foreign language is spoken

2. Face pt, and always speak to pt and their family directly and not to the interpreter

3. Try not to interrupt pt when speaking

4. Interviewing techniques (Table 12.4)

5. Pt history: chief complaint, history of present illness (HPI), past medical history (PMH), past surgical history (PSH), family history (FH), social history (SH), and allergies

6. Helpful Interviewing Mnemonic (**HEADSSS**)

a. Originally developed to interview adolescents but can be used for all ages as a way to break the ice of an initial interview and to cover major areas

b. **HEADSSS** assessment allows physicians to evaluate critical areas in each pt's life that may be detrimental to their health

(1) **H**ome environment: Who does pt live with? Any recent changes? Quality of family interaction (if applicable)?

(2) **H**ealth risks: Exposure to TB, Hepatitis, asbestos, cigarette smoke, radiation

Table 12.4   Interviewing Techniques

Technique	Description	Example
Empathy	Communicating an understanding of pt's feelings	"I can tell you must really be upset about this situation."
Paraphrasing	Communicates an understanding of content	"So, you have been waiting 3 hrs for your appointment."
Silence	A pause in a conversation is worth a thousand words. Doctor and pt can use this time to watch each other's nonverbal posturing and to take an inventory of how interview is going	"........................"
Open-ended questions	Allows pt and family to express themselves fully regarding the topic in question	"Why have you come to the hospital today?"
Questions for the doctor	Allows pt to express their concerns and to assure themselves of what has been discussed during the interview and what still has not been addressed	"Do you have any questions for me?"
Direct questioning	Allows the interviewer to focus on an important topic	"Now, tell me more about how you got that bruise on your arm."
Identifying/ validation	Allows pt's concerns to appear acceptable and worth discussing	"I am also afraid of doctors and hospitals; please tell me more about why you are here."

ETHICS/LAW/CLINICALS
STUDIES

(3) **E**mployment and **E**ducation: Is pt in school? Favorite subjects? Academic performance? Are friends in school? Any recent changes? Does pt have a job? Future plans?

(4) **A**ctivities: What does pt like to do in spare time? Who does pt spend time with? Involved in any sports/exercise: Hobbies? Attends parties or clubs?

(5) **D**rugs: Has pt ever used tobacco? Alcohol? Marijuana? Other illicit drugs? If so, when was the last use? How often? Do friends or family members use drugs? Who does the pt use these substances with?

(6) **S**exual activity: Sexual orientation? Is pt sexually active? Number of sexual partners? Does the pt use condoms or other forms of contraception? Any history of STDs or pregnancy?

(7) **S**uicide: Does the pt ever feel sad, tired, or unmotivated? Has the pt ever felt that life was not worth living? Any feelings of wanting to harm self? If so, does the pt have a plan? Has the pt ever tried to harm self in the past? Does the pt know anyone who has attempted suicide?

(8) **S**afety: Does the pt use a seat belt or bike helmet? Does the pt enter into high-risk situations? Does the pt have access to a firearm? Is the pt's home environment safe?

C. Identifying Abuse

1. Not necessarily physical in nature. Can be physical assault, sexual assault, psychological abuse, economic control, and/or progressive social isolation

2. Depending on state laws, certain potential abuse situations mandate reporting. Failure to report subjects practitioner to disciplinary action, fines, and/or liability

3. Department of Social Services should be made aware of suspected child abuse and elder abuse cases

4. Cameras and rape kits should be made available in all emergency departments to property handle potential evidence

5. Must know and understand cultural demographics of community served. Certain cultural medicine rituals may be misinterpreted by health practitioners:

   a. Cupping: Cupping, pinching, or rubbing (also known as coining). Thought to restore balance by releasing excessive "air"

   (1) Small cups are used; i.e., small shot glasses. A small amount of alcohol is put into the cup and ignited, and the cup is immediately pressed tight against the skin (forehead, abdomen, chest, or back). A vacuum is produced by the combustion of the alcohol and the evacuation of oxygen from the cup. The developing vacuum then sucks out noxious materials or excess energy into the cup from the body. A circular ecchymotic area is left on the skin

   (2) Pinching: Pressure is applied by pinching the skin between the thumb and index finger to the point of

producing a contusion. Done at the base of the nose, between the eyes, on the neck, chest, or back

(3) Rubbing is usually in the same areas as pinching and involves firmly rubbing lubricated skin with a spoon or a coin in order to bring toxic "air" to the body surface

a. Female genital mutilation carried out today in more than 30 countries across Africa and the Middle East. Awareness of this practice and its consequences is necessary to adequately treat these pts

D. Cultural Medicine

1. Hot and Cold Theory: Seen in Latin American cultures; illness is caused by an imbalance of hot and cold. Eating appropriately hot or cold type foods as needed can restore balance

2. Prominent among Mexican-American folk healers is the curandero, a type of shaman who uses white magic and herbs to effect cures

3. Five types of folk illness are most prominent:
   a. Mal de ojo (evil eye)
   b. Empacho (GI blockage due to excessive food intake)
   c. Susto (magically induced fright)
   d. Caida de la mollera (fallen fontanel, or opening in or between bones)
   e. Mal puesto (sorcery)

E. Interpreter

1. In order to provide best available pt services, all efforts should be made to facilitate communications with pt in their language, using an interpreter whenever possible

2. Physician must always face pt and speak directly to pt while discussion is translated

3. Have pt repeat instructions to you through interpreter to assure understanding

4. Whenever possible use a trained interpreter, and avoid using family members to prevent embarrassment and miscommunication of discussion

VI. Health Care Delivery

A. Hospitals

1. Tertiary Medical Center: Receives referrals from community, has latest technologies, including organ transplantation, Level 1 trauma, etc. Most academic medical centers

2. Intermediate Hospital: No organ transplantation, much of the same technology as a major medical center

3. Community Hospital: Provides basic services, lacks major staffing and technology of larger medical centers

B. Health Maintenance Organizations (HMOs)

1. Provide health care to people who have prepaid enrollment

2. Various Models Exist: Staff Model, Preferred Provider Organization (PPO), and Independent Practice Association (IPA)

   a. Staff Model: Physicians are salaried employees or contracted to provide medical services to members. All pts must be seen by a primary care physician prior to referral to most specialists

   b. PPOs: Occurs when an insurance company has established contracts with certain independent providers, allowing pts to choose physicians not normally on their list of providers for a surcharge

   c. IPAs: Physicians paid on an agreed upon fee-for-service whenever a member of the HMO uses their services

3. Capitation: Physicians are paid a certain amount per pt, per year, regardless of the amount of services provided to each of the pts assigned

C. Extended Care Facilities

1. Nursing Homes/Skilled Nursing Facilities (SNFs)

   a. Provide IV fluids, nutrition, and medications

   b. Nursing staff available 24 hr

2. Intermediate Care Facilities (ICF)

   a. Provide assistance mainly with activities of daily living

   b. Nursing not necessarily available 24 hr

D. Hospice

1. Specializes in providing terminal care to pts in their final moments of life

E. Medicare/Medicaid

1. Medicare: Authorized under the Social Security Act

   a. Provides health insurance to people >65 yrs old or who are disabled and receive social security, does not cover prescription medications

2. Medicaid: Also authorized under the Social Security Act

   a. Unlike medicare, it is provided to the very poor who usually receive other types of public assistance. Qualifications vary by state, does cover prescription medications

F. Hospital Personnel

1. Nurses: Many levels of training

   a. Nurse's Aid: Basic medical vocational training

   b. LPN/LVN: Licensed Practical Nurse/Licensed Vocational Nurse; undergo a 1 yr program of nursing vocational training followed by a state licensing exam

   c. Registered Nurse: May have a Bachelors degree or Associates degree, have passed state nursing board exams and have a registered state license

   d. Clinical Nurse Specialist: Usually Masters degree prepared nurse, has advanced training in a specific medical area; i.e., intensive care, cardiac care, enterostomal care, etc.

   e. Nurse Practitioner: Usually Masters degree prepared nurse, practice as a family nurse practitioner, pediatric nurse practitioner, nursing midwife

   f. Doctoral Nurses: Hold Doctorate degree in various areas, mainly work in academic nursing schools as professors and researchers

2. Physician Assistant: Usually Bachelors degree level of education and a state licensing exam. Function as independent practitioners under the supervision of a physician

APPENDIX

A. ZEBRAS AND SYNDROMES

Dz	Description/Sx
Achondroplasia	Autosomal dominant dwarfism due to early epiphyseal closure → shortening and thickening of bones Si/Sx = leg bowing, hearing loss, sciatica, infantile hydrocephalus. Pts can have nml lifespans
Adrenoleukodystrophy	X-linked recessive defect in long-chain fatty acid metabolism due to a peroxisomal enzyme deficiency. Causes rapidly progressing central demyelination, adrenal insufficiency, hyperpigmentation of skin, spasticity, seizures, death by age 12
Albers-Schönberg dz (osteopetrosis)	↑↑ Skeletal density because of osteoclastic failure → multiple fractures due to ↓ perfusion of thick bone, also causes anemia due to ↓ marrow space blindness, deafness and cranial nerve dysfunction because of narrowing, impingement of neural foramina
Alkaptonuria	Defect of phenylalanine metabolism causing accumulation of homogentisic acid. Presents with black urine, ochronosis (blue-black pigmentation of ear, nose, cheeks), arthropathy due to cartilage binding homogentisic acid
Alport's syndrome	X-linked hereditary collagen defect causing sensorineural hearing loss, lens dislocation, hematuria (glomerulonephritis)
Argyria	Dermal deposits of silver bound to albumin. Related to prolonged exposure or ingestion of silver-containing products. Dx = slate-gray skin color, including mucosa and sclera. Tx = psychosocial support, discoloration is irreversible (see Figure A.1)
Ataxia-telangiectasia	DNA repair defect affects B and T lymphocytes. Autosomal recessive dz usually appears by age 2. Physical signs include ataxia of gait, telangiectasias of skin and conjunctiva, recurrent sinus infxns
Banti's syndrome	"Idiopathic portal HTN." Splenomegaly and portal HTN following subclinical portal vein occlusion. Insidious onset, occurring yrs after initial occlusive event

Dz	Description/Sx

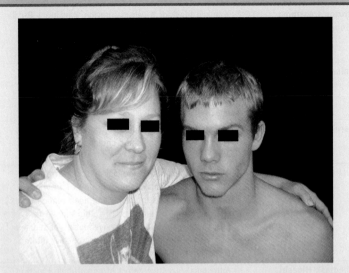

FIGURE A.1

Argyria. Note the slate-gray skin discoloration of the young man on the **right**, in contrast to the nml skin color of the woman on the **left**. (Courtesy of Scott C. Wickless, Tor Shwayder, Davide Iacobelli, and Susan Smolinske. From Greenberg MI, Hendrickson RG, Silverberg M, et al. *Greenberg's text-atlas of emergency medicine*. Philadelphia: Lippincott Williams & Wilkins, 2004, with permission.)

Bartter's syndrome	Kidney dz that causes Na, K, and Cl wasting. Despite ↑ levels of renin, BP remains low
Beckwith-Wiedemann syndrome	Autosomal dominant fetal overgrowth syndrome of macrosomia, microcephaly, macroglossia, organomegaly, omphalocele, distinctive lateral ear-lobe fissures, hypoglycemia associated with hyperin-sulinemia, ↑ incidence of Wilms' tumor
Bernard-Soulier syndrome	Autosomal recessive defect of platelet GPIb receptor (binds to von Willebrand factor), presents with chronic, severe mucosal bleeds and giant platelets on blood smear
Binswanger's dz	Subacute subcortical dementia caused by small artery infarcts in periventricular white matter. Usually seen in long-standing HTN but is rare

Dz	Description/Sx
Bruton's agamma-globulinemia	X-linked block of B-cell maturation, causing ↓ B-call levels and immunoglobulin (Ig)G levels. Presents with recurrent bacterial infxns in infants aged >6 mo
Caisson's dz	Decompression sickness ("the bends") caused by rapid ascent from deep-sea diving. Sx occur from 30 min–1 hr = joint pain, cough, skin burning/mottling
Caroli's dz	Segmental cystic dilation of intrahepatic bile ducts complicated by stones and cholangitis, can be CA precursor
Charcot-Marie-Tooth dz	Autosomal dominant peroneal muscular atrophy causing foot drop and stocking-glove ↓ in vibration/pain/temperature sense and deep tendon reflex (DTR) in lower extremities. Histologically → repeated demyelination and remyelination of segmental areas of the nerve. Pts may present as children (type 1) or adults (type 2)
Chédiask-Higashi syndrome	Autosomal recessive defect of microtubule function of neutrophils, leads to ↓ lysosomal fusion to phagosomes. Presents with recurrent *Staphylococcus* and *Streptococcus* infxns, albinism, peripheral and cranial neuropathies
Cheyne-Stokes respirations	Central apnea seen in congestive heart failure, ↑ intracranial pressure, or cerebral infxn/inflammation/trauma: cycles of central apnea followed by regular crescendo-decrescendo breathing (amplitude first waxes and then wanes back to apnea); Biot's is an uncommon variant seen in meningitis in which the cycles consist of central apnea followed by stead amplitude breathing that then shuts back off to apnea
Chronic Granulomatous Dz (CGD)	Phagocytes lack respiratory burst or NADPH oxidase, so can engulf bacteria but are unable to kill them. Presents with recurrent infxns with *Aspergillus* and *Staphylococcus aureus* infxns. Tx = recombinant interferon-g
Cystinuria	Autosomal recessive failure of tubular resorption of cystine and dibasic amino acids (lysine, ornithine, arginine), clinically see cystine stones. Tx = hydration to ↑ urine volume, alkalinization of urine with bicarbonate and acetazolamide

Dz	Description/Sx
de Quervain's tenosynovitis	Tenosynovitis causing pain on flexion of thumb (motion of abductor pollicis longus)
Diamond-Blackfan syndrome	"Pure red cell aplasia," a congenital or acquired deficiency in the RBC stem cell. Congenital disorder is sometimes associated with abnormal facies, cardiac, and renal abnormalities. Tx = steroids
DiGeorge's syndrome	Embryologic defect in development of pharyngeal pouches 3 and 4 → thymic aplasia that causes T cell deficiency and parathyroid aplasia. Most commonly presents with tetany due to hypocalcemia 2° to hypoparathyroidism and recurrent severe viral, fungal, or protozoal infxns
Dressler's syndrome	Acute pericarditis, develops within 2–4 wk after acute MI or heart surgery, may be due to autoimmune reaction to myocardial antigens
Ehlers-Danlos syndrome	Autosomal dominant defect in collagen synthesis, variable expressivity. Si/Sx = loose joints, pathognomonic ↑ **skin elasticity,** mitral regurgitation, genu recurvatum of knee (fixed in hyperextension), aortic dilation
Ellis-van Creveld	Syndrome of polydactyly + single atrium
Erb's paralysis	Waiter's tip—upper-brachial plexopathy (C5–6)
Evan's syndrome	(Ig)G autoantibody-mediated hemolytic anemia and thrombocytopenia, associated with collagen-vascular dz, thrombotic thrombocy topenic purpura, hepatic cirrhosis, leukemia, sarcoidosis, Hashimoto's thyroiditis. Tx = prednisone and IVIG.
Fabry's dz	X-linked defect in galactosidase, Sx = lower-trunk skin lesions, corneal opacity, renal/cardiac/cerebral dz that are invariably lethal in infancy or childhood
Fanconi's anemia	Autosomal recessive disorder of DNA repair. Presents with pancytopenia, ↑ risk of malignancy, short stature, birdlike facies, café-au-lait spots, congenital urogenital defects, retardation, absent thumb
Fanconi syndrome	Dysfunction of proximal renal tubules, congenital or acquired (drugs, multiple myeloma, toxic metals), presenting with ↓ reabsorption of glucose, amino acids, phosphate, and bicarbonate. Associated with renal tubular acidosis type II, clinically see glycosuria, hyperphosphaturia, hypophosphatemia (vitamin D-resistant rickets), aminoaciduria (generalized, not cystine specific), systemic acidosis, polyuria, polydipsia

Dz	Description/Sx
Farber's dz	Auto recessive defect in ceramidase, causing ceramide accumulation in nerves, onset within mo of birth, death occurs by age 2
Felty's syndrome	Rheumatoid arthritis plus splenomegaly and neutropenia, often with thrombocytopenia
Fibrolamellar CA	Variant of hepatocellular CA. Occurs in young people (20–40 yr), is not associated with viral hepatitis or cirrhosis. Has a good Px. Histologically shows nests and cords of malignant hepatocytes separated by dense collagen bundles
Fitz-Hugh-Curtis syndrome	Chlamydia or gonorrhea perihepatitis as a complication of pelvic inflammatory dz. Presents with right upper quadrant pain and sepsis
Galactosemia	Deficient galactose-1-phosphate uridyltransferase blocks galactose conversion to glucose for further metabolism, leading to accumulation of galactose in many tissues. Sx = failure to thrive, infantile cataracts, mental retardation, cirrhosis. Rarely due to galactokinase deficiency, blocking the same path at a different step
Gardner's syndrome	Familial polyposis syndrome with classic triad of desmoid tumors, osteomas of mandible or skull and sebaceous cysts
Gaucher's dz	Most frequent cause of lysosomal enzyme deficiency in Ashkenazi Jews. Autosomal recessive deficiency in β-glucocerebrosidase. Accumulation of sphingolipids in liver, spleen, and bone marrow. Can be fatal if very expensive enzyme substitute (alglucerase) not administered
Glanzmann's thrombasthenia	Autosomal recessive defect in GPIIb-IIIa platelet receptor that binds fibrinogen, inhibiting platelet aggregation, presents with chronic, severe mucosal bleeds
Glycogenoses	Genetic defects in metabolic enzymes causing glycogen accumulation. Si/Sx = hepatosplenomegaly, general organomegaly, exertional fatigue, hypoglycemia. Type I = von Gierke's dz; type II = Pompe's dz; type III = Cori's dz; type V = McArdle's dz
Hartnup's dz	Autosomal recessive defect in tryptophan absorption at renal tubule. Sx mimic pellagra = the **3 Ds: D**ermatitis, **D**ementia, **D**iarrhea (tryptophan is niacin precursor). Rash is on sun-exposed areas, can see cerebellar ataxia, mental retardation, psychosis. Tx = niacin supplements

Dz	Description/Sx
Hepatorenal syndrome	Renal failure without intrinsic renal dz, occurring during fulminant hepatitis or cirrhosis, presents with acute oliguria and azotemia, typically progressive and fatal
Hepatopulmonary syndrome	Development of intrapulmonary arteriovenous malformations (AVMs) in the setting of cirrhosis that causes pulmonary shunting with severe refractory hypoxia; pts present with platypnea, which is dyspnea when standing that improves with lying down; pathophysiology of AVM formation in the setting of cirrhosis is not understood, and the only Tx is liver transplantation, which may cause regression of AVMs
Holt-Oram syndrome	Autosomal dominant atrial septal defect in association with fingerlike thumb or absent thumb, cardiac conduction abnormalities, other skeletal defects
Homocystinuria	Deficiency in cystine metabolism. Sx mimic Marfan's = lens dislocation (downward in homocystinuria as opposed to upward in Marfan's), thin bones, mental retardation, hypercoagulability, premature atherosclerosis → strokes and MIs
Hunter's dz	X-linked lysosomal iduronidase deficiency, less severe than Hurler's syndrome. Sx = mild mental retardation, cardiac problems, micrognathia, etc
Hurler's dz	Defect in iduronidase, causing multiorgan mucopolysaccharide accumulation, dwarfism, hepatosplenomegaly, corneal clouding, progressive mental retardation, death by age 10
Incontinentia pigmenti	Rare X-linked, dominant defect of the NEMO gene (Nuclear factor κ B Essential MOdulator = IKBKG-IKK γ), resulting in excessive deposits of melanin in the body. Presents with neonatal erythematous skin rash, with spiral lines of small fluid-filled blisters transforming into rough, warty skin growths. Eventually areas of hyperpigmentation develop which later become atrophied and hypopigmented. Dental problems, alopecia with scarring, and seizures and muscle weakness can occur, and can be associated with a variety of anatomical defects (e.g., dwarfism, club foot, skull deformities). Extremely wooly or kinky hair and severe immune system dysfunction may also appear
Isovalinic acidemia	"Sweaty-foot odor" dz. Caused by a defect in leucine metabolism, leads to buildup of isovaline in the bloodstream, producing characteristic odor

Dz	Description/Sx
Job's syndrome	B-cell defect causing hyper-IgE levels but defects in other (Ig)G and immune functions. Presents with recurrent pulmonary infxns, dermatitis, excess teeth (pts unable to shed their baby teeth), frequent bone fractures, classic "gargoyle facies," IgE levels 10- to 100-fold higher than nml
Kasabach-Merritt	Expanding hemangioma trapping platelets, leading to systemic thrombocytopenia
Keshan's dz	Childhood cardiomyopathy 2° to selenium deficiency, very common in China
Klippel-Trénaunay Weber syndrome	Autosomal dominant chromosomal translocation → prematurity, hydrops fetalis, hypertrophic hemangioma of leg, Kasabach-Merritt thrombocytopenia
Klumpke's paralysis	Clawed hand—lower brachial plexopathy (C8, T1) affecting ulnar nerve distributions, often presents with Horner's syndrome as well
Leber's congenital amaurosis (LCA)	Autosomal Recessive disorder of photoreceptors appearing at birth or in infancy causing blindness, lack of papillary response, and nystagmus
Leigh's dz	Mitochondrially inherited dz → absent or ↓↓ thiamine pyrophosphate. Infants or children present with seizures, ataxia, optic atrophy, ophthalmoplegia, tremor
Lesch-Nyhan syndrome	Congenital defect in Hypoxanthine-Guanine Phosphoribosyl Transferase (HPRT) → gout, urate nephrolithiasis, retardation, choreiform spasticity, self-mutilation (pts bite off their own fingers and lips). Mild deficiency → Kelley-Seegmiller syndrome = gout without nervous system Si/Sx
Leukocyte adhesion deficiency	Type I due to lack of β_2-in tegrins (LFA-1), type II due to lack of fucosylated glycoproteins (selectin receptors). Both have plenty of neutrophils in blood but cannot enter tissues due to problems with adhesion and transmigration. Both present with recurrent bacterial infxns, **gingivitis, poor wound healing, delayed umbilical cord separation**
Lhermitte sign	Tingling down the back during neck flexion, occurs in any craniocervical disorder
Liddle's dz	Dz mimics hyperaldosteronism. Defect in the renal epithelial transporters. Si/Sx = HTN, hypokalemic metabolic alkalosis
Li-Fraumeni's syndrome	Autosomal dominant inherited defect of p53 leading to 1° CA of a variety of organ systems presenting at an early age

Dz	Description/Sx
Maple syrup urine dz	Disorder of branched-chain amino acid metabolism (valine, leucine, isoleucine). Sx include vomiting, and pathognomonic maplelike odor of urine
Marchiafava-Bignami syndrome	Overconsumption of red wine → demyelination of corpus callosum, anterior commissure, middle cerebellar peduncles. Possibly anoxic/ischemic phenomenon
Marfan's dz	Genetic collagen defect → tall, thin body habitus, long and slender digits, pectus excavatum, scoliosis, aortic valve dilation → regurgitation, aortic dissection, mitral valve prolapse, joint laxity, optic lens dislocations, blue sclera. Think about Abe Lincoln when considering this disease: tall and thin
Melanosis coli	Overzealous use of laxatives causing darkening of colon but no significant dz
MELAS & MERRF syndrome	Mitochondrial Encephalopathy and Lactic Acidosis (MELAS) syndrome and Myoclonic Epilepsy associated with Ragged Red Fibers (MERRF) syndrome are genetic, mitochondrial disorders (therefore maternally inherited) in which electron transport is disrupted, usually due to a mutation in the mitochondrial leucine–transfer RNA gene. Presentation and severity is variable, depending on the cellular distribution of defective mitochondria throughout the body. MELAS can involve Type 2 diabetes, seizures, psychosis, stroke, renal failure, heart failure, hearing loss. MERRF Sx include seizures, myopathy with ragged-red-fibers on Bx, including ptosis and ophthalmoparesis, cerebellar ataxia, dementia, or deafness. Screen with serum lactate/pyruvate ratio ($\geq$20:1 suggests Dx), confirm with muscle Bx or genetic test
Mendelson's syndrome	Chemical pneumonitis following aspiration of acidic gastric juice pt presents with acute dyspnea, tachypnea, and tachycardia, with pink and frothy sputum
Meralgia paresthetica	Condition common to truckers, hikers, and overweight individuals who wear heavy backpacks or very tight-fitting belts compressing inguinal area. This causes pts to have a diffuse unilateral pain and paresthesias along anterior portion of upper thigh, corresponding to lateral femoral cutaneous nerve. Typically self-limiting but can treat with steroids for refractory dz
Minamata dz	Toxic encephalopathy from mercury poisoning, classically described from fish eaten near Japanese mercury dumping site

Dz	Description/Sx
Mönckeberg's arteriosclerosis	Calcific sclerosis of the media of medium-size arteries, usually radial and ulnar. Occurs in people >50 yr, but it does NOT obstruct arterial flow because intima is not involved. Unrelated to other atherosclerosis and does not cause dz
Münchhausen's syndrome	Factitious disorder in which the pt derives gratification from feigning a serious or dramatic illness. In Münchhausen's by proxy, the pt derives gratification from making someone else ill (often a mother injures her child for attention)
Niemann-Pick's dz	Autosomal recessive defect in sphingomyelinase with variable age at onset (↑ severe dz in younger pt) → demyelination/neurologic Sx, hepatosplenomegaly, xanthoma, pancytopenia
Noonan's syndrome	Autosomal dominant with Sx similar to Turner's syndrome → hyperelastic skin, neck webbing, ptosis, low-set ears, short stature, pulmonary stenosis, atrial-septal (AS) defect, coarctation of aorta, small testes. Presents in males, X and Y are both present
Ortner's syndrome	Impingement of recurrent laryngeal nerve by the enlarging atrium in mitral regurgitation, leading to hoarseness
Osteogenesis imperfecta	Genetic disorder of diffuse bone weakness due to mutations resulting in defective collagen synthesis. Multiple fractures 2° to minimal trauma = brittle bone dz. Classic sign = blue sclera due to translucent connective tissue over choroid
Peliosis hepatis	Rare 1° dilation of hepatic sinusoids. Associated with exposure to anabolic steroids, oral contraceptives, danazol. Irregular cystic spaces filled with blood develop in the liver. Cessation of drug intake causes reversal of the lesions
Plummer-Vinson syndrome	Iron-deficiency syndrome with classic triad of esophageal web, spoon nail, and iron-deficiency anemia. Webs produce dysphagia, will regress with iron replacement
Polycystic kidney dz	Autosomal dominant bilateral dz; Si/Sx = onset in early or middle adult life with hematuria, nephrolithiasis, uremia, 33% of cases have cysts in liver, 10%–20% of pts have intracranial aneurysms, HTN is present in 70% of pts at Dx. Juvenile version is autosomal recessive, much rarer than adult type; almost all pts have cysts in liver and portal bile duct proliferation = "congenital hepatic fibrosis"

Dz	Description/Sx
Poncet's dz	Polyarthritis that occurs DURING active TB infxn but in which no organisms can be isolated from the affected joints; is thought to be autoimmune-mediated dz
Pott's dz	Tubercular infxn of vertebrae (vertebral osteomyelitis) leading to kyphoscoliosis 2° to pathologic fractures
Potter's syndrome	Bilateral renal agenesis; incompatible with fetal life, mother has oligohydramnios because fetus normally swallows large quantities of amniotic fluid and then urinates it out, but fetus cannot excrete swallowed fluid because it has no kidneys
Reflex sympathetic dystrophy (RSD) syndrome	Also known as complex regional pain syndrome (CRPS), a chronic neurologic syndrome characterized by severe burning pain, pathologic changes in bone and skin, excessive sweating, tissue swelling, extreme sensitivity to touch, usually 2° to an initiating noxious event or immobilization
Refsum's dz	Autosomal recessive defect in phytanic acid metabolism → peripheral neuropathy, cerebellar ataxia, retinitis pigmentosa, bone dz, ichthyosis (scaly skin)
Rett's syndrome	Congenital retardation 2° to ↑ serum ammonia levels, more common in females. Sx = autism, dementia, ataxia, tremors
Schafer's dz	Defect in hexosaminidase B, in contrast to the A component of the enzyme that is defective in Tay-Sachs. Px is better for Schafer's
Schindler's dz	Defect in *N*-acetylgalactosaminidase
Schmidt's syndrome	Hashimoto's thyroiditis with diabetes and/or Addison's dz (autoimmune syndrome)
Sweet's syndrome	Recurrent painful reddish-purple plaques and papules (see Figure A.2) associated with fever, arthralgia, neutrophilia. Occurs more commonly in women, possibly due to hypersensitivity reaction associated with *Yersinia* infxn. Can also be seen in following upper respiratory infxn or with leukemia. Tx = prednisone, antibiotics if associated with *Yersinia* infxn
Syndrome X	Angina relieved by rest (typical) with a nml angiogram. Caused by vasospasm of small arterioles, unlike Prinzmetal's angina, which is vasospasm of large arteries
Tay-Sachs dz	Autosomal recessive defect in hexosaminidase A, causing very early onset, progressive retardation, paralysis, dementia, blindness, cherry-red spot on macula, death by 3–4 yr. Common in Ashkenazi Jews

Dz	Description/Sx

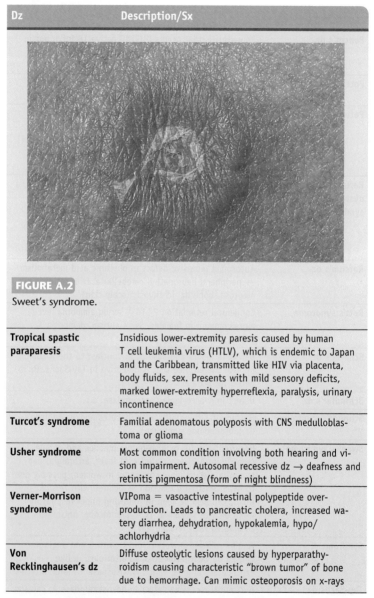

FIGURE A.2
Sweet's syndrome.

Tropical spastic paraparesis	Insidious lower-extremity paresis caused by human T cell leukemia virus (HTLV), which is endemic to Japan and the Caribbean, transmitted like HIV via placenta, body fluids, sex. Presents with mild sensory deficits, marked lower-extremity hyperreflexia, paralysis, urinary incontinence
Turcot's syndrome	Familial adenomatous polyposis with CNS medulloblastoma or glioma
Usher syndrome	Most common condition involving both hearing and vision impairment. Autosomal recessive dz → deafness and retinitis pigmentosa (form of night blindness)
Verner-Morrison syndrome	VIPoma = vasoactive intestinal polypeptide overproduction. Leads to pancreatic cholera, increased watery diarrhea, dehydration, hypokalemia, hypo/achlorhydria
Von Recklinghausen's dz	Diffuse osteolytic lesions caused by hyperparathyroidism causing characteristic "brown tumor" of bone due to hemorrhage. Can mimic osteoporosis on x-rays

Dz	Description/Sx
Wiskott-Aldrich syndrome	X-linked recessive defect in IgM response to capsular polysaccharides such as those of *Streptococcus pneumoniae,* but pts have ↑ IgA levels. Classic triad = recurrent pyogenic bacteria infxns, eczema, thrombocytopenia. Bloody diarrhea is often first Sx, then upper respiratory infxns; leukemia and lymphoma are common in children who survive to age 10
Xeroderma pigmentosa	Defect in repair of DNA damage caused by UV light (pyrimidine dimers). Pts highly likely to develop skin CA. Only Tx is avoidance of sunlight

QUESTIONS

1. A 44-yr-old man presents to the hospital complaining of atypical chest pain. He says he had similar Sx 3 wks ago, when the pain lasted for 4 hrs and was accompanied by nausea and vomiting. His pain did not radiate at that time. He does not like doctors and did not come to the hospital, and eventually the pain resolved with an aspirin. He has felt weak and fatigued since then. Now he has recurrent chest pain that feels like heartburn to him but is causing him to be short of breath. His wife forced him to come to the ER. His pain has been going on for 30 min without stopping at the time you evaluate him. Cardiac enzymes are pending. His initial ECG is shown below. What is this pt's risk category?
   A. Noncardiac chest pain
   B. Low-risk unstable angina
   C. Intermediate-risk unstable angina
   D. High-risk unstable angina
   E. ST-elevation myocardial infarction

2. Which of the following describes this pt's ECG:
   A. Ventricular escape rhythm with T-wave inversions
   B. Wandering pacemaker with ST elevations and T-wave inversions
   C. Nml sinus rhythm with type II Mobitz block and T-wave inversions
   D. Sinus rhythm with bifascicular block (right bundle-branch block + left anterior fascicular block), Q waves, T-wave inversions
   E. Atrial flutter with left bundle-branch block, T-wave inversions

3. A 40-yr-old white man presents to the hospital with crushing substernal chest pain for 45 min that is ongoing. He is diaphoretic and short of breath. An aspirin is administered, and the pt is started on O_2 and nitroglycerin without relief. His admission ECG is shown below. Cardiac enzymes are pending. What is the cause of the ST elevations on this pt's ECG?
   A. Early repolarization in a 40-yr-old man
   B. Acute pericarditis
   C. ST elevation myocardial infarction (STEMI)
   D. Ventricular aneurysm

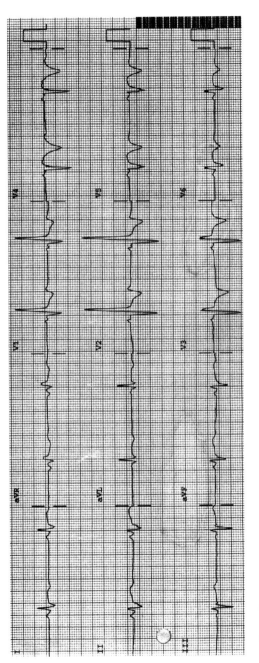

FIGURE 1 ECG Tracing for Questions 1 & 2

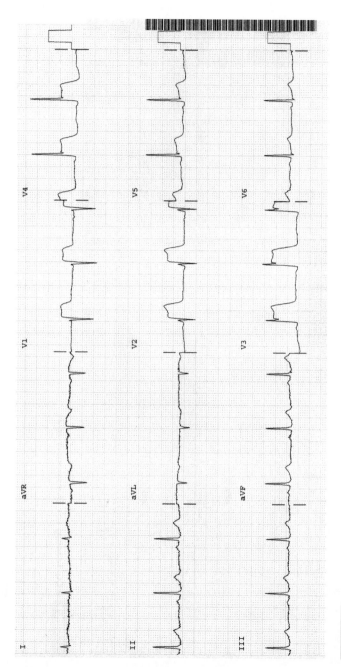

FIGURE 2 ECG Tracing for Question 3

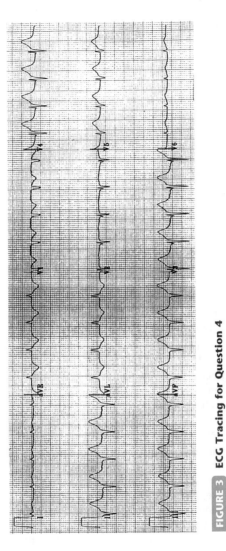

FIGURE 3 ECG Tracing for Question 4

4. A 56-yr-old diabetic woman presents to the hospital complaining of GI upset with mild midepigastric abd pain and nausea. She is also slightly short of breath. A series of tests are ordered, including routine chemistries, CXR, and ECG (shown on page 499). What does the ECG in question show?

A. Atrial flutter with 2:1 block and peaked T waves concerning for hyperkalemia
B. Ventricular tachycardia
C. Junctional tachycardia and an anteroinferior STEMI
D. Sinus tachycardia and an anterolateral STEMI
E. Atrial fibrillation with rapid response and an anterolateral STEMI

5. A 45-yr-old man presents to your office complaining of episodic palpitations and shortness of breath. He says these attacks come on randomly and without warning, and nothing specific triggers them. He feels like his heart begins to race during these attacks. You order an ECG (see Figure 4 on page 501). What is the most likely Dx?

A. Anxiety disorder
B. Malingering
C. STEMI
D. Hyperthyroidism
E. Wolff-Parkinson-White (WPW) syndrome

6. A 25-yr-old female presents to your urgent care clinic with her 4-year-old son. The mother tells you that her little boy has just fallen in the playground. You examine the child and notice that he has bruises that are bilateral, symmetric, and different colors. The bruises are on the back of his hands, buttocks, and back. You then take a better look at the mother and notice that she has her left arm in a cast. What do you do next?

A. You explain to her not to worry about her child's injuries because they are minor and will quickly heal
B. You ask to further examine the mother for the possibility of other broken bones
C. You explain to the mother that you suspect abuse in the family and that you are required by law to call children's protective services. You also advise her that there are shelters for battered women that can assist this family with a safe place to stay, and a social worker will soon be here to discuss her options
D. You allow her to leave after you have treated her child and then you look on the urgent care check-in sheet for her address and call the police to investigate her house for suspected child abuse

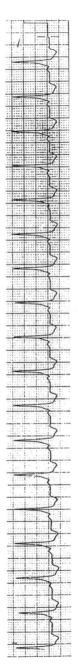

FIGURE 4 ECG Tracing for Question 5

7. A 16-yr-old female is brought into your pediatric clinic by her mother who thinks the daughter is pregnant. After a long discussion in which the mother explains how hard she has worked to properly raise this child, the mother tells you that her daughter has not had her menses in the past two months, throws up every morning, constantly complains of constipation, and is constantly wearing big sweaters to hide her belly. You ask your nurse to come in the room and explain to the mother that you must question her daughter privately first. The mother agrees and then you do which of the following?

A. Immediately ask the 16-yr-old female to tell you what this is all about and stop wasting your time

B. Inform her that whatever she tells you is confidential except if suicide, homicide, or abuse is concerned

C. Perform your exam and then immediately call in the mother and review your findings

D. Examine the mother for possible referral to a teen-daughter support group

8. After interviewing and examining the 16-yr-old female, you check labs and an EKG and note the following findings: emaciation, cardiac arrhythmia, tooth decay, anemia, and fluid and electrolyte abnormalities. You also verify her sexual hx, obtain a negative urine HCG, verify the Hx of amenorrhea and then ask her about her diet hx. You then inform both of them of the following potential Dx and Tx:

A. The 16-year-old is pregnant and possibly it is too early to detect with a urine pregnancy test. It is obvious she is suffering from morning sickness. You give her iron supplements and antiemetics that will not harm the fetus

B. This teenager probably has bulimia, as evidenced by poor dentition, vomiting, and poor body image. She will be referred to a child psychiatrist or psychologist for Tx after a short hospitalization to correct her electrolyte abnormalities

C. This teenager has no problems and the mother should be referred to a teen-daughter support group

D. This 16-year-old girl has all the classic findings of anorexia nervosa. She may need to be admitted to the hospital to correct her electrolyte abnormalities and to observe her eating habits. You will discuss this with the child psychiatrist

9. Match the following Si/Sx with the possible intoxicating substance. Each choice will be used only once:

1. Hypotension and bradycardia
2. Tachycardia, HTN, weight loss
3. GI complaints after eating barracuda
4. Rigid abd muscles, vomiting, pain in extremity
5. Flushed face, burning sensation in mouth after eating marine tuna
6. Microcytic anemia with basophilic stippling purple lines on teeth
7. Decreased consciousness, pinpoint pupils, respiratory depression

A. Ciguatera Toxin

B. Organophosphates

C. Scombroid

D. Opiods

E. Lead poisoning

F. Black widow spider

G. Ma huang

10. Match the following Si/Sx with the psychiatric Dx:

1. Depressive episodes with hypomanic episodes, no manic episodes disorder
2. Hallucinations, lack of affect, disorganized behavior lasting less than 6 mo
3. Continuous depressive Sx for at least 2 yrs
4. Socially withdrawn, recognizes reality, blunt affect
5. Hair pulling resulting in observable hair loss

A. Dysthymic

B. Bipolar II

C. Schizoid

D. Trichotillomania

E. Schitzophreniform

11. A 40-yr-old male comes into your community clinic and the nurse asks him to wait in your examining room. When you walk in you notice a large, obese man asleep in your examining chair, snoring loudly. You attempt to wake him but it proves to be very difficult. When he finally wakes up he tells you another doctor checked his blood and found his hematocrit to be elevated. The other doctor then advised him to have surgery to correct his snoring. What do you think this pt may have and is surgery indicated?

A. This pt obviously has narcolepsy as evidenced by his recurrent sleep attacks

B. He has central obstructive sleep apnea that can only be treated with surgery

C. This pt has the classic triad of Pickwickian Syndrome and the first-line Tx is weight loss

D. This pt has no need to have surgery or lose weight, a CPAP machine at night will solve all his problems

12. A 78-yr-old Chinese male comes into your office alone. He speaks only Mandarin and he is trying to explain to you something related to his knees and elbows. You graciously greet him and ask him to wait for the interpreter to arrive. Once the interpreter arrives, he explains to her that for 20 yrs he has used needles and herbs to treat his joint pains. He has heard of certain new medications that may be of some use and would like information. You then begin talking directly to the Mandarin interpreter and inform her of the anti-inflammatory cyclo-oxygenase inhibitors. You tell the translator that the pt should also have a prostate exam, PSA test, and sigmoidoscopy prior to starting these medicationss since he is >50 yrs old. After a lengthy discussion with the translator, you finally allow her to translate your entire set of recommendations. Upon hearing the translation, the pt begins shouting. The translator tells you the pt is upset because you insulted him by offering to examine his colon when all he wanted was arthritis medicine. How could this incident have been avoided?

A. Next time act out with your hands what you are describing to the translator so that the pt, if he is looking, can visualize the instructions

B. Next time face the pt, and explain all instructions carefully to him, allowing the translator time to translate by pausing frequently. Then ask the pt during the interview if he has any questions. Finally, ask the pt to repeat your instructions to assure that he fully understands

C. Next time, don't call for an interpreter and just prescribe strong narcotic medications for his pain

D. Next time, have the pt bring a family member to translate for him

13. Match the following terms with their corresponding definitions:

1. Sensitivity
2. Prevalence
3. Variance
4. Attributable risk
5. Specificity
6. Nonmalfeasance
7. Beneficence

A. Difference between incidence rates of exposed and nonexposed pts
B. Probability that a test result will be negative in pts without dz
C. Probability that a test result will be positive in pts with dz
D. The number of existing cases of a dz divided by the total population at a given time
E. An estimate of the variability of each individual data point from the mean
F. Trusted to act on behalf of the well being of pts
G. Above all, do no harm

14. A 24-yr-old female, who is contemplating conceiving with her husband, comes in for a prenatal screening physical. They both are monogamous. She is currently being treated for essential HTN with lisinopril. She also takes a daily prenatal vitamin per recommendation of her sister. There is no FHx Her remaining exam is unremarkable. What is the most appropriate management of her HTN?

A. Increase her lisinopril to 40 mg and check her renal function in 2 wks
B. No changes to current medications
C. Discontinue her lisinopril and start an alternative regimen of hypertensive TX
D. Recommend against conceiving
E. Discontinue her lisinopril and monitor her BP monthly

15. A 32-yr-old female with a 26 wks gestational age fetus presents to her physician for pregnancy monitoring. On routine urine dipstick she had 3+ glucose and no protein. A nonfasting finger stick reading was 142 mg/dL. What is the most appropriate next step in the management of this pt?

A. Provide reassurance and recheck her urine in 4 wks
B. Dx her with gestational diabetes because her finger stick was greater than 126 and start her on insulin
C. Have her return tomorrow for a fasting blood glucose analysis

D. Perform an oral glucose challenge test to screen her for gestational diabetes

E. Retest her urine on consecutive days and diagnose her with gestational diabetes if greater than 2+ glucose on subsequent measurements

16. A 27-yr-old female with Hx of gestational diabetes during her first pregnancy presents for follow-up. She is currently at 28 wks gestational age, and was just diagnosed as again having gestational diabetes based on a 3 hr glucose tolerance test. On examination, her pulse is 88 bpm, BP 98/68, respiratory rate of 18, and she is afebrile. Her examination is unremarkable with a fundal height of 30 cm. Recent labs revealed nml renal function. She would like to discuss Tx options for gestational diabetes. Appropriate recommendations at this time include:

A. Discuss the various Tx options with her including dietary Tx, strict blood glucose monitoring, and pharmacotherapy including insulin and potentially some oral agents

B. Inform her that her sibling should be screened for type I diabetes mellitus as well

C. Inform her that she will require life-long Tx for her diabetes

D. Begin insulin Tx as it is the only appropriate form of Tx for gestational diabetes

E. Provide reassurance and close monitoring of fetal size with potential Tx if the fetus develops macrosomia

17. A 32-yr-old female presents to her local emergency room with steady regular contractions. She estimates she is at 35 wks of gestation but is unsure, as she has had no prenatal care. She is admitted to the labor and delivery ward and is found to be in the first stage of labor. After laboring for 16 hours, she delivers an 8 lb 6 oz boy. Shortly after delivery, she becomes lightheaded and dizzy and calls for her physician. Her heart rate is 146 bpm, BP 78/44, respirations 22 breaths per min, and temperature is 100.2°F. On examination she appears to have lost approximately 750 cc of blood since delivery and a boggy uterus is felt. What is the next step in her management?

A. Take her to the OR for Caesarean delivery of her placenta

B. Call surgery to perform emergent hysterectomy

C. Begin IV fluids, blood transfusion, uterine massage, and oxytocin administration

D. Draw a stat CBC and DIC panel

E. Provide reassurance as this is expected in the postpartum period

18. A 32-yr-old female at 32 wks gestation presents for routine prenatal evaluation. She has had an unremarkable pregnancy and was healthy prior to conception. She has noticed increased swelling in both her feet as well as frothy urine. Her vitals are: BP 138/96, pulse 96, respirations 20, and is afebrile. On examination, she has 3+ pitting bilateral edema. Urine dipstick reveals 3+ proteinuria. What is the next step in her management?

A. Induction of labor to prevent fetal demise

B. Confirm the Dx by rechecking her BP tomorrow and obtaining a 24 hr urine protein level

C. Begin Tx with furosemide diuretics

D. Restrict her diet of magnesium as that will result in disease progression to eclampsia

E. Encourage her to elevate her legs and follow up at 36 wks

19. A 37-yr-old female presents to clinic for her annual pelvic exam and Pap smear. She would like to discuss birth control options during this visit. She is currently sexually active with multiple male partners. She has been previously tested for sexually transmitted illness and has always tested negative. She currently smokes one pack of cigarettes per day. Other than an isolated venous thrombosis event several years ago she has been healthy. She is undecided about having children in the future. What is the most appropriate form of birth control for her?

A. Start her on a combination estrogen-progestin oral contraceptive

B. Instruct her on natural family planning and recommend a calendar rhythm method to prevent pregnancy

C. Educate her on the practice of coitus interruptus and recommend this method to her

D. Refer her to an obstetrician to arrange a tubal ligation

E. Recommend that she and her partners use barrier contraceptive 100% of the time

20. A 45-yr-old female presents for her annual physical examination. After reviewing her chart you realize she has not had a Pap smear in 24 mo. She reports never having a previous abnormal test and this is confirmed in your records. Her last three Pap smears were performed once every 12 mo. She has had three children and only one lifetime sexual partner. She is not currently sexually active as her husband died 3 years previously. What is the most appropriate recommendation regarding her need for cervical CA screening?

A. Perform a Pap smear test today as she is high risk and overdue for cervical CA screening by 12 mo

B. Inform her that she likely has cervical CA since she has not had a Pap smear in 24 mo

C. Inform her that since her previous three Pap smears were nml and she is not currently sexually active, that she should be screened every 2–3 yrs

D. Since she is no longer sexually active there is no need for cervical CA screening; have her return if she becomes sexually active again

E. Since she has had only one lifetime sexual partner, there is no indication for cervical CA screening

21. A 63-yr-old Caucasian female presents for follow up after brief hospitalization for low back pain. Her pain was 2° to a non-pathologic L5 vertebral fracture. She had no ensuing traumatic event. She received kyphoplasty and her pain has improved. Following the Dx of her fracture, she underwent a bone density scan that was abnormal. She is 60 inches tall and weighs 95 lbs. She has a 30 pack/year Hx of tobacco. What is the Dx of this pt's bone dz?

A. Osteopenia
B. Vitamin D deficiency
C. Ehlers-Danlos syndrome
D. Osteoporosis
E. Metastatic lung CA

22. A 72-yr-old female who has not seen a physician in over 25 yrs presents to an urgent care facility with complaints of vaginal bleeding and malodorous discharge. She has been postmenopausal for 21 yrs. She is not currently sexually active and has never undergone cervical CA screening. A pelvic examination is performed and an atrophic vagina is seen but no cervical lesions. A Pap smear was completed and shows high-grade squamous intraepithelial lesion (HSIL). What is the next step in her management?

A. Begin Tx with chemotherapy and local radiation
B. Perform colposcopy with Bx
C. Schedule her for urgent total abd hysterectomy
D. Repeat the Pap smear in 6 mo
E. Enroll her into a local hospice facility

23. A 67-yr-old man presents to an urgent care clinic with complaints of left shoulder pain that has progressively worsened over the past 5 days. During this time, he was painting the walls of his newly purchased home. He denies any similar complaints in his right shoulder. On examination he is able to actively fully abduct his left shoulder but it elicits pain. He also has some weakness with

internal rotation and with Jobe's testing of this shoulder compared to the right shoulder. He states the pain is worse at night. What is the appropriate Tx of this pt's shoulder pain?

A. Conservative Tx with rest, NSAIDs, and ice
B. Perform anterior shoulder dislocation reduction
C. Arthroscopic shoulder surgery
D. Nothing, since osteoarthritis is a chronic condition treated with supportive measures
E. Inject corticosteroids into his deltoid muscle

24. A 38-yr-old male presents to his internal medicine physician with progressive right knee discomfort. He first noticed the pain while twisting to return a shot during a racquetball match 8 days ago. Initially, there was only mild pain and he was able to walk and return to work later that afternoon. By the next morning, his knee had become mildly swollen, and since then he has complained of pain with climbing stairs and squatting. On examination, McMurray's maneuver elicits severe discomfort. His Lockman's test was nml. He has nml passive range of motion and some discomfort with active flexion of the knee. There is no point tenderness of the patella or fibula. Distal pulses are present. What is the next step in diagnosing this pt?

A. Obtain standard series x-rays of his knee
B. Obtain an MRI of his knee
C. Obtain CT scan of his knee
D. Refer him to an orthopedic physician to make the accurate Dx
E. No further testing is indicated

25. A 25-yr-old female is seen by her primary care physician for evaluation of a rash that has been present for 6 wks. She denies ever having a previous similar rash and there is no FHx of rashes. Her mother does have psoriatic arthritis. On exam, symmetrically distributed plaques involving her extensor elbows are present. The rash is erythematous with sharply defined margins that are raised above the surrounding nml skin and a thick silvery scale is also present. Its greatest dimension is 8 cm in diameter. What is the Dx of this rash?

A. Eczema
B. Seborrheic keratosis
C. Vitiligo
D. Psoriasis
E. Lichen simplex chronicus

26. A 74-yr-old African American man presents to the emergency room with a 2-day Hx of diffuse abd pain, anorexia, nausea, and vomiting. He recalls no flatus for the past 12 hrs. He is relatively healthy and currently does not take any medications. He had an open cholecystectomy 15 yrs ago and right hemicolectomy 25 yrs ago. His examination reveals tachycardia to 113, respiratory rate of 20, BP of 88/64, and a temperature of 99.6°F. He has tympany to percussion and high pitched bowel sounds. This is accompanied by diffuse abd pain on deep palpation. His labs were remarkable for a creatinine of 1.8 (baseline 0.9) and BUN 41. Lipase was nml. His KUB is shown. What is his most likely Dx?

A. Small bowel obstruction
B. Perforated peptic ulcer
C. Colon adenoCA
D. Acute pancreatitis
E. Severe constipation

27. A 56-yr-old man with Hx of insulin dependent diabetes and HTN presents to his PMD office for routine follow up. The pt has no acute issues to address. Vital signs are: heart rate of 78, BP 158/88, and respirations 18. His glycohemoglobin was 7.1 and creatinine was 1.6. A urinanalysis was completed and it showed 3+ protein. What should to be done to prevent further progression of his renal dz?

A. Low protein diet
B. Improve glucose control
C. Improve blood pressure control
D. Refer for transplant evaluation
E. Renal Bx

28. A 68-yr-old female presents to her primary care provider with a 4 wk Hx of shortness of breath and a chronic productive cough for the past 3 mo. She also reports an episode last year were she had a similar cough that lasted for 4 mo. She is a current smoker and has a 45 pack/year Hx. What diagnostic study is required to make the likely Dx?

A. CT with contrast of lungs
B. Lung Bx
C. PA/Lateral CXR
D. Pulmonary function tests
E. Overnight sleep study

29. A 16-yr-old male who has lived in an urban environment for his entire life is seen in urgent care clinic for shortness of breath which has been present for several mo. His family has noticed audible wheezing, and he has frequent nighttime coughing episodes. Several mo ago, his family adopted a cat from the local

humane society. His mother suffers from atopic dermatitis, and he has a sister with seasonal allergies. What diagnostic study can confirm the Dx of asthma?

A. CT of the lungs
B. Peak flow measurements
C. PA/Lateral CXR
D. Pulmonary function tests with bronchodilator Tx
E. No additional studies

30. A 23-yr-old female presents to an urgent care clinic with complaint of shortness of breath that started earlier today. She denies any sick contacts or recent travel Hx. Her only medication is an estrogen oral contraceptive. She is currently in a monogamous relationship and has had four previous sexual partners. She also smokes one pack of cigarettes per day. Her heart rate is 112, BP 108/68, respiratory rate of 22, temperature of 100.1°F, and her oxygen saturation is 92%. She appears comfortable with some obvious increased work of breathing. Her lungs are clear in all fields, and her cardiac exam is remarkable for tachycardia only. CXR is nml. Her labs are nml including an arterial gas with PCO_2 of 40. What is her most likely DX?

A. Hyperventilation from anxiety
B. Community acquired pneumonia
C. Pulmonary emboli
D. Asthma exacerbation
E. Atypical pneumonia from Chlamydia pneumoniae

31. A 35-yr-old woman presents to a local emergency room with complaints of right flank pain with radiations to her groin. She describes the pain as a sharp cramping pain that waxes and wanes. She has never previously experienced this pain. She has noticed hematuria as well. She reports recently starting a rhubarb diet. She is in a monogamous relationship and uses barrier method for contraception. On exam, she is writhing in bed and clutching her knees to her chest. She is tachycardic at 122 bpm, and her BP is elevated to 156/88. Her abdomen is soft and tender to deep palpation in her right lower quadrant. Pelvic examination reveals no cervical motion tenderness or adnexal tenderness or masses. Her only medication is hydrochlorothiazide for her BP. What is her most likely Dx?

A. Nephrolithiasis
B. Ectopic pregnancy
C. Ovarian torsion
D. Acute diverticulitis
E. Pelvic inflammatory disease

32. A 73-yr-old man is brought to the emergency room by EMS after calling 911 with a headache and blurry vision. He appears somewhat confused upon arrival. His past medical Hx is significant for HTN and chronic kidney dz. He reports running out of his medications 2 wks ago. He also mentions not passing urine in last 24 hrs. His examination revealed a BP of 250/120, heart rate of 136, and respiratory rate of 18. On fundoscopic examination he has papilledema. What is the most appropriate management of his HTN?

A. Write a prescription for his previous anti HTN medications and have him follow up with his PMD

B. Start him on IV nitroprusside and titrate to ↓ his BP to 195/90

C. Start him on IV nitroglycerin and titrate to a nml BP of 120/80

D. Give him oral lisinopril and monitor for improvement before discharge

E. Mobilize the cardiac catherization team for his evolving myocardial infarction

33. A 78-yr-old man was brought to an urgent care clinic by his daughter 2° to confusion. He has a past medical Hx of benign prostate hypertrophy, HTN, urinary incontinence, and seasonal allergies. His medications include diphenhydramine and terazosin which he ran out of 2 wks ago. His daughter, who cares for him, has noticed no recent episodes of incontinence and he has not voided otherwise. On exam, there is suprapubic fullness. His laboratories showed a BUN of 78 and creatinine of 3.1 (baseline 1.2). What is the most likely explanation of his acute renal failure?

A. HTN nephropathy

B. Acute interstitial nephritis 2° to diphenhydramine

C. Urinary tract infxn for his incontinence

D. Prerenal azotemia from diphenhydramine

E. Postrenal azotemia 2° to his benign prostate hypertrophy

34. A mother presents to a pediatric clinic with her 36-hr newborn. The infant's grandmother noticed yellowing of the eyes and became quite concerned. The infant was born at 39 wks by an uncomplicated vaginal delivery. There is no clinic evidence of infxns at this time. Immediately after delivery there was no clinical evidence of jaundice. The mother had appropriate prenatal care and had no high risk behaviors. Other than scleral icterus there were no remarkable exam findings. What is the most likely explanation for the infant's jaundice?

A. Conjugated hyperbilirubinemia

B. Crigler-Najjar syndrome

C. Chlamydia trachomatis conjunctivitis

D. Physiologic jaundice
E. Kernicterus

35. A 33-yr-old woman presents to her primary care physician with complaints of urinary frequency, dysuria, and urgency. These Sx have been present for three days. She takes no medications, but she has been drinking cranberry juice. On examination, she is afebrile, pulse 88, and BP 108/82. On examination, she does not have flank or abd tenderness. Pelvic examination did not reveal cervical motion tenderness. Her cardiovascular and pulmonary examinations are unremarkable. Her laboratories reveal a mild leukocytosis to 12.1 and her urine analysis was remarkable for 25–50 WBCs, 2+ leukocyte esterase, and bacteria were present. What is the most appropriate Tx at this time?

A. Continue to encourage cranberry juice
B. Admit her to the hospital for management of pyelonephritis with IV antibiotics
C. Start oral antibiotics for an anticipated 10-day course
D. Start oral antibiotics for an anticipated 3-day course.
E. Obtain cervical culture to confirm DX of pelvic inflammatory dz

36. A 34-yr-old woman presents to her primary care physician with complaints of bilateral hand pain. It is present each morning and lasts for approximately 90 min. She also complains of some pains in her feet as well. She has a FHx of both osteoarthritis and Sjögren's syndrome in her father. Her examination reveals bilateral synovitis in her metacarpophalangeal (MCP) and proximal interphalangeal (PIP) joints. Radiography reveals erosions into the cortex of the bone. What is her most likely Dx?

A. Osteoarthritis
B. Rheumatoid arthritis
C. Sjogren's syndrome
D. Septic arthritis
E. Reactive arthritis

37. A 55-yr-old man is referred to a primary physician by a circuit court judge due to being involved in a automobile crash after falling asleep while driving his car. The man reports falling asleep while reading, watching television, riding in cars, and after eating lunch. Although this was his first car accident; he has been reprimanded several times for sleeping at work. On examination, he is obese with BMI of 45 and a neck circumference of 18 inches. His airway is clear with no appreciated abnormalities. The remainder of his examination was unremarkable. What diagnostics tests are indicated to make the Dx in the man?

A. The Dx can be made clinically
B. Pulmonary function test

C. Polysomnography (sleep study)

D. CT of the neck and chest

E. Improved Sx after trial of continuous positive airway pressure (CPAP)

38. A 78-yr-old man is seen in an emergency room for evaluation of a syncopal event that occurred 20 min earlier. For the past several mo, he has been experiencing lightheadedness and dizziness after standing up. He also becomes quite dyspneic with exertion of less than 40 ft. He currently is on an angiotensin converting enzyme inhibitor for his long-standing HTN. On examination his BP is 86/40, heart rate 90, and respirations 18. He currently is awake and oriented. His cardiac auscultation reveals a systolic crescendo-decrescendo murmur with radiations to his carotids. His rhythm was regular with no extra beats. His carotid pulses appear slow and sluggish. Lung auscultation reveals bibasilar crackles. An ECG is performed and reveals a stiff aortic valve with a valve area of 1.1 cm^2. What is the most appropriate next step in Tx for this man?

A. Referral to cardiothoracic surgeon for aortic valve replacement

B. Cardiac event monitor for 30 days

C. Close monitoring by his primary care physician for repeat events

D. Begin Tx with a β-blocker to slow his heart rate and increase contractility

E. Repeat echocardiogram in 6 mo to evaluate for dz progression

39. A 24-yr-old male is found at the scene of a motor vehicle crash after he ran his motorcycle into a tree. He is now unconscious. Witnesses estimate he was riding at least 60 miles per hour. He was not wearing a helmet. You are part of the initial response team to the accident site. In the initial assessment, he is placed in a cervical spine collar. The pt is breathing spontaneously at a rate of 12 and has equal breath sounds in both lung fields. His heart rate is 110 and his BP is 80/40. The pt does not open his eyes; he makes no verbal responses to questions. He withdraws to pain when pressing on the left upper quadrant of his abdomen. What is the most appropriate next step in the pt's management?

A. Establish 2 large bore peripheral IV lines and infuse nml saline

B. Check a serum ethanol and glucose

C. Perform a 2° survey

D. Place an endotracheal tube

E. Give dextrose, thiamine, and narcan

40. A 78-yr-old male with a Hx of chronic obstructive pulmonary dz, HTN, and hyperlipidemia presents to clinic for an annual physical. He is without complaints. He currently takes fomoterol, simvastatin, and hydrochlorothiazide. He has a 50 pack/yr Hx of tobacco use,

having quit 12 yrs ago. On physical examination, his BP is 120/80 with a pulse of 75. His lungs are clear and his heart is regular. His abd examination reveals a pulsatile mass in the right midline of his abdomen. Ultrasound scan of the abdomen reveals a 3.5 cm abd aortic aneurysm. What is the most appropriate management plan for the pt's abd aortic aneurysm?

A. Immediate referral to vascular surgery for an open repair
B. Follow up ultrasound in 6 mo
C. Follow up ultrasound in 12 mo
D. Order an abd CT scan with contrast
E. Change his hydrochlorothiazide to metoprolol

41. A 63-yr-old female with a Hx of peptic ulcer dz and myocardial infarction presents to the emergency department with chest pain. The pt describes the pain as sudden in onset, has been ongoing for the past hr, and is located below her sternum and radiating to her scapula. She notes a tearing and ripping sensation. Pain does not vary with food. She is not taking any prescription medications. She took 800 mg of ibuprofen for the pain, which did not help her Sx. On physical examination, her pulse is 110, BP is 175/110, oxygen saturation 100% room air. She appears uncomfortable and diaphoretic. On cardiovascular examination, she is tachycardic with a faint systolic murmur. Her lungs are clear. She has mild abd tenderness to deep palpation. Her EKG reveals sinus tachycardia with no ST segment changes. Chest radiograph shows no infiltrate and a widened mediastinum.

Labs

WBC: 9.0

Hgb: 10

Plt: 200

Na: 134

K: 4.0

Cl: 100

Hco3: 18

Cr: 1.6

What is the most likely Dx?

A. Recurrent myocardial infarction
B. Duodenal ulcer perforation
C. Gastric ulcer perforation

D. Aortic dissection

E. Pulmonary embolus

42. A 42-yr-old male presents to clinic to discuss CA screening. He is concerned as his older sister was just Dx with colon CA after undergoing an evaluation for anemia and weight loss. His sister is 54-yr-old and just underwent a subtotal colectomy. The pt reports that he is healthy. He takes one multivitamin a day. He does not smoke or drink alcohol. He runs between 10–15 miles a wk for exercise. He reports one daily bowel movement which is well formed and does not require straining.

His labs are as follows:

Hemoglobin: 15

Platelets: 300

Iron panel: Nml

What colon CA screening strategy would you recommend to the pt?

A. CEA level now

B. Colonoscopy now

C. Colonoscopy at age 50

D. Colonoscopy at age 44

E. CT colonography

The following vignette applies to questions 43 and 44:

A 90-yr-old female with advanced dementia presents from a nursing home with vomiting and moaning. She has not moved her bowels in 72 hr. At baseline, she is non verbal but is able to feed herself. She does not recognize relatives or friends. At the nursing home, she is on docusate and milk of magnesia for constipation. She appears obtunded. On abd examination she grimaces to light touch and guards with deep palpation. She is distended and has high pitched bowel sounds. On rectal examination, she has no stool in the vault and nml rectal walls. Abd radiographs reveal dilated loops of bowel with loss of haustra. She has a narrowing of the colon in her left lower quadrant that the radiologist describes as a "bird's beak."

43. What is the most likely Dx?

A. Sigmoid volvulus

B. Fecal impaction

C. Ogilvie's syndrome

D. Rectal CA

E. Nml progression of her dementia

44. How should this pt's underlying problem be managed?

A. Give a surgical bowel prep
B. Anal canal Bx
C. Colonoscopy
D. Manual disimpaction and suppositories
E. Start donepezil

45. A 58-yr-old male presents to clinic with insomnia. He reports that he has issues falling asleep at night and will stay up for 2 hrs after his bedtime watching television. He often drinks several glasses of wine with dinner in order to help expedite his sleep. He reports that his Sx started 9 mo ago after he lost his job, and ever since then he has felt things are hopeless. Associated with his loss of sleep, he has feelings of hopelessness given that he has been unsuccessful in finding new employment. His past medical Hx includes gout. He does not smoke. He has been married for 20 yrs; he reports things are stressful with his wife due to his fatigue and a lack of interest in sex. His physical examination is nml. Lab studies are nml. Which is the first choice of medical Tx for the pt's problem?

A. Electroconvulsive Tx
B. Paroxetine
C. Amitriptyline
D. Zolpidem
E. Temazepam

46. A 90-yr-old female with Alzheimer's dementia is admitted to the intensive care unit with shortness of breath, hypoxia, and an infiltrate on CXR. At baseline, she is unable to complete activities of daily living without assistance. She requires assistance with feeding, bathing, and toileting. She resides at home with her husband. For her pneumonia, she is treated with ceftriaxone and azithromycin. Her home medications are restarted in the hospital and include memantine and donepezil. While in the hospital, she is given milk of magnesia for constipation, as well as haloperidol for agitation when she pulls at her IV lines. While in the ICU, her telemetry monitor shows a prolonged QT interval. Electrocardiogram shows sinus rhythm with a rate of 60 beats per minute. Her corrected QT interval is 550 ms. Her admission EKG was nml. What is the most appropriate intervention for the pt's prolonged QT interval?

A. Defibrillate the pt
B. Cardiology consultation for electrophysiology study
C. Discontinue the haloperidol
D. Discontinue the donepezil
E. Discontinue the memantine

47. A 28-yr-old female presents to the emergency department after being found unconscious. First responders found her pulse to be 75, BP 120/70, and her blood glucose to be 22. She is given IV dextrose, and she is brought to the emergency department. On arrival to the ED, her blood glucose is 100 and she regains consciousness. She is admitted to the hospital; one hr after admission, her blood sugar is 40 and she is given more dextrose. Over the next 23 hrs of observation her blood sugars range from 90–110. Review of her medical records reveals that she takes no medications and has no prior Hx of chronic illnesses. She was admitted to the hospital three times in the past 6 wks for complaints of hematuria. Extensive diagnostic work up including CT scan of the abdomen, cystoscopy, and urine cultures were nml. The pt does not drink or smoke. She is a third yr medical student. Her mother is a diabetic and takes regular insulin with meals. You discuss the case with psychiatry as you suspect a Dx of facticious disorder. What is the most appropriate next step in the pt's management?

A. Notify the dean of the medical school of your suspicions
B. Notify the state medical board
C. Order an octreotide scan
D. Start fluoxetine
E. Order an insulin and c-peptide level

48. A 45-yr-old female presents to clinic for a new pt visit. While in the waiting room, she was heard telling other pts that you came highly recommended, that you were the best physician ever, and that you cared for important pts such as herself. Your receptionist asks her to keep her voice down and she becomes very angry and upset. When you enter the exam room she begins to tell you how incompetent the receptionist is and how wonderful and highly recommended you were to her. She notes to you that she has seen three other doctors in the past year and that they all were incredibly stupid and not nearly as talented as you are. What underlying personality disorder does this pt have?

A. Histrionic
B. Borderline
C. Narcissistic
D. Antisocial
E. Obsessive compulsive

49. A 10-yr-old male presents to clinic with his mother. He is currently suspended from school for kicking a teacher. He has had numerous altercations at school with other children. He was also suspended earlier in the month for throwing the class's hamster against the wall. He did not show any remorse for his actions. His mother states she does not know what to do with him. He has poor grades and does not listen to her at home. She has no help from the pt's father, as he has been in prison for 2 yrs. What is the most likely Dx?

A. Antisocial personality disorder
B. Attention-deficit hyperactivity disorder
C. Oppositional defiant disorder
D. Conduct disorder
E. Bipolar disorder

50. A 55-yr-old male presents to the outpt psychiatry clinic with complaints of anxiety and depression for the past 6 mo. He tells you that he has been having nightmares regarding his time in the Vietnam War. He has repeated dreams in which he sees one of his friends being shot in the chest. He has trouble sleeping through the night due to these dreams. He has constant thoughts about death. The pt works as an accountant. He is married and has two grown children. He reports that things at home and at work have been strained due to his lack of sleep. He does not smoke or use illicit drugs; he drinks 4 beers at night to try to help his sleep. You screen and diagnose the pt with posttraumatic stress disorder and refer him for psychotherapy. Which of the following medications should be used to treat the pt's sleep disturbance and PTSD?

A. Amitriptyline
B. Lithium
C. Gabapentin
D. Zolpidem
E. Lorazepam

51. A mother brings her 2-yr-old daughter to clinic with a fever. Her mother has noticed for the past 2 days that the pt has been pulling on her ears. She also notes a fair amount of thick rhinorrhea. The child has had a nml growth and development Hx. She has never been hospitalized and is up to date on her vaccinations. She has no allergies. She resides in a nonsmoking household and has an older brother who is 5 yrs old. On physical examination, she is febrile to 101.6°F. She has a bulging right tympanic membrane with a yellow fluid level. She has no palpable lymph nodes. Her heart and lungs are nml. Which is the most appropriate next step in management?

A. Start ciprofloxacin ear drops
B. Perform a myringotomy and place a tympanostomy tube in affected ear

C. Start oral amoxicillin
D. Start oral amoxicillin/clavulanate
E. Order a CXR

52. A couple presents for prenatal genetic counseling. They are currently 10 wks pregnant with their first child. The father of the child is 30; the mother is 28. The mother has never been pregnant before. Both parents are Caucasian and are healthy. The mother has no known FHx of genetic dz. The father's brother has cystic fibrosis. The parents are concerned about the possibility of their baby having cystic fibrosis. What is the probability of the baby having cystic fibrosis?

A. 1/4
B. 1/2
C. 1/25
D. 1/150
E. 1/250

53. A 30-yr-old male presents to clinic with complaints of depression and issues with his gait. He notes that he feels a general hopelessness about his life, with anhedonia. He states that his wife of 5 yrs feels that his personality has changed. In discussing his gait, he notes difficulty with standing from a chair and getting started with his gait. His past medical Hx includes migraine headaches. He does not drink or smoke. He has a paternal uncle who died of cirrhosis. On physical exam, he appears tired and older than his stated age. Heart and lung exam is nml. His abdomen is soft, nontender, and without fluid wave. He has a palpable nontender liver edge. His vision is nml, however he has dark copper colored rings encircling his iris on both eyes. On neurologic exam, he has a resting, pill rolling tremor. His gait is slow and shuffled.

Labs

AST:	100
ALT:	120
Bilirubin:	3.0
Alk Phos:	120
Hemoglobin:	10
Plt:	200
Creatinine:	1.2
Iron Panel:	Nml

Initial diagnostic evaluation should include testing for which of the following diseases?

A. Hemochromatosis
B. Wilson's Dz
C. Alcoholism
D. Parkinson's Dz
E. Depression

The follow vignette applies to questions 54 and 55:

A 45-yr-old female presents to clinic with complaints of an odd looking mole on her back. She is unsure how long it has been present. Her husband noticed it one wk ago while they were at the beach. The pt has no complaints of weight loss or other skin changes. The lesion does not itch or bleed. The pt has numerous moles on her back and legs. She tries to wear sunscreen. You examine the pt's back lesion.

54. Which of the following features of a skin lesion would be most concerning for a malignant melanoma?

A. Pearly translucent borders with fine telangietasias
B. Stuck-on-the-skin appearance
C. Black uniform color
D. A diameter of 2 mm
E. An asymmetric lesion with irregular borders

55. You examine the pt and you suspect a Dx of melanoma. What is the most appropriate first diagnostic test to order on the lesion?

A. Surgical excision
B. Shave Bx
C. Core Bx
D. PET scan
E. CT scan of the chest, abdomen, and pelvis

56. A 68-yr-old male with a Hx of alcoholic cirrhosis presents to the emergency department after an extensive drinking binge complaining of hematemesis. He notes three episodes of emesis with a bright red color. He feels dizzy and tired. His last drink was 2 hrs prior to presentation. The pt has a Hx of child's C alcoholic cirrhosis. He drinks approximately 1 liter of vodka a day and was recently admitted for alcohol withdrawal a month ago. On physical examination, his BP is 80/40 with a pulse of 120. He is disoriented to time and place. He is slurring his words and at times falls asleep during your physical examination. His skin exam is remarkable for palmar erythema and spider angiomata. He is

jaundiced. His abdomen is not tender. He wakes up as you are leaving the room and vomits about 200cc of red colored emesis.

Labs

Hemoglobin: 10

Platelets: 55

What is the most appropriate next step in the pt's management?
A. Start IV pantoprazole
B. Start IV octreotide
C. Intubate the pt
D. Start a wide open IV bolus of nml saline and cross and match for transfusion
E. Emergent esophogogastroduodenoscopy (EGD)

57. A 35-yr-old female presents complaining of generalized fatigue, weight loss, and amenorrhea. Her fatigue has been ongoing for several mo. She is unsure how much weight she has lost, however, her pants are fitting loosely. The pt notes that her last menstrual period was 3 mo ago, and prior to that it was regular with no unusual bleeding pattern. Her past medical Hx includes HTN and systemic lupus erythematosis. Both chronic illnesses are well controlled. She does not drink or smoke. She is not currently sexually active. On physical examination, she appears thin and tired. Her abd exam is remarkable for a palpable, enlarged, nontender liver. Her labs are as follows:

Basic chemistry panel:	Nml
Hemoglobin:	10.2
Platelets:	212
INR:	1.2
AST:	314
ALT:	432
Alkaline phosphatase:	120
Bilirubin:	0.7
Albumin:	3.2
ANA:	Positive
Antismooth muscle Ab:	Positive
Antimitochondrial Ab:	Negative

Hepatitis C Ab:	Negative
Hepatitis B core Ab:	Negative
Hepatitis B surface Ab:	Positive
Hepatitis B Surface Ag:	Negative
Serum hCG:	Negative

What is the most likely etiology of the pt's abnormal liver function tests and hepatomegaly?

A. Autoimmune hepatitis
B. 1° biliary cirrhosis
C. Hepatitis B infxn
D. Ectopic pregnancy

58. A 48-yr-old male with a Hx of amyotrophic lateral sclerosis is hospitalized for aspiration pneumonia. The pt was diagnosed with ALS 5 yrs ago and has been experiencing rapid neurological decline in the past 6 mo. Currently, the pt cannot walk or move his arms or hands. He is able to eat if somebody feeds him, however, he has been choking on his food lately and requires a thickened liquid diet. The pt mumbles in a low voice when he tries to communicate, however, he can clearly state "yes" or "no" to questions by blinking his eyes. The pt is divorced and is not in contact with his wife. He has a full-time caretaker who assists him. He has one son who lives in the same city and comes to visit him every day after work.

The pt has an advanced directive as well as a power of attorney for health care. His advanced directive states that he does not want cardiopulmonary resuscitation, intubation with mechanical ventilation, or feeding tubes. The document names his son as power of attorney for health care.

During his hospitalization, the pt continues to aspirate food and liquids. He is also noted to be malnourished. Discussions with the pt are held regarding placement of a percutaneous gastric feeding tube to improve his nutrition. Through blinking his eyes the pt states "no." He will not consent to the procedure. The pt's son becomes upset as he feels his father is going to starve.

What is the most appropriate next step in management?

A. Have the pt's son sign the consent for feeding tube
B. Have the pt's wife sign the consent for the feeding tube
C. Do not place the feeding tube
D. Obtain a court order for the feeding tube and place it
E. Place a temporary nasogastric feeding tube and reason with the pt

59. You are running a research trial on a new cardiac drug that is designed to prevent sudden cardiac death in pts with class IV congestive heart failure. The trial compares pts with heart failure on standard CHF Tx to pts with heart failure on standard CHF Tx plus your new drug. The mortality rate in people treated with standard Tx was 22% compared to a mortality rate of 12% in the people given your new drug. What is the number of people needed to treat with your new drug to prevent one death?

A. 12
B. 50
C. 8
D. 22
E. 10

60. A 25-yr-old male presents to clinic for a preemployment physical examination. He plans to work at a large tertiary referral hospital as a transport assistant. He was formerly working in a nursing home in a similar role. He is without complaints. He denies fevers, chills, nausea, cough, or weight loss. He has a Hx of seasonal allergies in the spring which are well controlled on loratadine as needed. He smokes half a pack of cigarettes a day and is trying to quit. For his employment, he has a number of requirements and screenings to be done including placement of a purified protein derivative (PPD). You place the test on his right forearm and he returns in 72 hrs with 7 mm of induration. What is the most appropriate next step in management?

A. Order a chest radiograph
B. Sputum culture for AFB
C. Isoniazid Tx for 9 mo
D. Isoniazid, rifampin, ethambutol, pyrazinamide for 6 mo
E. No further action needed

61. A 68-yr-old female presents to clinic with complaints of upset stomach for 3 wks. The pt was no prior Hx of similar Sx in the past. She describes the pain as a burning sensation in her chest that is worse when she eats. The pain is somewhat relieved by over the counter heartburn tablets. The pt has a Hx of HTN and gout. She takes indomethecin for her gout as needed, as well as metoprolol for her HTN. She does not note any diarrhea, abd pain, emesis, or change in bowel habits. She has lost 10 pounds in the past 2 mo. She attributes this to not eating as much due to her pain. Her physical examination is nml. What is the most appropriate next step in the pt's management?

A. Order an upper endoscopy
B. Order a serum h. pyolri antibody

C. Treat empirically with a proton pump inhibitor for 4 wks
D. Advise her to stop the indomethacin
E. Advise her to stop the metoprolol

62. A 30-yr-old male presents to clinic after being found to have an elevated BP at an employee health screening fair last week. The pt noted no prior Hx of HTN to you. He is without complaints of chest pain, headache, or shortness of breath. He has a past medical Hx of gonococcal urethritis 5 yrs ago. He does not smoke. His father is 60 yrs old and has HTN. He has no FHx of other medical problems. On physical examination, his BP is 130/82, heart rate is 67, body mass index is 23. His cardiovascular examination is nml. He has no Si of systemic dz. What is the most appropriate intervention for the pt's BP?

A. Start an ACE inhibitor
B. Start a thiazide diuretic
C. Start a β blocker
D. Advise him to exercise
E. Advise him to take potassium supplements

63. A 60-yr-old female presents to the emergency department with complaints of sudden onset right upper quadrant pain for the past 4 hrs. She has no prior Hx of similar Sx. Her pain is associated with nausea and two episodes of vomiting as well as weakness and chills. She has no prior Hx of surgeries or malignancies. She takes no medications. On physical examination, her temperature is 102.5°F, pulse 120, BP 90/45. She has scleral icterus. Her skin has a yellowish hue. Her abdomen is diffusely tender and she localizes pain to her right upper quadrant.

Labs

WBC:	15,000
Hgb:	12
Plt:	300
Na:	140
K:	4.0
HCO3:	18
Cr:	1.2
AST:	113
ALT:	230
Tbili:	9.4

Ultrasound of her abdomen shows dilation of her common bile duct. After starting antibiotics and IV fluids, what is the most appropriate definitive management for this pt?

A. Laparoscopic cholecysectomy
B. Open cholecysectomy
C. ERCP (Endoscopic Retrograde Cholangiopancreatography)
D. CT scan of the abdomen
E. Continue IV fluids and make the pt NPO

64. A 66-yr-old man with a Hx of diabetes mellitus type 2 and HTN presents with difficulty speaking for the last 6 hrs. His wife reports that 3 wks ago he was also having some difficulty with right arm weakness, but this resolved on its own after a couple of hrs. On examination today, the pt speaks fluently, but the words are incongruent with reasonable speech. He is able to follow commands. Cardiovascular examination reveals regular heart rate and rhythm with no murmurs. Carotid bruits are present bilaterally. A noncontrast head CT confirms the Dx of acute stroke. An electrocardiogram shows nml sinus rhythm. An echocardiogram reveals mild tricuspid regurgitation with nml cardiac function and no clots. Telemetry shows no arrhythmias. Which test is most likely to yield the origin of the pt's stroke?

A. Carotid ultrasound
B. CT of the chest, abdomen, and pelvis
C. Hemoglobin A1c
D. INR
E. ESR

65. After noticing a breast lump, a 52-yr-old woman, with no prior medical problems, visits her primary care physician. The pt reports the lump has changed in size with her menstrual period over the last 2 mo, but never resolved completely. She has no FHx of breast CA. On breast examination, a 1 cm, oval shaped mass is palpated. It is mobile and fluctuant. No adenopathy is palpated. A fine-needle aspiration (FNA) of mass is performed and yields no fluid. What is the next appropriate step?

A. Core Bx
B. CT scan of the chest
C. Reassurance and close follow up
D. Refer for chemotherapy
E. Repeat FNA

66. In the middle of the night at a small community hospital, a 73-yr-old woman hospitalized for congestive heart failure develops sudden weakness in the left arm and leg. Neurologic

examination is consistent with a stroke. Prior to giving tissue plasminogen activator (tPA), what test must be ordered first?

A. Carotid ultrasound
B. CT of the head without contrast
C. EEG
D. Lumbar puncture
E. MRI of the brain with and without contrast

67. A 21-yr-old woman with Down's syndrome is brought in by her family for evaluation of fevers and confusion occurring over the last 6 days. The pt has also had fatigue and weakness over the last 2 mo. On examination, the pt is lethargic, but has no focal neurologic abnormalities. Cardiovascular examination is also nml. Skin examination is notable for petechiae. A CXR is unremarkable. Her CBC reveals pancytopenia. What diagnostic study is most likely to yield the Dx?

A. Echocardiogram
B. Karotyping
C. MRI of the brain
D. Bone marrow Bx
E. PT/PTT

68. An annual H&P exam is scheduled for a healthy 14-yr-old girl prior to entering middle school. Vaccine Hx shows completion of the following: Hib (Haemophilus influnezae type b)—4th given at 15 mo; Hepatitis B series—3rd given at 15 mo; IPV (inactivated poliovirus)—4th given at 6 yr; DTaP (Diphtheria, tetanus, pertussis)—5th given at 6 yr; Varicella—given at 15 mo; MMR (measles, mumps, rubella) series—2nd given at 6 yr. Which of the following would be recommended at this visit?

A. Hepatitis B titer
B. Hib booster
C. Td booster
D. TB skin test
E. Varicella booster

69. A 48-yr-old deer hunter presents with concerns about Lyme dz, as one of his friends was recently diagnosed with the dz. The pt reports hunting and other outdoor activities during the spring and in endemic areas. Which of the following is appropriate advice?

A. Avoid wearing long pants as it may be difficult to find a tick
B. If a tick bite is found, apply permethrin cream to the area after removal of the tick
C. No advice, because Lyme dz cannot be prevented

D. Prophylactic penicillin on the days the pt is outdoors
E. Use DEET spray on the skin and clothes

70. In the emergency room, an 83-yr-old man with a Hx of prostate CA is brought in by family for confusion. The pt is also on coumadin for Hx of pulmonary embolus and has had multiple falls recently. The last fall occurred 5 days prior to presentation. His examination shows decreased range of motion of the left hip due to pain. The pt is drowsy and does not follow commands consistently. Labs include a WBC count of 6.0 and an INR of 3.4. Which of the following should be performed first?

A. CT angiogram of the head and neck
B. CT of the head without contrast
C. Left hip x-ray
D. Lumbar puncture
E. MRI of the brain with and without contrast

71. A 50-yr-old man presents for a routine H&P. He has a 30 pack/yr Hx of smoking and drinks 1–2 alcoholic beverages four times wkly. BP is 168/92. Fasting labs show: LDL 192, HDL 25, Triglycerides 225, and glucose 102. Which of the following are his risks of ischemic heart dz?

A. Alcohol use, smoking, HTN
B. Alcohol use, HTN, hypercholesterolemia
C. Diabetes mellitus, smoking, HTN.
D. Diabetes mellitus, smoking, hypercholesterolemia
E. Smoking, HTN, hypercholesterolemia

72. A 32-yr-old man, with no prior medical Hx, presents to his primary care doctor with complaints of blurry vision in his right eye. The pt has been having episodes of dark spots in his vision, which wax and wane, for the last 3 days. In addition, the pt is having pain in the eye. Since his last visit 6 mo ago, the pt also reports experiencing numbness and tingling in the hands, which is self-limited but recurs every few wks. He denies any travel, stating, "I've never left the great state of Minnesota in all of my life." On neurologic examination, the pt has horizontal nystagmus and ↓ vibratory sensation in the arms bilaterally. Remainder of examination is negative. A lumbar puncture is performed. Which test is likely to make the Dx?

A. Cytology
B. Glucose level
C. Gram stain and culture
D. HSV PCR
E. Protein electrophoresis

73. A 24-yr-old homeless man with a Hx of being imprisoned previously presented with fevers and a cough. He was recently diagnosed with pneumonia at an outside clinic and was given a prescription for azithromycin. The pt insists he has been taking his medication, however, his fever and cough have not resolved. The pt's CXR shows bilateral upper lobe infiltrates. On examination, the pt is alert and appropriate. Cardiovascular exam shows a regular rate and rhythm with no murmurs or gallops. No jugular venous distention or edema. Respiratory exam reveals coarse breath sounds with few crackles in the upper lobes bilaterally otherwise clear to auscultation. PPD skin test is negative. What is the most appropriate step next?

A. Add a third-generation cephalosporin for superior *S. pneumoniae* coverage
B. Check BNP (Brain Natriuretic Peptide) to rule out heart failure
C. CT scan of the chest with contrast to rule out pulmonary embolus
D. CT scan of the chest without contrast to rule out malignancy
E. Place pt in respiratory isolation and check sputum AFB smears

74. 27-yr-old woman presents with complaints of fever and facial rash. She has noted difficulty with performing her work since the rash began several weeks ago. She reports feeling "achy" in her hands and knees and thinks she may have caught the "flu." Her exam is notable for an erythematous rash over the cheeks, sparing her nasolabial folds. She also has a few shallow ulcers in the oral cavity. Joint exam is unremarkable, and respiratory exam reveals a harsh pleural rub at the left base. Lab tests are as follows:

Hemoglobin:	10.2 g/dL
WBC count:	15,600/uL
Sodium:	142 mEq/L
Potassium:	4.1 mEq/L
Bicarbonate:	23 mEq/L
Creatinine:	1.6 mg/dL

Which of the following would be the best test to confirm the Dx if ⊕?

A. Anti–double strand DNA
B. ANA
C. ESR
D. PTT
E. Rheumatoid factor

75. In the emergency room, a 22-yr-old man is brought in for evaluation and Tx after a witnessed grand mal seizure. His parents, who witnessed the event, report that the pt has had similar episodes in the past and is taking phenytoin for his Hx of seizures. Currently the pt appears drowsy, but is no longer having any involuntary movements. Which of the following is most appropriate first step?

A. Administer IV benzodiazepine
B. Change his medication from dilantin to ethosuximide
C. Check dilantin level
D. Order immediate EEG
E. Order immediate EKG

76. A 27-yr-old previously healthy woman presents with complaints of fatigue. She quit smoking 5 yrs ago, and other than heavy menses, has no other medical problems. Anemia is suspected as the cause of her Sx. Which of the following lab results would be consistent with the cause of anemia?

A. High MCV (mean corpuscular volume), low iron, high TIBC (total iron binding capacity)
B. High MCV, low vitamin B12, low MMA (methylmalonic acid)
C. Low MCV, low iron, low ferritin
D. Nml MCV, nml iron, low TIBC
E. Nml MCV, high bilirubin, high haptoglobin

ANSWERS

1. D. This pt has an ECG that is worrisome for cardiac dz. It is true that the pt's pain is slightly atypical in that he describes it as heartburn. Nevertheless, his ECG shows evidence of a prior myocardial infarction (note Q waves in leads V_1–V_4), indicating that the pt has problematic coronary artery dz. Furthermore, the other elements of his story are concerning. In particular, rest pain that lasts >20 min and is ongoing at the time of evaluation places this pt at high risk by definition (intermediate risk is rest pain lasting >20 minutes but which has resolved at the time of evaluation).

2. D. The ECG shows sinus bradycardia. The rate is approximately 50 bpm, and there is a p wave before every QRS and a QRS after every p wave. QRS width is >0.12 ms (>3 small boxes wide), indicating a bundle-brunch block. The potentially confusing aspect of this tracing is the lack of an RSR' (rabbit ears). The absence of an RSR' is explained by the fact that the pt has infarcted his septum and anterior wall, resulting in Q waves in leads V_1–V_4. The Q wave occupies where the R wave should be, so the pt has QSR' instead of RSR'. Note that the QSR' is in leads V_1 and V_2, indicating that the bundle-branch block is in the right bundle, not the left bundle. The other classic aspect of a right bundle-branch block is the deep S waves in the lateral leads (I, V_5, V_6). There are no ST elevations that would be characteristic of a left bundle-branch block. Finally, this pt has a leftward axis (I is upright, but aVF is mostly negative). An unexplained left-axis deviation defines the presence of a left anterior fascicular block. Therefore, this pt has a bifascicular block.

3. C. Please tell us you got this one! Look at those enormous tombstone signs in leads V_1–V_4, with a smaller version in V_5. This is a classic acute ST elevation myocardial infarction (STEMI). Early repolarization is a nml variant in a healthy, aSx pt, and it causes a gently concave upward sloping (smiley face) ST segment. These are flat (angry face) ST elevations, not consistent with early repolarization. The pt's Sx also are not consistent with acute pericarditis or ventricular aneurysm, nor is PR depression or electrical alternans present to support a Dx of pericarditis.

531

4. **C.** Again, did you spot the STEMI? First, this is junctional rhythm because there are no p waves to be seen anywhere on the tracing. The QRS complexes are narrow, so this is not ventricular tachycardia. There are ST elevations in inferior leads II, III, and aVF and in lateral leads V_3 and V_4, indicating an acute STEMI. There are no flutter waves, so this is not atrial flutter, and the rhythm is regular, so it is not atrial fibrillation.

5. **E.** This tracing is classic for WPW syndrome. Note the very short PR interval (approximately 0.06 second, or 1.5 small boxes) and the slurred delta wave, which is the R wave coming up off the P wave. There is no ST elevation. However, also noted is ST depression concerning for ischemia. The pt's episodic Sx likely are caused by the reentrant tachycardia that occurs as a result of the bypass pathway in WPW syndrome.

6. **C.** The law requires that all suspected cases of child abuse must be reported to child protective services. Depending on the state you practice in, spouse abuse may also require reporting. People who suffer from this type of abuse frequently hospital-shop so hospital personnel will not recognize the pattern of abuse. Therefore, it is very unlikely that they will give any factual information during their check in.

7. **B.** In order to establish trust, you must first assure the adolescent that your conversation is confidential. This is especially important in areas concerning sex or drugs. By removing the mother from the room, you can establish this trust and therefore gain more information to assist the pt and the family. The mother may still need a support group to deal with her daughter's possible Dx.

8. **D.** The classic Sx of amenorrhea (weight loss >15%, constipation, electrolyte and cardiac abnormalities) are all present in this female. This dangerous combination can be fatal. Therefore, hospitalization is indicated to better observe the pt and correct her electrolyte imbalance. Bulimic pts generally appear healthier and also have poor dentition from frequent self-induced vomiting episodes.

9. 1–**B**, 2–**G**, 3–**A**, 4–**F**, 5–**C**, 6–**E**, 7–**D**.

10. 1–**B**, 2–**E**, 3–**A**, 4–**C**, 5–**D**.

11. **C.** Pickwickian Syndrome describes the triad of somnolence, obesity, and erythrocytosis. Tx is weight loss. There is no such

thing as a central obstructive disorder. Central sleep apnea is related to lack of respiratory drive, whereas obstructive sleep apnea is related to mechanical obstruction of ventilation. Pts with narcolepsy have sudden uncontrolled drop attacks unlike our pt.

12. B. Effective pt–doctor communication requires sufficient time. An interpreter should be available to assist with communication. Family members and friends should not be used unless absolutely necessary. This places the pt in embarrassing situations and does not assure that what you are saying is fully understood by the person translating. You should always speak directly to the pt and ask questions frequently to avoid any misunderstandings.

13. 1–**C**, 2–**D**, 3–**E**, 4–**A**, 5–**B**, 6–**G**, 7–**F**.

14. C. When women are considering pregnancy or have become pregnant, complete review of their medications is warranted looking for teratogenic compounds. Lisinopril is an angiotensin converting enzyme inhibitor which carries a Class C label during first trimester and Class D during the second and third trimesters. Therefore, continuing it or ↑ it would not be appropriate. However, the pt has HTN so although discontinuing her lisinopril is appropriate, her HTN should be medically managed with an alternative regimen during pregnancy. Essential HTN is not an indication to recommend against conception.

15. D. Gestational diabetes is a serious illness that has major adverse effects on both the infant and the mother. Screening is recommended between 24–28 wk of pregnancy. However, it should be done as early as the first prenatal visit if there is a high degree of suspicion that the pregnant woman has undiagnosed type 2 diabetes. It is not appropriate to provide reassurance at this time 2° to the high risk of adverse outcomes with gestational diabetes. Moreover, a urine dipstick for glucose is not the recommended way to screen for gestational diabetes. A Dx of gestational diabetes can be accomplished several different ways. One way requires a random finger stick greater than 200mg/dL, fasting finger stick greater than 126mg/dL on subsequent days. or an oral glucose challenge test with 50g glucose load and a 1 hr serum glucose greater than 130mg/dL. The Dx is confirmed with a 3 hr GTT.

16. **A.** Tx of gestational diabetes (GDM) is critical to ↓ the risk of mother and fetal morbidity and mortality. An effective Tx regimen consists of dietary Tx, self blood glucose monitoring, and the administration of medications if target blood glucose values are not met with diet alone. Tx of GDM requires several different modalities. Carbohydrates should make up 33%–40% of daily calories. Insulin has been the mainstay of Tx for many yrs; however, recent studies have investigated the safety and efficacy of glyburide and metformin. These medications are now considered category B by the FDA and should not be used unless clearly needed. GDM is generally related to an ↑ in insulin resistance associated with hormonal changes during pregnancy. Very rarely is there a relationship with latent type I DM. There are no current recommendations to screen family members. Only approximately 30% of women with GDM will require Tx after the peripartum period. Although insulin Tx may be indicated, there is not enough information to determine if this pt requires pharmacotherapy at this time. Waiting until the fetus has macrosomia to start pharmacotherapy is not appropriate. The goal of Tx is to prevent macrosomia and other GDM-related morbidities.

17. **C.** Recognize the Si/Sx of postpartum hemorrhage. This is defined as >500cc of blood loss associated with delivery. There are several main causes including uterine atony, lacerations, and retained placenta. The first step in management is resuscitation. Although a retained placenta is a common cause of postpartum hemorrhage, initial resuscitation is indicated prior to any further management. It also is somewhat less likely as this pt has a boggy uterus. Once the pt has stabilized, then consider further definitive Tx. A hysterectomy is a last resort for Tx of uterine atony and should not be performed before other medical and less definitive surgical therapies. The first step in management includes basic resuscitation. The pt is able to speak and has a pulse, so fluids and blood products are reasonable. This should be followed by uterine massage to stimulate contractions. If unsuccessful then medical Tx to induce uterine contractions is appropriate. Although disseminated intravascular coagulation is a cause of postpartum hemorrhage, this pt requires resuscitative measures now.

18. **B.** Preeclampsia is defined as the new onset of HTN and proteinuria after 20 wks of gestation. The female must have previously been normotensive. Preeclampsia is divided into two categories: mild and severe. Confirmation of the dz and ruling out other potential Dx is appropriate with mild preeclampsia. Delivery of the fetus and placenta remains the only curative Tx and is recommended in the presence of severe dz. Induction of labor is appropriate after confirmation of Dx and if gestational age is >37 wks with a favorable cervix. If severe Sx are present including CNS Sx, thrombocytopenia, or liver damage, then immediate delivery is recommended. This pt likely has mild preeclampsia. Confirmation of the dz by 24 hr urine protein level or spot urine protein to creatinine ratio would also be appropriate. Repeating her BP is also required to confirm the Dx. The use of antihypertensive drugs to control mildly elevated BP in the setting of preeclampsia does not alter the course of the dz or diminish perinatal morbidity or mortality. Specifically, diuretics have no role in Tx. Current guidelines recommend seizure prophylaxis with magnesium sulfate. This dz has significant morbidity and mortality. Four-wk follow-up is not appropriate management.

19. E. In order to appropriately counsel women on various contraceptive methods, an understanding of both what methods are available and their contraindications, as well as the woman's lifestyle, is important to prevent unintended pregnancies. Combination hormonal oral contraceptive is contraindicated in this pt 2° to her age, smoking habits, and previous thrombotic event. Although natural family planning can be an effective means of contraception, it is less effective for people who are not in a stable relationship and does not prevent against sexually transmitted illnesses. Coitus interruptus occurs when the male partner ejaculates outside of the vaginal canal. There is a 15%–20% failure rate associated with this method, and, therefore, it should not be recommended. Tubal ligation is an effective means of contraception; however, it is not recommended for women who are still considering future childbirth. Moreover, it does not protect against sexually transmitted illnesses.

20. C. The Pap smear was designed as a screening tool to be used on aSx pts and not a diagnostic tool to confirm suspicion of dz. Certain strains of human papillomavirus have been associated with development of squamous cell CA as well as a broad spectrum of genital dz. Having one sexual partner does not put her at high risk for cervical CA. There is no clinical information provided that would suggest she has developed cervical CA. In addition, her Hx of no abnormal studies is reassuring. The current guidelines suggest she can be screened every 2–3 years based on her age (>30), three consecutive nml Pap smears, and no high risk behaviors. Although having multiple or new sexual partners does increase your risk of obtaining HPV, those who have previously had intercourse should be screened regularly. The frequency depends on age, previous tests, and other medical conditions. Current recommendations are to begin screening 3 yrs after first intercourse or at age 21, which ever comes first.

21. D. Unless a fracture is present, osteoporosis has no clinical manifestations. This makes screening an important tool in the early Dx of osteoporosis. Risk factors for low bone density and therefore fractures include: age, postmenopausal, smoking, low BMI, corticosteroid use, family history, and white race. This pt is Caucasian and has significant smoking Hx and small body frame. Screening is recommended at age 65 unless there are risk factors present, in which case screening should be initiated earlier. A lumbar fracture in absence of traumatic injury is an automatic qualifier for the Dx of osteoporosis. Vitamin D deficiency is associated with osteomalacia in adults and Rickets in children. Ehlers-Danlos syndrome is a group of rare genetic disorders affecting humans caused by a defect in collagen synthesis. She would have been symptomatic before entering her seventh decade of life. An abnormal bone density scan that meets qualifications for osteopenia, and a fracture is an automatic qualifier for the Dx of osteoporosis. Although she has a significant tobacco Hx, there is nothing to suggest lung CA.

22. B. This pt's clinical presentation is concerning for Dx of cervical CA. Further investigation is warranted based on the cytology results of her Pap smear. Colposcopic evaluation of the cervix and vagina increases the yield of visualizing tissue that is concerning for malignant and premalignant epithelium. The improved visualization of epithelial surfaces enhances the colposcopist's ability to obtain directed Bx from suspicious tissue. Women diagnosed with high-grade squamous intraepithelial lesions are at ↑ risk of having serious underlying pathology. Approximately 2% of HSIL contain invasive CA. Chemotherapy and radiation are not the appropriate Tx until a diagnosis of CA is confirmed. Colposcopy of the entire cervix and vagina is recommended at this time, with Bx of all visible lesions and endocervical curettage. If this procedure is nondiagnostic then a loop electrosurgical excision should be performed. Without appropriately pathology hysterectomy is not indicated at this time. With the potential of serious underlying pathology, repeating the Pap smear is not the appropriate management. She has not been diagnosed with a dz that has an expected mortality of six mo or less.

23. A. Shoulder pain is a very common complaint in the primary care setting. Pts with rotator cuff tendinopathy complain of shoulder pain with overhead activity, and often have localized pain to the lateral deltoid which may be worse at night. Rotator cuff disorders are common in repetitive motions and are a significant source of morbidity among manual laborers. Any of the four rotator cuff tendons may be involved, but the supraspinatus tendon is most frequently injured. The initial Tx for rotator cuff tendinopathy includes rest, NSAIDs, and ice. This can be followed by physical Tx. No additional imaging is required in this pt to make the Dx. The presentation of this pt is not consistent with a dislocated shoulder. Anterior shoulder dislocations generally involve a traumatic event or blow to an abducted, externally rotated arm. Arthroscopy is appropriate Tx for a complete rotator cuff tear in the acute period; however, this pt's presentation dose not support a rotator cuff tear. His examination finding of pain with active abduction but still having full range of motion is not consistent with a cuff tear. The acute nature of his Sx does not support a Dx of osteoarthritis. There is minimal evidence to support the use of corticosteroids for Tx of rotator cuff tendinopathy. Moreover, the injection should be in the subacromial space as opposed to the deltoid muscle.

24. E. A meniscus tear is a common cause of knee pain, and may be associated with a twisting injury; however, older individuals may develop tears from degenerative conditions with no associated trauma or injuries. The pain is generally not well localized with vague Sx. Knee x-rays may be helpful to Dx a fracture. The Ottawa Rules are guidelines used to determine who should have plain radiography done. These guidelines include age >55, isolated patella or fibula tenderness, inability to flex the knee great than 90 degrees, and inability to bear weight immediately after injury. Occasionally, MRIs are required to confirm the Dx of meniscus tear in difficult cases. This is a straightforward presentation and further imaging is not necessary. CT imaging is not as useful as MRI in evaluating the soft tissues of the lower extremity. Moreover, further imaging is not necessary 2° to the straightforward presentation. Referral to orthopedic physician may be necessary if initial conservative Tx is unsuccessful, but at this time there is no indication for referral to establish a Dx. His mechanism of injury and his exam findings support a Dx of meniscus tear, and no further imaging is required at this time.

25. D. Psoriasis is a common chronic skin disorder that is characterized by erythematous plaques containing a silver scale. Many cases are not severe enough to affect a person's general health and may never be treated in a medical setting. Eczema or atopic dermatitis is an inflammatory skin condition involving a complex interaction between environmental and genetic factors. It often occurs in pts with an atopic diathesis including eczema, asthma, and allergic rhinitis. Seborrheic keratosis is a common benign growth of unknown cause seen in the elderly due to a thickening of an area of the top skin layer. Vitiligo is an acquired depigmentation of the skin. Although lichen simplex chronicus may present with demarcated plaques it classically has a puritis component and is located in moist regions like the groin.

26. A. Small bowel obstructions are a common cause of abd pain and are generally associated with nausea and vomiting. The etiology is often from adhesions from previous surgeries or hernias. Less frequently tumors and strictures can cause obstructions. Labs are generally not helpful in securing the Dx but can aid in the determination dehydration. This is a typical presentation and findings are consistent with a small bowel obstruction. He should be managed with aggressive fluids, bowel rest, NG to low intermittent suction, and NPO diet order. Close monitoring is required and surgical intervention if evidence of bowel strangulation is present. A perforated peptic ulcer will have free air under the diaphragm on imaging and will often have Sx and exam findings of peritonitis. This is not a typical presentation for colon CA. A barium enema may show an "apple core" lesion which should increase the suspicion. Acute pancreatitis will often have epigastric pains that may radiate to the back. Etiology is often from gallbladder dz or alcohol abuse. It would be unusual to have a nml lipase with an acute presentation. In chronic pancreatitis, the pancreatic calcifications can be seen on abd series. Constipation typically does not have associated nausea and vomiting. This would be an alarming finding and should be further investigated. The x-ray would not show this amount of air in the small bowel.

27. C. Renal dz is a common finding in people with both diabetes and poorly controlled HTN. In fact, nearly 80% of chronic kidney dz can be attributed to these two dz. Dietary modifications would not be sufficient alone to alter the course of his dz progression, although, it may be recommended this pt will benefit from improved BP control. Glucose control is important in diabetics as poor control can lead to diabetic nephropathy; however, this pt's control is only slightly above the current recommendations. Moreover, improving his BP has been shown to have a greater impact on slowing progression. This pt will benefit the most from improved BP control. An angiotensin converting enzyme inhibitor can minimize progression of, or even prevent, glomerular dz in the absence of glycemic control. It may be appropriate for this pt to be seen by a nephrologist, but his renal function does not warrant transplantation at this time. Renal Bx is an invasive procedure that is unlikely to add any additional information in this setting. This pt's renal dz is consistent with long-standing HTN and diabetes.

28. D. This is a typical presentation of COPD and chronic bronchitis. It can be defined as a chronic productive cough for 3 mo in 2 successive yrs in a pt in whom other causes of chronic cough have been excluded. Pulmonary function tests are the diagnostic study of choice to confirm the Dx of COPD. They determine the severity of the airflow obstruction, and can be used to follow dz progression. The most important values measured are the FEV1 and the forced vital capacity. An FEV1/FVC ratio less than 0.70 indicates airway obstruction. A CT can be useful to evaluate lung tissue, but it is unable to make the Dx of COPD. Moreover, contrast would be helpful only to evaluate the vasculature. There is no role for a lung Bx to make the Dx of COPD. Although there are classic findings on a CXR of hyperinflated lung fields and flattened diaphragms, it is not a diagnostic tool used to make the Dx. A sleep study is used to evaluate for obstructive sleep apnea or other sleep related dz. It has no role in the Dx of COPD.

29. D. The classic presentation Sx of asthma are a triad of wheeze, cough, and shortness of breath. A FHx of allergies or atopic dz (specifically, atopic dermatitis, seasonal allergic rhinitis and conjunctivitis, or hives) favors a Dx of asthma in a pt with suggestive Sx. Pulmonary function tests should show obstructive lung dz, but with a ≥10% ↑ in FEV after administration of bronchodilator Tx. Asthma cannot be diagnosed by CT or CXR. A single peak flow determination made in the doctor's office while a pt is experiencing Sx is suggestive of asthma. However, it is not diagnostic, because a reduced peak flow is not specific for asthma and can be seen with other pulmonary processes.

30. C. This is a typical presentation for pulmonary emboli. She has several risk factors including oral contraceptives, specifically the estrogen component, and active smoking. Hormonal contraception is now contraindicated for her and she should be encouraged to stop smoking. There is nothing in her presentation that is suspicious for anxiety or panic attack. A nml PCO_2 makes hyperventilation unlikely. There is no mention of productive cough or significant fevers that would be consistent with pneumonia. She has several risk factors for PE including estrogen only oral contraceptive pill and smoking. Classically, a low-grade fever, tachycardia and tachypnea are present. The most common CXR reading is a nml. It is unlikely that she is experiencing an asthma exacerbation with clear lung fields on examination. Often Sx have been present for several mo prior to Dx.

31. A. This is a typical presentation for acute nephrolithiasis. It is generally associated with a sharp cramping pain that waxes and wanes. Hematuria is often frequently present. Rhubarb is high in oxalate which puts her at ↑ risk for an oxalate stone. Her abnormal vitals are 2° to the discomfort she is experiencing. This is a straightforward presentation. Imaging with helical CT scan with contrast should be obtained to identify complications and evaluate the size of her stone. Ectopic pregnancy may have peritoneal signs, amenorrhea, or vaginal bleeding which are not present in this pt. Also, her unremarkable pelvic examination makes ectopic pregnancy less likely. The unremarkable pelvic examination makes ovarian torsion less likely. The quality of pain generally does not wax and wane. Diverticulitis is far more common on the left side of the colon. It is typically associated with constant pain and Si of system infxns may be present. The lack of findings during the pelvic examination makes this less likely. A monogamous relationship and barrier method of contraception are practices less likely to be associated with sexually transmitted infxn.

32. **B.** This is an example of hypertensive emergency based on evidence of end-organ compromise. This is supported by his anuria, confusion, and papilledema. These findings distinguish this from hypertensive urgency which could be managed with oral antihypertensives. This pt requires IV medications with a short half-life that can be titrated quickly and discontinued if his BP drops too rapidly. The goal is to decrease his BP by 25%. IV nitroglycerin is less effective at lowering BP, but might be used in the setting of myocardial ischemia.

33. **E.** Acute renal failure is defined as the sudden loss of kidney function which results in the accumulation of urea and the dysregulation of volume and electrolytes. Urea is able to cross the blood brain barrier and may result in encephalopathy called uremia. Classically, acute renal failure is divided into three categories: prerenal, renal, and postrenal azotemia. This is based on the location of the underlying etiology for renal failure. His benign prostate hypertrophy and diphenhydramine use are associated with urethra obstruction and anticholinergic side effects which both frequently result in postrenal azotemia. HTN nephropathy is generally a chronic condition that develops over years of poorly controlled BP. Most episodes of acute interstitial nephritis (ANI) are associated with drug exposure, most commonly antibiotics. Although infxns in elderly often result in delirium there were no other Sx consistent with a urinary tract infxn. Generally, polyuria is a frequent Sx and this gentleman is anuric, which is less common.

34. **D.** Physiologic jaundice occurs in almost 50% of newborns and is a benign condition. It is an unconjugated hyperbilirubinemia that results from increased bilirubin production and low amounts of glucuronyl transferase 2° to immature livers. Physiologic jaundice is a very common condition that occurs 1–2 days post-partum. It requires no Tx and generally resolves as the infant's liver produces more glucuronyl transferase. Conjugated hyperbilirubinemia is generally caused by infxn with the ToRCH dz, congenital causes, anomalies, and metabolic causes. The clinical presentation and physical exam would be more revealing. Crigler-Najjar syndrome, or congenital nonhemolytic jaundice, is an autosomal recessive disorder caused by glucuronosyltransferase deficiency. It is generally present at time of birth Infants born vaginally to mothers with *Chlamydia trachomatis* genital infxns are at risk for acquiring *C. trachomatis*. This usually presents as conjunctivitis and/or pneumonia. Kernicterus is the chronic and permanent neurologic sequelae of bilirubin-induced neurologic dysfunction (BIND). It is too early to see such a manifestation.

35. D. Uncomplicated urinary tract infxns are common in women. There is weak evidence that cranberry juice might be effective in prevention of urinary tract infxns 2° to ↓ the urine pH. However, once infxn is present, antibiotic Tx should be administered. Pyelonephritis is an infxn of the renal pelvis. It classically presents with fevers, flank pain, nausea, and vomiting. This pt does not have a clinical picture consistent with a systemic pyelonephritis. Starting oral antibiotics is appropriate in this pt; Tx for an uncomplicated urinary tract infxn is for 3 days duration. The was no evidence of cervical motion tenderness on examination, making PID unlikely.

36. B. This is a classic presentation for rheumatoid arthritis. Pts will often complain of symmetrical distal polyarthritis and morning stiffness. In many cases, bone erosions are present on radiographic imaging. Osteoarthritis pain is present after extended use of the joint and presents with PIP and DIP joint dz, rather than MCP and PIP joint dz, which is typical of RA. Sjögren's syndrome is a chronic inflammatory disorder characterized by diminished lacrimal and salivary gland functions. It may occur in both a primary form which is not associated with other dz, or in a 2° form that complicates other rheumatic conditions. Septic arthritis is generally monoarticular and rarely affects the fingers. Reactive arthritis is used to refer to rheumatic disorders that appear following an episode of infxn. A triad of Sx is generally associated with it including: postinfectious arthritis, urethritis, and conjunctivitis. It was previously referred to as Reiter syndrome.

37. C. This pt has several Sx of obstructive sleep apnea (OSA). Although his clinical presentation is consistent with OSA, sleep study is required to confirm the Dx. OSA causes airway obstruction only when asleep, in contrast to obesity hypoventilation syndrome, in which hypoventilation occurs during awake periods. Therefore, pulmonary function testing may not reveal an abnormality in OSA since the pnt is awake during the test. If concerned for obesity hypoventilation syndrome, which may coexist with OSA, then a pulmonary function test may be useful. Radiographic imaging of the upper airway is not helpful in confirming or excluding OSA. CPAP may be useful in confirming a Dx, but it has a poor specificity. Although it is a relatively benign Tx, it generally is not recommended for chronic use without first confirming the Dx of OSA with polysomnography.

38. **A.** This is a typical presentation for aortic stenosis. Sx may include syncope, dyspnea, and/or angina. Severity is based on valve area, but anybody who is symptomatic is considered to have severe dz. Symptomatic aortic stenosis is an indication for valve replacement despite a valve area greater than 1 cm^2. Arrhythmias are uncommon in aortic stenosis, and thus monitoring would have limited benefit. Because this pt is already symptomatic, monitoring him would not be beneficial. In severe aortic stenosis, the peripheral vasculature is constricted to maintain blood pressure and perfusion. Starting a β blocker is contraindicated in this pt. In aSx individuals, following the valve area and dz progression through serial echocardiograms may be reasonable; however, this is not appropriate with Sx present.

39. **D.** Place an endotracheal tube. "GCS less than 8, intubate." Know the 1° and 2° surveys in the management of a trauma pt. Maintaining a pt's airway is the most essential first step in a trauma situation. Unconsciousness is an absolute indication for an endotracheal tube to protect the pt's airway. A Glascow Coma scale of less than 8 is also an absolute indication for intubation. In this case, the pt's GCS = 6 (eye opening, 1; verbal response, 1; motor response, 4). After securing the pt's airway in the 1° survey, breathing, circulation, disability, and exposure can be assessed. Establishing IV access and volume expansion is essential to prevent further circulatory compromise; however, securing the airway should not be delayed. Dextrose, thiamine, and naloxone are typically administered in the 1° survey in instances of loss of consciousness, however intubation should take place first. Labs such as serum ethanol should not delay intubation either.

40. **B.** Follow-up Utz in 6 mo. Understand the indications for screening and intervention in abd aortic aneurysm. Aneurysms >5 cm in diameter are at an elevated risk for rupture in all risk groups for pts, therefore aneurysms >5 cm are referred for operative intervention. Aneurysms that ↑ by >0.5 cm in size in 6 mo are also at high risk for rupture and should be surgically managed. Aneurysms <5 cm in size without Sx are typically monitored with serial Utz examinations every 6 mo to observe for expanding size. Urgent surgical repair is only indicated if the pt is unstable. 12 mo follow up would not accurately assess for expansion in size. CT scan is another modality to look at aneurysms, but would be of low utility in this case since the Dx is already confirmed. Optimizing BP, lipids, and quitting smoking all ↓ the risk of aneurysm rupture. In this case, the pt's BP is well-controlled and modifying Tx would not be necessary.

41. **D.** Aortic Dissection. Recognize the clinical Si/Sx of aortic dissection. Pts with aortic dissection classically present with a tearing chest pain radiating towards their back in the setting of HTN. On chest radiography, they will have mediastinal widening of >8 cm. Aortic dissection is the only answer choice that would cause a widened mediastinum. While the pt is at risk for a recurrent myocardial infarction given her Hx, her EKG findings are not indicative of active ischemia. While pts with peptic ulcer dz can present with chest pain in the setting of NSAID use, they would not typically have mediastinal widening on chest radiography; they may, however, have free air under the diaphragm from perforation. Pts with a pulmonary embolus can also present with chest pain and tachycardia, but they would typically have hypoxia and would not have a widened mediastinum.

42. **B.** Colonoscopy now. Know the colon CA screening guidelines in a high-risk pt. While the pt is in good health and has no signs of malignancy in his Hx and laboratory examination, he is at elevated risk for colon CA given his FHx. According to American Gastroenterological Association screening guidelines, pts with a first degree relative with a Dx of colon CA at an age <60 need to be screened at age 40 or 10 yrs earlier than the youngest Dx, whichever comes first. This pt should be screened now since he is already >40. CEA levels are used in tracking established colon CA and not for its Dx. CT colonography has not been completely established as an accurate screening examination in higher risk pts.

43. **A.** Sigmoid Volvulus. Recognize the abd radiograph findings of a volvulus. Volvulus is the rotation of the large intestine along its mesenteric axis. It commonly occurs in elderly, institutionalized pts. X-ray reveals dilated loops of bowel and a "bird beak" appearance at the site of the bowel rotation. Fecal impaction would present with stool in the rectum or visible on radiography. Ogilvie's syndrome features right-sided colon dilatation in the absence of an obstruction. Rectal CA would present with a rectal mass. Progression of dementia as an etiology for change in baseline mental status is a Dx of exclusion and would not feature change in abd exam findings or bowel dilatation on abd films.

44. **C.** Colonoscopy. Know the management of a volvulus. A sigmoid volvulus can be managed with either a colonoscopy or sigmoidoscopy to decompress the rotated bowel. If this is not successful, or if the pt progresses to perforation or becomes ischemic, the pt should undergo a laparotomy with a surgical resection.

45. **B.** Paroxetine. Recognize the clinical features of depression and know the first line medical Tx. The pt's insomnia Sx have been ongoing for 9 mo and are associated with feelings of hopelessness and anhedonia. This is consistent with a Dx of depression and not simple insomnia. SSRIs such as paroxetine would be first line Tx for depression given their tolerable side effect profile. Amitryptiline is a tricyclic antidepressant which would be second line. Electroconvulsive Tx is for refractory cases of depression. Zolpidem and temazepam are used as sleep aides; this would not be addressing the pt's underlying 1° problem.

46. **C.** Discontinue the haloperidol. Recognize the adverse effects of antipsychotic medications. Atypical antipsychotics such as haloperidol can have serious side effects such as QT prolongation and torsades de pointes. Use of these medications should be avoided if possible in pts with possible underlying cardiac dz. Discontinuing the haloperidol is the correct answer as it can help to prevent a potentially fatal arrhythmia in this pt. Memantine and donepezil are medications used in the Tx of dementia and do not have arrythmogenic side effects. Defibrillation is used in the setting of ventricular fibrillation or pulseless ventricular tachycardia. The pt is not in one of these rhythms, however she is at a risk for an arrhythmia if the haloperidol is not stopped. Electrophysiology study to evaluate for cardiac conduction system dz is not necessary at this point since there is a new inciting factor for the pt's QT prolongation.

47. **E.** Order an insulin and C-peptide level. Judiciously use diagnostic testing in the setting of possible facticious disorder. If a pt is using exogenous insulin, they will have high serum insulin levels and the absence of serum C-peptide levels in the presence of hypoglycemia. This is a relatively simple diagnostic test if the pt is suspected of giving herself insulin. Neither the state medical board nor the medical school should be notified if there is no actual confirmation of a Dx. This would also be inappropriate as the pt should be screened for depression or other psychiatric comorbidities. Antidepressants such as fluoxentine are not effective in facticious disorder; it would also be inappropriate to start fluoxetine without diagnosing the pt with depression. Octreotide scanning is used in the work up of neuroendocrine tumors. Excessive diagnostic tests should not be ordered in cases of facticious disorder.

48. **B.** Borderline. Recognize different personality disorders. Personality disorders are pervasive patterns of maladaptive behaviors that often create disruptions in the health care setting. This pt exhibits borderline personality disorder as she is widely emotional and sees people as either very good or very bad. Histrionic personality would exhibit more attention seeking behavior. Narcissistic would feel that everyone is inferior. Antisocial violates the rights of others and breaks the law. Obsessive-compulsives are preoccupied with rules, regulations, and neatness.

49. **D.** Conduct Disorder. Differentiate conduct disorder from other psychiatric diagnoses. Children with conduct disorder are often bullies who will show physical cruelty to people and animals; they often have an unsettled home life as the pt in this case has. Antisocial personality disorder is an adult Dx and would not apply to a 10-yr-old. Attention-deficit hyperactivity disorder can also be associated with poor school performance, however it does not typically feature violent behavior. Oppositional defiant disorder will have features of argumentativeness, but will not act out their aggressions. Bipolar disorder features episodes of mania alternating with bouts of depression.

50. **A.** Amitriptyline. Know the therapeutic options for PTSD. Tricyclic antidepressants as well as SSRIs have been shown in clinical trials to be effective in the Tx of PTSD. When taken at night, amitriptyline can also have a sleep aid effect. Medications are combined with psychotherapy. While benzodiazepines and sleep aids such as zolpidem and lorazepam can help with the pt's anxiety Sx, they have a high potential for abuse given his alcohol use. Lithium and gabapentin are mood stabilizers utilized in bipolar disorder.

51. **C.** Start oral amoxicillin. Based on the pt's physical exam, she has acute otitis media. Amoxicillin has activity against all of the common otitis media pathogens. Amoxicillin/clavulanate would be unnecessary in the first isolated episode of otitis media. It has broader spectrum activity than amoxicillin alone,

and should be reserved for suspected cases of amoxicillin-resistant infxns. Ear drops are not used in otitis media as the infxn is behind the tympanic membrane. Surgical drainage and tympanostomy tubes are used in recurrent otitis media infxns; they would not be placed after one isolated episode. A chest radiograph is unnecessary in the setting of a nml pulmonary examination.

52. **D.** 1/150. Be able to apply basic statistics and a 2×2 table to genetic counseling. Cystic fibrosis is an autonomic recessive genetic disorder. For inheritance to be passed, it requires transmission of the gene to the fetus from 2 carrier parents. In Caucasian populations, the probability of being a carrier for CF is 1/25. This is the mother's odds of being a carrier. The father's brother has CF, which means that both of his parents are carriers of the recessive gene. When the father was born, he had a 25% chance of inheriting a CF gene from both parents, a 50% chance of inheriting a CF gene from one parent, and a 25% chance of not inheriting any CF genes. Because the father does not have dz, we know he does not have 2 CF genes. That means he either inherited one copy of the CF gene from one parent and is a carrier (2/3 chance of this) or inherited no CF genes (1/3 chance of this). If both parents are carriers, there is a 1/4 chance that the baby will receive both copies of the gene and therefore have the dz. Thus, the odds of the baby having CF are 2/3 (the father's odds of carrier status) $\times$ 1/25 (the mother's odds of carrier status) $\times$ 1/4 (the odds of getting both copies of a recessive gene) = 1/150.

53. **B.** Wilson's Dz. Recognize ocular signs of systemic dz. This pt exhibits many Si/Sx of Wilson's Dz, a deficiency in copper metabolism. Wilson's dz commonly presents with basal ganglia type neurologic Sx as exhibited by his Parkinson's-like exam findings as well as depression or psychosis. Pts will also have liver dysfunction and elevated transaminases. Kayser-Fleischer rings are dark rings around the irises that are from copper deposits. This finding is indicative of underlying Wilson's dz; it would not be found in any of the other dz processes. Hemochromatosis and alcoholism both cause liver dz. Alcoholism would not cause basal ganglia-like neurologic Sx; it can cause Wernicke's encephalopathy from thiamine deficiency. Hemochromatosis also causes cirrhosis, however the pt would have excess stores of iron. Parkinson's dz alone would not cause elevated liver enzymes, and neither would depression.

54. E. An asymmetric lesion with irregular borders. Recognize the clinical features of melanoma. Clinical suspicion for a malignant melanoma is raised by the following features of a skin lesion, the ABCDEs. A = asymmetry. B = irregular border. C = multicolored. D = diameter >6mm. E = Enlargement in size. Basal cell CAs will feature pearly translucent borders with fine telangiectasias (bad, but not as bad Melanoma). Seborrheic keratosis are benign and are brown or black plaques with a stuck on appearance.

55. A. Surgical excision. Know how to manage the initial Dx of melanoma. The preferred management of a suspected melanoma is excision of the lesion with a 1–2mm margin of healthy surrounding tissue to ensure complete excision of the lesion. All layers of skin are needed as part of the excision. A shave Bx will not obtain all layers of skin. Core Bx could be considered if the lesion were on the face and could potentially be disfiguring; however, if the Dx of melanoma is confirmed, complete excision would be required. Imaging studies such as PET scan and CT are used for staging and looking for metastatic dz. They would not be ordered prior to an excision of the lesions and a pathologic Dx.

56. C. Bolus; the pt and cross match for transfusion. The pt is hypotensive and requires volume resuscitation. Immediately begin a nml saline bolus and cross and match for transfusion in case the hemoglobin falls from volume equilibration and/or further bleeding. IV pantoprazole is used in the setting of upper GI bleeding when ulcer dz is suspected; it should be given after volume resuscitation. IV octreotide is used when esophageal varcies as suspected. In this case the pt has underlying liver dz which puts him at an elevated risk for variceal hemorrhage, and octreotide should be given, but again, after volume resuscitation. EGD should be performed in this pt, however diagnostic procedures should be held until the pt's hemodynamic status stabilizes. Endoscopy requires sedation as well as procedural intervention, therefore the pt must be stabilized prior to the performance of an EGD.

57. A. Autoimmune Hepatitis. Be able to interpret liver function tests. In order to interpret liver function abnormalities, an appropriate Hx must be taken and then applied to supplemental tests. In this case, the most common causes of a chronically elevated AST and ALT, viral hepatitis and alcohol use, are unlikely based on the history. Autoimmune hepatitis is typically seen in pts with known autoimmune dz, such as systemic lupus erythematosis. A positive antinuclear antibody and a positive antismooth muscle antibody are diagnostic for autoimmune hepatitis. Primary biliary cirrhosis would feature an elevated alkaline phosphatase as well as a ⊕ antimitochondrial antibody. The pt has hepatitis B immunity as her surface antibody is ⊕, but not the antigen. Ectopic pregnancy would not cause hepatomegaly.

58. **C.** Do not place the feeding tube. Understand the meaning of an advance directive. An advance directive is a document filled out by a pt while they are of sound mind that directs their health care wishes. A power of attorney is a document which grants decision making to a surrogate in the event of incapacitation. A power of attorney should direct the plan of care in accordance to the pt's pre-stated wishes. A power of attorney is not acti-vated until the pt is unable to make his own health care deci-sions. In this case, the pt is able to clearly communicate "no" in regards to a feeding tube, therefore it would be inappropriate to place the tube. Since the pt can communicate his wishes his power of attorney is not active. The pt's "no" is also consistent with his prior advance directives stating no feeding tubes. Placing the tube under these circumstances would be unethical.

59. **E.** 10. Understand the number needed to treat. The number needed to treat is the number of pts that need to be exposed to an intervention in order to achieve the desired outcome. In this case, the desired outcome is prevention of death. The number needed to treat is 1/absolute risk reduction. Absolute risk reduction is the difference in death rates between the placebo group and the new drug group. In this case: ARR = 22% − 12% = 10%; NNT = 1/ARR; NNT = 1/0.1 = 10.

60. **E.** No further action needed. Interpret a ⊕ test for TB. The PPD skin test is a screening test for latent TB infxn. Its results are based upon the pt's characteristics and the size of induration. Greater than 15 mm is the cut-off size for a ⊕ test in the general popula-tion. Greater than 10mm is the cut-off size for a ⊕ test for peo-ple who work in health care settings or who have chronic illness. Greater than 5 mm is the cut off for a ⊕ test in immunocompro-mised hosts. The pt's induration is 7 mm which would fall below the 10 mm cut off for a health care worker, therefore no action is needed. Chest radiograph and sputum culture for AFB would only be ordered if the pt's Hx and Sx were suspicious for TB.

Isoniazid for 9 mo is Tx for latent TB. Isoniazid, rifampin, ethambutol, and pyrazinamide is Tx for active TB infxn.

61. **A.** Order an upper endoscopy. Recognize alarming Sx in pts with dyspepsia. The DDx for pts with dyspepsia is broad and includes ulcers, reflux, and malignancy. Pts >65 who have Sx such as weight loss are at ↑ risk for malignancy and peptic ulcer dz and should be referred for endoscopy without delay. This pt falls in this category given her weight loss. *H. pylori* is strongly associated with peptic ulcer dz; testing for its presence should be done in the setting of known ulcers. *H. pylori* in the absence of an ulcer does not warrant Tx; an endoscopy would be needed first to confirm an ulcer. Empiric Tx with PPIs is indicated in dyspepsia without alarm Sx such as weight loss. Stopping indomethacin is advisable if the pt has an ulcer. Metoprolol is not known to cause upper GI disorders.

62. **D.** Advise him to exercise. Know the indications to initiate Tx in essential HTN. According to the JNC-7 (Joint National Committee on Prevention-Seventh Report) criteria, HTN is defined as a BP greater than 140/90 in a healthy pt without diabetes, renal dz, or underlying cardiac dz. This pt does not meet criteria for HTN, however he does have pre-HTN and a discussion about lifestyle modification may slow his progression towards HTN. Starting medications for HTN is only indicated if the BP is elevated, and a pt has failed lifestyle modification. While a potassium-rich diet has been shown to ↓ BP, potassium supplements have not.

63. **C.** Endoscopic Retrograde Cholangiopancreatography (ERCP). Know the Tx for ascending cholangitis. Cholangitis results from obstruction in the biliary tree leading to a bacterial infxn. Relief of the obstruction via ERCP will decompress the biliary tree by removing gallstones or strictures. Cholangitis is a medical emergency that causes sepsis, jaundice, and RUQ pain. Cholecysectomy is the Tx of choice for cholecystitis; in cholangitis the problem is in the common bile duct, so removing the gallbladder will not solve the problem. CT scan is not necessary in this case since the Utz examination confirms the common bile duct dilation. IV fluids will not provide a definitive Tx for the pt's underlying problem.

64. **A.** This pt has Wernicke's aphasia and, with weakness on the right, has a stroke involving the left temporal lobe. His prior TIA also involved the left (contralateral to affected side) side of

the brain. This would suggest an embolic phenomena and with carotid bruits present; the most likely source would be the carotid artery. Carotid Utz would identify significant stenosis or clot. CT scans of the chest, abdomen, or pelvis are not likely to identify the source of this pt's stroke. Neither the hemoglobin A1c, INR, or ESR would identify the source of the pt's stroke.

65. A. After initial unsuccessful FNA, the most appropriate step would be core Bx given her age. If the pt were younger (<35 yrs old) and no FHx, reassurance and close follow up could be considered. CT scans are not indicated in evaluation of a breast mass. No Dx has been established, so chemotherapy would be inappropriate. After the initial failed FNA, performing a repeat FNA is unlikely to be helpful.

66. B. tPA can be administered to treat embolic stroke, but the presence of hemorrhage is an absolute contraindication and must be excluded prior to administration of the drug. Based on the rapidity with which it can be obtained and the sensitivity for detecting hemorrhage, a noncontrast head CT is the study of choice. A carotid Utz is part of the diagnostic work-up for a suspected embolic stroke, but it is not relevant to determining tPA candidacy. An EEG is used for diagnostic evaluation of a pt who presents with Sx of stroke to rule out a seizure if the history or exam suggests that possibility. This pt does not exhibit any signs of seizure. An LP is not routinely performed prior to administering tPA. Time is important for tPA use, and an MRI typically is not available for evaluation in the acute setting. In addition, the test itself will take longer to complete.

67. D. Down's syndrome pts are at increased risk of a few conditions, and it is increasingly important to be aware of these as the life expectancy continues to increase. This pt has Si/Sx suggestive of a hematologic malignancy, and Down's syndrome pts are at ↑ risk of leukemia. A bone marrow Bx must be performed to confirm the Dx. Down's syndrome pts are also at ↑ risk of cardiac defects, however a cardiac defect would not explain fever or pancytopenia. Karotyping is used to identify chromosomal abnormalities and has no role in diagnosing the current complaints. An MRI could be considered for evaluation of the pt's confusion, but is unlikely to shed light on the cause of the cytopenias. A PT/PTT may reveal evidence of DIC, consistent with acute myelogenous leukemia, but a bone marrow Bx would need to be conducted to confirm the Dx.

68. C. A tetanus booster is required again at 11–16 yrs old and then should be given every 10 yrs. None of the other vaccinations are required after the age of 6 yrs if the pt is healthy and has a nml immune system. Routine screening by tuberculin skin testing is not indicated for healthy children.

69. E. Lyme dz is transmitted via tick bite. Prevention can occur if steps are taken to limit exposure and monitoring during times of high transmission. Using DEET will decrease tick exposure due to its repellant properties. Pts should be encouraged to wear long pants as this will decrease the likelihood of tick bites. If possible, pant legs should be tucked into boots or shoes, preventing further chance of tick exposure. Permethrin is used for preventative purposes prior to tick bites. Tx after tick bites requires monitoring the bite site and possible oral or IV antibiotics.

70. B. This pt has two potential emergencies—an intracranial bleed and hip fracture. He will need to have evaluation of his head injuries prior to any Tx for the left hip (if the hip does need surgery, the pt will need DVT prophylaxis postop). The elevated INR increases this pt's risk of intracranial bleeding and his mental status indicates possible Sx related to this condition. The most likely cause of his bleed is due to trauma and given the time of presentation from his fall, a subdural bleed is most likely. This can be evaluated with the CT of the head. An angiogram can be used to identify bleeding AVMs or berry aneurysms, which are not likely the cause of the pt's current problem. A hip x-ray should be performed, but the possibility of a head bleed takes precedence. A lumbar puncture can demonstrate evidence of a subarachnoid bleed by the presence of xanthochromia. However, an LP would be contraindicated given the pt's INR, and would also be contraindicated without first obtaining a noncontrast CT scan to rule out impending herniation given the pt's altered mental status. An MRI takes too long to complete; CT is the test of choice.

71. E. Ischemic heart dz is the leading cause of death and knowing the risk factors is important in assessing pt's risk and potential Tx. This pt is a smoker and that is one of the major risks for heart dz. His BP is also above nml, and this would be another risk factor. In addition, his LDL cholesterol is elevated and he has a total cholesterol/HDL ratio above 5.0. Alcohol is not a risk factor for coronary artery dz. This pt has a fasting blood sugar which would not be considered diagnostic of diabetes mellitus (>125). Further testing would be required to make this Dx.

72. E. This pt is presenting with Sx concerning for multiple sclerosis. The pt lives in a northern climate, which increases his risk. The Sx involving his hands are relapsing, another hallmark of MS, and both eye and hand Sx suggest neurologic pathology. The CSF can be sent for protein electrophoresis to look for oligoclonal bands, which would support the Dx. The pt's Sx are not consistent with a CNS malignancy, which would present with headache and signs of elevated intracranial pressure, so cytology is unlikely to be helpful. There is no evidence of infxn. Pt has had no fever and has had a course of illness which is too long for meningitis or encephalitis. Also the waxing and waning character of the illness is not consistent with infxn. Therefore, CSF glucose, Gram stain and culture, and HSV PCR are not likely to be helpful.

73. E. The pt in question is homeless, has a Hx of being in prison, and has a pneumonia not responding to appropriate antibiotics. His Hx of imprisonment and homelessness are risk factors for TB, and his bilateral upper lobe infiltrates are in the appropriate location for reactivation TB. A PPD test cannot be used to rule out active infxn, and instead is used to screen for latent infxn in aSx pts. Macrolides have excellent pneumococcal coverage. Failure of macrolide Tx for community acquired pneumonia should raise suspicion for TB. Pts with congestive heart failure will have bilateral infiltrates, however, they will usually occur at the bases. No other information is provided to suggest heart failure, which would be less likely in a pt at this age. The pt has a low risk for pulmonary embolus. It would also be an unusual presentation on CXR. Given the pt's age, a malignancy would be less likely. In any event, TB should be ruled out first.

74. A. This pt has fever, malar rash, oral ulcers, possible pleural rub, and elevated creatinine. All of these could be explained by a possible Dx of systemic lupus erythematous (SLE). Her age and gender would also support this Dx. The most specific test to rule-in SLE is the anti-ds-DNA. ANA has excellent sensitivity for SLE, and can help rule SLE out if negative. However, its specificity is low, and it is often ⊕ even in pts without SLE. ESR can but a supportive diagnostic test, but lacks specificity. The PTT is prolonged in the presence of a "lupus anticoagulant" antibody, but the test is not as specific as a ds-DNA. Rheumatoid factor has no role in evaluation of lupus, but is used in the diagnostic work up of a pt with rheumatoid arthritis. The pt's nml joint exam makes this Dx unlikely.

75. **C.** Any pt who presents with Sx of recurrent seizure should have their level of medication checked. This will ensure compliance with medication and also check if therapeutic dosing was achieved. As many of the medications have side effects, compliance can be difficult, especially in younger adults. Before switching medications, achievement of therapeutic levels should be investigated. IV benzodiazepines are used for pts with active seizures. This pt is postictal and would not benefit from this Tx. Ethosuximide is used for absence seizures, which the pt does not have. Also blood levels should be checked before changing medications. An EEG can be helpful in identifying seizure, however, this pt already has been diagnosed and Sx are unchanged. There is no role at this time for EKG.

76. **C.** A pt with a Hx of heavy menses is most likely to have iron deficiency as the cause of her anemia. In this condition, the pt's iron and ferritin are low and TIBC is elevated. The MCV is low due to ↓ hemoglobin production. Elevated MCV's result from inadequate DNA synthesis within the RBC, which is usually caused by folate or vitamin B_{12} deficiency, or by medications (e.g., azathioprim, AZT, etc.). In cases of low vitamin B_{12}; however, one would expect to find increased MMA levels. In anemia of chronic dz, the MCV is nml, and iron levels may be nml to low, with low TIBC levels (option D). Nml MCV and high bilirubin suggest hemolysis as a cause for anemia. The haptoglobin in this condition, however, would be expected to be low. No history supports hemolysis as a cause for the pt's anemia.

Index

Page numbers followed by *f* refer to figures; page numbers followed by *t* refer to tables.

A

AAA. *See* Abdominal aortic aneurysm
Abandonment, 475*t*
ABCDE diagnosis, 147–150, 148*f*, 408*t*, 410*f*
Abdomen surgery, 156–157, 156*f*–158*f*, 159*t*–162*t*
Abdominal aortic aneurysm (AAA), 162*t*
Abortion, 242–243, 244*t*
   chromosomal abnormalities causing, 242
   occurrence of, 242
   risk factors for, 242
   spontaneous, 248
   types of, 244*t*
   vaginal bleeding with, 243
Abscess, 374
   bacterial, 448*t*
   Bezold's, 277
   dermatology, 391
   hepatic, 65
   peritonsillar, 318–319
   retropharyngeal, 319
   subperiosteal, 277
Absence, 378, 379*t*
Abuse. *See also* Child abuse; Drug abuse
   identifying, 480–481
   sexual, 304
Acantholysis, 383
Acanthosis nigricans, 405, 407*f*
Acetaminophen, 463*t*
Achalasia, 158, 163
Achilles tendonitis, 336
Achondroplasia, 484
Acid-base disorder, 128
ACL. *See* Anterior cruciate ligament tear
Acne, 390
Acoustic neuroma, 313*t*
Acquired immunodeficiency syndrome (AIDS), 326–329
Acromegaly, 78
ACS. *See* Acute coronary syndrome
Acting out, 353
Acute coronary syndrome (ACS), 5, 7*t*
Acute dystonia, 350*t*
Acute lymphoblastic leukemia (ALL), 119–120
Acute myelogenous leukemia (AML), 120–121
Acute renal failure (ARF), 68–69, 68*t*
Acute tubular necrosis (ATN), 69
Adenoiditis, 283, 285*f*
Adenoma sebaceum (Angiofibromas), 298*f*
Adenomyosis, 254
Adenovirus pharyngitis, 318*t*
ADHD. *See* Attention-deficit hyperactivity disorder
Adjustment disorder, 365
Adolescence, 305–307. *See also* Child and adolescent psychiatry
   anorexia nervosa, 306
   confidentiality, 306–307
   eating disorders, 306
   epidemiology, 305–306
   injuries, 305–306
   screening, 307
   sex, 306
   substance abuse, 306
   suicide, 306
Adrenal cortical hyperfunction, 82
Adrenal disorders, 80–82, 81*f*
   adrenal cortical hyperfunction, 82
   adrenal insufficiency, 80, 82
   adrenal medulla, 82
   Cushing's syndrome, 80, 81*f*
Adrenal hyperplasia, 260*t*
Adrenal insufficiency, 80, 82
Adrenal medulla, 82
Adrenergics, 443*t*
Adrenoleukodystrophy, 484
Adult respiratory distress syndrome (ARDS), 41, 43, 44*f*, 449*t*
Advance directives, 477
Agoraphobia, 350–351
AIDS. *See* Acquired immunodeficiency syndrome
Akathisia, 350*t*
Albers-Schönberg disease, 484
Albinism, 398–399
Albumin-cytologic dissociation, 376
Alcohol, 363*t*
Alkali agents, 463*t*
Alkaptonuria, 484
ALL. *See* Acute lymphoblastic leukemia
Allergic conjunctivitis, 430*t*
Alport's syndrome, 313–314, 426, 484
ALS. *See* Amyotrophic lateral sclerosis
Altruism, 353
Alzheimer's disease, 379–380
Amaurosis fugax, 369*t*
Amblyopia, 424
Amebiasis, 451*t*
Amenorrhea
   causes of, 257–258
   definitions, 257
   post-pill, 251
   pregnancy causing, 257
   treatment of, 258
AML. *See* Acute myelogenous leukemia
Amphetamine, 363*t*
Amyloidosis, 450*t*
Amyotrophic lateral sclerosis (Lou Gehrig's disease), 381–382
Anal cancer, 183
Anal fissure, 183
Anemia, 109–115, 111*f*, 112*t*, 113*f*, 113*t*, 114*t*, 115*t*, 116*t*, 117*f*
   hemolytic, 116*t*, 117*f*, 290–291
   hypoproliferative, 115*t*
   megaloblastic, 114–115, 114*f*
   microcytic, 109–113, 111*f*, 112*t*, 113*f*, 113*t*
   normocytic, 115, 115*t*, 116*t*, 117*f*
   sickle cell, 112–113, 113*f*, 437
   sideroblastic, 110
   thalassemias, 112, 112*t*, 113*t*

Anesthetics, 442t
Aneurysms, 209–210, 211f, 212f
  abdominal aortic, 162t
  ventricular, 22t
Angina
  pectoris, stable, 3–4, 4t
  Prinzmetal's, 9
  unstable, 5, 6t
Angiofibromas. See Adenoma sebaceum
Angiotensin-converting enzyme inhibitor, 221t
Angle-closure glaucoma, 431t, 438
Anhedonia, 344
Ankle injuries, 336
Ankle sprains, 336
Anorexia nervosa, child/adolescent, 306, 362
Anovulation, 261
Anterior cruciate ligament tear (ACL), 201t
Antibacterials, 443t
Anticholinergics, 443t, 463t
Antipsychotic-associated movement disorders, 350t
Antisocial personality disorder, 354t
Antiviral, 443t
Anus surgery. See Rectum and anus surgery
Anxiety disorders, 349–352. See also
      Separation anxiety
  agoraphobia, 350–351
  generalized anxiety disorder, 352
  obsessive-compulsive disorder, 351, 355t
  panic disorder, 349–350
  posttraumatic stress disorder, 351–352
Aortic dissection, 210, 212
Aortic regurgitation (AR), 31, 32t, 33t, 34
Aortic stenosis (AS), 32t, 33t, 34–35
Aphasia, 369, 369t, 370
Appendicitis, 160t
Apple core lesion, 452t
AR. See Aortic regurgitation
ARDS. See Adult respiratory distress syndrome
ARF. See Acute renal failure
Argyll-Robertson pupil, 426
Argyria, 484, 485f
Aripiprazole, 350t
Arnold-Chiari malformation, 295
Arrest disorders, 238
Arsenic, 463t
Arthritis. See also Rheumatoid arthritis
  monoarticular, 104
  osteoarthritis, 98, 99f
  septic, 105, 107, 286t
Arthropathies and connective tissue disorders, 94f, 95–107, 97f, 99f–101f, 105f, 106f
  Behçet's syndrome, 98
  gout, 104–107, 105f, 106f
  mixed connective tissue disease, 103
  rheumatoid arthritis, 94f, 95
  sarcoidosis, 102, 103f
  scleroderma (progressive systemic sclerosis), 100–102, 101f
  seronegative spondyloarthropathy, 98–100, 99f, 100f
  Sjögren's syndrome, 97–98
  systemic lupus erythematous, 95–97, 97f

Artificial tears, 444t
AS. See Aortic stenosis
ASD. See Atrial septal defect
Aseptic avascular necrosis, 286t
Asherman's syndrome, 258
Asperger's syndrome, 359–360
Aspirin, 463t
Assault, 475t
Asterixis, 377
Asthma, 40t
Ataxia-telangiectasia, 484
Ataxic cerebral palsy, 382
Athetoid cerebral palsy, 382
Athlete's foot. See Tinea pedis
ATN. See Acute tubular necrosis
Atopic dermatitis, 396, 396
Atrial fibrillation, 16t, 25, 27
Atrial flutter, 16t, 25, 27–28
Atrial septal defect (ASD), 299
Atrophic gastritis. See Chronic gastritis
Attention-deficit hyperactivity disorder (ADHD), 361
Audiogram, 314–315
Auricular hematoma, 469t
Auspitz sign, 396
Autism, 359–360
A-V nicking, 437

B

B_1 (Thiamine), 340t, 377
B_2 (Riboflavin), 340t
B_3 (Niacin), 340t
B_5 (Pantothenate), 340t
B_6 (Pyridoxine), 340t
B_{12} (Cyanocobalamin), 340t, 377
Bacillary angiomatosis (Peliosis hepatis), 417
Bacterial abscess, 448t
Bacterial conjunctivitis, 430t
Bacterial tracheitis, 279t
Banti's syndrome, 484
Barbiturates, 364t
Barrett's esophagus, 320–321, 321f
Bartonella henselae, 417
Bartonella quintana, 417
Bartter's syndrome, 485
Basal cell carcinoma, 408t, 409f
Basilar skull fractures, 205, 206f
Bat's-wing shadow, 449t
Battery, 475t
Beckwith-Wiedemann syndrome, 485
Bee/wasp sting, 467t
Behçet's syndrome, 98
Bell's palsy, 126t
Bence-Jones proteinuria, 91
Beneficence, 477
Benign cysts, 267t
Benign positional vertigo, 313t
Benign prostatic hyperplasia (BPH), 330
Benzodiazepine, 364t, 463t
Benzodiazepines, panic disorder treated with, 349
Bereavement, 345
Berger's disease, 74t

Bernard-Soulier syndrome, 485
Beta-blockers, 444t, 463t
Bezold's abscess, 277
Bifid uvula, 293
Bilaterally elevated diaphragm, 451t
Biliary colic, 159t, 168
Binswanger's disease, 485
Biofeedback, 352
Biostatistics, 471, 471t–472t
Biotin, 340t
Bipolar disorder (Manic-depression), 346
Birth defects, drug influencing, 221t, 222t
Bishop score, 238, 239t
Bitemporal hemianopsia, 424, 425f
Bites/stings, 467t–468t
    bee/wasp, 467t
    black widow spider, 467t
    brown recluse spider, 467t
    cats, 467t
    dogs, 468t
    human, 468t
    snake, 467t
Bitot's spots, 430t
Black widow spider bite, 467t
Blastomyces dermatitidis, 54t
Bleeding
    dysfunctional uterine, 258–259
    flame hemorrhages, 437
    gastrointestinal hemorrhage, 179–180, 179f
    intracranial, 370
    postpartum hemorrhage, 239–241
    preoperative evaluation of, 141
    retrobulbar hemorrhage, 442t
    subarachnoid hemorrhage, 308, 310t, 311t
    subconjunctival hemorrhage, 427, 431t
    third-trimester, 245, 245t
    vaginal, 222
Blepharitis, 428t
Blistering disorders, 407–417
    bullous pemphigoid, 410, 415f
    erythema multiforme, 416, 416f
    pemphigus vulgaris, 407, 410, 414f
    porphyria cutanea tarda, 417
Blood dyscrasias, 346
Blood product replacement, surgery, 137, 141–143, 142t
    bleeding disorders, preoperative evaluation of, 141
    normal hemostasis, 137, 141
    transfusions, 142–143, 142t
Blowout fracture, 441t
Blue sclera, 433
Blunt laryngeal trauma, 469t
Body dysmorphic disorder, 358
Boil. See Furuncle
Bone tumors, 91–95, 92t, 93f, 94f, 454f
"Bone within bone" sign, 448t
Borderline personality disorder, 354t
Botulism, infant, 270
BPH. See Benign prostatic hyperplasia
Bradycardia, 24
Bradykinesia, 381

Branchial cleft cyst, 154t
Braxton Hicks contractions, 235
Breast surgery, 184–192, 187f, 188f, 190f, 191f, 193f
    cancer risks, 184–185
    gynecomastia, 184
    mammography, 192
    mastalgia, 184
    tumors, 185–192, 187f, 188f, 190f, 191f, 193f
Breast-feeding, 241
Breech presentation, 239, 240f
Broca's aphasia, 369
Bronchiectasis, 40t–41t
Bronchiolitis, 277
Bronchitis, 125t
    chronic, 40t
Bronze diabetes, 405
Brown recluse spider bite, 467t
Brudzinski's sign, 372
Brushfield spots. See Speckled irises
Bruton's agammaglobulinemia, 486
Budd-Chiari syndrome, 66
Buffalo hump, 80, 81f
Bulimia nervosa, 362
Bulla, 383, 388f
Bullous myringitis, 277
Bullous pemphigoid, 410, 415f
Bunting of costophrenic angles, 450t, 455f, 456f
Burns, surgery, 152, 153f, 153t

C

CABG. See Coronary artery bypass graft
CAD. See Ischemic heart disease
Café-au-lait spots, 412t, 413f
CAH. See Congenital adrenal hyperplasia
Caisson's disease, 486
Cancer, 169, 408t
    anal, 183
    basal cell carcinoma, 408t, 409f
    bone tumors, 91–95, 92t, 93f, 94f, 454f
    breast
        risks, 184–185
        tumors, 185–192, 187f, 188f, 190f, 191f, 193f
    cervical carcinoma, 266
    colon, 181–182
    cutaneous T-cell lymphoma, 408t
    endometrial carcinoma, 264–265
    esophageal tumors, 163
    gastric tumors, 163
    hepatic tumors, 166–167
    Kaposi's sarcoma, 328, 408t, 411f
    kidney tumors, 77
    malignant melanoma, 408t, 410f
    medullary, 89
    neurosurgery for, 206–207, 207t
    orbital tumors, 438–439
    papillary, 88
    parenchymal lung, 45, 46t
    rectal, 183
    renal cell, 77

Cancer (continued)
    respiratory tract, 45–48, 46t, 47f
    squamous cell carcinoma, 408t, 409f
    thyroid malignancy, 88–89
    vulvar and vaginal carcinoma, 266,
        268–269
    Wilms' tumor, 77
Candida, 254, 256f, 422t, 423f
CAP. See Community acquired pneumonia
Capillary hemangioma, 439
Carbamazepine
    bipolar disorder treated with, 346
    birth defects due to, 221t
    seizure therapy with, 379t
Carbon monoxide, 463t
Carbon monoxide poisoning, 376
Carbonic anhydrase inhibitors, 444t
Carbuncle, 392
Carcinoid syndrome, 58
Cardiac disease, pregnancy with, 228
Cardiology, 1–37
    acute coronary syndrome, 5, 7t
    angina pectoris, stable, 3–4, 4t
    arrhythmias, 9, 10f–23f, 24–29
    cardiomyopathy, 31t
    congestive heart failure, 29–30
    EKG findings, 9, 10f–23f, 24–29
    Goldman cardiac risk index, 144t
    hypertension, 1–2, 1t–3t
    ischemic heart disease, 2–9, 4t, 6t, 7t, 8f
    perioperative review of, 144, 144t
    Prinzmetal's angina, 9
    unstable angina, 5, 6t
    valvular disease, 30–37, 32t, 33t
Cardiomyopathy, 31t
Cardiopulmonary resuscitation (CPR), 477
Caroli's disease, 486
Carotid atheroma, 369
Carotid body tumor, 154t
Carotid Doppler ultrasound, 446t
Carotid vascular disease, 216–217
Carpal tunnel syndrome, 197–198
Case control study, 471, 472
Cat bite, 467t
Cataract, 433
Catheterization, 7t
Cat-scratch disease, 417
Cauda equina syndrome, 333, 334t
Causation, 475t
Cavity, 451t, 459f
Cellulitis, 391
Central alveolar hypoventilation.
            See Pickwickian syndrome
Central pontine myelinolysis, 376
Cerebral infarction, 371f
Cerebral palsy, 382
Cerebrospinal fluid (CSF), 372t
Cervical carcinoma, 266
Cervical lymphadenitis, 157t
CGD. See Chronic granulomatous disease
Chalazion, 428t
Charcot-Marie-Tooth disease, 486
Chédiak-Higashi syndrome, 486

Chemical burns, 440t
Cherry-red spot on macula, 378, 437
Cheyne-Stokes respirations, 486
Chicken pox. See Varicella
Child abuse, 301–304, 302f
    burns, 303
    diagnosis of, 304
    epidemiology of, 303
    head injury, 303–304
    reporting requirements for, 303
    sexual abuse, 304
    signs/symptoms of, 303
    skeletal survey, 302f
    treatment of, 304
Child and adolescent psychiatry, 358–362,
        358t, 359t
    anorexia, 362
    Asperger's syndrome, 359–360
    attention-deficit hyperactivity disorder,
        361
    autism, 359–360
    bulimia nervosa, 362
    conduct disorder, 360–361
    depression, 360
    developmental theories, 358t
    oppositional defiant, 360–361
    psychological testing, 359t
    separation anxiety, 360
    Tourette's disorder, 361–362
Chlamydia, 220, 277
Chlamydia psittaci, 53t
Chlamydophila pneumoniae, 53t
Chloasma. See Melasma
Chlorpromazine, 349t
Cholangitis, 125t, 159t
    ascending, 169
Cholecystitis, 159t, 168
Choledocholithiasis, 159t, 168–169
Cholelithiasis, 167
Chromium, 340t
Chronic gastritis (Atrophic gastritis), 56
Chronic granulomatous disease (CGD), 486
Chronic lymphoblastic leukemia (CLL),
        121–123, 122f
Chronic myelogenous leukemia (CML), 121
Chronic obstructive pulmonary disease
        (COPD), 40t–41t, 41
    asthma, 40t
    bronchiectasis, 40t–41t
    chronic bronchitis, 40t
    emphysema, 40t
Chronic renal failure, 71
Ciguatera, 465t
Ciprofloxacin, 443t
Cirrhosis, 61, 64–65, 64t
Clavicle fracture, 335
Cleft lip, 293, 294f
Cleft palate, 293, 294f
Clinical studies, 471–483
    biostatistics, 471, 471t–472t
    study types, 472
Clinical trial, 471, 472
CLL. See Chronic lymphoblastic leukemia

Clonazepam, seizure therapy with, 379t
Clozapine, 349t
Cluster headache, 309t, 311t
CML. See Chronic myelogenous leukemia
CMV. See Cytomegalovirus
Coagulation disorders, 115, 117–118, 118t, 119t
Coarctation of aorta, 301
Cocaine, 363t
Coccidioides, 374
Coccidioides immitis, 54t
Coffee bean sigmoid volvulus, 452t, 461f
Cog-wheel rigidity, 381
Cohort study, 471, 472
Cold-agglutinin disease, 116t
Collagen vascular disease, 285–289, 289t
Collateral ligament tear, 201t
Colon, surgery, 175–182, 177f, 179f
    cancer, 181–182
    colonic polyps, 175–176, 177f
    diverticular disease, 176–178
    GI hemorrhage, 179–180, 179f
    large intestine obstruction, 180
    volvulus, 180–181
Colonic polyps, 175–176, 177f
Colposcopy, 253
Common good, 475t
Community acquired pneumonia (CAP), 52–55, 53t–55t
Comparative negligence, 475t
Computed tomography (CT)
    ground glass opacities on lung, 449t
    MRI v., 446t
    multiple contrast-enhancing lesions, 448t, 453f
    pleural fluid, 456f
Conduct disorder, 360–361
Confidentiality, 476–477
Congenital adrenal hyperplasia (CAH), 84t, 260t
Congenital heart disease, 299–301, 300f
Congenital hyperbilirubinemia, 58, 59t
Congenital hypothyroidism, 290
Congenital pyloric stenosis, 298
Congestive heart failure, 29–30, 449t
Conjugated hyperbilirubinemia, 291, 291t
Connective tissue disorders. See Arthropathies and connective tissue disorders
Consent, 475t
Contact dermatitis, 396
Contraception, 250–251, 251t–253t
Contractions, 222
Conversion disorder, 357
COPD. See Chronic obstructive pulmonary disease
Copper, 340t
Copper wiring, 437
Corneal abrasion, 431t
Coronary artery bypass graft (CABG), 7
Courvoisier's law, 169
Coxsackie A virus, 274t
CPR. See Cardiopulmonary resuscitation
Crabs. See Pediculosis pubis

Craniofacial abnormalities, 293–294, 294f
CRASH mnemonic, 287
Creeping eruption. See Cutaneous larva migrans
CREST syndrome, 101–102, 101f
Croup (Laryngotracheobronchitis), 278t, 280f
Cryptococcus neoformans, 54t
CSF. See Cerebrospinal fluid
CT. See Computed tomography
Cultural medicine, 481
Cupping, 480–481
Cushing's syndrome, 80, 81f
Cutaneous larva migrans (Creeping eruption), 419, 421f
Cutaneous T-cell lymphoma, 408t
Cyanide, 463t
Cyanocobalamin. See B$_{12}$
Cystic fibrosis, 449t
Cystic hygroma, 154t
Cysticercosis, 375t, 448t
Cystinuria, 486
Cysts, 383
    benign, 267t
    branchial cleft, 154t
    dermoid, 154t
    hydatid, 452t
    thyroglossal duct, 154t
Cytomegalovirus (CMV), 272t

D

Dacryocystitis (Tear duct inflammation), 433, 435f
Damages, 475t
DCIS. See Ductal carcinoma in situ
De Quervain's tenosynovitis, 487
Death, 477
Decongestants, 443t
Degenerative disease, 379–382, 380t
Delirium, 348t, 379, 380t
Delivery, 235–241, 236f, 239t, 240f
    abnormal labor, 237–239, 239t, 240f
        arrest disorders, 238
        management of, 238
        passage, 238
        passenger, 237
        power, 237
    Bishop score to quantify, 238, 239t
    Braxton Hicks contractions, 235
    breech presentation, 239, 240f
    initial presentation, 235
    postpartum hemorrhage in, 239–241
    preterm labor, 246–247
    stages of labor, 235–237, 236f
Delusional disorder, 348t
Dementia, delirium v., 379, 380t
Demyelinating disease, 374–376, 448t
Denial, 353
Dependent personality disorder, 355t
Depo-Provera contraception, 252t
Deposition, 475t
Depression, 360. See also Major depressive disorder

Dermatology, 383–423
  blistering disorders, 407–417
  cancer, 408t
  common disorders, 396–407, 395f–399f,
      401f–404f, 406f, 407f
  fungal cutaneous disorders, 422t, 423f
  infections, 390–393, 391f, 393f
  neurocutaneous syndromes
      (phakomatoses), 412t
  parasitic infection, 418–421, 419f–421f
  terminology, 383, 384f–389f
  topical steroids, 390t
  vector-borne disease, 417–418
Dermatomyositis, 405
Dermographism, 397
Dermoid cyst, 154t
Diabetes, 2, 78–80, 310
Diabetic retinopathy, 435, 436f
Diagnostic & Statistical Manual of Manual of
      Mental Disorders fourth Ed.
      See DSM-IV
Diamond-Blackfan syndrome, 487
Diarrhea, 321–325, 322t–325t
DIC. See Disseminated intravascular
      coagulation
Diflorasone, 390t
DiGeorge's syndrome, 487
Digoxin, 464t
Dilated small bowel, 452t, 460f, 461f
Diphtheria, immunization for, 275f, 276f
Dishydrotic eczema, 396
Displacement, 353
Disproportionate means, 475t
Disseminated intravascular coagulation (DIC),
      118t
  postpartum, 241
Dissociative amnesia, 365
Dissociative disorder (Multiple personality
      disorder), 365
Dissociative fugue, 365
Diverticular disease, 176–178
Diverticulitis, 161t, 178
Diverticulosis, 176, 178
Dizygotic twins, 247
DNI. See Do not intubate
DNR. See Do not resuscitate orders
Do not intubate (DNI), 478
Do not resuscitate orders (DNR), 477–478
Doctoring, 476t, 478–481
  cultural medicine, 481
  identifying abuse, 480–481
  interpreter, 481
  interview technique, 476t, 478–480
  trust in patient doctor relationship, 478
Dog bite, 468t
Double-wall sign on abdominal plain
      film, 451t
Down's syndrome, 295, 296f, 379
Dressler's syndrome, 487
Drop attack, 369t
Drospirenone and ethinyl estradiol
      contraception, 252t
Drug abuse, 363, 363t–364t. See also
      Substance abuse

Drug-induced mania, 346–347
DSM-IV (Diagnostic & Statistical Manual of
      Manual of Mental Disorders fourth
      Ed.), 343, 343t
Duchenne's muscular dystrophy, 107
Ductal carcinoma in situ (DCIS), 189, 190f
Due care, 475t
Duodenal ulcer (Peptic ulcer), 57, 161t,
      162t
Durable power of attorney, 477
Duty, 475t
Dyschezia, 255
Dysfibrinogenemia, 119t
Dysfunctional uterine bleeding, 258–259
Dyskinetic cerebral palsy, 382
Dysmenorrhea, 255
Dyspareunia, 255
Dyspepsia, 319–320
Dysphonia. See Hoarseness
Dyssomnias, 367
Dysthymic disorder, 344–345
Dystocia, 237–239, 239t, 240f
Dystonia, 350t

E
"Early repolarization," 21t
Ears, nose, and throat (ENT), 308–319, 312f,
      313t, 316t, 317f, 318t
  Alport's syndrome, 313–314
  epistaxis, 315–316
  hearing loss, 313–315
  inner ear disease, 311, 313t
  Lemierre's syndrome, 319
  otitis externa, 308–310, 312f
  peritonsillar abscess (quinsy), 318–319
  pharyngitis, 318t
  retropharyngeal abscess, 319
  sinusitis, 316–317, 316t, 317f
  tinnitus, 311
  trauma, 468t–470t
  vertigo, 311, 313t
Ebstein-Barr virus. See Mononucleosis
ECC. See Endocervical curettage
Eclampsia, 227t
ECT. See Electroconvulsive therapy
Ectopic pregnancy, 160t, 161t, 243–245
  differential diagnosis of, 243
  signs/symptoms of, 243
  treatment for, 243–245
Eczema (Eczematous dermatitis), 396,
      396, 397f
Eczematous dermatitis. See Eczema
EDC. See Estimated date of confinement
Edward's syndrome, 295
Ego defenses, 353, 355–356
  acting out, 353
  altruism, 353
  denial, 353
  displacement, 353
  humor, 355
  identification, 355
  introjection, 355
  projection, 355

rationalization, 355
reaction formation, 355
regression, 355
sublimation, 356
suppression, 356
Ehlers-Danlos syndrome, 487
EKG findings, 9, 10f–23f, 24–29
acute pericarditis, 22t
atrial fibrillation, 16t, 25, 27
atrial flutter, 16t, 25, 27–28
"early repolarization," 21t
heart blocks, 12t–15t, 24–25
hyperkalemia related, 124t
ischemia, 19t, 26
left ventricular hypertrophy, 18t, 26
multifocal atrial tachycardia, 28
P-QRS-T complex, 9, 10f–11f
rate, 24
rhythm, 24
ST elevation myocardial infraction, 20t
supraventricular tachycardia, 28
ventricular aneurysm, 22t
ventricular fibrillation, 12t, 24, 29
ventricular tachycardia, 11t, 28–29
wandering pacemaker, 17t, 25
Wolff-Parkinson-White syndrome, 17t, 25
Elbow injuries, 335–336
Electroconvulsive therapy (ECT), 344
Ellis-van Creveld, 487
Emergency medicine, 463–470
bites/stings, 467t–468t
ENT trauma, 468t–470t
fish/shellfish toxins, 465t–466t
toxicology, 463t–465t
Emphysema, 40t
Encephalitis, 126t, 374, 375t
Endocarditis, 35–36, 36t, 125t
Libman-Sacks, 35
Endocervical curettage (ECC), 253
Endocrine pancreatic neoplasm, 173
Endocrinology, 77–89
adrenal disorders, 80–82, 81f
diabetes, 2, 78–80, 310
gonadal disorders, 82–84, 83t, 84t
hypothalamic pituitary axis, 77–78
multiple endocrine neoplasia syndromes, 89, 89t
perioperative review of, 145–146
thyroid disorders, 85–89, 85f, 87f
Endometrial carcinoma, 264–265
Endometrioma, 254
Endometriosis, 254–257
Endoscopic retrograde
cholangiopancreatography (ERCP), 446t
ENT. See Ears, nose, and throat
Eosinophilic granuloma, 289
Ephelis. See Freckle
Epicanthal folds, 295
Epicondylitis (Tendinitis), 335
Epididymitis, 192, 194
Epiglottitis (Supraglottitis), 279t, 281f, 282, 282f
Epistaxis, 315–316

Epithelial cell tumors, 267t, 268t
Erb's paralysis, 487
ERCP. See Endoscopic retrograde
cholangiopancreatography
Erysipelas, 391
Erythema infectiosum (Fifth disease), 274t
Erythema multiforme, 416, 416f
Erythema nodosum, 404–405, 404f
Erythematous maculopapular rash, 417
Erythrasma, 393, 393f
Erythromycin, 443t
Esophageal diverticula (Zenker's diverticulum), 163
Esophageal tumors, 163
Esophagus surgery, 157–158, 163
Estimated date of confinement (EDC), 220
Estrogen, 250–251
dysfunctional uterine bleeding from stimulation of, 258
Ethics and law, 471–483
abandonment, 475t
advance directives, 477
assault, 475t
battery, 475t
beneficence, 477
causation, 475t
common good, 475t
comparative negligence, 475t
confidentiality, 476–477
consent, 475t
damages, 475t
death, 477
deposition, 475t
disproportionate means, 475t
do not resuscitate orders, 477–478
doctoring, 476t, 478–481
due care, 475t
duty, 475t
fiduciary, 476t
futility, 476t
good Samaritan law, 476t
health care delivery, 481–483
human dignity, 476t
informed consent, 476, 476t
malpractice, 474, 476
nonmaleficence, 477
persistent vegetative state, 477
primum non nocer, 477
privilege, 476t
settlement, 476t
terms, 475t–476t
wrongful death, 476t
Ethosuximide, 379t
Ethylene glycol, 464t
Evan's syndrome, 487
Evil eye. See Mal de ojo
Ewing's sarcoma, 92t
Exanthem subitum. See Roseola infantum
Exanthems, 274t
Exposure desensitization, 351
Extended care facilities, 482
Extrapulmonary disease, 42t
Extrinsic hemolysis, 116t
Eyelid laceration, 440t

F

FA. *See* Fibroadenoma
Fabry's disease, 487
Facial fracture, 470*t*
Factitious disorder, 356
Failure to thrive (FTT), 292–293
Familial adenomatous polyposis (FAP), 175
Familial polyposis syndromes, 175
Family medicine. *See* Outpatient medicine
Fanconi syndrome, 487
Fanconi's anemia, 487
FAP. *See* Familial adenomatous polyposis
Farber's disease, 488
Febrile seizures, 292
Felty's syndrome, 488
Femoral hernia, 165*f*, 166
Fetal alcohol syndrome, 297–298
Fetal assessment/intrapartum surveillance, 229–234, 232*f*
FEV. *See* Forced expiratory volume
Fibroadenoma (FA), 185–186, 186*f*
Fibrocystic disease, 186–189, 187*f*, 188*f*
Fibroids. *See* Uterine leiomyomas
Fibrous dysplasia, 90–91, 439, 448*t*
Fibrous histiocytoma, 439
Fibrous pseudo-lump, 189
Fiduciary, 476*t*
Fifth disease. *See* Erythema infectiosum
Filling defects in stomach on upper GI series, 451*t*
Fingernail pitting, 396, 395*f*
Fish/shellfish toxins, 465*t*–466*t*
    ciguatera, 465*t*
    neurotoxic shellfish, 466*t*
    paralytic shellfish, 466*t*
    scombroid, 465*t*–466*t*
    tetrodotoxin, 466*t*
Fistula-in-ano, 182–183
Fitz-Hugh-Curtis syndrome, 159*t*, 488
Flaccid epidermal bullae, 407
Flame hemorrhages, 437
Fluid and electrolytes, surgery with, 136–137, 137*f*, 138*t*–139*t*
    common disorders, 138*t*–139*t*
    fluid management, 136
    hydration of patient, 136–137
    physiology, 136, 137*f*
Fluocinonide (Lidex), 390*t*
Folic acid, 340*t*
Folk illness, 481
Follicle-stimulating hormone (FSH), 248–250
Folliculitis, 390–391
Forced expiratory volume (FEV), 41
Forced vital capacity (FVC), 41
Foreign body, 468*t*
Foreign body orbital trauma, 440*t*
Foreign-body aspiration, 279*t*
Fournier's gangrene, 194
Fractures, 196–197, 196*f*, 197*f*
Fragile X syndrome, 295
Freckle (Ephelis), 400
FSH. *See* Follicle-stimulating hormone

FTT. *See* Failure to thrive
Fungal cutaneous disorders, 422*t*
    Candida, 254, 256*f*, 422*t*, 423*f*
    onychomycosis, 422*t*
    tinea, 422*t*
    tinea versicolor, 422*t*
Fungal pharyngitis, 318*t*
Furuncle (Boil), 392
Futility, 476*t*
FVC. *See* Forced vital capacity

G

Galactosemia, 488
Gallbladder surgery, 167–169
    ascending cholangitis, 169
    biliary colic, 168
    cancer, 169
    cholecystitis, 168
    choledocholithiasis, 168–169
    cholelithiasis, 167
Gangrene
    dry, 213, 213*f*
    Fournier's, 194
Gardnerella, 254, 256*f*
Gardner's syndrome, 488
Gas in portal vein, 452*t*
Gasless abdomen on abdominal plain film, 451*t*, 460*f*
Gastric tumors surgery, 163
Gastric ulcer (GU), 56
Gastritis, chronic, 56
Gastroenteritis, 125*t*, 162*t*, 376
Gastroenterology and hepatology, 56–68
    gastroesophageal disease, 56
    large intestine, 58, 59*t*
    liver, 58–68, 59*t*, 62*t*, 63*f*, 64*t*
    small intestine, 57–58
Gastroesophageal disease, 56
Gastroesophageal reflux disease (GERD), 162*t*, 320–321, 321*f*
Gastrointestinal complaints, outpatient
    Barrett's esophagus, 320–321, 321*f*
    diarrhea, 321–325, 322*t*–325*t*
    dyspepsia, 319–320
    gastroesophageal reflux disease, 320–321, 321*f*
Gastrointestinal hemorrhage, 179–180, 179*f*
Gaucher's disease, 488
Generalized anxiety disorder, 352
Genetic and congenital disorders, pediatrics, 292–301, 294*f*, 296*f*–298*f*, 300*f*
    Arnold-Chiari malformation, 295
    atrial septal defect, 299
    bifid uvula, 293
    cleft lip, 293, 294*f*
    cleft palate, 293, 294*f*
    coarctation of aorta, 301
    congenital heart disease, 299–301, 300*f*
    congenital pyloric stenosis, 298
    craniofacial abnormalities, 293–294, 294*f*
    Down's syndrome, 295, 296*f*
    Edward's syndrome, 295

failure to thrive, 292–293
fetal alcohol syndrome, 297–298
Fragile X syndrome, 295
macroglossia, 294
neural tube defects, 297
Patau's syndrome, 295
patent ductus arteriosus, 301
tetralogy of Fallot, 299–301, 300f
transposition of great arteries, 301
tuberous sclerosis, 298, 298f
Turner's syndrome, 295, 297f
ventricular septal defect, 299
GERD. See Gastroesophageal reflux disease
Germ cell tumors, 267t, 268t
German measles. See Rubella
Gestational diabetes mellitus, pregnancy with,
224–225
Gestational trophoblastic neoplasia (GTN),
269
GFR. See Glomerular filtration rate
Giant cell tumor, 92t
Glanzmann's thrombasthenia, 488
Glasgow coma scale, 150t
Glaucoma, 437–438
    angle-closure, 431t, 438
    open angle, 437–438
Glomerular disease, 72–75, 72t–75t
    nephritic syndrome, 73, 74t–75t
    nephrotic syndrome, 72–73, 72t, 73t, 75t
    urinalysis in, 75t
Glomerular filtration rate (GFR), 221
Glycogenoses, 488
GnRH. See Gonadotropin-releasing hormone
Goiter, 157t
Goldman cardiac risk index, 144t
Golfer's elbow. See Medial epicondylitis
Gonadal disorders, 82–84, 83t, 84t
Gonadotropin-releasing hormone (GnRH), 248
Good Samaritan law, 476t
Gout, 104–107, 105f, 106f
Gradenigo syndrome, 310
Grand mal seizure, 378, 379t
Grasp reflex, 369t
Grave's disease, 85, 85f
Gravidity, 219
Ground glass opacities on lung CT, 449t
Group A Strep throat, 318t
Group B Streptococcus, 277
    pregnancy with, 228
GTN. See Gestational trophoblastic neoplasia
GU. See Gastric ulcer
Guillain-Barré syndrome, 376
Guttate psoriasis, 396
Gynecology, 248–269
    amenorrhea, 257–258
    benign, 248–257, 249f, 250t–253t, 255t,
    256f
    contraception, 250–251, 251t–253t
    dysfunctional uterine bleeding, 258–259
    endometriosis, 254–257
    hirsutism, 259, 260t
    human papilloma virus vaccine, 254
    infertility, 261–262
    menopause, 259–261
    menstrual cycle, 248–250, 249f, 250t
    oncology, 264–269, 267t–268t
    pap smear, 251, 253–254
    reproductive endocrinology,
    257–262, 260t
    urogynecology, 262–264, 263f
    vaginitis, 254, 255t, 256f
    virilization, 259, 260t
Gynecomastia, 184

H

HAART. See Highly active antiretroviral
    treatment
Haemophilus influenzae, immunization
    for, 275f
Hairy cell leukemia, 121–123, 122f
Haloperidol, 349t
Hampton's hump, 45
Hand, foot, and mouth disease, 274t
Hand-Schüller-Christian disease, 290
Hartnup's disease, 488
HCAP. See Health care associated pneumonia
Head injury, 200–201, 203t, 204f, 205f
Head louse. See Pediculosis capitis
Headache, 308, 309t–311t
HEADSSS assessment, 307
HEADSSS interviewing mnemonic, 478–480
Health care associated pneumonia (HCAP),
    55–56
Health care delivery, 481–483
    extended care facilities, 482
    health maintenance organizations, 482
    hospice, 482
    hospital personnel, 482
    hospitals, 481–482
    medicare/medicaid, 482
Health maintenance organizations
    (HMO), 482
Hearing loss, 313–315
    Alport's syndrome, 313–314
    conductive, 314
    diagnostic hearing tests, 314–315
    sensorineural, 313
Helicobacter pylori, 320
HELLP syndrome, pregnancy with, 227
Hemangioma, 400–401, 401f
Hemangiosarcoma, 167
Hematology, 108f, 109–124
    anemia, 109–115, 111f, 112t, 113f, 113t,
    114f, 115t, 116t, 117f
    coagulation disorders, 115, 117–118,
    118t, 119t
    leukemia, 119–123, 122f
    lymphoma, 122f, 123–124
    myeloproliferative disease, 119, 120t
    perioperative review of, 145
Hematuria, 329–330
Hemiplegia, 369t
Hemolytic anemia, 116t, 117f, 290–291
Hemolytic-uremic syndrome (HUS), 118t
Hemophilia, 117

Hemophilus influenzae, 53*t*
Hemorrhoids, 182
Henoch-Schönlein purpura (HSP), 75*t*, 288–289
Heparin, 464*t*
Hepatic abscess, 65
Hepatic encephalopathy, 377
Hepatic tumors surgery, 166–167
Hepatitis, 61, 62*t*, 63*f*, 159*t*
Hepatitis A, immunization for, 275*f*, 276*f*
Hepatitis B, 275*f*, 276*f*
Hepatocellular cancer, 167
Hepatolenticular degeneration. *See* Wilson's
        disease
Hepatology. *See* Gastroenterology and
        hepatology
Hepatopulmonary syndrome, 489
Hepatorenal syndrome, 489
Hernia surgery, 164–166, 165*f*, 165*t*
Herniation compressing spinal nerves.
        See Radiculopathy
Heroin (Opioids), 364*t*
Herpangina, 318*t*
Herpes simplex virus (HSV), 273*t*, 327*t*, 375*t*
        vesicle of, 387*f*
Herpes zoster, 126*t*, 431*t*, 432*f*, 433*f*
Hiatal hernia, 157–158
Hidradenitis suppurative, 393
Highly active antiretroviral treatment (HAART),
        328
Hilar adenopathy, 450*t*
Hip and thigh injuries, 198–200, 200*f*
Hirsutism, 259, 260*t*
Histiocytosis X, 289–290, 449*t*, 450*t*
Histoplasma capsulatum, 54*t*
Histrionic personality disorder, 355*t*
HIV. *See* Human immunodeficiency virus
Hives. *See* Urticaria
HMO. *See* Health maintenance organizations
Hoarseness (Dysphonia), 341–342
Hodgkin's lymphoma, 122*f*, 123–124
Hollenhorst plaque, 437
Holt-Oram syndrome, 489
Homocystinemia, 119*t*
Homocystinuria, 489
Homonymous hemianopia, 369*t*
Homosexuality, 365
Honeycomb lung, 449*t*
Hordeolum (Stye), 428*f*, 428*t*
Hormone replacement therapy (HRT), 260
Horner's syndrome, 46, 47*f*
Hospice, 482
Hospital personnel, 482
Hospitals, 481–482
Hot and cold theory, 481
HPV. *See* Human papilloma virus
HRT. *See* Hormone replacement therapy
HSP. *See* Henoch-Schönlein purpura
HSV. *See* Herpes simplex virus
HTN. *See* Hypertension
Human bite, 468*t*
Human dignity, 476*t*
Human immunodeficiency virus (HIV), 326,
        328, 417

Human papilloma virus (HPV), 327*t*–328*t*
        immunization for, 276*f*
        vaccine against, 254
        verrucae with, 405
Humor, 355
Hunter's disease, 489
Huntington's chorea, 381
Hurler's disease, 489
HUS. *See* Hemolytic-uremic syndrome
Hydatid cyst, 452*t*
Hydatidiform mole, 269
Hydrocephalus, 207–209, 208*f*
Hydrocortisone, 390*t*
Hydrops fetalis, 233–234
Hyperbilirubinemia
        conjugated, 291, 291*t*
        unconjugated, 290
Hypercholesterolemia
        CAD risk with, 2
        initiation of therapy for, 4*t*
Hypercoagulable disease, 119*t*
Hyperdense tissue, 445
Hyperemesis gravidarum, pregnancy with,
        228–229
Hyperkalemia, 124*t*, 127*t*, 135, 142
Hyperkeratosis, 383
Hypernatremia, 133, 140
Hyperparathyroidism, 448*t*
Hyperpigmentation, 400–405, 401*f*–404*f*,
        406*f*, 407*f*
        acanthosis nigricans, 405, 407*f*
        bronze diabetes, 405
        dermatomyositis, 405
        erythema nodosum, 404–405, 404*f*
        freckle (ephelis), 400
        hemangioma, 400–401, 401*f*
        lentigo, 400
        melasma (chloasma), 400
        Mongolian spot, 400
        nevocellular nevus, 400
        pityriasis rosea, 401, 403*f*, 404
        seborrheic keratosis, 405, 406*f*
        xanthoma, 401, 402*f*
Hypersomnia, 367
Hypertension (HTN), 1–2, 1*t*–3*t*
        CAD risk with, 2
        causes of, 1
        causes of secondary, 2*t*
        definitions, 1, 1*t*
        malignant, 1–2
        portal, 65–66, 66*t*, 67*f*
        pregnancy-induced, 225–226, 226*t*
        pulmonary, 45
        renovascular, 217–218
        treatment, 2, 3*t*
Hypertensive emergency, 1
Hypertensive urgency, 1
Hyperthyroidism, 85–87, 85*f*
Hypertrophic subaortic stenosis, 32*t*, 33*t*
Hyperviscosity syndrome, 91
Hyphema, 430*t*, 432*f*, 441*t*
Hypochondriasis, 357
Hypodense tissue, 445

Hypokalemia, 127t, 134, 141
Hyponatremia, 132
Hypopigmentation, 398–399, 399f
   albinism, 398–399
   pityriasis alba, 399
   vitiligo, 398, 399f
Hypoproliferative anemia, 115t
Hypothalamic deficiency, amenorrhea caused
      by, 258
Hypothalamic pituitary axis, 77–78
   acromegaly, 78
   prolactinoma, 77–78
Hypothyroidism, 87–88, 87f
Hypotonia, 295
Hypoxemia, 37–39, 38t, 41

I

"Ice-cream scoop falling off cone," 287t
ICF. See Intermediate care facilities
IDC. See Invasive ductal carcinoma
Identification, 355
Idiopathic thrombocytopenic purpura (ITP),
      118t
Immunization, 275f–276f
Impetigo, 390, 391f
Impingement syndrome. See Rotator cuff
      injury
Impotence, 331–332
Impulse-control disorders, 366
   intermittent explosive disorder, 366
   kleptomania, 366
   pyromania, 366
   trichotillomania, 366
Incontinentia pigmenti, 489
Independent practice association (IPA), 482
Infant botulism, 270
Infection, 372–374, 372t, 373t, 375t.
      See also Abscess; Parasitic infection;
      Vector-borne disease
   Coxsackie A virus, 274t
   cytomegalovirus, 272t
   dermatology, 390–393, 391f, 393f
   empiric antibiotic treatment for,
      125t–127t, 128–135
   encephalitis, 126t, 374, 375t
   erythema infectiosum (fifth
      disease), 274t
   hand, foot, and mouth disease, 274t
   herpes simplex virus, 273t
   hoarseness with, 341
   immunization recommendations,
      275f–276f
   infant botulism, 270
   low back pain with, 333, 334t
   measles (rubeola), 274t
   meningitis, 125t, 126t, 372–374, 372t,
      373t
   Mycoplasma, 277
   paramyxovirus, 274t
   parvovirus B19, 274t
   pediatric, 270, 272t–274t, 275f–276f
   perioperative review of, 145

   postpartum uterine, 242
   roseola infantum (exanthem subitum),
      274t
   rubella (German measles), 272t, 274t
   syphilis, 273t
   togavirus, 274t
   ToRCHS, 272t–273t
   toxoplasmosis, 272t
   urinary tract, 325
   varicella (chicken pox), 274t
   varicella zoster virus, 274t
   viral exanthems, 274t
Inferior surface rib notching, 449t
Infertility, 261–262
   anatomic disorder, 262
   anovulation, 261
   causes of, 261
   defined, 261
   treatment, 262
Inflammation, 372–374, 372t, 373t, 375t.
      See also Abscess
   encephalitis, 126t, 374, 375t
   meningitis, 125t, 372–374, 372t, 373t
Inflammatory carcinoma, 192
Influenza, immunization for, 275f, 276f
Informed consent, 476, 476t
Inguinal hernia, 164–166, 165f
Inner ear disease, 311, 313t
   tinnitus, 311
   vertigo, 311, 313t
Insomnia, 367
Intermediate care facilities (ICF), 482
Intermittent explosive disorder, 366
Internal medicine
   cardiology, 1–37
   endocrinology, 77–89
   gastroenterology and hepatology, 56–68
   hematology, 108f, 109–124
   musculoskeletal disorders, 89–109
   nephrology, 68–77
   pulmonary, 37–56
   treatment for infections, 125t–127t,
      128–135
Internuclear ophthalmoplegia, 424
Interpreter, 481
Interstitial fibrosis, 42t
Interview technique, 476t, 478–480
Intestinal lymphangiectasia, 324t
Intracranial bleeding, 370
Intraductal hyperplasia, 189
Intraductal papilloma, 189
Intrahepatic cholestasis, 60
Intrapartum surveillance, 229–234, 232f
   fetal growth, 229
   fetal well-being, 229–230
   genetic testing, 234
   intrapartum fetal assessment,
      230–233, 232f
   isoimmunization, 233–234
   tests of fetal maturity, 230
Intrauterine device contraception, 252t
Intravenous pyelogram (IVP), 446t
Intrinsic hemolysis, 116t

Introjection, 355
Intussusception, 160*t*
Invasive ductal carcinoma (IDC), 190, 191*f*
Invasive lobular carcinoma, 192
Inverse psoriasis, 396
Iodine, 340*t*
IPA. *See* Independent practice association
Iron, 340*t*, 464*t*
Ischemia, 19*t*, 26
Ischemic heart disease (CAD), 2–9, 4*t*, 6*t*, 7*t*, 8*f*
    acute coronary syndrome, 5
    angina pectoris, stable, 3–4, 4*t*
    NSTEMI, 5, 6*t*
    Prinzmetal's angina, 9
    risk factors for, 2
    ST elevation MI, 5–9
    unstable angina, 5, 6*t*
Isoimmunization, 233–234
Isoniazid, 464*t*
Isovalinic academia, 489
ITP. *See* Idiopathic thrombocytopenic purpura
Ivory vertebral body, 449*t*
IVP. *See* Intravenous pyelogram

J

Janeway lesions, 35
Jaundice, 58–61, 59*t*
Job's syndrome, 490
Juvenile polyposis syndrome, 176
Juvenile rheumatoid arthritis, 285–287, 289*t*

K

Kallmann's syndrome, 84*t*
Kaposi's sarcoma, 328, 408*t*, 411*f*
Kasabach-Merritt, 490
Kawasaki's disease (Mucocutaneous lymph
        node syndrome), 287–288
Kayser-Fleischer ring, 377, 378*f*, 426
Keflex, 433
Keloid, 383, 389*f*
Keratitis, 431*t*, 432*f*–434*f*
Keratoconjunctivitis (Sjögren's disease), 430*t*
Kerley B lines, 450*t*, 457*f*
Kernig's sign, 372
Keshan's disease, 490
Kidney, ureter, bladder x-ray (KUB), 446*t*
Klebsiella pneumoniae, 53*t*
Kleptomania, 366
Klinefelter's syndrome, 83*t*
Klippel-Trénaunay Weber syndrome, 490
Klumpke's paralysis, 490
Knee injuries, 201*t*, 202*f*
Köbner's phenomenon, 396
KUB. *See* Kidney, ureter, bladder x-ray

L

Labor/delivery, 235–241, 236*f*, 239*t*, 240*f*
    abnormal, 237–239, 239*t*, 240*f*
        Bishop score to quantify, 238, 239*t*
    Braxton Hicks contractions, 235
    breech presentation, 239, 240*f*
    initial presentation, 235
    postpartum hemorrhage in, 239–241
    preterm, 246–247
    stages, 235–237, 236*f*
Labyrinthitis, viral, 313*t*
Lactase deficiency, 324*t*
Lactation, 241
Lacunar infarct, 369
Lambert-Eaton syndrome, 48, 109
Large intestine disorders, 58, 59*t*
Large intestine obstruction, 180
Larva currens, 421
Laryngomalacia, 284*f*
Laryngotracheobronchitis. *See* Croup
Larynx, 342
Lateral decubitus chest plain film, 446*t*
Laurence-Moon-Biedl syndrome, 84*t*
LBBB. *See* Left bundle branch block
LCA. *See* Leber's congenital amaurosis
LCIS. *See* Lobular carcinoma in situ
Lead, 464*t*
Lead pipe sign on barium enema, 452*t*, 462*f*
Leber's congenital amaurosis (LCA), 490
Left bundle branch block (LBBB), 14*t*, 25
Left ventricular hypertrophy, 18*t*, 26
Legal issues, 474–478, 475*t*–476*t*
    abandonment, 475*t*
    advance directives, 477
    assault, 475*t*
    battery, 475*t*
    beneficence, 477
    causation, 475*t*
    common good, 475*t*
    comparative negligence, 475*t*
    confidentiality, 476–477
    consent, 475*t*
    damages, 475*t*
    death, 477
    deposition, 475*t*
    disproportionate means, 475*t*
    do not resuscitate orders, 477–478
    due care, 475*t*
    duty, 475*t*
    fiduciary, 476*t*
    futility, 476*t*
    good Samaritan law, 476*t*
    human dignity, 476*t*
    informed consent, 476, 476*t*
    malpractice, 474, 476
    nonmaleficence, 477
    persistent vegetative state, 477
    primum non nocer, 477
    privilege, 476*t*
    settlement, 476*t*
    wrongful death, 476*t*
Legg-Calvé-Perthes disease, 286*t*, 288*f*
Legionella pneumoniae, 53*t*
Leigh's disease, 490
Leiomyosarcoma, 266
Lemierre's syndrome, 319
Lens dislocation, 426
Lentigo, 400
Leriche's syndrome, 213
Lesch-Nyhan syndrome, 490
Letterer-Siwe disease, 289

Leukemia, 119–123, 122f, 439
Leukocoria, 437
Leukocyte adhesion deficiency, 490
LH. See Luteinizing hormone
Lhermitte sign, 490
Libman-Sacks endocarditis, 35
Lichenification, 383, 389f
Liddle's disease, 490
Lidex. See Fluocinonide
Li-Fraumeni's syndrome, 490
Limp, pediatric, 285, 286t–287t, 288f
Listeria monocytogenes, 373t
Lithium
    bipolar disorder treated with, 346
    birth defects due to, 221t
Liver calcifications, 452t
Liver disorders, 58–68, 59t, 62t, 63f, 64t
    Budd-Chiari syndrome, 66
    cirrhosis, 61, 64–65, 64t
    hepatic abscess, 65
    hepatitis, 61, 62t, 63f
    jaundice, 58–61, 59t
    portal hypertension, 65–66, 66t, 67f
    veno-occlusive disease, 68
Living will, 477
Lobular carcinoma in situ (LCIS), 190
Loteprednol, 442t
Lou Gehrig's disease. See Amyotrophic lateral
        sclerosis
Low back pain, 332–333, 334t, 335f
    muscle strains with, 332
    red flags with, 333, 334t
    treatment for, 333
LSD. See Lysergic acid diethylamide
Lucent lesions, 445
Lung cancer, parenchymal, 45, 46t
Lung nodules, 450t, 458f
Luteinizing hormone (LH), 250
Lyme disease, 417–418
Lymphangioma, 439
Lymphangitis carcinomatosa, 450t
Lymphoid tumors, 439
Lymphoma, 122f, 123–124, 448t, 450t, 451t
Lysergic acid diethylamide (LSD), 364t

M

Macroglossia, 294
Macula, cherry-red spot on, 378, 437
Macular degeneration, age-related, 435
Macule, 383, 384f
Magnetic resonance imaging (MRI)
    bone tumors, 454f
    CT v., 446t
    multiple contrast-enhancing lesions, 448t,
        453f
Major depressive disorder (MDD), 344, 345t
    pharmacologic therapy for, 345t
Mal de ojo (Evil eye), 481
Malabsorption diarrhea, 322, 323t, 324t
Malignant melanoma, 408t, 410f
Malpractice, 474, 476
Mammography, 192
Mandible fx, 470t

Manic-depression. See Bipolar disorder
MAOI. See Monoamine oxidase inhibitors
Maple syrup urine disease, 491
Marchiafava-Bignami syndrome, 491
Marcus-Gunn pupil, 424
Marfan's disease, 491
Marfan's syndrome, 426
Mask-like facies, 381
Mastalgia, 184
MCTD. See Mixed connective tissue disease
MDD. See Major depressive disorder
Measles (Rubeola), 274t
    immunization for, 275f, 276f
Meckel's diverticulum, 160t
Medial epicondylitis (Golfer's elbow), 335
Mediastinal tumors, 48f, 48t
Medicare/medicaid, 482
Medullary cancer, 89
Megaloblastic anemia, 114–115, 114f
Melanocytes, 398
Melanoma, malignant, 408t, 410f
Melanosis coli, 491
MELAS syndrome. See Mitochondrial
        encephalopathy and lactic acidosis
        syndrome
Melasma (Chloasma), 400
Membranous pharyngitis, 318t
Mendelson's syndrome, 449t, 491
Ménière's disease, 313t
Meningismus, 372
Meningitis, 125t, 372–374, 372t, 373t
    acute, 372
    bacterial, 373t
    cerebrospinal fluid findings in, 372t
    empiric therapy by age for, 373t
    pediatric, 126t
    signs of, 372
    subacute/chronic, 372, 374
Meningococcal, immunization for, 275f, 276f
Meniscus tear, 201t
Menopause, 259–261
    defined, 259
    signs/symptoms of, 259
    treatment of, 260–261
Menstrual cycle, 248–250, 249f, 250t
Mental retardation, 295
Meralgia paresthetica, 491
Mercury, 464t
MERRF syndrome. See Myoclonic epilepsy
        associated with ragged red fibers
        syndrome
Mesenchymal tumor, 439
Mesenteric ischemia, 218
Metabolic acidosis, 129
Metabolic alkalosis, 130
Metabolic and nutritional disorders, 376–378,
        378f
    B_{12} deficiency, 377
    carbon monoxide poisoning, 376
    hepatic encephalopathy, 377
    pediatrics, 290–292, 291t
    Tay-Sachs disease, 377–378
    thiamine deficiency, 377
    Wilson's disease (Hepatolenticular
        degeneration), 377, 378f

Metabolic bone disease, 89–90
  osteomalacia, 90
  osteoporosis, 89–90
  Paget's bone disease (osteitis deformans),
      90
  rickets, 90
  scurvy, 90
Methanol, 464t
MG. See Myasthenia gravis
Microcytic anemia, 109–113, 111f, 112t,
      113f, 113t
Migraine headache, 309t, 311t
Minamata disease, 491
Minnesota Multiphasic Personality Inventory
      (MMPI), 359t
Mitochondrial encephalopathy and lactic
      acidosis syndrome (MELAS
      syndrome), 491
Mitral stenosis (MS), 30–31, 32t, 33t
Mitral valve prolapse (MVP), 30, 32t, 33t
Mitral valve regurgitation (MVR), 30–31, 32t,
      33t
Mixed connective tissue disease (MCTD), 103
MMPI. See Minnesota Multiphasic Personality
      Inventory
Molar pregnancy, 269
Mongolian spot, 400
Monoamine oxidase inhibitors (MAOI), 345t
Monoarticular arthritis, 104
Mononucleosis (Ebstein-Barr virus), 318t
Monozygotic twins, 247
Mood disorders, 344–347
  bereavement, 345
  bipolar disorder, 346
  drug-induced mania, 346–347
  dysthymic disorder, 344–345
  major depressive disorder, 344, 345t
Moon facies, 80, 81f
Moraxella catarrhalis, 53t
Motor neuron disease. See Amyotrophic lateral
      sclerosis
MRI. See Magnetic resonance imaging
MS. See Mitral stenosis; Multiple sclerosis
Mucocele, 439
Mucocutaneous lymph node syndrome.
      See Kawasaki's disease
Multifocal atrial tachycardia (MFAT), 28
Multi-infarct dementia, 380
Multiple contrast-enhancing lesions, 448t, 453f
Multiple endocrine neoplasia syndromes, 89,
      89t
Multiple gestations, 247–248
  congenital anomalies with, 248
  dizygotic twins, 247
  incidence of, 247
  monozygotic twins, 247
  spontaneous abortions with, 248
  twin-twin transfusion syndrome with, 248
Multiple lung small soft tissue, 450t
Multiple myeloma, 75t, 91, 93f, 448t
Multiple personality disorder. See Dissociative
      disorder
Multiple sclerosis (MS), 374, 376
  internuclear ophthalmoplegia with, 424
  retrobulbar neuritis with, 427

Mumps, immunization for, 275f, 276f
Münchhausen's syndrome, 492
Muscle disease, 107–109, 108f
  Duchenne's muscular dystrophy, 107
  myasthenia gravis, 109
  polymyositis, 107–108, 108f
Musculoskeletal disorders, 89–109
  arthropathies and connective tissue
      disorders, 94f, 95–107, 97f,
      99f–101f, 105f, 106f
  bone tumors, 91–95, 92t, 93f, 94f
  metabolic bone disease, 89–90
  muscle disease, 107–109, 108f
  nonneoplastic bone disease, 90–91
  pediatric, 285–290
MVP. See Mitral valve prolapse
MVR. See Mitral valve regurgitation
Myasthenia gravis (MG), 109
Mycoplasma infection, 277
Mycoplasma pneumoniae, 53t
Myeloproliferative disease, 119, 120t
Myocardial infarction, 161t, 162t
Myoclonic epilepsy associated with ragged
      red fibers syndrome (MERRF
      syndrome), 491
Myoclonic seizure, 379t

N

Nägele's rule, 220
Naphazoline hydrochloride, 443t
Narcissistic personality disorder, 355t
Nasal fx, 469t
Neck mass differential diagnosis, 154t–157t
Necrotizing fasciitis, 392
Neer's sign, 198
Neisseria gonorrhea, 220
Nephritic syndrome, 73, 74t–75t
Nephrolithiasis, 76–77
Nephrology, 68–77
  glomerular disease, 72–75, 72t–75t
  nephrolithiasis, 76–77
  renal artery stenosis, 76
  renal tubular and interstitial disorders,
      68–71, 68t, 70t
  tumors of kidney, 77
  urinary tract obstruction, 76–77
Nephrotic syndrome, 72–73, 72t, 73t, 75t
Neural tube defects, 297
Neuroblastoma, 439
Neurocutaneous syndromes (Phakomatoses),
      412t
  neurofibromatosis, 412t, 413f
  Sturge-Weber syndrome, 400, 401f, 412t
  tuberous sclerosis, 298, 298f, 412t, 412t
  Von Hippel-Lindau syndrome, 412t
Neurofibromatosis, 412t, 413f, 449t
Neuroleptic malignant syndrome, 350t
Neurology, 369–382
  degenerative disease, 379–382, 380t
  demyelinating disease, 374–376
  infection and inflammation, 126t,
      372–374, 372t, 373t, 375t
  metabolic and nutritional disorders,
      376–378, 378f

perioperative review of, 144
seizures, 378–379, 379t
stroke, 369–371, 369t, 371f
Neurosurgery, 200–209, 203t, 204f–206f, 207t, 208f
basilar skull fractures, 205, 206f
head injury, 200–201, 203t, 204f, 205f
hydrocephalus, 207–209, 208f
temporal bone fractures, 201, 205
tumors, 206–207, 207t
Neurotoxic shellfish, 466t
Nevocellular nevus, 400
Newborn jaundice, 290–291, 291t
Niacin. See B₃
Niemann-Pick's disease, 492
Night terror, 368
Nightmares, 368
Nikolsky's sign, 410, 414f
Nocturnal penile tumescence, 331
Non-bizarre delusions, 348t
Non-Hodgkin's lymphoma, 122f, 123
Nonmaleficence, 477
Nonneoplastic bone disease, 90–91
Non-rapid eye movement sleep (NREM), 366, 366t
Nonsclerotic skull lucency, 448t
Non-ST elevation myocardial infraction (NSTEMI), 5, 6t
Non-steroidal anti-inflammatory drugs (NSAID), 444t
birth defects due to, 221t
Noonan's syndrome, 492
Normocytic anemia, 115, 115t, 116t, 117f
Norplant contraception, 252t
Norwalk virus, 322t, 324t
NREM. See Non-rapid eye movement sleep
NSAID. See Non-steroidal anti-inflammatory drugs
NSTEMI. See Non-ST elevation myocardial infraction
Nursemaid's elbow, 335
Nutrition. See also Metabolic and nutritional disorders
assessment, 338–340
nutritional supplements, 339, 340t–341t
vitamins, 340t–341t

O

Obsessive-compulsive disorder (OCD), 351, 355t
Obstetrics, 219–248
accelerations in, 231–233, 232f
complications, 242–248, 244t, 245t
contractions with, 222
drug influencing, 221t, 222t
fetal assessment in, 229–234, 232f
gestational week, height of uterus with, 222t
glomerular filtration rate with, 221
intrapartum surveillance in, 229–234, 232f
labor/delivery in, 235–241, 236f, 239t, 240f
postpartum care, 241–242

pregnancy, physiologic changes in, 223–224
prenatal care in, 219–223, 220t–222t
rupture of membranes with, 222
terminology, 219
umbilical cord compression in, 230
uteroplacental insufficiency in, 230
vaginal bleeding with, 222
OCD. See Obsessive-compulsive disorder
Ocular melanoma, 442t
Olanzapine, 349t
Olecranon bursitis, 336
Olecranon fracture, 335
Onychomycosis, 422t
Opaque eye, 433
Open angle glaucoma, 437–438
Open globe injury. See Ruptured globe
Ophthalmology, 424–444
classic syndromes/symptoms, 424–428, 425f–427f
dacryocystitis (tear duct inflammation), 433, 435f
eye colors, 433
glaucoma, 431t, 437–438
medications, 442t–444t
orbital trauma, 440t–442t
orbital tumors, 438–439
palpebral inflammation, 428f, 428t
red eye, 428, 430t–431t
retina, 435–437, 436f
Opioids, 464t. See also Heroin
Oppositional defiant, 360–361
Optic neuritis, 427–428
Oral contraceptives, 250–251, 251t–253t
alternatives to, 252t–253t
contraindications to use of, 251
risks/benefits of, 251t
Orbital cellulitis, 428f, 428t
Orbital trauma, 440t–442t
blowout fracture, 441t
chemical burns, 440t
eyelid laceration, 440t
foreign body, 440t
hyphema, 441t
ocular melanoma, 442t
retinal detachment, 441t
retrobulbar hemorrhage, 442t
ruptured globe (open globe injury), 441t
traumatic optic neuropathy, 442t
Orbital tumors, 438–439
adult, 438
capillary hemangioma, 439
fibrous dysplasia, 439
fibrous histiocytoma, 439
leukemia, 439
lymphangioma, 439
lymphoid tumors, 439
mesenchymal tumor, 439
metastases, 438
mucocele, 439
neuroblastoma, 439
pediatric, 439
rhabdomyosarcoma, 439
schwannoma, 439

Organophosphate, 464t
Orthopedic surgery, 196–200, 196f, 197f,
        199f, 200f, 201t, 202f
    hip and thigh injuries, 198–200, 200f
    knee injuries, 201t, 202f
    shoulder injuries, 198, 199f
    wrist injuries, 196–198, 196f, 197f
Ortner's syndrome, 492
Osler's nodes, 35
Osteitis deformans. See Paget's bone disease
Osteoarthritis, 98, 99f
Osteochondroma, 92t
Osteogenesis imperfecta, 492
Osteomalacia, 90
Osteomyelitis, 91, 126t, 287t, 448t
Osteopetrosis, 448t, 484
Osteoporosis, 89–90
Osteosarcoma, 92t
Otitis externa, 308–310, 312f
    bacterial, 308
    diabetes with, 310
    fungal, 308
    viral, 310
Otitis media, 270, 277
Outpatient medicine, 308–342
    ears, nose, and throat, 308–319, 312f,
        313t, 316t, 317f, 318t
    gastrointestinal complaints, 319–325,
        321f, 322t–325t
    headache, 308, 309t–311t
    hoarseness, 341–342
    nutrition, 338–340, 340t–341t
    sports medicine complaints, 332–337,
        334t, 335f
    urogenital complaints, 325–332,
        327t–328t
Ovarian dysfunction, amenorrhea caused by,
        258
Ovarian neoplasms, 267t–268t
Ovarian torsion, 160t, 161t

P

Paget's bone disease (Osteitis deformans), 90
Paget's breast disease, 192
Paget's disease, 448t, 449t
Palpebral inflammation, 428t
    blepharitis, 428t
    chalazion, 428t
    hordeolum (stye), 428f, 428t
    orbital cellulitis, 428f, 428t
Pancoast tumor. See Superior sulcus tumor
Pancreas disease, 324t
Pancreas surgery, 170–173, 171t, 172f
    acute pancreatitis, 170, 171t
    endocrine pancreatic neoplasm, 173
    pancreatic cancer, 171, 172f
    pancreatic pseudocyst, 170–171
Pancreatic cancer, 171, 172f
Pancreatic pseudocyst, 162t, 170–171
Pancreatitis, 162t, 170, 171t, 451t
Panic disorder, 349–350
Pantothenate. See B5

Pap smear, 251, 253–254
Papillary cancer, 88
Papilledema, 437
Papule, 383, 385f
Paraganglioma, 154t
Parakeratosis, 383
Paralytic shellfish, 466t
Paramyxovirus, 274t
Paranoid personality disorder, 354t
Parasitic infection
    cutaneous larva migrans (creeping
        eruption), 419, 421f
    dermatology, 418–421, 419f–421f
    larva currens, 421
    pediculosis capitis (head louse), 418, 420f
    pediculosis pubis (crabs), 418–419
    scabies, 418, 419f
Parasomnias, 368
parasympathomimetics, 444t
Parenchymal disease, 42t
Parenchymal lung cancer, 45, 46t
Parinaud's syndrome, 424
Parity, 219
Parkinsonism, 350t
Parkinson's disease, 381
Paronychia, 392
Parvovirus B19, 274t
Pastia's lines, 392
Patau's syndrome, 295
Patch contraception, 252t
Patent ductus arteriosus (PDA), 301
Pathognomonic palpable purpura, 289
PCL. See Posterior cruciate ligament tear
PCP. See Phencyclidine
PDA. See Patent ductus arteriosus
Pediatric painful limp, 285, 286t–287t, 288f
    aseptic avascular necrosis, 286t
    Legg-Calvé-Perthes disease, 286t, 288f
    osteomyelitis, 287t
    septic arthritis, 286t
    slipped capital femoral epiphysis, 287t
    toxic synovitis, 286t
Pediatrics, 270–307. See also Adolescence
    child abuse, 301–304, 302f
    developmental milestones, 271t
    genetic and congenital disorders,
        292–301, 294f, 296f–298f, 300f
    immunization recommendations,
        275f–276f
    infant botulism, 270
    infections, 270, 272t–274t, 275f–276f
    meningitis, 126t
    metabolic disorders, 290–292, 291t
    musculoskeletal, 285–290
    orbital tumors, 439
    poisonings, 304–305, 305t
    respiratory disorders, 270–285
    Tanner stages, 271t
    ToRCHS, 272t–273t
    toxicology, 305t
    trauma and intoxication, 301–305, 302f,
        305t
    viral exanthems, 274t

Pediculosis capitis (Head louse), 418, 420f
Pediculosis pubis (Crabs), 418–419
Peliosis hepatis, 492. See also Bacillary
    angiomatosis
Pelvic inflammatory disease (PID), 327t
Pelvic relaxation, 262–264, 263f
Pemphigus vulgaris (PG), 407, 410, 414f
Peptic ulcer. See Duodenal ulcer
Percutaneous transluminal coronary (PTCA), 7
Pericardial disease, 37
Pericarditis, acute, 22t
Peripartum cardiomyopathy, 228
Peripheral vascular disease, 212–214, 213f
Peritonsillar abscess (Quinsy), 318–319
Persistent vegetative state (PVS), 477
Personality disorders, 353–356, 354t–355t
    antisocial, 354t
    borderline, 354t
    characteristics, 353
    clusters, 353
    dependent, 355t
    ego defenses, 353, 355–356
    histrionic, 355t
    narcissistic, 355t
    obsessive-compulsive, 355t
    paranoid, 354t
    schizoid, 354t
    schizotypal, 354t
Pertussis, 278t
    immunization for, 275f, 276f
Pervasive developmental disorder, 359
Petechiae, 383
Peutz-Jeghers syndrome, 176, 177f
PG. See Pemphigus vulgaris
Phakomatoses. See Neurocutaneous
    syndromes
Phalen's test, 198
Pharyngitis, 126t, 318t, 430t
Phencyclidine (PCP), 364t
Phenobarbital, 464t
Phenylephrine hydrochloride, 443t
Phenytoin, seizure therapy with, 379, 379t
Phrenic nerve palsy, 451t
Pick's disease, 381
Pickwickian syndrome (Central alveolar
        hypoventilation), 367
PID. See Pelvic inflammatory disease
Pinching, 480–481
Pinguecula, 427, 427f
Pityriasis alba, 399
Pityriasis rosea, 401, 403f, 404
Placenta abruption, 245, 245t
Placenta previa, 245, 245t
Plantar fasciitis, 332
Plaque, 383, 386f
Pleural effusion, 41, 42t, 43t, 44f
Plummer's disease, 86
Plummer-Vinson syndrome, 492
PML. See Progressive multifocal
    leukoencephalopathy
Pneumococcal, immunization for, 275f, 276f
Pneumocystis jiruveci, 54t
Pneumonia, 52–56, 53t–55t, 159t, 277, 280

community acquired, 52–55, 53t–55t
    health care associated, 55–56
Pneumoperitoneum, 451t
Poisonings, pediatric, 304–305, 305t
Polycystic kidney disease, 492
Polycystic ovarian disease, 260t
Polymyalgia rheumatica, 107
Polymyositis, 107–108, 108f
Poncet's disease, 493
Porphyria cutanea tarda, 417
Portal hypertension, 65–66, 66t, 67f
Port-wine hemangioma of face, 401f, 412t
Post-coital contraception, 253t
Posterior cruciate ligament tear (PCL), 201t
Postpartum care, 241–242
    breast-feeding, 241
    contraception, 241
    depression, 241–242
    immunizations, 241
    lactation, 241
    uterine infection, 242
Postpartum depression, 241–242
Postpartum hemorrhage, 239–241
Post-pill amenorrhea, 251
Posttraumatic stress disorder (PTSD), 351–352
Potter's syndrome, 493
Pott's disease, 493
Power of attorney, 477
PPO. See Preferred provider organization
P-QRS-T complex, 9, 10f–11f
Prader-Willi syndrome, 84t
Prednisolone, 442t
Preeclampsia, 227t
Preferred provider organization (PPO), 482
Pregnancy, 451t
    amenorrhea caused by, 257
    diastolic murmurs not normal in, 223
    disease, 219–220
    ectopic, 160t, 161t, 243–245
    medical conditions in, 224–229, 226t
    molar, 269
    physiologic changes in, 223–224
    test, 219
Pregnancy-induced hypertension, 225–226,
        226t
Premature delivery, 219
Premature rupture of membranes
        (PROM), 247
Prenatal care, 219–223, 220t–222t
    contraceptive history in, 220
    drug influencing, 221t, 222t
    estimated date of confinement in, 220
    first trimester visits for, 221–222
    first visit for, 219–221
    medical history in, 220, 220t, 221t
    obstetrical history in, 220
    pregnancy disease in, 219–220
    second trimester visits for, 222
    third trimester visits for, 222
    ultrasound in, 219
Preoperative care, 143–146, 144t
Preterm labor, 246–247
Preterm labor (PTL), 222

Pretibial myxedema, 85–86
Primum non nocer, 477
Prinzmetal's angina, 9
Privilege, 476t
Progestin, 250–251
Progestin-only pills contraception, 252t
Progressive multifocal leukoencephalopathy (PML), 375t
Progressive optic neuropathy, 437
Progressive systemic sclerosis (PSS). *See* Scleroderma
Projection, 355
Prolactinoma, 77–78
PROM. *See* Premature rupture of membranes
Proparacaine hydrochloride, 442t
Prostate, 330
Prostate cancer, 330–331
Prostatitis, 330
Pruritus, 430t
Pseudogout, 104
Psoriasis, 396, 395f, 396f
    Auspitz sign with, 396
    fingernail pitting with, 396, 395f
    guttate, 396
    inverse, 396
    Köbner's phenomenon with, 396
    pustular, 396, 396f
    treatment, 396
PSS. *See* Scleroderma
Psychiatry, 343–368
    adjustment disorder, 365
    antipsychotic-associated movement disorders, 350t
    anxiety disorders, 349–352
    child and adolescent, 358–362, 358t, 359t
    dissociative disorders, 365
    drug abuse, 363, 363t–364t
    DSM-IV classifications of, 343, 343t
    factitious disorder, 356
    impulse-control disorders, 366
    mood disorders, 344–347
    personality disorders, 353–356, 354t–355t
    principles for USMLE of, 343
    prognosis of disorders of, 343, 344t
    psychosis, 347–349, 348t, 349t
    sexuality/gender identity disorders, 365
    sleep, 366–368, 366t
    somatoform disorders, 356–358
Psychological testing, child/adolescent, 359t
Psychosis, 347–349, 348t, 349t
    diagnosis of, 348t
    prognosis for, 347
    signs/symptoms of, 347
    treatment of, 347, 349t
PTCA. *See* Percutaneous transluminal coronary
Pterygium, 426–427, 426f
PTL. *See* Preterm labor
PTSD. *See* Posttraumatic stress disorder
Pulmonary disorders, 37–56. *See also* Respiratory disorders, pediatric
    chronic obstructive pulmonary disease, 40t–41t, 41
    hypoxemia, 37–39, 38t, 41

    mediastinal tumors, 48f, 48t
    perioperative review of, 144
    pleural effusion, 41, 42t, 43t, 44f
    pneumonia, 52–56, 53t–55t
    pulmonary vascular disease, 41, 43–45, 44f
    respiratory tract cancer, 45–48, 46t, 47f
    restrictive lung disease, 41, 42t, 43t, 44f
    tuberculosis, 48–52, 50f, 51f
Pulmonary edema, 41, 43, 449t
Pulmonary embolism, 43, 45, 451t
Pulmonary hypertension, 45
Pulmonary hypoplasia scoliosis, 451t
Pulmonary regurgitation, 33t, 35
Pulmonary stenosis, 33t, 35
Pulmonary vascular disease, 41, 43–45, 44f
Pustular psoriasis, 396, 396f
PVS. *See* Persistent vegetative state
Pyridoxine. *See* B₆
Pyromania, 366

Q

Quetiapine, 349t
Quinidine, 464t
Quinsy. *See* Peritonsillar abscess

R

RA. *See* Rheumatoid arthritis
Radiculopathy (Herniation compressing spinal nerves), 333, 334t
Radiology, 445–462
    chest x-ray, approach to, 446, 447f
    common findings, 446, 448t–452t
    studies, 446t
    terms and concepts, 445
Raloxifene, menopause treatment with, 260–261
Rapid eye movement sleep (REM), 366, 366t
Rationalization, 355
RBBB. *See* Right bundle branch block
Reaction formation, 355
Rectal cancer, 183
Rectum and anus surgery, 182–183
    anal cancer, 183
    anal fissure, 183
    fistula-in-ano, 182–183
    hemorrhoids, 182
    rectal cancer, 183
Red eye, 428, 430t–431t
    allergic conjunctivitis, 430t
    angle-closure glaucoma, 431t, 438
    bacterial conjunctivitis, 430t
    corneal abrasion, 431t
    hyphema, 430t, 432f
    keratitis, 431t, 432f–434f
    subconjunctival hemorrhage, 431t
    uveitis, 431t, 434f
    viral conjunctivitis, 430t
    xerophthalmia, 430t
5-α-Reductase deficiency, 83t

Reflex sympathetic dystrophy syndrome (RSD), 493
Refsum's disease, 493
Regression, 355
Relaxation, 352
REM. *See* Rapid eye movement sleep
Renal artery stenosis, 76
Renal cell cancer, 77
Renal tubular and interstitial disorders, 68–71, 68*t*, 70*t*
   acute renal failure, 68–69, 68*t*
   acute tubular necrosis, 69
   chronic renal failure, 71
   drug-induced allergic interstitial nephritis, 69
   renal tubular functional disorders, 69–71, 70*t*
Renovascular hypertension, 217–218
Reproductive endocrinology, 257–262
   amenorrhea, 257–258
   dysfunctional uterine bleeding, 258–259
   hirsutism, 259, 260*t*
   infertility, 261–262
   menopause, 259–261
   virilization, 259, 260*t*
Respiratory acid-base differential, 131
Respiratory disorders, pediatric, 270–285
   adenoiditis, 283, 285*f*
   bronchiolitis, 277
   bullous myringitis, 277
   epiglottitis (supraglottitis), 279*t*, 281*f*, 282, 282*f*
   otitis media, 270, 277
   pneumonia, 277, 280
   stridor, 282–283, 283*f*, 284*f*
   upper respiratory disease, 278*t*–279*t*, 280*f*, 281*f*
Respiratory syncytial virus (RSV), 277
Respiratory tract cancer, 45–48, 46*t*, 47*t*
Restrictive lung disease, 41, 42*t*, 43*t*, 44*f*
Retained placenta, 240–241
Retina, 435–437, 436*f*
   age-related macular degeneration, 435
   diabetic retinopathy, 435, 436*f*
   physical findings of, 437
   retinal detachment, 437
   retinitis pigmentosa, 437
Retinal detachment, 437, 441*t*
Retinitis pigmentosa, 437
Retinoic acid, birth defects due to, 221*t*
Retrobulbar hemorrhage, 442*t*
Retrobulbar neuritis, 427
Retropharyngeal abscess, 319
Rett's syndrome, 493
Reye syndrome, 291–292
Rhabdomyosarcoma, 439
Rheumatic fever/heart disease, 36–37
Rheumatoid arthritis (RA), 94*f*, 95, 449*t*
   hoarseness with, 341
   juvenile, 285–287, 289*t*
Rheumatoid lung disease, 451*t*
Riboflavin. *See* B$_2$
RICE (Rest, Ice, Compression, Elevation), 336

Rickets, 90
Right bundle branch block (RBBB), 15*t*, 25
Rimexolone, 442*t*
Ring enhancement, 445
Rinne's test, 314
Risperidone, 349*t*
Rocky mountain spotted fever, 418
ROM. *See* Rupture of membranes
Rorschach, 359*t*
Roseola infantum (Exanthem subitum), 274*t*
Rotator cuff injury (Impingement syndrome), 198
Rotavirus, immunization for, 275*f*
Roth spots, 35, 437
RSD. *See* Reflex sympathetic dystrophy syndrome
RSV. *See* Respiratory syncytial virus
Rubbing, 481
Rubella (German measles), 272*t*, 274*t*
   immunization for, 275*f*, 276*f*
Rubeola. *See* Measles
Rupture of membranes (ROM), 222
Ruptured globe (Open globe injury), 441*t*

S

Salpingitis, 161*t*
Sarcoidosis, 102, 103*f*, 449*t*, 450*t*
Scabies, 418, 419*f*
Scarlet fever, 392–393
Schafer's disease, 493
Schindler's disease, 493
Schirmer test, 430*t*
Schizoaffective disorder, 348*t*
Schizoid personality disorder, 354*t*
Schizophrenia, 348*t*
Schizotypal personality disorder, 354*t*
Schmidt's syndrome, 493
Schwannoma, 439
Scleroderma, 449*t*
Scleroderma (Progressive systemic sclerosis), 100–102, 101*f*
Sclerotic bone lesions, 448*t*, 454*f*
Sclerotic lesions, 445
Scombroid, 465*t*–466*t*
Scurvy, 90
"Sea fan" neovascularization, 437
Seborrheic dermatitis, 396, 397*f*
Seborrheic keratosis, 405, 406*f*
Seizures, 378–379, 379*t*
   presentation, 378
   status epilepticus, 379
   terminology, 378
   treatment, 379, 379*t*
Selective serotonin reuptake inhibitors (SSRI)
   depression treated with, 345*t*
   panic disorder treated with, 349
Selenium, 340*t*
Senile dementia of Alzheimer type, 379
Separation anxiety, 360
Septic arthritis, 105, 107, 286*t*
Septic shock, 126*t*

Seronegative spondyloarthropathy, 98–100, 99f, 100f
Serotonin-norepinephrine reuptake inhibitors (SNRI), depression treated with, 345t
Serpiginous threadlike lesion, 419, 421f
Sertoli-Leydig cell tumor, 260t
Settlement, 476t
Sexual abuse, 304
Sexuality/gender identity disorders, 365
Sexually transmitted disease (STD), 327t–328t
    herpes simplex virus, 273t, 327t
    human papilloma virus, 254, 276f, 327t–328t
    pelvic inflammatory disease, 327t
    syphilis, 273t, 327t–328t
Sézary syndrome, 408t
Shellfish toxins. See Fish/shellfish toxins
Shock
    septic, 126t
    trauma surgery, 151, 151t
Shoulder dislocation, 333–335
Shoulder injuries, 198, 199f
Shuffling gait, 381
Sickle cell anemia, 112–113, 113f, 437
Sideroblastic anemia, 110
Sigmoid volvulus, 161t
Sinusitis, 316–317, 316t, 317t
Sjögren's syndrome (SS), 97–98
Skilled nursing facilities (SNF), 482
Skin elasticity, 487
SLE. See Systemic lupus erythematous
Sleep, 366–368, 366t
    disorders, 367–268
    NREM, 366, 366t
    REM, 366, 366t
    stages of, 366t
Sleep apnea, 367
Sleep walking (Somnambulism), 368
Slipped capital femoral epiphysis, 287t
Small intestine disorders, 57–58
    carcinoid syndrome, 58
    Crohn's disease (inflammatory bowel disease), 57–58, 59t
    duodenal ulcer (peptic ulcer), 57
Small intestine surgery, 173–174, 174f
    small bowel neoplasm, 174
    small bowel obstruction, 173, 174f
Smoking, CAD risk with, 2
Smooth philtrum of lip, 298
Snake bite, 467t
SNF. See Skilled nursing facilities
SNRI. See Serotonin-norepinephrine reuptake inhibitors
Somatoform disorders, 356–358
    body dysmorphic disorder, 358
    conversion disorder, 357
    factitious disorder v., 356
    hypochondriasis, 357
Somnambulism. See Sleep walking
Spaghetti and meatball appearance, 422t
Spastic cerebral palsy, 382
Speckled irises (Brushfield spots), 295
Spherocytosis, 116t

Spinal stenosis, 333, 334t
Splenic rupture, 161t
Splinter hemorrhages, 35
Spongiosis, 383
Sports medicine complaints, 332–337, 334t, 335f
    ankle injuries, 336
    clavicle fracture, 335
    elbow injuries, 335–336
    low back pain, 332–333, 334t, 335f
    plantar fasciitis, 332
    shoulder dislocation, 333–335
Squamous cell carcinoma, 408t, 409f
SS. See Sjögren's syndrome
SSRI. See Selective serotonin reuptake inhibitors
ST elevation myocardial infraction (STEMI), 5–9, 20t
"Staccato cough," 277
Staphylococcus aureus, 53t
Status epilepticus, 379
STD. See Sexually transmitted disease
Steeple sign, 451t
"Steeple sign," 278t, 280f
STEMI. See ST elevation myocardial infraction
Steroids, topical, 390t, 442t–443t
Stevens-Johnson syndrome, 416, 416f
Stings, 467t–468t
Strawberry tongue, 392
Streptococcus agalactiae, 277, 373t
Streptococcus aureus, 373t
Streptococcus pneumoniae, 53t, 373t
Stress echocardiogram, 7t
Stress incontinence, 262, 263f
Stress treadmill, 7t
Striae, 80, 81f
Stridor, 282–283, 283f, 284f
String of beads on renal arteriogram, 452t
String sign on barium swallow, 452t
Stroke, 369–371, 369t, 371f
    diagnosis, 370
    presentation of, 369–370, 369t
    prognosis, 370
    signs/symptoms of, 369t
    terminology, 369
    treatment, 370
Stromal cell tumors, 267t, 268t
Sturge-Weber syndrome, 400, 401f, 412t
Stye. See Hordeolum
Subarachnoid hemorrhage, 308, 310t, 311t
Subclavian steal syndrome, 217
Subconjunctival hemorrhage, 427, 431t
Subcutaneous infection, 391–392
Sublimation, 356
Subperiosteal abscess, 277
Substance abuse, 306
Suicide, 480
    adolescence, 306
Sulfacetamide, 443t
Superior sulcus tumor (Pancoast tumor), 46, 47f, 48
Superior vena cava syndrome, 48
Suppression, 356
Supraglottitis. See Epiglottitis

Supraventricular tachycardia, 28
Surgery, 136–218
    abdomen, 156–157, 156f–158f,
        159t–162t
    blood product replacement, 137,
        141–143, 142t
    breast, 184–192, 187f, 188f, 190f, 191f,
        193f
    burns, 152, 153f, 153t
    colon, 175–182, 177f, 179f
    esophagus, 157–158, 163
    exocrine pancreas, 170–173, 171t, 172f
    fluid and electrolytes, 136–137, 137f,
        138t–139t
    gallbladder, 167–169
    gastric tumors, 163
    hepatic tumors, 166–167
    hernia, 164–166, 165f, 165t
    neck mass differential diagnosis,
        154t–157t
    neurosurgery, 200–209, 203t, 204f–206f,
        207t, 208f
    orthopedics, 196–200, 196f, 197f, 199f,
        200f, 201t, 202f
    preoperative care, 143–146, 144t
    rectum and anus, 182–183
    small intestine, 173–174, 174f
    trauma, 146–151, 148f, 150t, 151t
    urology, 192–194, 195f
    vascular diseases, 209–218, 211f–213f,
        215f, 216f
Sweet's syndrome, 493, 494f
Swinging flashlight test, 426
Sympathomimetics, 444t
Syndrome of tremor, 381
Syndrome X, 493
Syphilis, 273t, 327t–328t, 375t, 426, 448t
Systemic lupus erythematous (SLE),
    95–97, 97f

T

Tachycardia, 24
Tanner stages, 271t
Tardive dyskinesia, 350t
Tay-Sachs disease, 377–378, 437, 493
TB. See Tuberculosis
TCA. See Tricyclic antidepressants
Tear duct inflammation. See Dacryocystitis
Temporal arteritis, 308, 309t, 311t
Temporal bone fractures, 201, 205
Temporal mandibular joint disorders,
    310t, 311t
Tendinitis. See Epicondylitis
Tension headache, 309t, 311t
Teratogens, 220t
Term delivery, 219
Testicular feminization syndrome, 83t
Testicular torsion, 192
Tetanus, immunization for, 275f, 276f
Tetracaine, 442t
Tetrahydrozoline hydrochloride, 443t
Tetralogy of Fallot, 299–301, 300f
Tetrodotoxin, 466t

Thalassemias, 112, 112t, 113t
Theophylline, 465t
Thiamine. See B1
Thigh injuries. See Hip and thigh injuries
Third-trimester bleeding, 245, 245t
Thrombocytopenia, 115, 117–118, 118t
Thromboembolic disease, pregnancy
    with, 225
Thrombotic thrombocytopenic purpura (TTP),
    118t
Thumb sign, 281f, 282, 451t
Thyroglossal duct cyst, 154t
Thyroid disorders, 85–89, 85f, 87f
    hyperthyroidism, 85–87, 85f
    hypothyroidism, 87–88, 87f
    thyroid malignancy, 88–89
Thyroid malignancy, 88–89
TIA. See Transient ischemic attack
Tinea, 422t
Tinea pedis (Athlete's foot), 422t
Tinea versicolor, 422t
Tinel's sign, 197
Tinnitus, 311
Tissue plasminogen activator (TPA), 370
TLC. See Total lung capacity
TM. See Tympanic membrane
TM perforation, 468t
Tobramycin, 443t
Togavirus, 274t
Tonic seizure, 378
Topical steroids, 390t
ToRCHS, 272t–273t
Torticollis, 154t
Total lung capacity (TLC), 41
Tourette's disorder, child/adolescent,
    361–362
Toxic synovitis, 286t
Toxicology, 463t–465t. See also
        Fish/shellfish toxins
    acetaminophen, 463t
    alkali agents, 463t
    anticholinergics, 463t
    arsenic, 463t
    aspirin, 463t
    benzodiazepine, 463t
    beta-blockers, 463t
    carbon monoxide, 463t
    cyanide, 463t
    digoxin, 464t
    ethylene glycol, 464t
    heparin, 464t
    iron, 464t
    isoniazid, 464t
    lead, 464t
    mercury, 464t
    methanol, 464t
    opioids, 464t
    organophosphate, 464t
    pediatric, 305t
    phenobarbital, 464t
    quinidine, 464t
    theophylline, 465t
    tricyclics, 465t
    warfarin, 465t

Toxoplasmosis, 272t, 375t, 448t
TPA. *See* Tissue plasminogen activator
Transfusions, 142–143, 142t
Transient ischemic attack (TIA), 369
Transposition of great arteries, 301
Trauma, 301–305, 302f, 305t
    auricular hematoma, 469t
    blunt laryngeal trauma, 469t
    child abuse, 301–304, 302f
    ears, nose, and throat, 468t–470t
    facial fracture, 470t
    foreign body, 468t
    mandible fx, 470t
    nasal fx, 469t
    surgery, 146–151, 148f, 150t, 151t
    TM perforation, 468t
Trauma, orbital, 440t–442t
    blowout fracture, 441t
    chemical burns, 440t
    eyelid laceration, 440t
    foreign body, 440t
    hyphema, 441t
    ocular melanoma, 442t
    retinal detachment, 441t
    retrobulbar hemorrhage, 442t
    ruptured globe (open globe injury), 441t
    traumatic optic neuropathy, 442t
Traumatic optic neuropathy, 442t
Trench fever, 417
Treponema pallidum. *See* Syphilis
Triamcinolone, 390t
Trichomonas, 254, 256f
Trichotillomania, 366
Tricuspid regurgitation, 32t, 33t, 35
Tricuspid stenosis, 32t, 33t, 35
Tricyclic antidepressants (TCA)
    depression treated with, 345t
    panic disorder treated with, 349
Tricyclics, 465t
Trifluridine, 443t
Trigeminal neuralgia, 308, 310t, 311t
Trisomy 13, 295
Trisomy 18, 295
Trisomy 21, 295
Tropical spastic paraparesis, 494
Truncal obesity, 80, 81f
TTP. *See* Thrombotic thrombocytopenic
    purpura
Tuberculosis (TB), 48–52, 50f, 51f
    diagnosis and treatment, 49–52
    miliary (disseminated), 49, 51f
    1°, 48–49
    2°, 49
Tuberous sclerosis, 298, 298f, 412f, 412t,
    448t, 449t
Tumors of kidney, 77
    renal cell cancer, 77
    Wilms' tumor, 77
Turcot's syndrome, 494
Turner's syndrome, 295, 297f
Twin-twin transfusion syndrome, 248
Tympanic membrane (TM), erythema of,
    270

U

Ulcer, 451t
Ulcerative colitis, 58, 59t
Ultrasound, 446t
Umbilical cord compression, 230
Unconjugated hyperbilirubinemia, 290
Unilaterally cystic renal mass, 452t
Unilaterally elevated diaphragm, 451t, 460f
Unstable angina, 5, 6t
Upper respiratory disease, pediatric,
    278t–279t, 280f, 281f
    bacterial tracheitis, 279t
    croup (laryngotracheobronchitis),
        278t, 280f
    epiglottitis (supraglottitis), 279t, 281f,
        282, 282f
    foreign-body aspiration, 279t
    pertussis, 278t
Up-slanted palpebral fissures, 295
Urge incontinence, 263, 263f
Urinalysis, 325
Urinary incontinence, 262–264, 263f, 369t
Urinary tract infection (UTI), 325
Urinary tract obstruction, 76–77
Urination, burning during, 325
Urogenital complaints, 325–332, 327t–328t
    acquired immunodeficiency syndrome,
        326–329
    benign prostatic hyperplasia, 330
    hematuria, 329–330
    impotence, 331–332
    prostate, 330
    prostate cancer, 330–331
    prostatitis, 330
    sexually transmitted disease, 327t–328t
    urinary tract infection, 325
Urogynecology, 262–264, 263f
Urology surgery, 192–194, 195f
    prostate cancer, 194, 195f
    scrotal emergencies, 192, 194
Urticaria (Hives), 383, 387f, 397–398, 398f
Usher syndrome, 494
Uterine atony, 239–240
Uterine bleeding, 258–259
Uterine infection, postpartum, 242
Uterine leiomyomas (Fibroids), 265–266
Uteroplacental insufficiency, 230
UTI. *See* Urinary tract infection
Uveitis, 431t, 434f

V

Vaccinations. *See* Immunization
Vaginal bleeding, 222
Vaginal carcinoma, 266, 268–269
Vaginal contraceptive ring
    contraception, 253t
Vaginitis, 254, 255t, 256f
    Candida, 254, 256f
    diagnosis, 255t
    Gardnerella, 254, 256f
    Trichomonas, 254, 256f

Valproate
 bipolar disorder treated with, 346
 birth defects due to, 221t
 seizure therapy with, 379t
Valvular disease, 30–37, 32t, 33t
 aortic regurgitation, 31, 32t, 33t, 34
 aortic stenosis, 32t, 33t, 34–35
 endocarditis, 35–36, 36t
 hypertrophic subaortic stenosis, 32t, 33t
 mitral stenosis, 30–31, 32t, 33t
 mitral valve prolapse, 30, 32t, 33t
 mitral valve regurgitation, 30–31, 32t, 33t
 pericardial disease, 37
 pulmonary regurgitation, 33t, 35
 pulmonary stenosis, 33t, 35
 rheumatic fever/heart disease, 36–37
 tricuspid regurgitation, 32t, 33t, 35
 tricuspid stenosis, 32t, 33t, 35
Varicella (Chicken pox), 274t
 immunization for, 275f, 276f
Varicella zoster virus (VZV), 274t
Vascular diseases, surgery, 209–218,
  211f–213f, 215f, 216f
 aneurysms, 209–210, 211f, 212f
 aortic dissection, 210, 212
 carotid vascular disease, 216–217
 mesenteric ischemia, 218
 peripheral vascular disease, 212–214, 213f
 renovascular hypertension, 217–218
 subclavian steal syndrome, 217
 vessel disease, 214–217, 215f, 216f
Vector-borne disease, 417–418
 bacillary angiomatosis (peliosis hepatis), 417
 Lyme disease, 417–418
 rocky mountain spotted fever, 418
Veno-occlusive disease, 68
Ventricular aneurysm, 22t
Ventricular fibrillation, 12t, 24, 29
Ventricular septal defect (VSD), 299
Ventricular tachycardia, 11t, 28–29
Verner-Morrison syndrome, 494
Verrucae (Warts), 405, 407
 human papilloma virus, 405
 verruca plana (flat wart), 405
 verruca vulgaris, 405
Vertigo, 311, 313t, 369t
Vesicle, 383, 387f
Vessel disease, 214–217, 215f, 216f
Vidarabine, 443t
Viral conjunctivitis, 430t
Viral exanthems, 274t
Viral labyrinthitis, 313t
Virchow's triad, 43
Virilization, 259, 260t
Visceral hernia, 166
Vitamin A, 340t–341t
Vitamin C, 341t
Vitamin D, 341t
Vitamin E, 341t
Vitamin K, 341t
Vitamins/minerals, 340t–341t
 B₁ (thiamine), 340t
 B₂ (riboflavin), 340t

 B₃ (niacin), 340t
 B₅ (pantothenate), 340t
 B₆ (pyridoxine), 340t
 B₁₂ (cyanocobalamin), 340t
 biotin, 340t
 chromium, 340t
 copper, 340t
 folic acid, 340t
 iodine, 340t
 iron, 340t
 selenium, 340t
 vitamin A, 340t–341t
 vitamin C, 341t
 vitamin D, 341t
 vitamin E, 341t
 vitamin K, 341t
 zinc, 341t
Vitiligo, 398, 399f
Volvulus, 180–181
Von Hippel-Lindau syndrome, 412t
Von Recklinghausen's disease, 494
Von Willebrand factor deficiency, 117
VSD. See Ventricular septal defect
Vulvar carcinoma, 266, 268–269
VZV. See Varicella zoster virus

W

WAIS-R. See Wechsler Adult Intelligence
  Scale - Revised
Wandering pacemaker, 17t, 25
Warfarin, 465t
 birth defects due to, 221t
Warts. See Verrucae
Wasp sting, 467t
Water-bottle-shaped heart on PA plain film,
  449t
Waterhouse-Friderichsen, 80
Watershed infarct, 369
Weber's test, 314
Wechsler Adult Intelligence Scale - Revised
  (WAIS-R), 359t
Wechsler Intelligence Scale for
  Children - Revised (WISC-R), 359t
Wechsler Preschool and Primary Scale of
  Intelligence (WPPSI), 359t
Wegener's disease, 450t
Wernicke's aphasia, 369
Wheal, 383, 387f
Whipple's disease, 324t
Wide-Range achievement Test (WRAT), 359t
Wilms' tumor, 77
Wilson's disease (Hepatolenticular
  degeneration), 377, 378f, 426
WISC-R. See Wechsler Intelligence Scale for
  Children - Revised
Wiskott-Aldrich syndrome, 495
Withdrawal, drug, 363, 363t–364t
Withdrawal headache, 310t, 311t
Wolff-Parkinson-White syndrome, 17t, 25
WPPSI. See Wechsler Preschool and Primary
  Scale of Intelligence

WRAT. *See* Wide-Range achievement Test
Wrist injuries, 196–198, 196f, 197f
Wrongful death, 476t

X

Xanthelasma, 398
Xanthoma, 401, 402f
Xeroderma pigmentosa, 495
Xerophthalmia, 430t
XYY syndrome, 83t

Y

Yellow eye (Icterus), 433
Yellow vision, 433
Yersinia enterocolitis, 160t

Z

Zenker's diverticulum. *See* Esophageal diverticula
Zinc, 341t
Ziprasidone, 349t

DAVID WEBER

MORE THAN

HONOR

DAVID DRAKE

S. M. STIRLING

BAEN

A Baen Books Original

Baen Publishing Enterprises
P.O. Box 1403
Riverdale, NY 10471

ISBN: 0-671-87857-3

Cover art by David Mattingly

First printing, January 1998

Distributed by Simon & Schuster
1230 Avenue of the Americas
New York, NY 10020

Typeset by Windhaven Press, Auburn, NH
Printed in the United States of America

Contents

A *Beautiful Friendship*, by David Weber 1

A *Grand Tour*, by David Drake 133

A *Whiff of Grapeshot*, by S. M. Stirling 243

The Universe of Honor Harrington,
    by David Weber 289

A Beautiful Friendship

David Weber

I

Climbs Quickly scurried up the nearest trunk, then paused at the first cross-branch to clean his sticky true-hands and hand-feet with fastidious care. He *hated* crossing between trees now that the cold days were passing into those of mud. Not that he was particularly fond of snow, either, he admitted with a bleek of laughter, but at least it melted out of his fur—eventually—instead of forming gluey clots that dried hard as rock. Still, there *were* compensations to warming weather, and he sniffed appreciatively at the breeze that rustled the furled buds just beginning to fringe the all-but-bare branches. Under most circumstances, he would have climbed all the way to the top to luxuriate in the wind fingers ruffling his coat, but he had other things on his mind today.

He finished grooming himself, then rose on his rear legs in the angle of the cross-branch and trunk to scan his surroundings with grass-green eyes. None of the two-legs were in sight, but that meant little; two-legs were full of surprises. Climbs Quickly's own Bright Water Clan had seen little of them until lately, but other clans had observed them for twelve full turnings of the seasons, and it was obvious they had tricks the People had never mastered. Among those was some way to keep watch from far away— so far, indeed, that the People could neither hear nor taste them, much less see them. Yet Climbs Quickly detected no sign that *he* was being watched, and he flowed smoothly to the adjacent trunk, following the line of cross-branches deeper into the clearing.

His clan had not been too apprehensive when the first flying thing arrived and the two-legs emerged to create the clearing, for the clans whose territory had already been invaded had warned them of what to expect. The two-legs could be dangerous, and they kept *changing* things, but they weren't like death fangs or snow hunters, who all too often killed randomly or for pleasure, and scouts and hunters like Climbs Quickly had watched that first handful of two-legs from the cover of the frost-bright leaves, perched high in the trees. The newcomers had spread out carrying strange things—some that glittered or blinked flashing lights and others that stood on tall, skinny legs—which they moved from place to place and peered through, and then they'd driven stakes of some equally strange not-wood into the ground at intervals. The Bright Water memory singers had sung back through the songs from other clans and decided that the things they peered through were tools of some sort. Climbs Quickly couldn't argue their conclusion, yet the two-leg tools were as different from the hand axes and knives the People made as the substance from which they were made was unlike the flint, wood, and bone the People used.

All of which explained why the two-legs must be watched most carefully . . . and secretly. Small as the People were, they were quick and clever, and their axes and knives and use of fire let them accomplish things larger but less clever creatures could not. Yet the shortest two-leg stood more than two People-lengths in height. Even if their tools had been no better than the People's (and Climbs Quickly knew they were much, *much* better) their greater size would have made them far more effective. And if there was no sign that the two-legs intended to threaten the People, there was also no sign they did *not*, so no doubt it was fortunate they were so easy to spy upon.

Climbs Quickly slowed as he reached the final cross-branch. He sat for long, still moments, cream and gray coat blending into invisibility against trunks and branches veiled in a fine spray of tight green buds, motionless but for a single true-hand which groomed his whiskers reflexively. He listened carefully, with ears and thoughts alike, and those ears pricked as he tasted the faint mind glow that indicated the presence of two-legs. It wasn't the clear, bright communication it would have been from one of the People, for the two-legs appeared to be mind-blind, yet there was something . . . nice about it. Which was odd, for whatever else they were, the two-legs were *very* unlike the People. The memory singers of every clan had sent their songs sweeping far and wide when the two-legs first appeared twelve season-turnings back. They'd sought any song of any other clan which might tell them something—*anything*—about these strange creatures and whence they had come . . . or at least why.

No one had been able to answer those questions, yet the memory singers of the Blue Mountain Dancing Clan and the Fire Runs Fast Clan had remembered a very old song—one which went back almost two hundred turnings. The song offered no clue to the two-legs' origins or purpose, but it did tell of the very first time the People had ever seen two-legs and how the long ago scout who'd brought it back to his singers had seen their egg-shaped silver thing come down out of the very sky in light and fire and a sound more terrible than any thunder.

That had been enough to send the People of that time scurrying into hiding, and they'd watched from the shadows and leaves—much as Climbs Quickly did now. The first scout to see the masters of that silver egg emerge from it had been joined by others, set to watch the fascinating creatures from a safe distance, but no one had approached the intruders. Perhaps they might have, had not a death fang attempted to eat one of the two-legs.

People didn't like death fangs. The huge creatures looked much like outsized People, but unlike People, they were far from clever. Not that something their size really *needed* to be clever. Death fangs were the biggest, strongest, most deadly hunters in all the world. Unlike People, they often killed for the sheer pleasure of it, and they feared nothing that lived . . . except the People. They never passed up the opportunity to eat a single scout or hunter if they happened across one stupid enough to be caught on the ground, but even death fangs avoided the heart of any clan's range. Individual size meant little when an entire clan swarmed down from the trees to attack.

Yet the death fang who attacked one of the two-legs had discovered something new to fear. None of the watching People had ever heard anything like the ear shattering "*Craaack!*" from the tubular thing the two-leg carried, but the charging death fang had suddenly somersaulted end-for-end, crashed to the ground, and lain still, with a bloody hole blown clear through it.

Once they got over their immediate shock, the watching scouts had taken a fierce delight in the death fang's fate, but anything that could kill a death fang with a single bark could certainly do the same to one of the People, and so the decision had been made to avoid the two-legs until the watchers learned more about them. Unfortunately, the scouts were still watching from hiding when, after perhaps a quarter turning, they dismantled the strange, square living places in which they had dwelt, went back into their egg, and disappeared once more into the sky.

All of that had been long, long ago, and Climbs Quickly regretted that no more had been learned of them before they left. He understood the need for caution, yet he wished the Blue Mountain

Dancing scouts had been just a *little* less careful. Perhaps then the People might have been able to decide what the two-legs wanted—or what the People should do about them—between their first arrival and their reappearance.

Personally, Climbs Quickly thought those first two-legs had been scouts, as he himself was. Certainly it would have made sense for the two-legs to send scouts ahead; any clan did the same when expanding or changing its range. Yet if that was the case, why had the rest of their clan delayed so long before following them? And why did the two-legs spread themselves so thinly? The living place in the clearing he'd come to watch had required great labor by over a dozen two-legs to create, even with their clever tools, and it was large enough for a full clan. Yet its builders had simply gone away when they finished. It had stood completely empty for over ten days, and even now it housed only three of the two-legs, one of them—unless Climbs Quickly was mistaken—but a youngling. He sometimes wondered what had happened to the youngling's litter mates, but the important point was that the way in which the two-legs dispersed their living places must surely deprive them of any communication with their fellows.

That was one reason many of the watchers believed two-legs were unlike People in *all* ways, not just their size and shape and tools. It was the ability to communicate with their fellows which made People *people*, after all. Only unthinking creatures—like the death fangs, or the snow hunters, or those upon whom the People themselves preyed—lived sealed within themselves, so if the two-legs were not only mind-blind but chose to avoid even their own kind, they could not be people. But Climbs Quickly disagreed. He couldn't fully explain why, even to himself, yet he was convinced the two-legs were, in fact, people—of a sort, at least. They fascinated him, and he'd listened again and again to the song of the first two-legs and their egg, both in an effort to understand what it was they'd wanted and because even now that song carried overtones of something he thought he had tasted from the two-legs *he* spied upon.

Unfortunately, the song had been worn smooth by too many singers before Sings Truly first sang it for Bright Water Clan. That often happened to older songs or those which had been relayed for great distances, and *this* song was both ancient and from far away. Though its images remained clear and sharp, they had been subtly shaped and shadowed by all the singers who had come before Sings Truly. Climbs Quickly knew what the two-legs of the song had *done*, but he knew nothing about *why* they'd done it, and the interplay of so many singers' minds had blurred any mind glow the long ago watchers might have tasted.

Climbs Quickly had shared what he thought he'd picked up from "his" two-legs only with Sings Truly. It was his duty to report to the memory singers, of course, and so he had. But he'd implored Sings Truly to keep his suspicions only in her own song for now, for some of the other scouts would have laughed uproariously at them. Sings Truly hadn't laughed, but neither had she rushed to agree with

him, and he knew she longed to travel in person
to the Blue Mountain Dancing or Fire Runs Fast
Clan's range to receive the original song from their
senior singers. But that was out of the question.
Singers were the core of any clan, the storehouse
of memory and dispensers of wisdom. They were
always female, and their loss could not be risked,
whatever Sings Truly might want. Unless a clan was
fortunate enough to have a surplus of singers, it
must protect its potential supply of replacements
by denying them more dangerous tasks. Climbs
Quickly understood that, but he found its implications a bit harder to live with than the clan's other
scouts and hunters did. There could be disadvantages to being a memory singer's brother when she
chose to sulk over the freedoms her role denied her
. . . and allowed *him*.

Climbs Quickly gave another soft chitter of laughter (it was safe enough; Sings Truly was too far away
to taste his thoughts), then crept stealthily out to
the last trunk. He climbed easily to its highest fork
and settled down on the comfortable pad of leaves
and branches. The cold days' ravages required a few
repairs, but there was no hurry. It remained ser-
viceable, and it would be many days yet before the
slowly budding leaves could provide the needed
materials, anyway.

In a way, he would be unhappy when the leaves
did open. In their absence, bright sunlight spilled
through the thin upper branches, pouring down with
gentle warmth, and he stretched out on his belly
with a sigh of pleasure. He folded his true-hands
under his chin and settled himself for a long wait.

Scouts learned early to be patient. If they needed help with that lesson, there were teachers enough—from falls to hungry death fangs—to drive it home. Climbs Quickly had never needed such instruction, which, even more than his relationship to Sings Truly, was why he was second only to Short Tail, Bright Water Clan's chief scout . . . and why he'd been chosen to keep watch on these two-legs since their arrival.

So now he waited, motionless in the warm sunlight, and watched the sharp-topped stone living place the two-legs had built in the center of the clearing.

II

"I mean it, Stephanie!" Richard Harrington said. "I don't want you wandering off into those woods again without me or your mom along. Is that clear?"

"Oh, *Daaaddy*—" Stephanie began, only to close her mouth sharply when her father folded his arms. Then the toe of his right foot started tapping the carpet lightly, and her heart sank. This wasn't going well at all, and she resented that reflection on her . . . negotiating skill almost as much as she resented the restriction she was trying to avoid. She was eleven T-years old, smart, an only child, a daughter, and cute as a button. That gave her certain advantages, and she'd become an expert at wrapping her father around her finger almost as soon as she could talk. She rather suspected that much of her success came from the fact that he was perfectly willing to be so wrapped, but that was all right as long as it worked.

13

Unfortunately, her mother had always been a tougher customer . . . and even her father was unscrupulously willing to abandon his proper pliancy when he decided the situation justified it.

Like now.

"We're not going to discuss this further," he said with ominous calm. "Just because you haven't *seen* any hexapumas or peak bears doesn't mean they aren't out there."

"But I've been stuck inside with nothing to do all *winter*," she said as reasonably as she could, easily suppressing a twinge of conscience as she neglected to mention snowball fights, cross-country skiing, sleds, and certain other diversions. "I want to go outside and *see* things!"

"I know you do, honey," her father said more gently, reaching out to tousle her curly brown hair. "But it's dangerous out there. This isn't Meyerdahl, you know." Stephanie rolled her eyes and looked martyred, and his expression showed a flash of regret at having let the last sentence slip out. "If you really want something to do, why don't you run into Twin Forks with Mom this afternoon?"

"Because Twin Forks is a complete *null*, Daddy." Exasperation colored Stephanie's reply, even though she knew it was a tactical error. Even above average parents like hers got stubborn if you disagreed with them *too* emphatically, but *honestly!* Twin Forks might be the closest "town" to the Harrington homestead, but it boasted a total of *maybe* fifty families most of whose handful of kids were zork brains. None of *them* were interested in xeno-botany or biosystem hierarchies. In fact, they were such nulls they spent most of their free time trying to catch anything small enough to keep as a pet, however much damage they might do to their intended "pets" in the process, and Stephanie was pretty sure any effort to enlist *those* zorks in her explorations would have led to words—or a fist or two in the eye—in fairly short order. Not, she thought darkly, that *she* was to blame for the situation. If Dad and Mom hadn't insisted on dragging her away from Meyerdahl just when she'd been accepted for the junior forestry program, she'd have been on her first internship field trip by now. It wasn't *her* fault she wasn't, and the least they could do to make up for it was let her explore their own property!

"Twin Forks is *not* a 'complete null,'" her father said firmly.

"Oh yes it is," she replied with a curled lip, and Richard Harrington drew a deep breath.

He made himself step back mentally, reaching for patience, that most vital of parental qualities. The edge of guilt he felt at Stephanie's expression made it a little easier. She hadn't wanted to leave everyone she'd ever known behind on Meyerdahl, and he knew how much she'd looked forward to becoming a forestry intern, but Meyerdahl had been settled for over a thousand years . . . and Sphinx hadn't. Not only had Meyerdahl's most dangerous predators been banished to the tracts of virgin wilderness reserved for them, but its Forestry Service rangers nursemaided their interns with care, and the nature parks where they ran their junior studies programs were thoroughly "wired" with satellite com interfaces, surveillance, and immediately available emergency services. Sphinx's endless forests were not only *not* wired or watched over, but home to predators like the fearsome, five-meter-long hexapuma (and scarcely less dangerous peak bear) and totally unexplored. Over two-thirds of their flora was evergreen, as well, even here in what passed for the semi-tropical zone, and the best aerial mapping could see very little through that dense green canopy. It would be generations before humanity even began to get a complete picture of the millions of other species which undoubtedly lived in the shade of those trees.

All of which put any repetition of yesterday's solo exploration trip completely out of the question. Stephanie swore she hadn't gone far, and he believed her. Headstrong and occasionally devious she might be, but she was an honest child. And she'd taken her wrist com, so she hadn't really been out of communication and they would have been able to home in on her beacon if she'd gotten into trouble. But that was beside the point. She was his daughter, and he loved her, and all the wrist coms in the world wouldn't get an air car there fast enough if she came face to face with a hexapuma.

"Look, Steph," he said finally, "I know Twin Forks isn't much compared to Hollister, but it's the best I can offer. And you know it's going to grow. They're even talking about putting in their own shuttle pad by next spring!"

Stephanie managed—somehow—not to roll her eyes again. Calling Twin Forks "not much" compared to the city of Hollister was like saying it snowed "a little" on Sphinx. And given the long, dragging, *endless* year of this *stupid* planet, she'd almost be *seventeen T-years old* by the time "next spring" got here! She hadn't quite been ten when they arrived . . . just in time for it to start snowing. And it hadn't *stopped* snowing for the next fifteen T-months!

"I'm sorry," her father said quietly, reading her thoughts. "I'm sorry Twin Forks isn't exciting, and I'm sorry you didn't want to leave Meyerdahl, and I'm sorry I can't let you wander around on your own. But that's the way it is, honey. And—" he gazed sternly into her brown eyes, trying not to see the tears which suddenly filled them "—I want your word that you'll do what your Mom and I tell you on this one."

Stephanie squelched glumly across the mud to the steep-roofed gazebo. *Everything* on Sphinx had a steep roof, and she allowed herself a deep, heart-felt groan as she plunked herself down on the gazebo steps and contemplated the reason that was true.

It was the snow, of course. Even here, close to Sphinx's equator, annual snowfall was measured in meters—*lots* of meters, she thought moodily—and houses needed steep roofs to shed all that frozen water, especially on a planet whose gravity was over a third higher than Old Earth's. Not that Stephanie had ever seen Old Earth . . . or *any* world which wasn't classified as "heavy grav" by the rest of humanity.

She sighed again, with an edge of wistful misery,

and wished her great-great-great-great-whatever grandparents hadn't volunteered for the Meyerdahl First Wave. Her parents had sat her down to explain what that meant shortly after her eighth birthday. She'd already heard the word "genie," though she hadn't realized that, technically at least, it applied to her, but she'd only started her classroom studies four T-years before. Her history courses hadn't gotten to Old Earth's Final War yet, so she'd had no way to know why some people still reacted so violently to any notion of modifications to the human genotype . . . and why they considered "genie" the dirtiest word in Standard English.

Now she knew, though she still thought anyone who felt that way was silly. Of *course* the bioweapons and "super soldiers" whipped up for the Final War had been bad ideas, and the damage they'd done to Old Earth had been horrible. But that had all happened five hundred T-years ago, and it hadn't had a thing to do with people like the Meyerdahl or Quelhollow first waves. She supposed it was a good thing the original Manticoran settlers had left Sol before the Final War. Their old-fashioned cryo ships had taken over six T-centuries to make the trip, which meant they'd missed the entire thing . . . and the prejudices that went with it.

Not that there was anything much to draw anyone's attention to the changes the geneticists had whipped up for Meyerdahl's colonists. Mass for mass, Stephanie's muscle tissue was about twenty-five percent more efficient than that of "pure strain" humans, and her metabolism ran about twenty percent faster to fuel those muscles. There were a few minor changes to her respiratory and circulatory systems and some skeletal reinforcement, as well, and the modifications had been designed to be dominant, so that all her descendants would have them. But her kind of genie was perfectly interfertile with pure-strainers, and as far as she could see all the changes put together were no big deal. They just meant that because she and her parents needed less muscle mass for a given strength, they were ideally suited to colonize high gravity planets without turning all stumpy and bulgy-muscled. Still, once she'd gotten around to studying the Final War and some of the anti-genie movements, she'd decided Daddy and Mom might have had a point in warning her not to go around telling strangers about it. Aside from that, she seldom thought about it one way or the other . . . except to reflect somewhat bitterly that if they *hadn't* been genies, the heavy gravities of the Manticore Binary System's habitable planets might have kept her parents from deciding they simply *had* to drag her off to the boonies like this.

She chewed her lower lip and leaned back, letting her eyes roam over the isolated clearing in which she'd been marooned by their decision. The tall, green roof of the main house was a cheerful splash of color against the still-bare picket wood and crown oaks which surrounded it, but she wasn't in the mood to be cheerful, and it took very little effort to decide green was a stupid color for a roof. Something dark and drab—brown, maybe, or maybe even black—would have suited her much better. And while she was on the subject of inappropriate building materials, why couldn't they have used something more colorful than natural gray stone? She knew it had been the cheapest way to do it, but getting enough insulating capacity to face a Sphinx winter out of natural rock required walls over a meter thick. It was like living in a dungeon, she thought . . . then paused to savor the simile. It fitted her present mood perfectly, and she stored it away for future use.

She considered it a moment longer, then shook herself and gazed at the trees beyond the house and its attached greenhouses with a yearning that was almost a physical pain. Some kids knew they wanted to be spacers or scientists by the time they could pronounce the words, but Stephanie didn't want stars. She wanted . . . green. She wanted to go places no one had ever been yet—not through hyper-space, but on a warm, living, breathing planet. She wanted waterfalls and mountains, trees and animals who'd never heard of zoos. And she wanted to be the first to see them, to study them, under-stand them, protect them. . . .

Maybe it was because of her parents, she mused, forgetting to resent her father's restrictions for the moment. Richard Harrington held degrees in both Terran and xeno-veterinary medicine. They made him far more valuable to a frontier world like Sphinx than he'd ever been back home, but he'd occasion-ally been called upon by Meyerdahl's Forestry Service. That had brought Stephanie into far closer contact with her birth world's animal kingdom than most people her age ever had the chance to come, and her mother's background as a plant geneticist—

another of those specialties new worlds found so necessary—had helped her appreciate the beautiful intricacies of Meyerdahl's flora, as well.

Only then they'd brought her way out here and dumped her on *Sphinx*.

Stephanie grimaced in fresh disgust. Part of her had deeply resented the thought of leaving Meyerdahl, but another part had been delighted. However much she might long for a Forestry Service career, the thought of starships and interstellar voyages had been exciting. And so had the thought of immigrating on a sort of rescue mission to help save a colony which had been almost wiped out by plague. (Although, she admitted, *that* part would have been much less exciting if the doctors hadn't found a *cure* for the plague in question.) Best of all, her parents' specialities meant the Star Kingdom had agreed to pay the cost of their transportation, which, coupled with their savings, had let them buy a huge piece of land all their own. The Harrington homestead was a rough rectangle thrown across the steep slopes of the Copperwall Mountains to overlook the Tannerman Ocean, and it measured twenty kilometers on a side. Not the twenty *meters* of their lot's frontage in Hollister, but twenty *kilo*meters, which made it as big as the entire city had been back home! And it backed up against an area already designated as a major nature preserve, as well.

But there were a few things Stephanie hadn't considered in her delight. Like the fact that their homestead was almost a thousand kilometers from anything that could reasonably be called a city.

Much as she loved wilderness, she wasn't used to being *that* far from civilization, and the distances between settlements meant her father had to spend an awful lot of time in the air just getting from patient to patient. At least the planetary datanet let her keep up with her schooling and enjoy some simple pleasures—in fact, she was first in her class (again), despite the move, and she stood sixteenth in the current planetary chess competition, as well— and she enjoyed her trips to town (when she wasn't using Twin Forks' dinkiness in negotiations with her parents). But none of the few kids her age in Twin Forks were in the accelerated curriculum, which meant they weren't in any of her classes, and the settlement was totally lacking in all the amenities of a city of almost half a million people.

Yet Stephanie could have lived with that if it hadn't been for two other things: snow, and hexapumas.

She dug a booted toe into the squishy mud beyond the gazebo's bottom step and scowled. Daddy had warned her they'd be arriving just before winter, and she'd thought she knew what that meant. But "winter" had an entirely different meaning on Sphinx. Snow had been an exciting rarity on warm, mild Meyerdahl, but a Sphinxian winter lasted almost *sixteen T-months*. That was over a tenth of her entire *life*, and she'd become well and truly sick of snow. Daddy could say whatever he liked about how other seasons would be just as long. Stephanie believed him. She even understood, intellectually, that she had the better part of four full T-years before the snow returned. But she hadn't *experienced* it yet, and all she had right now was mud. Lots and lots and *lots* of mud, and the bare beginning of buds on the deciduous trees, and boredom.

And, she reminded herself with a scowl, she also had the promise not to do anything *about* that boredom which Daddy had extracted from her. She supposed she should be glad he and Mom worried about her, but it was so . . . so *underhanded* of him to make her promise. It was like making Stephanie her own jailer, and he knew it!

She sighed again, rose, shoved her fists into her jacket pockets, and headed for her mother's office. She doubted she could get Mom to help her change Daddy's mind about grounding her, but she could try. And at least she might get a little understanding out of her.

Dr. Marjorie Harrington stood by the window and smiled sympathetically as she watched Stephanie trudge toward the house. Dr. Harrington knew where her daughter was headed . . . and what she meant to do when she got there. In a general way, she disapproved of Stephanie's attempts to enlist one parent against the other when edicts were laid down, but she understood her daughter too well to resent it in this case. And one thing about Stephanie: however much she might resent a restriction or maneuver to get it lifted, she always honored it once she'd given her word to do so.

Dr. Harrington turned from the window and headed back to her desk terminal. Her services had become much sought after in the seventeen T-months she and Richard had been on Sphinx, but

unlike Richard, *she* seldom had to go to her clients.
On the rare occasions when she required physical
specimens rather than simple electronic data, they
could be delivered to her small but efficient lab and
supporting greenhouses here on the homestead as
easily as to any other location, and she loved the
sense of freedom that gave her. In addition, all three
habitable planets of the Manticore Binary System
had remarkably human-compatible biosystems. So
far, she hadn't hit any problems she couldn't find
answers for fairly quickly—aside from the disappearing celery mystery, which was hardly in her area of
specialization anyway—and she had a sense of
helping to build something new and special here
which she hadn't had on long-settled Meyerdahl.
She loved that, but for now she put her terminal
on hold and leaned back in her chair while she
considered the rapidly looming interview with
Stephanie.

There were times when she thought it might have
been nice to have a child who wasn't quite so gifted.
Stephanie knew she was much further along in
school than other children her age, just as she knew
her IQ was considerably higher than most. What
she did *not* know—and what Marjorie and Richard
had no intention of telling her just yet—was that
her scores placed her squarely in the top tenth of
a percent of the human race. Even today, tests
became increasingly unreliable as one reached the
stratosphere of intelligence, which made it impossible to rank her any more positively, but Marjorie
had firsthand experience of just how difficult it
could be to win an argument with her. In fact, her

parents, faced with an endless and inventive series of perfectly logical objections (logical, at least, from *Stephanie's* perspective) often found themselves with little option but to say "because we *said* so, that's why!" Marjorie hated using that discussion-ender, but, to her credit, Stephanie usually took it better than Marjorie had when *she* was a child.

But gifted or not, Stephanie was only eleven. She truly didn't grasp—yet—all that Sphinx's slow seasons meant. The next several weeks, Marjorie estimated, would be marked by long, dark sighs, listlessness, draggy steps (when anyone was looking, at least), and all those time-honored cues by which offspring showed uncaring parents how cruelly oppressed they were. But assuming that all concerned survived long enough for spring to get underway, Stephanie was going to find that Sphinx without snow was a far more interesting place, and Marjorie made a firm mental note to take some time away from the terminal. There was no way she could spend as many hours in the woods as Stephanie wanted to, but she could at least provide her only child with an adult escort often enough for Stephanie's habit to get a minimum fix.

Her thoughts paused, and then she smiled again as another idea occurred to her. They couldn't let Stephanie rummage around in the woods by herself, no, but there might just be another way to distract her. Stephanie had the sort of mind that enjoyed working the *Yawata Crossing Times* crossword puzzles in permanent ink. She was constitutionally incapable of resisting a challenge, so with just a little prompting . . .

Marjorie let her chair slip upright and drew a sheaf of hardcopy closer as she heard boots moving down the hall towards her office. She uncapped her stylus and bent over the neatly printed sheets with a studious expression just as Stephanie knocked on the frame of the open door.

"Mom?" Dr. Harrington allowed herself one more sympathetic smile at the put-upon pensiveness of Stephanie's tone, then banished the expression and looked up from her paperwork.

"Come in, Steph," she invited, and leaned back in her chair once more.

"Could I talk to you a minute?" Stephanie asked, and Marjorie nodded.

"Of course you can, honey," she said. "What's on your mind?"

III

Climbs Quickly perched in his observation post once more, but the sunlit sky of three days earlier had turned to dark, gray-black charcoal, and a stiff wind whipped in from the mountains to the west. It brought the tang of rock and snow, mingled with the bright sharpness of thunder, but it also blew across the two-legs' clearing, and he slitted his eyes and flattened his ears, peering into it as it rippled his fur. There was rain, as well as thunder, on that wind. He didn't look forward to being soaked, and lightning could make his present perch dangerous, yet he felt no temptation to seek cover, for other scents indicated his two-legs were up to something interesting in one of their transparent plant places.

Climbs Quickly cocked his head, lashing the tip of his prehensile tail as he considered. He'd come to think of this clearing's inhabitants as "his" two-legs, but there were many other two-legs on the planet, most with their own scouts keeping watch over them. Those scouts' reports, like his own, were circulated among the memory singers of all the clans, and they included something he felt a burning desire to explore for himself.

One of the cleverest of the many clever things the two-legs had demonstrated to the People were their plant places, for the People weren't *only* hunters. Like the snow hunters and the lake builders (but not the death fangs), they ate plants as well, and they required certain kinds of plants to remain strong and fit.

Unfortunately, some of the plants they needed couldn't live in ice and snow, which made the cold days a time of hunger and death, when too many of the very old or very young died. Although there was usually prey of some sort, there was less of it, and it was harder to catch, and the lack of needed plants only made that normal hunger worse. But that was changing, for the eating of plants was yet another way in which two-legs and People were alike . . . and the two-legs had found an answer to the cold days, just as they had to so many other problems. Indeed, it often seemed to Climbs Quickly that two-legs could never be satisfied with a single answer to *any* challenge, and in this case, they had devised at least two.

The simpler answer was to make plants grow where *they* wanted during the warm days, but the more spectacular one (and the one that most intrigued Climbs Quickly) were their transparent plant places. The plant places' sides and roofs, made of yet another material the People had no idea how to make, let the sun's light and heat pass through, forming little pockets of the warm days amid even the deepest snow, and the two-legs made the plants they ate grow inside that warmth all turning long. Nor did they grow them only during the cold days. There were fresh plants growing in these plant places even now, for Climbs Quickly could smell them through the moving spaces the two-legs had opened along the upper sides of the plant places to let the breeze blow in.

The People had never considered making things grow in specific places. Instead, they gathered plants wherever they grew of their own accord, either to eat immediately or to store for future need. In some turnings, they were able to gather more than enough to see them through the cold days; in less prosperous turnings, hunger and starvation stalked the clans, yet that was the way it had always been and the way it would continue. Until, that was, the People heard their scouts' reports of the two-leg plant places.

The People weren't very good at it yet, but they, too, had begun growing plants in carefully tended and guarded patches at the hearts of their clans' ranges. Their efforts had worked out poorly for the first few turnings, yet the two-legs' success proved it was possible, and they'd continued watching the two-legs and the strange not-living things which tended their open plant places. Much of what they observed meant little or nothing, but other lessons were clearer, and the People had learned a great deal. They had no way to duplicate the enclosed, transparent plant places, of course, yet this last

turning, Bright Water Clan had found itself facing
the cold days with much more white root, golden
ear, and lace leaf than it had required to survive
them. Indeed, there had been sufficient surplus for
Bright Water to trade it to the neighboring High
Crag Clan for additional supplies of flint, and
Climbs Quickly wasn't the only member of the clan
who realized the People owed the two-legs great
thanks (whether the two-legs ever knew it or not).

But what made his whiskers quiver with antici-
pation was something *else* the other scouts had
reported. The two-legs grew many strange plants
the People had never heard of—a single sharp-nosed
tour of any of their outside plant places would prove
that—yet most were *like* ones the People knew. But
one wasn't. Climbs Quickly had yet to personally
encounter the plant the other scouts had christened
cluster stalk, but he was eager to do so. Indeed,
he knew he was a bit *too* eager, for the bright
ecstasy of the scouts who'd sampled cluster stalk
rang through the relayed songs of their clans'
memory singers with a clarity that was almost stun-
ning. It wasn't simply the plant's marvelous taste,
either. Like the tiny, bitter-tasting, hard to find fruit
of the purple thorn, cluster stalk sharpened the
Peoples' mind voices and deepened the texture of
their memory songs. The People had known the
virtue of purple thorn for hundreds upon hundreds
of turnings—indeed, People who were denied its
fruit had actually been known to lose their mind
voices entirely—yet there had never been enough
of it, and it had always been almost impossible to
find in sufficient quantities. But the cluster stalk

was even better than purple thorn (if the reports were correct), and the two-legs seemed to grow it almost effortlessly.

And unless Climbs Quickly was mistaken, that scent blowing from the two-legs' plant places matched the cluster stalk's perfume embedded in the memory songs.

He crouched on his perch, watching the sky grow still darker and heavier, and made up his mind. It would be full dark soon, and the two-legs would retire to the light and warmth of their living place, especially on a night of rain such as this one promised to be. He didn't blame them for that. Indeed, under other circumstances, he would have been scurrying back to his own snugly-roofed nest's water-shedding woven canopy. But not tonight.

No, tonight he would stay, rain or no, and when the two-legs retired, he would explore more closely than he'd ever yet dared approach their living place.

Stephanie Harrington turned up the collar of her jacket and wiggled her toes in her boots for warmth. This part of Sphinx had officially entered Spring, but nights were still cold (though far, *far* warmer than they had been!), and Stephanie was grateful for her thick, warm socks and jacket as she sat in the darkened gazebo sniffing the ozone-heavy wind. The weather satellites said the Harrington homestead was in for a night of thunder, lightning, rain, and violent wind, and cold or not, Stephanie intended to savor it to the full. She'd always liked thunderstorms. She knew some kids were frightened by them, but Stephanie thought that was stupid. She had no intention of running out into the storm with a lightning rod—or, for that matter, standing under a tree—but the spectacle of all that fire and electricity crashing about the sky was simply too exhilarating and wonderful to miss . . . and this would be the first thunderstorm she'd seen in over a T-year.

Not that she'd mentioned her intention to observe it from the gazebo to her parents. She estimated that there was an almost even chance that they would have agreed to let her stay up to enjoy the storm, but she *knew* they would have insisted that she watch it from inside. Thoughts of fireplace-popped popcorn and the hot chocolate Mom would undoubtedly have added to the experience had almost tempted her into announcing her plans, but a little further thought had dissuaded her. Popcorn and hot chocolate were nice, but the only *proper* way to enjoy her first storm in so long was from out in the middle of it where she could feel and taste its power.

And, of course, there was that other little matter.

She smiled in the dark and patted the camera in her lap as thunder growled louder and lightning lashed the mountaintops to the west. She knew her mother had trolled the disappearing crops mystery in front of her as a distraction, but that hadn't made the puzzle any less fascinating. She didn't really expect to solve it, yet she could have fun trying, and if it just happened that she *did* find the answer, well, she was sure she could accept the credit with becoming modesty.

Her smile curled up in urchin glee at the

thought. The original idea might have been her mother's, and Dr. Harrington might have lent her enthusiastic support to Stephanie's approach to the problem, but Stephanie hadn't made her mother privy to *every* facet of her plan. Part of that was to avoid embarrassment if it didn't work, but most of it came from the simple knowledge that her parents wouldn't approve of her . . . hands-on approach. Fortunately, knowing what they would have said—had the occasion arisen—was quite different from actually having them say it when the occasion *hadn't* arisen, which was why she'd carefully avoided bringing the matter up at all.

For the past year or so, a mounting number of homesteads had reported vanishing crops. At first, people had been inclined to think it was some kind of hoax, especially since only one plant ever took missing. Personally, Stephanie couldn't imagine why anyone would want to steal *celery*, which she ate only under parental insistence, but it was obvious *someone* was.

The question was who. Logically, since celery was a Terran import, humans were the only people on Sphinx who should be interested in it, but the very limited evidence available suggested otherwise. Whoever was behind it must be fiendishly clever, for they seemed able to get in and out of places no human should have been able to sneak through, and they left very little in the way of clues. But Stephanie had noticed a pattern. First, the celery was always stolen from one of the more isolated homesteads, not from any of the farm plots or greenhouses near a town. And, second, whoever was stealing it operated only at night and, if possible, under cover of bad weather. For the most part, that had meant waiting to strike a greenhouse during a snow storm, when the blizzard would blot out any tracks they might leave, but Stephanie rather suspected that the bandits would find it hard to pass up the opportunity of a good, heavy thunderstorm. And if the raiders were not, in fact, simply a bunch of humans playing adolescent pranks—if, as she suspected, something *native* to Sphinx was behind it—then lurking out here in the dark might actually prove as interesting as the solo excursions into the woods which had been denied her.

Climbs Quickly clung to his pad as groaning branches lashed the night to protest the wind that roared among them. The rumbling thunder had drawn closer, barking more and more loudly, and lightning forks had begun to play about the mountain heads to the west. The storm was going to be even more powerful than he'd thought, and he smelled cold, wet rain on its breath. It would be here soon, he thought. Very soon, which meant it was time.

He climbed down the trunk more slowly and cautiously than was his wont, for he felt the sturdy tree quivering and shivering under his claws. It took him much longer than usual to reach the ground, and he paused, still a half dozen People-lengths up the tree, to survey his surroundings. The People were quick and agile anywhere, but true safety lay in their ability to scamper up into places where things like death fangs couldn't follow. Unfortunately, Climbs

Quickly's plans required him to venture into an area without handy trees, and while it was unlikely to hold any death fangs, either, he saw no harm in double-checking to be certain of that.

But scan the night though he might, he detected no dangers other than those of the weather itself, and he dropped the last distance to the ground. The mud, he noted, had begun to dry—on the top, at least—but the rain would change that. He felt the faint, pounding vibration of raindrops through the ground, coming steadily nearer, and his ears flattened in resignation. If the reports about cluster stalk proved true, getting soaked would be small enough cost for this evening's excursion, but that didn't mean he would enjoy it, and he flirted his tail and scampered quickly towards the nearest plant place.

In planning her own approach to the disappearing celery mystery, Stephanie had studied everything she could get her hands on about previous thefts. Not that there'd been much to study; the mysterious thieves didn't strike often, and their first known raids had completely surprised the colonists. Since no one had seen any reason to take precautions against celery thefts, whoever the thieves were had been able to simply walk into the fields or greenhouses, scarf up their prizes, and disappear. Given that ease of operation, Stephanie had been surprised to discover how small the original thefts had been. With so clear a field of operations, the bandits should have been able to take as much as they pleased, yet their known hauls were so small that she suspected they'd been pilfering for quite a while before anyone even noticed.

It had taken a long time for anyone to take the reports seriously, and even when the colonists finally moved to put precautions in place, they'd started by trying the predictable—and simplest—measures. But locking greenhouse doors or fencing outdoor garden plots had failed miserably. Despite the unlikeliness that any Sphinxian creature could have a taste for a Terran vegetable, opinion (among those who didn't still think it was all a hoax, at least) had hardened in favor of some clever local animal. Had whatever it was shown an interest in anything but celery, that might have been a cause for alarm; as it was, most of those who'd been raided seemed to take it as a challenge, not a threat. Whatever the pest was, it had to be small, agile, fast, and sneaky, and they were determined to figure out what it was, but they had to act within the limits of the Elysian Rule. With no clear idea what they were after, it was impossible to be sure even capture traps would be nonlethal, and the Elysian Rule absolutely forbade the use of lethal means against a complete unknown without evidence that whatever it was posed a physical danger to humans.

That rule had been adopted over a thousand years before, after a disastrous clutch of mistakes had devastated the ecology of the colony world of Elysian, and no administration on a planet in the early stages of settlement would even consider its violation without a reason far more compelling than the minuscule economic loss thefts of *celery* represented. But that hadn't ruled out trip wires, photoelectric detectors, and pressure plates. They were attached to lights or alarms or passive camera systems, but somehow the celery thieves always seemed to avoid them. There *had* been that one time when someone—or, Stephanie thought deliciously, some*thing*—had tripped a camera over in Jefferies Land in the middle of a howling blizzard. Unfortunately, all the exterior camera had recorded was a lot of swirling snow.

Given how hard others had been working on the mystery, Stephanie was willing to admit that it was unlikely *she* would be the one to solve it. But that wasn't the same as impossible, and she'd been very careful to leave the ventilation louvers open on the greenhouse which contained her mother's celery. The odds were against anything coming along to take advantage of the opportunity, but it wasn't as if Stephanie had a lot of other things to do just now, and she settled back in her chair, camera in her lap, as the first spatters of rain began to fall.

Climbs Quickly paused, head and shoulders rising as he stood high on his true-feet and hand-feet like—had he known (or cared)—an Old Terran prairie dog to peer into the night. This was the closest he'd ever come to his two-legs' living place, and his eyes glowed as he realized he'd been right. He *had* been tasting a mind glow from them, and he stood motionless in the darkness as he savored the texture.

It was unlike anything he'd ever tasted from another of the People . . . and yet it *wasn't* unlike. It was . . . was . . .

He sat down, curling his tail about his toes, and rubbed one ear with a true-hand while he tried to put a label on it. It *was* like the People, he decided after long, hard moments of thought, but without words. It was only the emotions, the feelings of the two-legs, without the shaping that turned those into communication, and there was a strange drowsiness to it, as if it were half-asleep. As if, he thought slowly, the mind glow rose from minds which had never even considered that anyone else might be able to taste or hear them and so had never learned to use it to communicate. Yet even as he thought that, it seemed impossible, for the glow was too strong, too powerful. Unformed, unshaped, it blazed like some marvelous flower, brighter and taller than any of the People had ever produced in Climbs Quickly's presence, and he shivered as he wondered what it would have been like if the two-legs *hadn't* been mind-blind. He felt the brightness calling to him, tempting him closer like a memory singer's song, and he shook himself. This would be a very important part of his next report to Sings Truly and Short Tail, but he certainly had no business exploring it on his own *before* he reported it. Besides, it wasn't what he'd come for.

He shook himself again, stepping back from the mind glow, but it was hard to distance himself from it. In fact, he had to make a deliberate, conscious decision not to taste it and then close his mind to it, and that took much longer to manage than he'd expected.

Yet he did manage it, eventually, and drew a deep breath of relief as he pulled free. He flipped his ears, twitched his whiskers, and began sliding once more through the darkness as the first raindrops splashed about him.

The rain came down harder, drumming on the gazebo roof. The air seemed to dance and shiver as incessant lightning split the night and thunder shook its halves, and Stephanie's eyes glowed as wind whipped spray in through the gazebo's open sides to spatter the floor and kiss her eyelashes and chilled cheeks. She felt the storm crackling about her and hugged it to herself, drinking in its energy.

But then, suddenly, a tiny light began to flash on her camera, and she froze. It couldn't be! But the light *was* flashing—*it really was!*—and that could only mean—

She pressed the button that killed the warning light, then snatched the camera up to peer through the viewfinder. Visibility was poor through the rain cascading off the gazebo roof. There was too much water in the air for a clear view, even with the camera's light-gathering technology, and the lightning didn't help as much as one might have expected. The camera adjusted to changing light levels more quickly than any human eye, but the contrast between the lightning's split-second, stroboscopic fury and the darkness that followed was too extreme.

Stephanie knew that, and she hadn't really expected to see anything just yet, anyway. Since the celery bandits had proved so clever at avoiding mechanical devices like trip wires, most of those working on the problem had opted for more subtle approaches. Photoelectric beams had been the next obvious approach, but whoever it was actually

seemed to avoid them even more readily than he—
or they—avoided mechanical barriers.

But Stephanie had a theory about why that was.
In every case she'd been able to research, the photoelectric system used had employed infrared. Well,
obviously visible light wouldn't work for something
like that, and people had used infrared for such systems just about forever. But Stephanie's discussions
with her father about his work with the fledgling
Sphinx Forestry Service had led her to suspect that
the people setting up those systems here had failed
to adequately analyze their problem. From what
Daddy said, relatively new evidence suggested that
Sphinx wildlife used much more of the lower end
of the spectrum than human eyes. That meant a
Sphinxian animal might actually see the infrared
light a human couldn't, and that, in turn, would
make the photoelectric beams relatively easy to
avoid, so *Stephanie's* alarms used the *other* end of
the spectrum.

It hadn't been hard for her and Daddy to tinker
them up in his workshop, and he'd helped her
weave a solid wall of ultraviolet beams to cover the
opened louvers. But while he and Mom knew all
about her sensors, they thought she'd connected
them to the data terminal in her room. Which she
had. She just hadn't mentioned that for tonight she'd
disabled the audible alarm on her data terminal and
set up a silent relay to her camera, instead. Mom
and Daddy were smart enough to guess why she
might have done that, but since they hadn't specifically asked, she hadn't had to tell them, and that
meant they hadn't gotten around to forbidding her

to lurk in the gazebo tonight, which was certainly the most satisfactory outcome for all concerned.

If pressed, Stephanie would have conceded that her parents might have quibbled with that last conclusion, but what mattered at this particular moment was that something had just climbed through the open louver. Whatever was stealing celery was inside the greenhouse right this minute, and she had a chance to be the very first person on Sphinx to get actual pictures of it!

She stood for a moment, biting her lip and wishing she had better visibility, then shrugged. Mom and Dad wouldn't be a *lot* madder at her for getting soaked than they'd be over her having snuck out at all, and she needed to get closer to the greenhouse. She took a second to clip the rain shield onto the camera, then dragged her hat down over her ears, drew a deep breath, and splashed down the gazebo steps into the rain-whipped night.

Climbs Quickly found it even harder to ignore the two-leg mind glows as he dropped to the soft, bare earth of the plant place's floor. The rich smells of unknown growing things filled his nostrils, and his tail twitched as he absorbed them. The transparent material of the plant place seemed far too thin to resist the rain beating upon it, yet it did, and without a single drop leaking through! The two-legs were truly clever to design a marvel like that, and he sat for a moment luxuriating in the enfolding warmth that was made somehow even warmer and more welcoming by the furious splashing of the icy, lightning-laced rain.

But he hadn't come here to be dry, he reminded himself, and his true-hands untied the carry net wrapped about his middle while he followed his nose and resolutely ignored the background mind glows of the two-legs.

Ah! There was the cluster stalk scent from Sings Truly's song! His eyes lit, and he swarmed easily up the side of the raised part of the plant place, then paused as he came face to face with cluster stalk for the very first time.

The growing heads were bigger than the ones from Sings Truly's song, and he wondered if the scout who first brought that song to his clan had sampled his first cluster stalk before it was fully grown. Whether that was true or not, each of *these* plants was two-thirds as long as Climbs Quickly himself, and he was glad he'd brought the carry net. Still, net or not, he would have to be careful not to take too much if he expected to carry it all the way home. He sat for another long moment, considering, then flipped his ears in decision. Two heads, he decided. He could manage that much, and he could always come back for more.

But even as he decided that, he realized he'd used the need to decide to distract him from the marvelous scent of the cluster stalk. It was like nothing he'd ever smelled before, and he felt his mouth water as he drew it deep into his lungs. He hesitated, then reached out and tugged gently on an outer stalk.

It responded with a springy resistance, like the top of a white root, and he tugged harder. Still it held out, and he tugged still harder, then bleeked in triumph as the stalk came loose in his true-hand. He raised it to his nose, sniffing deeply, then stuck out his tongue.

Magic filled his mouth as he licked delicately. It was like hot, liquid sunlight on a day of frozen ice. Like cold mountain water on a day of scorching heat, or the gentle caress of a new mother, just ruffling her first kitten's delicate fur while her mind promised him welcome and warmth and love. It was—

Climbs Quickly shook his head. It wasn't actually like any of those things, he realized, except that each of them, in its own way, was wonderful and unique. It was just that he didn't have anything else he could really compare that first blissful taste to, and he nibbled gently at the end of the stalk. It was hard to chew—People didn't really have the right kind of teeth to eat plants—but it tasted just as wonderful as that first lick had promised, and he crooned in pleasure as he devoured it.

He finished the entire stalk and reached quickly for another, then made himself stop. Yes, it tasted wonderful, and he wanted more, but he was no ground burrower to gorge himself into insensibility on yellow stalk. He was a scout of the Bright Water Clan, and it was his job to carry this home for Short Tail, Bright Claw, Broken Tooth, and the memory singers to judge it for themselves. Even if they hadn't been the leaders of his clan, they were his friends, and friends shared anything this marvelous with one another.

It was actually easier to get an entire head out of the soft earth in which it grew than it had been to peel off that single stalk, and Climbs Quickly soon had two of them rolled up in his carry net. They made an awkward bundle, but he tied the net as neatly as he could and slung it onto his back, reaching up to hold the hand loops with his mid-limbs' hand-feet while he used true-feet and true-hands to climb back down to the floor. Getting to the opening to the outer world would be more difficult with his burden than it had been coming in, but he could manage. He might not be very fast or agile, but not even a death fang would be out on a night like this!

Stephanie was glad her jacket and trousers were waterproof, and her broad-brimmed hat kept her head and face dry. But holding the camera on target required her to raise her hands in front of her, and ice-cold rain had flooded down the drain pipes of her nice, waterproof jacket sleeves. She felt it puddling about her elbows and beginning to probe stealthily towards her shoulders—just as her forearms were raised, her upper arms were parallel to the ground, providing an all too convenient channel for the frigid water—but all the rain in the world couldn't have convinced her to lower her camera at a moment like this.

She stood no more than ten meters from the greenhouse, recording steadily. Her camera's storage chip was good for over ten hours, and she had no intention of missing any of this for the official record. Excitement trembled inside as the minutes passed in the splashing, lightning-slivered darkness. Whatever it was had been inside the greenhouse for nine minutes now, *surely* it would be coming back out pretty s—

Climbs Quickly reached the opening with a profound sense of relief. He'd almost dropped his carry net twice, and he decided to catch his breath before leaping down into the rain with his prize. After all, he had plenty of ti—

A whisker-fringed muzzle and prick-eared head poked out of the opening, green eyes glowing emerald as lightning stuttered, and the universe seemed to stop as their owner found himself staring into the glassy eye of a camera in the hands of an eleven-year-old girl. Excitement froze Stephanie's breath, even though she'd known this moment was coming, but Climbs Quickly *hadn't* known. His surprise was total, and he went absolutely motionless in astonishment.

Seconds ticked past, and then he shook himself mentally. Showing himself to a two-leg was the one thing he'd been most firmly instructed *not* to do, and he cringed inwardly at how Short Tail would react to this. He knew he could claim distraction on the basis of the storm and his first experience with cluster stalk, but that wouldn't change his failure into success, and he stared down at the two-leg while his mind began to work once more.

It was the youngling, he realized, for it was smaller than either of its parents. He didn't know what it was pointing at him, but from all reports, he would have been dead already if the two-leg had intended to kill him. Yet deciding the thing aimed his way wasn't a weapon didn't tell him what it *was*. Those thoughts flashed through his brain in a heartbeat, and then, without really thinking about it, he reached out to the two-leg's mind glow in an effort to judge its intentions.

He was totally unprepared for the consequences. It was as if he'd looked straight up into the sun expecting to see only the glow of a single torch, and his eyes flared wide and his ears flattened as the intensity of the two-leg's emotions rolled over him. The glow was far brighter than before, and he wondered distantly if that was simply because he was closer and concentrating upon it, or if the cluster stalk he'd sampled might have something to do with it. But it didn't really matter. What mattered was the excitement and eagerness and wonder that blazed so brightly in the two-leg's mind. It was the first time any of the People had ever come face-to-face with a two-leg, and nothing could have prepared Climbs Quickly for the sheer delight with which Stephanie Harrington saw the marvelous, six-limbed creature crouched in the ventilation louver with the woven net of purloined celery slung over its back.

The representatives of two intelligent species, one of which had never even suspected the other's existence, stared at one another in the middle of a howling thunderstorm. It was a moment which could not last, yet neither wanted it to end. Stephanie felt her sense of triumph and excited discovery flow through her like a fountain, and she had no idea that Climbs Quickly felt those emotions even more clearly than he would have felt them from another of his own kind. Nor could she have guessed how very much he wanted to *continue* feeling them. She knew only that he crouched there, gazing at her for what seemed like forever, before he shook himself and leapt suddenly down and outward.

Climbs Quickly pulled free of the two-leg's mind glow. It was hard—possibly the hardest thing he'd ever done—yet he had his duty, and so he made himself step back from that wonderful, welcoming furnace. Or, rather, he stepped *away* from it, for it was too strong, too intense, actually to disconnect from. He could turn his eyes away from the fire, but he could not pretend it did not blaze.

He shook himself, and then he launched outward into the rain and darkness. He was slow and clumsy with the net of cluster stalk on his back, but he knew as surely as he'd ever known anything in his life that this young two-leg meant him no harm. The secret of the People's existence was already revealed, and haste would change nothing, so he sat upright in the rain for a moment, gazing up at the two-leg, who finally lowered the strange thing it had held before its face to look down at him with its own eyes. He met those odd, brown, round-pupiled eyes for a moment, then flicked his ears, turned, and scampered off.

Stephanie watched the intruder vanish with a sense of wonder which only grew as the creature disappeared. It was small, she thought, no more than sixty or seventy centimeters long, though its tail would probably double its body length. An arboreal, her mind went on, considering its tail and the well-developed hands and the claws she'd seen as it clung to the lip of the louver. And those hands, she thought slowly, might have had only three fingers each, but they'd also had fully opposable thumbs. She closed her eyes, picturing it once more, seeing the net on its back, and knew she was right.

The celery snatcher might *look* like a teeny-tiny hexapuma, but that net was incontrovertible evidence that the survey crews had missed the most important single facet of Sphinx. But that was all right. In fact, that was just *fine*. Their omission had abruptly transformed this world from a place of exile to the most marvelous, exciting place Stephanie Harrington could possibly have been, for she'd just done something which had happened only eleven other times in the fifteen centuries of mankind's diaspora to the stars.

She'd just made first contact with a tool-using, clearly sentient, alien race.

The only question now was what to do about it.

IV

Climbs Quickly lay on his back outside his nest, belly fur turned to the sun, and did his best to convince the rest of his clan he was asleep. He knew he wasn't fooling anyone who cared to taste his mind glow, but good manners required them to pretend he was.

Which was just as well, for blissful as it was, the comfort of the drowsy sunlight was far too little to distract him from the monumental changes in his life. Facing his clan leaders and admitting that he'd let one of the two-legs actually see him—and even worse, see him in the very process of raiding their plant place—had been just as unpleasant as he'd feared.

People seldom physically attacked other People. Oh, there were squabbles enough, and occasional serious fights—usually, though not always, limited to younger scouts or hunters—and even rarer

situations in which entire clans found themselves
feuding with one another or fighting for control of
their ranges. No one was particularly proud of such
situations, but the ability to hear one another's
thoughts and taste one another's emotions didn't
necessarily make other People any easier to live with
or fill a clan's range with prey when it was needed.
But a clan's leaders normally intervened before anything serious could happen *within* a clan, and it was
rare indeed for one member of a clan to deliberately attack another unless there was something fundamentally wrong with the attacker. Climbs Quickly
himself could remember an occasion on which High
Crag Clan had been forced to drive out one of its
scouts, a rogue who *had* attacked other People. The
exile had crossed into the Bright Water range, killing
prey not just to live but for the sheer joy of killing, and raided Bright Water's storage places. He'd
even attacked and seriously injured a Bright Water
scout while attempting to steal a mother's kittens
. . . for purposes Climbs Quickly preferred not to
consider too deeply. In the end, the clan's scouts
and hunters had been forced to hunt him down and
kill him, a grim necessity none had welcomed.

So Climbs Quickly hadn't expected any of the
Bright Water leaders to assault him, and they hadn't.
But they *had* left him feeling as if they'd skinned
him and hung his hide up to dry. It wasn't even
the things they'd said so much as the way they'd
said them.

Climbs Quickly's ears flicked, and he squirmed,
turning to catch the sun more fully, as he recalled
his time before Bright Water's leaders. Sings Truly

had been present as the clan's second singer and the obvious heir to the first singer's position when Song Spinner died or surrendered her authority, but even Sings Truly had been shocked by his clumsiness. She hadn't scolded him the way Short Tail or Broken Tooth had, yet tasting his sister's wordless reproach had been harder for Climbs Quickly to bear than all of Broken Tooth's cutting irony.

He'd tried to explain, as clearly and undefensively as possible, that he'd never *meant* to let the two-leg see him, and he'd suggested the possibility that somehow the two-leg had known he was in the plant place even before seeing him. Unfortunately, his suspicion rested on the mind glow of the two-leg, and although none of the others had actually said so, he knew they found it difficult to believe a two-leg's mind glow could tell one of the People so much. He even knew why they thought that way, for no other scout had ever come close enough to— or concentrated hard enough upon—a two-leg to realize how wonderfully, dreadfully powerful that mind glow truly was.

<I believe that you believe the two-leg had some way of knowing you were there,> Short Tail had told him judiciously, his mind voice grave, <yet I fail to see how it could have. You saw none of the strange lights or tool things the two-legs have used to detect other scouts, after all.>

<True,> Climbs Quickly had replied as honestly as possible, <yet the two-legs are very clever. I saw none of the tool things I knew to look for, but does that prove the two-legs have no tool things we have not yet learned of?>

<*You hunt for ground runners in the upper branches, little brother,*> Broken Tooth, the most senior of Bright Water's elders, had put in sternly. <*You allowed the two-leg not simply to see you but to see you raiding its range. I do not doubt you tasted its mind glow, but neither do I doubt that you tasted within that mind glow that which it was most important for you to taste.*>

Much as Broken Tooth's charge had angered Climbs Quickly, he'd been unable to counter it effectively. The feelings of the mind glow were always much easier to misinterpret, even among the People, than thoughts which were formed into words, and it was only reasonable for Broken Tooth, who'd never tasted a two-leg mind glow, to assume that it would be even more difficult to interpret those of a totally different creature. Climbs Quickly knew—didn't think; *knew*—that the two-leg's mind glow had been so strong, so vibrant, that he literally *could not* have read it wrongly, yet when he couldn't explain how he knew that even to himself, he could hardly blame the clan's leaders for failing to grasp the same fact.

And so, because he couldn't explain, he'd accepted his scolding as meekly as possible. The cluster stalk he'd brought home had muted that scolding to some extent, for it had proved just as marvelous as the songs from other clans had indicated, but not even that had been enough to deflect the one consequence he truly resented.

He had been relieved of his responsibility to watch over his two-legs, and Shadow Hider, another scout (who just happened to be a grandson of

Broken Tooth), had been assigned that task in his place. He understood why, however much he disliked it, for the People had only to watch them cutting down trees with their whining tools that ate through the trunks of trees large enough to hold whole clans of the People or using the machines that gouged out the deep holes in which they planted their living places to recognize the potential danger the two-legs represented. They need not decide to kill the People or destroy a clan's entire range to accomplish the same end by accident, and so the People had decided that their only true safety lay in avoiding them entirely. The clans must stay undetected, observing without being observed, until they decided how best to respond to the strange creatures who so confidently and competently reshaped the world.

Unfortunately, Climbs Quickly had come to doubt the wisdom of that policy. Certainly caution was necessary, yet it seemed to him that many People—such as Broken Tooth and his like among the other clans—had become too aware of the potential danger and too *un*aware of the possible advantages the two-legs presented. Perhaps without even realizing it, they had decided deep down inside that the time for the two-legs to learn of the People's existence would never come, for only thus could the People be safe.

But though Climbs Quickly had too much respect for his clan's leaders to say so, the hope that the two-legs would never discover the People was foolishness. There were more two-legs with every turning, and their flying things and long-seeing things

and whatever the young two-leg had used to detect
his own presence were too clever for the People
to hide forever. Even without his encounter with
the two-leg, the People would have been found
sooner or later. And when that happened—or perhaps, more accurately, now that it *had* happened—
the People would have no choice but to decide how
they would interact with the two-legs . . . assuming, of course, that the two-legs *allowed* the People
to make that decision.

All of that was perfectly clear to Climbs Quickly
and, he suspected, to Sings Truly, Short Tail, and
Bright Claw, the clan's senior hunter. But Broken
Tooth, Song Spinner, and Digger, who oversaw the
clan's plant places, rejected that conclusion. They
saw how vast the world was, how many hiding places
it offered, and believed they *could* avoid the two-
legs forever, even now that the two-legs knew the
People existed.

He sighed again, and then his whiskers twitched
with wry amusement as he wondered if the young
two-leg was having as many difficulties getting its
elders to accept *its* judgment. If so, should Climbs
Quickly be grateful or unhappy? He knew from its
mind glow that the youngling had felt only wonder and delight, not anger or fear, when it saw him.
Surely if its elders shared its feelings, the People
had nothing to fear. Yet the fact that one two-leg—
and one perhaps little removed from kittenhood—
felt that way might very well mean no more to the
rest of the two-legs than *his* feelings meant to
Broken Tooth.

Climbs Quickly lay basking in the sunlight,

considering all that had happened—and all that still threatened to happen—and understood the fear of Broken Tooth and his supporters. Indeed, a part of him shared their fear, but another part knew events had already been set in motion. The two-legs knew of the People's existence now. They would react to that, whatever the People did or didn't do, and all Broken Tooth's scolding could never prevent it.

Yet there was one thing Climbs Quickly hadn't reported, something he had yet to come to grips with himself and something he feared might actually panic Bright Water's leaders into abandoning their range and fleeing deep into the mountains. Perhaps that flight would actually be the path of wisdom, he admitted, but it might also cast away a treasure such as the People had never before encountered. It was scarcely the place of a single scout to make choices affecting his entire clan, yet no one else *could* make this decision, for he alone knew that somehow, in a way he couldn't begin to understand, he and the young two-leg now shared something.

He wasn't certain what that "something" was, but even now, with his eyes closed and the two-legs' clearing far away, he knew *exactly* where the youngling was. He could feel its mind glow, like a far-off fire or sunlight shining red through his closed eyelids. It was too distant for him to taste its emotions, yet he knew it wasn't his imagination. He truly *did* know the direction to the two-leg, even more clearly than the direction to Sings Truly, who was no more than twenty or thirty People-lengths away at this very moment.

Climbs Quickly had no idea at all what that might mean or where it might lead, but two things he did know. His connection, if such it was, to the young two-leg might—*must*—hold the key, for better or for worse, to whatever relationship People and two-legs might come to share. And until *he* decided what that connection meant in his own case, he dared not even suggest its existence to those who felt as Broken Tooth.

V

Stephanie leaned back in the comfortable chair, folded her hands behind her head, and propped her sock feet on her desk in the posture which always drew a scold from her mother. Her lips were pursed in a silent, tuneless whistle that was an all but inevitable complement to the vague dreaminess of her eyes . . . and which would, had she let her parents see it, instantly have alerted them to the fact that their darling daughter was Up To Something.

The problem was that for the first time in a very, very long time, she had only the haziest idea of precisely what she was up to. Or, rather, of how to pursue her objective. Uncertainty was an unusual feeling for someone who usually got into trouble by being too positive about things, yet there was something rather appealing about it, too. Perhaps because of its novelty.

She frowned, closed her eyes, tipped her chair further back, and thought harder.

She'd managed to evade detection on her way to bed the night of the thunderstorm. Oddly—though it hadn't occurred to her that it *was* odd until much later—she hadn't even considered rushing to her parents with her camera. The knowledge that humanity shared Sphinx with another sentient species was *her* discovery, and she'd felt strangely disinclined to share it. Until she did, it was not only her discovery but her secret, and she'd been almost surprised to realize she was determined to learn all she possibly could about her unexpected neighbors before she let anyone else know they existed. She wasn't certain when she'd decided that, but once she had, it had been easy to find logical reasons for her decision. For one thing, the mere thought of how some of the kids in Twin Forks would react was enough to make her shudder. Given their determination to catch everything from chipmunks (which didn't look at *all* like Meyerdahl's—or, for that matter, Old Terra's—chipmunks) to near-turtles as pets, they'd be almost certain to pursue these new creatures with even greater enthusiasm and catastrophic results.

She'd felt rather virtuous once she got that far, but it didn't come close to solving her main problem. If she didn't tell anybody, how did she go about learning more about them on her own? Stephanie knew she was brighter than most, but she also knew someone else would eventually catch a celery thief in the act. When that happened her secret would be out, and she was determined to learn everything she possibly could about them before that happened.

And, she thought, she was starting with a clean slate. She'd accessed the datanet without finding a single word about miniature hexapumas with hands. She'd even used her father's link to the Forestry Service to compare her camera imagery to known Sphinxian species, only to draw a total blank. Whatever the celery snatcher was, no one else had ever gotten pictures of one of his—or had it been *her*?— relatives or even uploaded a verbal description of them to the planetary database, and that said as much about their intelligence as the raider's woven net had. A planet was a big place, but from the pattern of celery thefts, these creatures must be at least as widely distributed as Sphinx's colonists. The only way they could have gone undetected for over fifty T-years was by deliberately avoiding humans . . . and that indicated a reasoned response to the colonists's presence *and* the existence of a language. Hiding so successfully had to indicate a deliberate, conscious, *shared* pattern of activity, and how could they coordinate that well without the ability to talk to one another? So they were not only tool-users but language-users, and their small size made that even more remarkable. The one Stephanie had seen couldn't have had a body length of more than sixty centimeters or weighed more than thirteen or fourteen kilos, and no one had ever before encountered a sentient species with a body mass that low.

Stephanie got that far without much difficulty. Unfortunately, that was as far as she *could* get without more data, and for the first time she could recall, she didn't know how to get any more. She might be first in her class, and she might have made it into the final round of the planetary chess championship, and she might approach most problems with complete confidence, but this time she was stumped. She'd exhausted the available research possibilities, so if she wanted more information, she had to get it for herself. That implied some sort of field research, but how did an eleven year old—and one who'd promised her parents she wouldn't tramp around the woods alone—investigate a totally unknown species without even telling anyone it existed?

In a way, she was actually grateful that her mother had found herself too tied down by her current projects to go for those nature hikes she'd promised to try to make time for. Stephanie had been grateful when her mother made the offer, though she'd realized even then that with her mom along her hikes could hardly have offered the sort of intensive investigation for which she'd longed. Now, however, her mother's presence would have posed a serious obstacle for any attempt to pursue private research in secret.

It was perhaps unfortunate, however, that her father, in an effort to make up for her "disappointment" over her mother's schedule, had decided to distract her by resuming the hang-gliding lessons their departure from Meyerdahl had interrupted. Stephanie loved the exhilaration of flight, even if Daddy did insist that she take along an emergency countergrav unit "just in case," and no one could have been a better teacher than Richard Harrington, who'd made it into the continental hang-gliding finals on Meyerdahl three times. But the time she spent on gliding lessons was time she didn't spend investigating her fascinating discovery, and if she *didn't* spend time on the lessons—and obviously enjoy them—her parents would suspect she had something else on her mind. Worse, Daddy insisted on flying into Twin Forks for her lessons. That made sense, since unlike her mom he had to be "on call" twenty-five hours a day and Twin Forks was the central hub for all the local homesteads. He could reach any of them quickly from town, and teaching the lessons there let him enlist the two or three other parents with gliding experience as assistant teachers and offer the lessons to all the settlement's other kids, as well. That was exactly the sort of generosity Stephanie would have expected of him, but it also meant her lessons were not only eating up an enormous amount of her free time but taking her over eighty kilometers away from the place where she was more eager than ever to begin the explorations she'd promised her parents she wouldn't undertake.

She hadn't found a way around her problems yet, but she was determined that she *would* find one—and without breaking her promise, however much that added to her difficulties. But at least it hadn't been hard to give the species a name. It looked like an enormously smaller version of a "hexapuma," and like the hexapuma, there was something very (or perhaps inevitably) *feline* about it. Of course, Stephanie knew "feline" actually referred only to a very specific branch of Old Terran evolution, but it had become customary over the centuries to apply Old Terran names to alien species (like the

Sphinxian "chipmunks" or "near-pine"). Most claimed the practice originated from a sort of racial homesickness and a desire for familiarity in alien environments, but Stephanie thought it was more likely to stem from laziness, since it let people avoid thinking up new labels for everything they encountered. Despite all that, however, she'd discovered that "treecat" was the only possible choice when she started considering names, and she hoped the taxonomists would let it stand when she finally had to go public with her discovery, though she suspected rather glumly that her age would work against her in that regard.

And if she hadn't figured out how to go about investigating the treecats without breaking her promise—which was out of the question, however eager she might be to proceed—at least she knew the direction in which to start looking. She had no idea how she knew, but she was absolutely convinced that she would know exactly where to go when the time came.

She closed her eyes, took one arm from behind her head, and pointed, then opened her eyes to see where her index finger was aimed. The direction had changed slightly since the last time she'd checked, and yet she knew beyond a shadow of a doubt that she was pointing directly at the treecat who'd raided her mother's greenhouse.

And that, she reflected, was the oddest—and most exciting—part of the whole thing.

VI

Marjorie Harrington finished writing up her latest microbe-resistant strain of squash, closed the file, and sat back with a sigh. Some of Sphinx's farmers had argued that it would be much simpler (and quicker) just to come up with something to swat the microbe in question. That always seemed to occur to the people who faced such problems, and sometimes, Marjorie was prepared to admit, it was not only the simplest but also the most cost effective and ecologically sound answer. That was especially true when the parasite in question was itself a new strain, a new mutation rather than an old, established part of the ecosystem. But in this case, she and the planetary administration had resisted firmly, and her final solution—which, she admitted, had taken longer than a more aggressive one might have—had been to select the least intrusive of three possible genetic modifications to the plant rather than going after the microbe. It was always a good idea for people on a planet whose biosystem they were still in the process of exploring to exercise the greatest possible care to limit the impact of their actions *on* that biosystem, and she expected the agricultural cartels and Interior Ministry officials to be quite pleased with her solution, despite the cost of all the additional hours she'd put into the project.

She made a wry face at the thought of the bureaucrats. She had to admit that the local varieties were far less intrusive—and more reasonable—than their equivalents on Meyerdahl, but the Star Kingdom was barely sixty T-years old. No doubt it would have all the entrenched bureaucracies the least imaginative, most procedure-loving clerical tyrant could desire by the time it was Meyerdahl's age.

Her wry expression turned into a grin remarkably like her daughter's, then faded as she turned her mind from squash to other matters. Her work load had grown much heavier over the past weeks as Sphinx's southern hemisphere moved steadily towards planting time, and now that the squash project was out of the way her nagging sense of guilt returned full force. It was hardly her fault that the press of assignments had kept her from finding the time for long hikes with Stephanie, but she hadn't even been able to free up the time to help her daughter explore possible answers to the celery pilferage which had finally reached the Harrington Homestead.

She was thankful that Richard had at least resumed Stephanie's hang-gliding lessons as a combination diversion and compensation. It had been a brilliant idea on his part, and Stephanie had responded with enthusiasm. Marjorie could only be grateful that she seemed to enjoy it so much—she'd started spending hours in the air, checking in periodically over her wrist com—and, despite the vocal worry of some of the Twin Folks parents whose kids were also learning to glide, Marjorie wasn't especially worried by the risks involved in her daughter's new hobby. She'd never pursued the sport herself, but it had been quite popular on Meyerdahl, where she'd known dozens of avid practitioners. And unlike some parents, she'd learned—not without difficulty, she admitted—that it was impossible to keep her only child wrapped in cotton wool. Children might not be indestructible, but they came far closer to it than most adults were prepared to admit, and a certain number of bumps, scrapes, contusions, bruises, or even broken bones were among the inevitable rites of childhood, whether or not parents liked that fact.

Yet if Marjorie had no particular qualms over Stephanie's new interest, she was still unhappily certain that Stephanie had embraced it mainly as a diversion from her disappointment in other directions. Appearances might suggest Stephanie had forgotten all about her hunger to explore the homestead's endless forests, but appearances could be deceiving, and Marjorie knew her daughter too well to believe she had, in fact, relinquished her original ambitions, however outwardly cheerful her acceptance of an alternate activity.

Marjorie rubbed her nose pensively. She had no

doubt Stephanie understood—at least intellectually—how important her own work was and why it had precluded the other activities they'd discussed, but that only made it almost worse. However bright Stephanie might be, she was also only eleven, and understanding and acceptance were too often two completely different things even for adults. Besides, whether Stephanie *accepted* it or not, the situation was grossly unfair to her, and "fairness" was of enormous importance to children . . . even going-on-twelve geniuses. Although Stephanie seldom sulked or whined, Marjorie had expected to hear quite a bit of carefully reasoned comment on the subject of fairness, and the fact that Stephanie hadn't complained at all only sharpened Marjorie's sense of guilt. It was as if Stephanie—

The hand rubbing Dr. Harrington's nose suddenly stopped moving as a fresh thought struck her, and she frowned, wondering why it hadn't occurred to her before. It wasn't as if she didn't know her daughter, after all, and this sort of sweet acceptance was very unlike Stephanie. No, she *didn't* sulk or whine, but neither did she give up without a fight on something to which she'd truly set her mind. And, Marjorie thought, while Stephanie had *enjoyed* hang-gliding back on Meyerdahl, it had never been the passion for her that it seemed to have become here. It was certainly possible that she'd simply discovered that she'd underestimated its enjoyment quotient on Meyerdahl, but Marjorie's abruptly roused instincts said something else entirely.

She ran her memory back over her more recent

conversations with her daughter, and her suspicion grew. Not only had Stephanie not complained about the unfairness of her grounding or the "zorkiness" of the younger citizens of Twin Forks who shared her gliding lessons, but it was over two weeks since she'd even referred to the mysterious celery thefts, and Marjorie scolded herself harder for falling into the error of complacency. She understood exactly how it had happened—given the pressures of her current projects, she'd been too grateful for Stephanie's restraint to adequately consider its roots—but that was no excuse. All the signs were there, and she should have realized that the only thing which could produce such a tractable Stephanie was a Stephanie who was Up To Something and didn't want her parents to notice.

But what *could* she be up to? And *why* didn't she want them to notice? The only thing she'd been forbidden was the freedom to explore the wilderness on her own, and Marjorie was confident that, however devious she might sometimes be, Stephanie would never break a promise. Yet if she was using her sudden interest in hang-gliding as a cover for something else, then whatever she was up to must be something she calculated would arouse parental resistance. Her daughter, Marjorie thought with affection-laced exasperation, was entirely too prone to figure that anything which hadn't been specifically forbidden was legal . . . whether or not the *opportunity* to forbid it had ever been offered.

On the other hand, Stephanie wasn't the sort to prevaricate in the face of specific questions. If

Marjorie sat her down and asked her, she'd open up about whatever she was up to. She might not want to, but she'd do it, and Marjorie made a firm mental note to set aside enough time to explore the possibilities—thoroughly.

VII

Stephanie whooped in sheer exuberance as she rode the powerful updraft. Wind whipped her short, curly hair, and she leaned to one side, banking the glider as she sliced still higher. The countergrav unit on her back could have taken her higher yet—and done it more quickly—but it wouldn't have been anywhere near as much *fun* as this was!

She watched the treetops below her and felt a tiny stir of guilt buried in her delight. She was safely above those trees—not even the towering crown oaks came anywhere near her present altitude—but she also knew what her father would have said had he known where she was. The fact that he *didn't* know, and thus *wouldn't say* it wasn't quite enough for her to convince herself her actions weren't just a *bit* across the line, but she could always say— truthfully—that she hadn't broken her word. She wasn't walking around the woods by herself, and no hexapuma or peak bear could possibly threaten her at an altitude of two or three hundred meters.

For all that, innate self-honesty forced her to admit that she knew her parents would instantly have countermanded her plans if they'd known of them. But Daddy had been forced to cancel today's lesson because of an emergency house call, and he'd commed Mr. Sapristos, the Twin Forks' mayor who usually subbed for him in the gliding classes. Mr. Sapristos had agreed to take over for the day, but Daddy hadn't specifically told him Stephanie would be there. The autopilot in Mom's air car could have delivered her under the direction of the planetary air traffic computers, and he'd apparently assumed that was what would happen. Unfortunately—or fortunately, depending on one's viewpoint—his haste had been so great that he hadn't asked Mom to arrange transportation. (Stephanie was guiltily certain that he'd expected *her* to tell her mother. But, she reminded herself, he hadn't actually *told* her to, had he?)

All of which meant Daddy thought she was with Mr. Sapristos but that Mr. Sapristos and Mom both thought she was with *Daddy*. And that just happened to have given Stephanie a chance to pick her own flight plan without having to explain it to anyone else.

It wasn't the first time the same situation had arisen . . . or that she'd capitalized upon it. But it wasn't the sort of opportunity an enterprising young woman could expect to come along often, either, and she'd jumped at it. She'd had to, for the long Sphinxian days were creeping past, and none of her previous unauthorized flights had given her big enough time windows. Avoiding parental discovery had required her to turn back short of the point at which she *knew* her treecats lurked, and if *she* didn't find out more about them soon, someone else was bound to. Of course, she couldn't expect to learn much about them flying around overhead, but that wasn't really what she was after. If she could just pinpoint a location for them, she was sure she could get Daddy to come out here with her, maybe with some of his friends from the Forestry Service, to find the physical evidence to support her discovery. And, she thought, her ability to tell them where to look would also be evidence of her strange link with the celery thief—a link, she was certain, which would require a *lot* of evidence before anyone else was prepared to accept it.

She closed her eyes, consulting her inner compass once more, and smiled. It was holding steady, which meant she was headed in the right direction, and she opened her eyes once more.

She banked again, very slightly, adjusting her course to precisely the right heading, and her face glowed with excitement. She was on track at last. She *knew* she was, just as she knew that this time she had enough flight time to reach her goal, and she was quite correct. Unfortunately, she was also very young, and for all her brilliance, she'd made one small mistake.

Climbs Quickly paused, one true-hand stopped in mid-reach for the branch above, and his ears flattened. He'd become accustomed to his ability to

sense the direction to the two-leg youngling, even
if he still hadn't mentioned it to anyone else. He'd
even become used to the way the youngling sometimes seemed to move with extraordinary speed—
no doubt in one of the two-legs' flying things—but
this was different. The youngling *was* moving
quickly, though not as quickly as it sometimes had,
but it was headed directly towards Climbs Quickly—
and already far closer than it had come since he'd
been relieved of his spying duties—and he felt a
sudden chill.

There was no question. He recognized exactly
what the youngling was doing, for he'd done much
the same thing often enough in the past. True, *he*
usually pursued his prey by scent, but now he
understood how a ground runner must have felt
when it realized he was on its trail, for the two-
leg was using the link between them in exactly the
same way. It was *tracking* him, and if it found him,
it would also find Bright Water Clan's central nesting
place. For good or ill, its ability to seek out Climbs
Quickly would result in the discovery of his entire
clan!

He stood for one more moment, heart racing, ears
flat with mingled excitement and fear, then decided.
He abandoned his original task and bounded off
along an outstretched limb, racing to meet the
approaching two-leg well away from the rest of his
clan.

Stephanie's attention was locked on the trees
below her now. Her flight had lasted over two hours,
but she was drawing close at last. She could feel

the distance melting away—indeed, it almost seemed the treecat was coming to meet her—and excitement narrowed the focus of her attention even further. The crown oak had thinned as she moved higher into the foothills. Now the woods below her were a mix of various evergreens and the crazy-quilt geometry of picket wood.

Of course they were, she thought, and her eyes brightened. The rough-barked picket wood would be the perfect habitat for someone like her little celery thief! Each picket wood system radiated from a single central trunk which sent out long, straight, horizontal branches at a height of between three and ten meters. Above that, branches might take on any shape; below it, they always grew in groups of four, radiating at near-perfect right angles from one another for a distance of ten to fifteen meters . . . at which point, each sent a vertical runner down to the earth below to establish its own root system and, in time, become its own nodal trunk. A single picket wood "tree" could extend itself for literally hundreds of kilometers in any direction, and it wasn't uncommon for one "tree" to run into another and fuse with it. When the lateral branches of two systems crossed, they merged in a node which put down its own runner.

Stephanie's mother was fascinated by the picket woods. Plants which spread by sending out runners weren't all that rare, but those which spread *only* via runner were. It was also more than a little uncommon for the runner to spread out through the air and grow down to the earth rather than the reverse, but what truly fascinated her was the tree's anti-disease defense mechanism. The unending network of branches and trunks should have made a picket wood system lethally vulnerable to diseases and parasites, but the plant had demonstrated a sort of natural quarantine process. Somehow—and Dr. Harrington had yet to discover how—a picket wood system was able to sever its links to afflicted portions of itself. Attacked by disease or parasites, the system secreted powerful cellulose-dissolving enzymes that ate away the connecting cross-branches and literally disconnected them at intervening nodal trunks, and Dr. Harrington was determined to locate the mechanism which made that possible.

But at the moment, her mother's interest in picket wood meant very little to Stephanie beside her realization of the same plant's importance to treecats. Picket wood stopped well short of the tree line, but it crossed mountains readily through valleys or at lower elevations, and it could be found in almost every climate zone. All of which meant it would provide treecats with the equivalent of aerial highways that could literally run clear across a continent! They could travel for hundreds—thousands!—of kilometers without ever once having to touch the ground where larger predators like hexapumas could get at them!

She laughed aloud at her deduction, but then her glider slipped abruptly sideways, and her laughter died as she stopped thinking about the sorts of trees beneath her and recognized instead the speed at which she was passing over them. She raised her head and looked around quickly, and a fist of ice seemed to squeeze her stomach.

The clear blue skies under which she had begun her flight still stretched away in front of her to the west. But the eastern sky *behind* her was no longer clear. A deadly looking line of thunderheads marched steadily west, white and fluffy on top but an ominous purple-black below, and even as she looked over her shoulder, she saw lightning flicker below them.

She should have seen it coming sooner, she thought numbly, hands aching as she squeezed the glider's grips in ivory-knuckled fists. She should have kept an eye out for it! But she was used to having other people—*adult* people—check the weather before she went gliding, and then she'd let herself get so excited, focus so intently on what she was doing, pay so little attention—

A harder fist of wind punched at her glider, staggering it in mid-air, and fear became terror. The following wind had been growing stronger for quite some time, a small, logical part of her realized. No doubt she would have noticed despite her concentration if she hadn't been gliding in the same direction, riding in the wind rather than across or against it where the velocity shift would *have* to have registered. But the thunderheads behind were catching up with her quickly, and the outriders of their squall line lashed through the airspace in front of them.

Daddy! She had to com Daddy—tell him where she was—tell him to come get her—tell him—!

But there was no time. She'd messed up, and for the first time in her life, Stephanie Harrington confronted her own mortality. All the theoretical discussions of what to do in bad weather, all the stern warnings to avoid rough air, came crashing in on her, and they were no longer theoretical. She was in deadly danger, and she knew it. Countergrav unit or no, a storm like the one racing up behind her could blot her out of the air as casually as she might have swatted a fly, and with just as deadly a result. She could die in the next few minutes, and the thought terrified her, but she didn't panic.

Yes, she had to com Mom and Daddy, but it wasn't as if she didn't know exactly what they'd tell her to do if she did. She had to get out of the air, and she couldn't afford the distraction of trying to explain where she was while she tried to get down safely . . . especially through that solid-looking green canopy below her.

She banked again, shivering with fear, eyes desperately seeking some opening, however small, and the air trembled as thunder rumbled behind her.

Climbs Quickly reared up on true-feet and hand-feet, lips wrinkling back from needle-sharp white fangs as a flood of terror crashed over him. It pounded deep into him, waking the ancient fight-or-flight instinct which, had he but known it, his kind shared with humanity, but it wasn't *his* terror at all.

It took him an instant to realize that, yet it was true. It wasn't his fear; it was the two-leg youngling's, and even as the youngling's fear ripped at him, he felt a fresh surge of wonder. He was still too far from the two-leg. He could never have felt another of the People's mind glow at this distance, and he knew it, but this two-leg's mind glow raged through him like a forest fire, screaming for his aid without even realizing it could do so, and it struck him like a lash. He shook his head once, and then flashed down the line of what humans called picket wood like a cream and gray blur while his fluffy tail streamed straight out behind him.

Desperation filled Stephanie. The thunderstorm was almost upon her—the first white pellets of hail rattled off her taut glider covering—and without the countergrav she would already have been blotted from the sky. But not even the countergrav unit could save her from the mounting turbulence much longer, and—

Her thoughts chopped off as salvation loomed suddenly before her. The black, irregular scar of an old forest fire ripped a huge hole through the trees, and she choked back a sob of gratitude as she spied it. The ground was dangerously rough for a landing in conditions like this, but it was infinitely more inviting than the solid web of branches tossing and lashing below her, and she banked towards it.

She almost made it.

Climbs Quickly ran as he'd never run before. Somehow he knew he raced against death itself, though it never occurred to him to wonder what someone his size could do for someone the size of even a two-leg youngling. It didn't matter. All that mattered was the terror, the fear—the danger—which confronted that other presence in his mind, and he ran madly towards it.

✧   ✧   ✧

It was the strength of the wind which did it. Even then, she would have made it without the sudden downdraft that hammered her at the last instant, but between them, they were too much. Stephanie saw it coming in the moment before she struck, realized instantly what was going to happen, but there was no time to avoid it. No time even to feel the full impact of the realization before her glider crashed into the crown of the towering evergreen at over fifty kilometers per hour.

VIII

Climbs Quickly slithered to a stop, momentarily frozen in horror, but then he gasped in relief. The sudden silence in his mind wasn't—quite—absolute. His instant fear that the youngling had been killed eased, but something deeper and darker, without the same bright panic but with even greater power, replaced it. Whatever had happened, the youngling was now unconscious, yet even in its unconsciousness, he was still linked to it . . . and he felt its pain. It was injured, possibly badly—possibly badly enough that his initial fear that it had died would prove justified after all. And if it was injured, what could *he* do to help? Young as it was, it was far larger than he—much *too* large for him to drag to safety.

But what one of the People couldn't do, many of them often *could*, he thought, and closed his eyes, lashing his tail while he thought. He'd run too far to feel the combined mind glow of his clan's central nest place. His emotions couldn't reach so far, but his mind voice could. If he cried out for help, Sings Truly would hear, and if she failed to, surely some hunter or scout between her and Climbs Quickly would hear and relay. Yet what words could he cry out with? How could he summon the clan to aid a two-leg—the very two-leg he had allowed to see him? How could he expect them to abandon their policy of hiding from the two-legs? And even if he could have expected that of them, what right had he to demand it?

He stood irresolute, tail flicking, ears flattened as the branch beneath him creaked and swayed and the first raindrops lashed the budding leaves. Rain, he thought, a flicker of humor leaking even through his dread and uncertainty. Was it *always* going to be raining when he and his two-leg met?

Strangely, that thought broke his paralysis, and he shook himself. All he knew so far was that the two-leg was hurt and that he was very close to it now. He had no way of knowing how bad its injuries might actually be, nor even if there were any *reason* to consider calling out for help. After all, if there was nothing the clan could do, then there was no point in trying to convince it to come. No, the thing to do was to continue until he found the youngling. He had to see what its condition was before he could determine the best way to help—assuming it required his help at all—and he scurried onward almost as quickly as before.

✧   ✧   ✧

Stephanie recovered consciousness slowly. The world swayed and jerked all about her, thunder rumbled and crashed, rain lashed her like an icy flail, and she'd never hurt so much in her entire life.

The pounding rain's chill wetness helped rouse her, and she tried to move, only to whimper as the pain in her left arm stabbed suddenly higher. She blinked, rubbing her eyes with her right palm, and felt a sort of dull shock as she realized part of what had been blinding her was blood, not simply rainwater.

She wiped again and felt a sliver of relief as she realized there was much less blood than she'd thought. It seemed to be coming from a single cut on her forehead, and the cold rain was already slowing the bleeding. She managed to clear her eyes well enough to look about her, and her relief vanished.

Her glider was smashed. Not broken: *smashed*. Its tough composite covering and struts had been specially designed to be crash survivable, but it had never been intended for the abuse to which she'd subjected it, and it had crumpled into a mangled lacework of fabric and shattered framing. Yet it hadn't quite failed completely, and she hung in her harness from the main spar, which was jammed in the fork of a branch above her. The throbbing ache where the harness straps crossed her body told her she'd been badly bruised by the abrupt termination of her flight, and one of her ribs stabbed her with a white burst of agony every time she breathed, but without the harness—and the forked branch which had caught her—she would have smashed straight into the massive tree trunk directly in front of her, and she shuddered at the thought.

But however lucky she might have been, there'd been bad luck to go with the good. Like most colony world children, Stephanie had been through the mandatory first-aid courses . . . not that any training was needed to realize her left arm was broken in at least two places. She knew which way her elbow was *supposed* to bend, and there was no joint in the middle of her forearm. That was bad enough, but there was worse, for her com had been strapped to her left wrist.

It wasn't there anymore.

She turned her head, craning her neck to peer painfully back along the all too obvious course of her crashing impact with the treetops, and wondered where the com was. The wrist unit was virtually inde-structible, and if she could only find it—and *reach* it—she could call for help in an instant. But there was no way she was going to find it in that mess. It was almost funny, she thought through the haze of her pain. *She* couldn't find it, but Mom or Daddy could have found it with ridiculous ease . . . if they'd only known to use the emergency override code to activate the locator beacon function. Or, for that matter, if *she'd* thought to activate it when the storm first came up. Unfortunately, she'd been too preoc-cupied finding a landing spot to bring the beacon up, and even if she had, no one would have found it until they thought to look for it.

And since I can't even find it, I can't com any-one to tell them to start looking for it, she thought fuzzily. *I really messed up this time. Mom and Daddy are going to be really,* really *pissed. Bet they ground me till I'm sixteen for* this *one!*

Even as she thought it, she knew it was ridiculous to worry about such things at a time like this. Yet there was a certain perverse comfort—a sense of familiarity, perhaps—to it, and she actually managed a damp-sounding chuckle despite the tears of pain and fear trickling down her face.

She let herself hang limp for another moment, but badly as she felt the need to rest, she dared do no such thing. The wind was growing stronger, not weaker, and the branch from which she hung creaked and swayed alarmingly. Then there was the matter of lightning. A tree this tall was all too likely to attract any stray bolt, and she had no desire to share the experience with it. No, she had to get herself down, and she blinked away residual pain tears and fresh rain to peer down at the ground.

It was a good twelve-meter drop, and she shuddered at the thought. Her gymnastics classes had taught her how to tuck and roll, but that wouldn't have helped from this height even with two good arms. With her left arm shattered, she'd probably finish herself off permanently if she tried it. But the way her supporting branch was beginning to shake told her she had no option but to get down *somehow*. Even if the branch held, her damaged harness was likely to let go . . . assuming the even more badly damaged spar didn't simply snap first. But how—?

Of course! She reached up and around with her right arm, gritting her teeth as even that movement

shifted her left arm ever so slightly and sent fresh
stabs of anguish through her. But the pain was worth
it, for her fingers confirmed her hope. The countergrav unit was still there, and she felt the slight,
pulsating hum that indicated it was still operating.
Of course, she couldn't be certain how long it would
go *on* operating. Her cautiously exploring hand
reported an entire series of deep dents and gouges
in its casing. She supposed she should be glad it
had protected her back by absorbing the blows
which had left those marks, but if the unit had taken
a beating anything like what had happened to the
rest of her equipment, it probably wouldn't last all
that long. On the other hand, it only had to hold
out long enough to get her to the ground, and—

Her thoughts chopped off, and she jerked back
around, in a shock spasm fast enough to wrench a
half-scream of pain from her bruised body and broken arm, as something touched the back of her
head. It wasn't that the touch *hurt* in any way, for
it was feather gentle, almost a caress. Only its totally
unexpected surprise produced its power, and all the
pain she felt was the result of her *response* to it.
Yet even as she bit her pain sound back into a
groan, the hurt seemed far away and unimportant
as she stared into the treecat's slit-pupiled green
eyes from a distance of less than thirty centimeters.

Climbs Quickly winced as the two-leg's peaking
hurt clawed at him, yet he was vastly relieved to
find it awake and aware. He smelled the bright,
sharp smell of blood, and the two-leg's arm was

clearly broken. He had no idea how it had managed to get itself into such a predicament, but the bits and pieces strewn around it and hanging from its harness of straps were obviously the ruin of some sort of flying thing. The fragments didn't look like the other flying things he'd seen, yet such it must have been for the two-leg to wind up stuck in the top of a tree this way.

He wished fervently that it could have found another place to crash. This clearing was a place of bad omen, shunned by all of the People. Once it had been the heart of the Sun Shadow Clan's range, but the remnants of that clan had moved far, far away, trying to forget what had happened to it here, and Climbs Quickly would have much preferred not to come here himself.

But that was beside the point. He was here, and however little he might like this place, he knew the two-leg had to get down. The branch from which it hung was not only thrashing with the wind but trying to split off the tree—he knew it was, for he'd crossed the weakened spot to reach the two-leg—and that didn't even consider the way green-needle trees attracted lightning. Yet he could see no way for a two-leg with a broken arm to climb like one of the People, and *he* was certainly too small to carry it!

Frustration bubbled in the back of his mind as he realized how little he could do, but it never occurred to him not to try to help. This was one of "his" two-legs, and he knew that it was the link to *him* which had brought it here. There were far too many things happening for him to begin to

understand them all, yet understanding was strangely
unimportant. This, he realized suddenly, wasn't "one"
of his two-legs after all; it was *his* two-leg. Whatever the link between them was, it cut both ways.
They weren't simply linked; they were *bound* to one
another, and he could no more have abandoned this
strange-looking, alien creature than he could have
walked away from Sings Truly or Short Tail in time
of need.

Yet what could he *do?* He leaned out from his
perch, clinging to the tree with hand-feet and one
true-hand, prehensile tail curled tight around the
branch, as he extended the other true-hand to stroke
the two-leg's cheek and croon to it, and he saw it
blink. Then its hand came up, so much smaller than
a full grown two-leg's yet so much bigger than his
own, and he arched his spine and crooned again—
this time in pleasure—as the two-leg returned his
caress.

Even in her pain and fear, Stephanie felt a sense
of wonder—almost awe—as the treecat reached out
to touch her face. She'd seen the strong, curved
claws the creature's other hand had sunk into the
evergreen's bark, but the wiry fingers that touched
her cheek were moth-wing gentle, claws retracted,
and she pressed back against it. Then she reached
out her own good hand, touching the rain-soaked
fur, stroking it as she would have stroked an Old
Terran cat, and the creature arched with a soft
sound of pleasure. She didn't begin to understand
what was happening, but she didn't have to. She
didn't know exactly what the treecat was doing, but

she dimly sensed the way it was soothing her fear—
even her pain—through that strange link they
shared, and she clung to the comfort it offered.

But then it drew back, sitting higher on its four
rear limbs. It cocked its head at her for a long
moment while wind and rain howled about them,
and then it raised one front paw—no, she reminded
herself, one of its *hands*—and pointed downward.

That was the only possible way to describe its
actions. It *pointed* downward, and even as it pointed,
it made a sharp, scolding sound whose meaning was
unmistakable.

"I *know* I need to get down," she told it in a
hoarse, pain-shadowed voice. "In fact, I was working
on it when you turned up. Just give me a minute,
will you?"

Climbs Quickly's ears shifted as the two-leg made
noises at him. For the first time, thanks to the link
between them, he had proof the noises were actually
words, and he felt a stab of pity for the two-leg and
its fellows. Was that the *only* way they knew to communicate with one another? But however crude and
imperfect the means might be compared to the
manner in which the People spoke, at least he could
now prove that they *did* communicate. That should
go a long way towards convincing the rest of the
clan leaders that two-legs truly were People in their
own fashion. And at least the noises the hurt
youngling was making, coupled with the taste of its
mind glow, were proof that it was still thinking. He
felt a surge of strange pride in the two-leg, comparing its reaction to how some of the People's

younglings might have reacted in its place, and bleeked at it again, more gently.

"I know, I know, I *know!*" Stephanie sighed, and reached back to the countergrav's controls. She adjusted them carefully, then bit her lower lip as a ragged pulsation marred its smooth vibration.

She gave the rheostat one last, gentle twitch, feeling the pressure of the harness straps ease as her apparent weight was reduced to three or four kilos, but that was as far as it would go. She would have preferred an even lower value—had the unit been undamaged, she could have reduced her apparent weight all the way to zero, in which case she would actually have had to pull herself down against its lift. But the rheostat was all the way over now. It wouldn't go any further . . . and the ragged pulsation served notice that the unit was likely to pack up any minute, even at its current setting. Still, she told herself, doggedly trying to find a bright side, maybe it was just as well. Any lighter weight would have been dangerous in such a high wind, and getting her lightweight self smashed against a tree trunk or branch by a sudden gust would hardly do her broken arm any good.

"Well," she said, looking back at the treecat, "here goes."

The two-leg looked at him and said something else, and then, to Climbs Quickly's horror, it unlatched its harness with its good hand and let itself fall. He reared up in protest, ears flattened, yet his horror vanished almost as quickly as it had come, for the youngling didn't actually *fall* at all. Instead, its good hand flashed back out, catching hold of a dangling strip of its broken flying thing, and he blinked. That frayed strip looked too frail to support even *his* weight, yet it held the two-leg with ease, and the youngling slid slowly down it from the grip of that single hand.

The countergrav unit's harsh, warning buzz of imminent failure clawed at Stephanie's ears, and she muttered a word she wasn't supposed to know and slithered more quickly down the broken rigging stay. It was tempting to simply let herself fall, but the countergrav unit only reduced her apparent *weight*. It didn't do a thing about her *mass*, and any object fell at over thirteen meters per second per second in Sphinx's gravity, which meant she would hit the ground just as fast and with just as much momentum as if she'd had no countergrav at all. But what she *could* do was let herself down the stay, whose torn anchorage would never have supported her normal weight.

She was only two meters up when the unit decided to fail, and she cried out, clutching at the stay as her suddenly restored weight snatched at her. She plummeted to the ground, automatically tucking and rolling as her gym teacher had taught her, and she would have been fine if her arm hadn't been broken.

But it *was* broken, and her scream was high and shrill as her rolling weight smashed down on it and the darkness claimed her.

IX

Climbs Quickly leapt down through the branches with frantic haste. His sensitive hearing had detected the sound of the countergrav unit, and though he'd had no idea what it was, he knew its abrupt cessation must have had something to do with the youngling's fall. No doubt it had been another two-leg tool which, like the youngling's flying thing, had broken. In an odd sort of way, it was almost reassuring to know two-leg tools *could* break, but that was cold comfort at the moment, and his whiskers quivered with anxiety as he hit the ground and scuttled quickly over to the youngling.

It lay on its side, and he winced as he realized its fall had ended with its broken arm trapped under it. He tasted the shadow of pain even through the murkiness of its unconscious mind glow, and he dreaded what the youngling would experience when it regained its senses. Worse, he sensed a new pain source in its right knee. But aside from the arm, the knee, and another bump swelling on its forehead, the young two-leg appeared to have taken no fresh damage, and Climbs Quickly settled back on his haunches in relief.

He might not understand what had happened to forge the link between him and this two-leg, but that was no longer really important. What mattered was that the link existed and that for whatever reason the two of them had somehow been made one. There was an echo to it much like that in the mind glows of mated couples, but this was different, without the overtones of physical desire and bereft of the mutual communication of ideas. It was a thing of pure emotion—or *almost* pure emotion, at any rate; he felt frustratingly certain that he had touched the very edge of the youngling's actual thoughts a time or two and wondered if perhaps another of the People and another two-leg might someday reach further than that. For that matter, perhaps he and *his* two-leg would manage that someday, for if this was in fact a permanent link, they would have turnings and turnings in which to explore it.

That prompted another thought, and he groomed his whiskers with a meditative hand while he wondered just how long two-legs lived. The People were much longer lived than large creatures like the death fangs and snow hunters. Did that mean they lived longer than two-legs? The possibility woke an unexpected pain, almost like a presentiment of grief for the loss of the youngling's—*his* youngling's—glorious mind glow. Yet it *was* a youngling, he reminded himself, while *he* was a full adult. Even if its natural span was shorter than his, the difference in their ages might give them an equal number of remaining turnings. That thought was oddly comforting, and he shook himself and looked around.

The battering rain had already eased as the squall line passed through, and much of the wind's strength had died away, as well. He was glad his two-leg had gotten down before the wind could knock it out of the tree, yet every instinct insisted that the ground was not a safe place to be. That was certainly true for the People, but perhaps the youngling had one of the weapons with which its elders sometimes slew the death fangs which threatened them. Climbs Quickly knew those weapons came in different shapes and sizes, but he'd never seen the small ones some two-legs carried, and so he had no way to tell if the youngling had one.

Yet even if it did, its injured condition would leave it in poor shape to defend itself, and it certainly couldn't follow him up into the trees if danger threatened. Which meant it was time to scout around. If there *was* danger here, best he should know about it now. Once the young two-leg reawakened, it might have ideas of its own about how to proceed; until then, he would simply have to do the best he could on his own.

He turned away from the two-leg and began to circle it, moving out in an ever-widening spiral while nose and ears probed alertly. This early in the season there was little undergrowth beneath the trees to obscure his lines of sight, though it was a different matter in the old forest fire's clearing, which low-growing scrub and young trees were beginning to reclaim, and the rain hadn't been hard enough or fallen long enough to wipe away scents. Indeed, the moist air actually made them sharper and richer, and his muzzle wrinkled as he tested them.

But then, suddenly, he froze, whiskers stiff and fluffy tail belled out to twice its normal diameter. He made himself take another long, careful scent, yet it was no more than a formality. No clan scout could *ever* mistake the smell of a death fang lair, and this one was close.

He turned slowly, working to fix the location clearly in his mind, and his heart fell. The scent came from the clearing, where the undergrowth would offer the lair's owner maximum concealment when it returned and scented the two-leg. And it *would* return, he thought sinkingly, for he smelled something more, now. The death fang was a female, and it had recently littered. That meant it must be out hunting food for its young . . . and that it would be back sooner rather than later.

Climbs Quickly stood a moment longer, then raced back to the two-leg. He touched its face with his muzzle, willing it to awaken with all his might, but there was no response. It would wake when it woke, he realized. Nothing he did would speed that moment, and that left but one thing he *could* do.

He sat upright on his four rearmost limbs, curling his tail neatly about his true-feet and hand-feet, and composed his thought carefully, then sent it soaring out through the dripping forest. He shaped and drove it with all the urgency in him, crying out to his sister, and somehow his link to the two-leg lent his call additional strength.

<Climb's Quickly?> Even from here he tasted the shock in Sings Truly's mind voice. *<Where are you? What's wrong?>*

<I am near the old fire scar to sun-rising of our range,> Climbs Quickly replied as calmly as he could, and felt a fresh surge of astonishment from his sister. No one from Bright Water Clan would soon forget the terrible day Sun Shadow Clan had lost control of a fire and seen its entire central nesting place—and all too many of its kittens—consumed in dreadful flame and smoke.

<Why?> she demanded. *<What could possibly take you there?>*

<I—> Climbs Quickly paused, then drew a deep breath. *<It would take too long to explain, Sings Truly. But I am here with an injured youngling . . . and so also is a death fang lair filled with young.>*

Sings Truly knew her brother well, and the oddness in his reply was obvious to her. But so was the unusual strength and clarity of his mind voice. He had always had a strong voice for a male, but today he had reached almost to the strength of a memory singer, and she wondered how he'd done it. Some scouts and hunters gained far stronger voices when they mated, as if their mates' minds somehow harmonized with theirs at need, but that couldn't explain Climbs Quickly's new power. Yet those thoughts were but a fleeting background for the chill horror she felt at the thought of any injured youngling trapped so near a death fang.

She started to reply once more, then stopped, tail kinking and ears cocking in sudden consternation and suspicion. No, surely not. Not even Climbs Quickly would dare *that*. Not after the way the clan elders had berated him! Yet try as she might, she could think of no way any Bright Water youngling would have strayed so far, and no other clan's range bordered on the fire scar. And Climbs Quickly had named no names, had he? But—

She shook herself. There was, of course, one way to satisfy her suspicion. All she had to do was ask . . . but if she did, then she would know her brother was violating the edicts of his clan heads. If she didn't ask, she could only suspect—not *know*—and so she kept that particular question to herself and asked another.

<*What do you wish of me, brother?*>

<*Sound the alarm,*> he replied, sending a burst of gratitude and love with the words, for he knew what she'd considered, and her choice of question told him what she'd decided.

<*For the "injured youngling."*> Sings Truly's flat statement was a question, and he flicked his tail in agreement even though she could not see it.

<*Yes,*> he returned simply, and felt her hesitation. But then her answer came.

<*I will,*> she said with equal simplicity—and the unquestionable authority of a memory singer. <*We come with all speed, my brother.*>

Stephanie Harrington awoke once more. A weak, pain-filled sound leaked from her—less words than the mew of an injured kitten—and her eyelids fluttered. She started to sit up, and her mew became a breathless, involuntary scream as her weight shifted on her broken arm. The sudden agony was literally blinding, and she screwed her eyes shut once more, sobbing with hurt as she made herself sit up anyway. Nausea knotted her stomach as the anguish in her arm and shoulder and broken rib vibrated through her, and she sat very still, as if the pain were some sort of hunting predator from which she could hide until it passed her by.

But the pain didn't pass her by. It only eased a bit, and she blinked on tears, scrubbing her face with her good hand and sniffling as she smeared mud and the blood from her mashed nose across her cheeks. She didn't need to move to know she'd smashed her knee, as well as her bad arm, in her fall, and she felt herself shuddering, quivering like a leaf as hopelessness and pain crushed down on her. The immediacy of the need to get down out of the tree had helped carry her to this point, but she was on the ground now. That gave her time to think—and feel.

Fresh, hot tears brimmed, dripping down her face, and she whined as she made herself gather her left wrist in her right hand and lift it into her lap. Just moving it twisted her with torment, but she couldn't leave it hanging down beside her like it belonged to someone else. She thought about using her belt to fasten it to her side, but she couldn't find the energy—or courage—to move that shattered bone again. It was too much for her. Now that the immediate crisis was over, she knew how much she hurt, how totally lost she was, how desperately she wanted—needed—her parents to come take her home, how *stupid* she'd been to get herself into this mess . . . and how very little she could do to get herself out of it.

She huddled there at the foot of the tree, crying hopelessly for her mother and father. The world had proved bigger and more dangerous than she'd ever quite believed, and she wanted them to come find her. No scold they could give her, however ferocious, could match the one she gave herself, and she whimpered as the sobs she couldn't stop shook her broken arm and sent fresh, vicious stabs of pain through her.

But then she felt a light pressure on her right thigh and blinked furiously to clear her eyes. She looked down, and the treecat looked back. He stood beside her, one hand resting on her leg, ears flattened with concern, and she heard—and felt—his soft, comforting croon. She gazed down at him for a moment, mouth quivering in exhaustion, despair, pain, and physical shock, and then she held out her good arm to him, and he didn't even hesitate. He flowed up her leg to stand on his rearmost limbs in her lap and place his hands—those strong, wiry, long-fingered hands with the carefully sheathed claws—on either side of her neck. He pressed his whiskered muzzle to her cheek, the power of his croon quivering through him as if he were a dynamo, and she locked her right arm around him. She held him close, almost crushing him, and buried her face in his soft, damp fur, sobbing as if her heart would break, and even as she wept, she felt him somehow taking the worst hurt, the worst despair and helplessness from her.

❖   ❖   ❖

Climbs Quickly accepted the two-leg's tight embrace. People's eyes didn't shed water as the two-leg's did, but only the mind-blind could possibly have mistaken the grief and fear and pain in the youngling's mind glow, and he felt a vast surge of protective tenderness for it. For *her*, he realized now, though he wasn't quite certain how he knew. Perhaps it was just that he was becoming more accustomed to the taste of her mind glow. One could almost always tell whether one of the People was male or female from no more than that, after all. Of course, this youngling was totally unlike the People, but still—

He pressed more firmly against her, stroking her cheek with his muzzle and patting her good shoulder with his right true-hand while he settled more deeply into fusion with her. It wasn't as it would have been with another of his own kind, for she was unable to anchor the fusion properly from her end, but it was enough to let him draw off the worst of her despair. He felt the burden of her fear and pain ease and sensed her surprised awareness that he was somehow responsible, and a deep, buzzing purr replaced his croon. He nudged her cheek more firmly, then pulled back just far enough to touch his nose to hers, staring deep into her eyes, and her good hand caressed his ears. She said something—another of those mouth noises which so far meant nothing—but he felt her gratitude and knew the meaningless sounds thanked him for being there.

She leaned back against the tree, easing her broken arm carefully, and he settled down in her lap, wishing with what he hoped was concealed desperation that there was some way to get her away from this place. He knew she remained confused and frightened, and he had no desire to undo all the soothing he'd achieved, yet the scent of the death fang seemed to clog his nostrils. If not for her injured knee, he would have done his best to get her on her feet despite her broken arm. But the tough covering she wore over her legs had torn when she hit the ground, and the gashed knee under it was swollen and purpling. He needed no link to know she could move neither fast nor far, and he turned his mind once more towards his sister.

<*Does the clan come?*> he asked urgently, and her reply astounded him.

<*We come,*> Sings Truly repeated with unmistakable emphasis, and he blinked. Surely she didn't mean—? But then she sent him a brief burst of her own vision, and he realized she did. She was leading every male adult of the clan herself. A *memory singer* was leading the clan's fighting strength into battle with a death fang! That wasn't merely unheard of—it was un*thinkable*. Yet it was happening, and he poured a flood of gratitude towards her.

<*There is no choice, little brother,*> she told him dryly. <*The clan may protect your "youngling" from the death fang, but without me, there will be no one to protect you from Broken Tooth and Digger . . . or Song Spinner! Now leave me in peace, Climbs Quickly. I cannot run properly with you nattering at me.*>

He pulled in his thought, basking in his sister's love and trying not to think about the implications of her warning. From the glimpse he'd shared through her eyes, she and the others were making excellent speed. They would be here soon, and only a very stupid death fang would risk attacking anything with an entire clan of People perched protectively in the trees above it. It would not be long until—

Stephanie had fallen into a half doze, leaning back against the tree, but her head snapped up instantly as the treecat came to his feet in her lap with a harsh, rippling snarl like shredding canvas. She'd never heard anything like it, yet she knew instantly what it meant. It was as if the link between them transmitted that meaning to her, and she felt his fear and fury . . . and fierce determination to protect her.

She looked around wildly, trying to find the danger, then gasped, eyes huge in a parchment face, as the hexapuma flowed out of the undergrowth like a gray, six-legged shadow of death. Its lips wrinkled back, baring bone-white canines at least fifteen centimeters long, and its ears flattened as it sent its own rippling snarl—this one voiced in deep, basso thunder—to meet the treecat's. Terror froze Stephanie, but the treecat leapt from her lap. He sprang up onto a low-lying limb and crouched there, threatening his gargantuan foe from above, and his claws were no longer sheathed. For some reason, the hexapuma hesitated, twisting its head around and staring up at the trees, almost as if it were afraid of something. But that couldn't last, and she knew it.

"No," she heard herself whisper to her tiny protector. "No, it's too big! Run away. Oh, *please*—please! *Run away!*"

But the treecat ignored her, his green eyes locked on the hexapuma, and despair mixed with her terror. The hexapuma was going to get them both, because the treecat *wouldn't* run away. Somehow she knew, beyond any possibility of question, that the only way the hexapuma would reach her would be through him.

There was very little to sense in a death fang's brain, but Climbs Quickly understood its hesitation. This was an old death fang, and it had not lived this long without learning some hard lessons. Among those lessons must have been what a roused clan could do to its kind, for it had the wit to look for the others who should have been there to support him.

But Climbs Quickly knew what the death fang couldn't. There *were* no other People—not yet. They were coming, tearing through the treetops with frantic, redoubled speed, but they would never arrive in time.

He glared down at the death fang, sounding his challenge, and knew he couldn't win. No single scout or hunter could encounter a death fang and live, yet he could no more abandon his two-leg youngling than he could have abandoned a kitten of the People. He felt her desperate emotions urging him to flee and save himself despite her own terror, even as he felt his sister's mind voice screaming the same, but it didn't matter. It didn't even matter that the death fang would kill the two-leg the moment he himself was dead. What mattered was that his two-leg—his *person*—must not die alone and abandoned. He would buy her every moment of life he could, and perhaps, just perhaps, it would be long enough for Sings Truly to arrive. He told himself that firmly, fiercely, trying to pretend he didn't know it was a lie, and then the death fang charged.

Stephanie watched the motionless confrontation as treecat and hexapuma glared and snarled at one another, and the tension tore at her like knives. She couldn't stand it, yet neither could she escape it, and the treecat's utter, hopeless gallantry ripped at her heart. He could have run away. He could have escaped the hexapuma *easily*, but he'd refused, and deep inside, under the panic of an exhausted, hurt, terrified child face-to-face with a murderous menace she should never have encountered, his fierce defiance touched something in *her*. She didn't know what it was. She didn't even realize what was happening. But even as the treecat was determined to protect her, she felt an equally fierce, equally unyielding determination to protect *him*.

Her right hand fell to her belt and closed on the hilt of her vibro blade survival knife. It was only a short blade—barely eighteen centimeters long, which was nothing compared to the sixty-centimeter bush knives Forestry Service rangers carried. But that short blade had a cutting "edge" less than a molecule wide, and it whined alive in her hand as she somehow shoved herself to her feet. She leaned back against the trunk, left arm dangling while terror rose like bile in her throat, and knew her knife was too puny. It would slice through the hexapuma effortlessly, cutting bone as easily as tissue, yet it was too short. The huge predator would tear her apart before she could cut it at all, and even if she somehow did manage to cut it as it charged, even inflict a mortal wound, it was so big and powerful it would kill her before it died. But the knife was all she had, and she stared at the hexapuma, hardly daring to breathe, waiting.

And then it charged.

Climbs Quickly saw the death fang move at last. He had time to send out one more urgent message to Sings Truly, to feel her raging despair and fury at the knowledge she would come too late, and then there was no more time to think. There was no time for anything but speed and violence and ferocity.

Stephanie couldn't believe it. The hexapuma was terrifyingly quick for so huge a creature, yet the treecat sprang from his perch, catapulting through the air in a cream-and-gray streak that somehow evaded the hexapuma's slashing forepaws. He landed on the back of its neck, and it screamed as centimeter-long claws ripped at thick fur and tough skin. It whirled, both rear pairs of limbs planted firmly, forequarters rising up as it twisted to snap and claw at the treecat, but its furious blows missed. The treecat had executed his flashing attack only to race further down his enemy's spine and fling himself back up onto another branch, and the hexapuma forgot about

Stephanie. It wheeled, charging the tree in which the treecat waited, rising up on its rear legs and spreading its front and mid-limbs wide to claw at the thick trunk. It dragged itself as high as it could, slashing and snarling, and Stephanie suddenly understood what the treecat was trying to do.

He was *distracting* the hexapuma. He knew he couldn't kill it or even truly fight it. His attack had been intended to hurt it, to make it angry and direct that anger at *him* and away from her, and it was working. But it was a desperate, ultimately losing game, for he must keep up the attacks, keep stinging the hexapuma, and he couldn't be lucky forever.

Climbs Quickly felt a fierce exultation, unlike anything he'd ever imagined. This was a fight he couldn't win, yet he was eager for it. He *wanted* it, and the blood-red taste of his own fury filled him with fire. He watched the death fang lunge up the tree and timed his response perfectly. Just as the death fang reached the very top of its leap, he dropped to meet it, slashing and ripping, and the death fang howled as he shredded its muzzle and tore an ear to pieces, but again its counter-striking forepaws missed him as he sprang away once more.

It charged after him, and he came to meet it yet again. He danced in and out of the trees, pitting blinding speed and skill and intelligence against the death fang's brute power and cunning. It was a dance which could have only one ending, yet he spun it out far longer than even he would have believed possible before it began.

❖   ❖   ❖

"No!"

Stephanie screamed in useless denial as the treecat finally made a mistake. Perhaps he slipped, or perhaps he'd simply begun to tire at last. She didn't know. She only knew that she'd felt a wild, impossible hope as the fight raged on and on. Not that he could win, but that he might not *lose*. Even as she'd let herself hope, she'd known it was in vain, but the suddenness of the end hit her with the cruelty of a hammer.

The treecat was a fraction of a second too slow, lingered to slash at the hexapuma's shoulders for just an instant too long, and a mid-limb paw flashed up savagely. Ten-centimeter claws gleamed like scimitars, and she heard—and *felt*—the treecat's scream of agony as that brutal blow landed.

It didn't hit squarely, but it was square enough. It stripped him away from the hexapuma's neck, flicking him aside like a toy, and he screamed again as he slammed into the trunk of a tree. He tumbled down it in a broken, bloody ball of fur, and the hexapuma rose on its rearmost limbs. It hovered there, howling its rage and triumph, and then it lowered all six feet to the ground and crouched to spring and rend and tear and crush its tiny enemy.

Stephanie saw it, understood it, knew what it intended . . . and that she couldn't possibly stop it. But the treecat—*her* treecat—had known he couldn't stop it from killing *her*, either, and that hadn't kept him from trying. A part of her knew it was only a pathetic gesture, no more than the hiss and spit of a kitten in the instant before hungry jaws closed on it forever, but it was a gesture she simply could not *not* make.

She lunged, ignoring her snapped rib, the agony in her wounded knee and broken arm. In that moment, she wasn't just an eleven-year-old girl. There was no time for her to fully grasp all that was happening, but something inside her had changed forever when the treecat offered his life to save hers, and her scream was a war cry as she brought the vibro blade slashing forward and offered *her* life for his.

The hexapuma shrieked as the high-tech blade sliced into it. It had forgotten about Stephanie, narrowed all its intention to Climbs Quickly, and it was totally unprepared for the unadulterated agony of that blow. The blade caught it on its right flank, so "sharp" that even an eleven-year-old's arm could drive it hilt-deep. The creature's own frantic lunge to escape the pain did the rest, and blood sprayed across the fallen leaves of winters past as its movement dragged the unstoppable blade through muscle, tendons, arteries, and bone.

Stephanie staggered and almost fell as the huge predator squirmed frantically away. Her hand and arm were soaked in its blood, more steaming blood had gouted across her face and eyes, and if she'd had time for it, she would have been nauseated. But she didn't have time, and she staggered further forward, putting herself between the treecat and the hexapuma.

It was all she could do to stay on her feet. She shook like a leaf, her blood-coated face streaked with tears while terror yammered within her, yet somehow she stayed upright and raised the humming blade between them as the hexapuma stared at her in animal disbelief. Its right rear leg trailed helplessly while blood pulsed from the huge, gaping wound in its flank, but the very sharpness of the vibro blade worked against Stephanie in at least one respect. That wound was fatal, but the hexapuma didn't know it. It would take time to bleed out, and the knife was so sharp, the wound inflicted so quickly, that the creature had no idea of the catastrophic damage it had just received. It only knew it was hurt, that the injured prey it had expected to take so easily had inflicted more agony than any enemy it had ever faced, and it howled its fury.

It paused for just a moment, hissing and spitting, the ears Climbs Quickly had shredded flat to its skull, and Stephanie knew it was going to charge. She had no more idea than the hexapuma that she'd already inflicted a mortal wound, and she tried to hold her knife steady. It was going to come right over her, but if she could get the knife up, stick it into its chest or belly and let its charge do there what its lunge away had done to its hindquarters, then maybe at least the treecat would—

The hexapuma howled again, and Stephanie wanted desperately to close her eyes. But she couldn't, and she saw it lunge—saw it spring forward in the first of the two leaps it would take to reach her, dragging its crippled leg, fang-studded maw agape.

Only it never completed that lunge, and Stephanie's head jerked up as a dreadful noise filled the forest. She'd heard a single echo of it from the treecat who'd fought to protect her, but this wasn't the defiant cry of one hopelessly gallant defender. This was the rippling snarl of dozens—scores—of treecats, filled with hate and vengeance, and its challenge pierced even the hexapuma's rage. Its head snapped up, as Stephanie's had done, and its yowl was filled with as much panic as fury as the trees exploded above it.

A cream-and-gray avalanche thundered down with a massed, high-pitched scream that seemed to shake the forest. It engulfed the hexapuma in an unstoppable flood of slashing ivory claws and needle-sharp fangs, and Stephanie Harrington collapsed beside a dreadfully wounded Climbs Quickly as the scouts and hunters of his clan literally ripped their foe to pieces.

X

"I'm home!" Richard Harrington called out as he walked into the living room.

"About time," Marjorie replied from her office. She was at the end of a section anyway, so she hit the save key and closed the report, then rose and stretched.

"Hey, don't give me a hard time," her husband told her severely as he walked down the short hall and poked his head in her door. "You may be able to do a full day's work without going anywhere, but *some* of us have patients who require our direct, personal attendance . . . not to mention a superb bedside manner."

"'Bedside manner,' right!" Marjorie snorted, and Richard grinned as he leaned close to kiss her cheek. She put an arm around him and hugged him briefly. "Did Steph have a good day with Mr. Sapristos?" she went on.

"What?" Richard pulled back with a strange expression, and she cocked an eyebrow.

"I asked if Stephanie had a good day with Mayor Sapristos," she said, and Richard frowned.

"I didn't drop her off in Twin Forks," he said. "I didn't have time, so I left her home. Didn't I tell you I was going to?"

"Left her home?" Marjorie repeated. "Here? On the homestead?"

"Of course! Where else would I—" Richard broke off as he recognized his wife's incomprehension. "Are you saying you haven't seen her all day?"

"I certainly haven't! Would I have asked you about Mr. Sapristos if I *had?*"

"But—"

Richard broke off again, and his frown deepened. He stood for a moment, thinking hard, then turned and half-ran down the hall. Marjorie heard the front door open and close—then it opened and closed again, seconds later, and Richard was back.

"Her glider's gone," he told Marjorie grimly.

"But you said you didn't take her to town," Marjorie protested.

"I didn't," he said even more grimly. "So if her glider's gone, she must've gone off on a flight of her own—without telling either of us."

Marjorie gazed at him, her own mind filled with a cascade of chaotic thoughts and sudden, half-formed fears. Then she took a firm mental grip on herself and cleared her throat.

"If she went out on her own, she should be back by now," she said as calmly as she could. "It's getting dark, and she would've wanted to be home before that happened."

"Absolutely," Richard agreed, and the tension in their locked gazes was just short of panic. An inextricable brew of fear for their daughter, guilt for not having watched her more closely, and—hard though they tried to suppress it—*anger* at her for evading their watchfulness, flowed through them, but there was no time for that. Richard shook himself, then raised his left wrist and keyed Stephanie's combination into his com.

He waited, right forefinger and second finger drumming anxiously on the com's wrist band, and his face went bleak as the seconds oozed past with no reply. He waited a full minute, in which his eyes became agate and the last expression leached from his face, and Marjorie caught his upper right arm and squeezed tightly. She said nothing, for she too understood what that lack of reply meant.

It took a painful act of will for Richard Harrington to accept the silence, but then his forefinger moved again. He keyed in another combination, and inhaled sharply as a red light began to flash almost instantly on the com. In one way, the light was almost worse than the total lack of response had been; in another, it was an enormous relief. At least it gave them a beacon to track—one which should guide them to their daughter. But if the emergency beacon was working the rest of the com unit should also be functional. And if it was— if it had produced the high-pitched buzz which was guaranteed to be audible from a distance of over thirty meters—then Stephanie should have answered it. If she hadn't, there had to be a reason, and neither Harrington had the courage to voice what that reason might well be.

"Grab the emergency med-kit," Richard said instead, his voice harsh. "I'll get my car back out of the garage."

Stephanie Harrington couldn't hear the signal from the lost com that hung on the stub of a limb more than fifty meters above her. Nor was she even thinking about coms, for she was surrounded by over two hundred treecats. They perched on branches, clung to trunks, and crouched with her on the wet leaves. Two actually sat pressed against her sides, and they—like all the rest—crooned a deep, soft harmony to the bloody, mauled ball of fur in her lap.

She was grateful for their presence, and she knew those scores of guardians could—and would—protect her from any other predators. Yet she had little attention to spare them, for every scrap of her attention was fixed with desperate strength on *her* treecat, as if somehow she could keep him alive by sheer force of will. The pain in her arm and knee and ribs and her residual, quivering terror still filled her, but those things scarcely mattered. They were there, and they were real, but nothing—literally *nothing*—was as important as the treecat she cuddled with fierce protectiveness in the crook of her good arm.

Her memory of what had happened after the other treecats poured down from the trees was vague. She recalled switching off the vibro knife, but she hadn't gotten it back into its sheath. She must have dropped it somewhere, but it didn't matter. All that had mattered was getting to her treecat.

She'd known he was alive. There was no way she could *not* know, but she'd also known he was desperately hurt, and her stomach had knotted as she fell to her good knee beside him. Her own pain had made her whimper as she moved with injudicious speed, yet she'd hardly noticed as she touched her protector—her *friend*, however he'd become that— with fearful fingers.

Blood matted his right side, and she'd felt fresh nausea as she saw how badly his right forelimb was mangled. The blood flow was terrifying, without the spurt of a severed artery, but far too thick and heavy. She had no idea how his internal anatomy was arranged, but her frightened touch had felt what had to be the jagged give of broken ribs, and his mid-limbs' pelvis was clearly broken, as well. She'd cringed at the thought of the damage all those broken bones could have done inside him, but there was nothing she could do about them. That shattered forelimb needed immediate attention, however, and she plucked the drawstring from the left cuff of her flying jacket. Tying it into a slip noose with only her teeth and one working hand was impossibly difficult, yet she managed it somehow, and slipped it up the broken, bloodsoaked limb. She settled it just above the ripped and torn flesh and drew it tight, bending close to use her teeth again, then worked a pocket stylus under the improvised tourniquet and tightened it carefully. She'd never done anything like this herself, but she knew the theory, and she'd once seen her father do the same thing for an Irish setter who'd lost most of a leg to a robotic cultivator.

It worked, and she sagged in relief as the blood flow slowed, then stopped. She knew that cutting off all blood from the damaged tissues would only damage them worse in the long run, but at least he wouldn't bleed to death now. Unless, of course, she thought, fighting a suddenly resurgent panic, there *was* internal bleeding.

She didn't really want to move him, but she couldn't leave him lying on the cold, wet ground. He needed warmth, and she lowered herself with a groan to sit beside him and lift him as carefully as she could with only one hand. She flinched when he twisted with a sound like the mewl of a broken kitten, but she didn't put him back down. Instead, she tucked him inside her unsealed flying jacket and tugged the loose flaps closed around him as well as her single working arm could manage. Then she leaned back, whimpering with her own pain, holding him against her and trying to fight his shock and blood loss with the warmth of her own body.

She didn't think about her missing com, or her parents, or her own pain. She didn't think of anything. She only sat there, cuddling her defender's broken body against her own, and thought of nothing at all, for that was all she had the strength to do.

The elders of Bright Water Clan sat in a circle about the young two-leg. *All* of them, even Song

Spinner, who had come after the others for the sole purpose of berating Sings Truly for her incredible folly in risking herself in such a fashion. But no one was berating anyone now. Instead, the other elders watched in confusion and uncertainty as Sings Truly and Short Tail crept closer to the two-leg. The chief scout and the clan's second ranking memory singer crouched on either side of the two-leg, quivering noses scarcely a handspan's distance from it. They sniffed it carefully, and then reached out to touch the link between it and Climbs Quickly.

Sings Truly's ears went flat in shock that, even for her, even now, was honed by disbelief. Despite the alienness of the two-leg, Climbs Quickly's link to it was *at least* as strong as that of any mated pair she'd ever encountered. More than that, the link clearly had yet to reach its maximum strength. That couldn't possibly happen—not with a creature as obviously and completely mind-blind as the two-leg. Yet it *had* happened, and Sings Truly's mind whirled as she tried to imagine the ramifications of that simple fact.

The rest of her clan's adult fighting strength sat or crouched or hung behind and above and all about her and the two-leg. As she, they'd watched the youngling, tasting its pain like their own, as it dragged its gravely injured body to Climbs Quickly. As Sings Truly, they had tasted its fear for him, its tenderness and frantic concern, its . . . love. And, as Sings Truly, they had watched the youngling— surely no more than a kitten itself—tighten the string that stopped Climbs Quickly's bleeding before he died. And then they watched the two-leg gather him against itself, hugging him, giving of its own body heat to him, and the massed music of the clan's soft, approving croon had risen about the two-leg. The clan had reached out, able to touch the two-leg, albeit indirectly, through its link to Climbs Quickly, and their massed touch had soothed the youngling's fear and pain and eased it tenderly into a gentle mind haze. The People of Bright Water took its hurt upon themselves and soothed it into something very like sleep, and it was safe for them to do so, for nothing that walked the world's forest could threaten or harm Climbs Quickly or his two-leg through their watchful ring of claws and fangs.

Sings Truly saw all that, understood all that, and deep inside, she wanted—as she had never wanted anything before—to hate the two-leg. Climbs Quickly might live. His mind glow was weak, yet it was there, and even now she felt his awareness creeping slowly, doggedly back towards the surface. But he was terribly hurt, and those hurts were the two-leg's fault. It was the two-leg which had drawn him here. It was the two-leg for whom he'd fought his impossible battle, risked—and all too possibly lost—his life. Even if he lived, he would have only one true-hand, and that, too, was the two-leg's fault.

Yet badly as Sings Truly wished to hate the two-leg, she knew Climbs Quickly had *chosen* to come. Or perhaps not. Perhaps the strength of his link to this alien creature had left him no choice *but* to come, yet if that was true, then it was equally true that the two-leg had been given no choice, either. They were one, as tightly bound as any mated pair, and Sings Truly knew it . . . just as she knew her brother, as she herself, would have fought to the death to protect his mate.

And so would this two-leg. Youngling or no, despite broken bones and legs which would scarcely bear it, this barely weaned kitten had attacked a *death fang* single-handed. Climbs Quickly had done the same, but he had been an adult—and uninjured. The two-leg had been neither, but it had risen above its wounds and terror to fight the same terrible foe for Climbs Quickly. No youngling of the People, and all too few of the People's adults, could have done that, and without the two-leg, Climbs Quickly would already be dead, so—

<How shall we untangle this knot, Sings Truly?> The question came from Short Tail, and though it was directed to Sings Truly, the chief scout had thought it loudly enough to be certain all of the elders heard him.

<We should leave while we still can!> Broken Tooth replied sharply, before Sings Truly could. *<The danger of this is far too great! Sooner or later, this two-leg's fellows will come seeking it, and we must not be here when they do.>*

<And Climbs Quickly?> Short Tail asked bitingly, and the People's ability to taste one another's emotions was not a useful thing at the moment. Broken Tooth felt the scout's searing contempt as clearly as if Short Tail had shouted it aloud—which, indeed, he had, in a way—and his own mind voice was hot when he replied.

<Climbs Quickly chose *to come here!>* he snapped. *<He was told to stay away from the two-legs—that*

Shadow Chaser would have that duty—yet he dis-obeyed. Not content with that, he summoned the clan to save the two-leg from a death fang, despite the danger. Many of us might have been killed or hurt by such an enemy, and you know it! I am sorry for his wounds, and I wish him no evil, but what happens to him stems from his own decisions. Our task is to safeguard our entire clan, and to do that we must be far away when the other two-legs arrive. If that requires us to leave Climbs Quickly to his fate, it cannot be helped.>

<It was not Climbs Quickly who summoned the clan,> Song Spinner observed with frigid disapproval. *<Or not directly. It was you, Sings Truly, and you knew he was trying to protect the two-leg!>*

<It was, and I did.> The calmness of Sings Truly's reply surprised even her. *<Oh, I didn't know, but that was only because I had declined to ask him. So, yes, senior singer. I knew what Climbs Quickly desired. Perhaps I was even wrong to give it to him. But even if I was wrong, he most certainly was not.>* The other elders stared at her in consternation, and she turned from her contemplation of the young two-leg and her brother to face them.

<Climbs Quickly and this two-leg are linked,> she told them. *<I have tasted that link, and so can any of you, if you doubt me. He was defending . . . not his "mate," precisely, but something very close to it. This is his two-leg, and he is its. He could no more have failed to protect it than he could have failed to protect me or I him.>*

<Prettily said,> Song Spinner said acidly when none of the males would meet Sings Truly's eyes

or refute her words. *<Perhaps even true . . . for Climbs Quickly. But Broken Tooth speaks for the rest of the clan. We have no link to this two-leg, and surely this is only fresh proof of the danger of hasty contact with them. Look at your brother, memory singer, and tell me risking further contact with these creatures is not the path of madness!>*

<Very well, senior singer,> Sings Truly said, still with that same astounding calm and clarity of mind voice, *<if you wish, I will tell you exactly that. Indeed, what has happened here is the clearest proof that we must seek out more contact with the two-legs, for we must learn if more of the People can establish such bonds with the two-legs.>*

<More bonds?> Broken Tooth gasped. He and Digger gawked in horror, but Song Spinner stared at her in shock too profound for any other emotion. Short Tail, on the other hand, crouched beside her, radiating fierce agreement, and they were joined—albeit with less certainty—by Fleet Wind, the elder charged with the instruction of young scouts and hunters, and by Stone Biter, who led the clan's flint shapers.

<More bonds,> Sings Truly replied levelly, and Broken Tooth hissed—not in anger, for no male would ever show challenge to a senior memory singer, whatever the provocation, but in utter rejection. *<No, hear me out!>* Sings Truly commanded. *<Right or wrong, I am a singer. You will hear me, and the clan—the clan, Broken Tooth, not simply the elders—will judge between us on this!>*

Broken Tooth settled back, and Song Spinner twitched in even greater shock. As the clan's second

ranking singer, Sings Truly had every right to make
that demand, yet by making it, she had in effect
challenged Song Spinner's own position. She had
appealed to the entire clan, seeking the judgment
of the majority of its adults, when all knew that
Song Spinner opposed her. If the clan chose to
support Sings Truly, *she* would become Bright
Water's senior singer, while if the clan chose to
reject her, she would be stripped of all authority.

But the challenge had been issued, and the clan
adults drew closer.

<*What my brother has done was not of his
choice,*> Sings Truly said quietly but clearly. <*It
could not have been his choice, for none of the
People even guessed such a thing was possible. Nor
could he, or any of us, have known how to establish such a link with a two-leg even had we desired
to do so. But he did establish the link, and though
the two-leg is mind-blind and clearly fails to understand, it shares the link. It is as linked to him as
he is to it. Is this not true, senior singer?*>

Sings Truly looked directly at Song Spinner, and
Bright Water's senior singer could only flick her ears
in curt agreement, for it was obvious to all, singer
and non-singer alike, that it *was* true.

<*Very well,*> Sings Truly continued. <*We didn't
know—then—that such links were possible. We do
know now, however, just as all of us have seen proof
of the link's depth and power. Climbs Quickly fought
the death fang for his two-leg, but the two-leg also
fought the death fang for him, and by the standards
of its own kind, this two-leg is but a kitten. We dare
not judge all two-legs by its actions, yet we dare*

not reject its example, either. We must learn more about them and their tools and their purpose in being here. They are too dangerous, and there are too many of them, and their numbers increase too quickly for us not to learn those things. Climbs Quickly was right in that . . . and the very things which make them so dangerous could also make them powerful allies.>

Not a whisper rose among her listeners. Every eye was fixed upon her, and even Broken Tooth's tail had stopped its lashing, for it had never occurred to him to consider what the two-legs could do *for* the People. He had been too aware of all the threats the intruders posed *to* them, and Sings Truly felt her hope rise higher as she tasted the shifting emotions of his mind glow.

<If others of the People can—and choose to— form such links, we will learn much. If they go with those they link with to live among the two-legs, they will see far more than we can ever see spying upon them from the shadows. They can report to us, tell us of all they learn, help us to understand the two-legs. And remember the nature of such links. The two-legs do, indeed, appear to be mind-blind. Certainly this one is. Yet for all its blindness, it senses the link. It feels and recognizes Climbs Quickly's love for it . . . and returns that love. I think it is clear from Climbs Quickly's original report that this two-leg thought him no more clever than the ground runners or lake builders when first it met him. It knows better now, yet it cannot know how much more clever the People are. Perhaps it would be as well if we do not let it or its elders know just how

clever we are, for it is always wise to let others underestimate us. But let us also build more links with the two-legs, if such we can. Let us learn, and let those of the People who share such links with them teach them that we do not threaten them. There is much room in the world, surely enough for us to share it with the two-legs if we can make them our friends.>

The mental silence lingered, hovering in the wet, rapidly darkening woods. And then, in the way of the People, it was broken by mind voices in ones and twos, choosing their course.

XI

Richard Harrington's face was white as the air car's powerful lights picked the wreckage trail from the darkness. The icon of Stephanie's emergency beacon glowed in the dead center of his HUD, indicating that it lay directly below him, but he didn't really need it. Bits and pieces of a mangled hang glider were strewn through the tops of three different trees, and the continued silence from his daughter's end of the com link was suddenly even more terrifying.

He didn't know what Stephanie had been doing out here, but she'd clearly been trying to reach the clearing ahead when she went down, and he sent the air car scudding forward. Marjorie sat tense and silent beside him, twisting the control that swept the starboard spotlight in a wide half-circle on her side of the car. Richard was just reaching for the control to the port light, when Marjorie gasped.

"Richard! *Look!*"

His head snapped around at his wife's command, and his jaw dropped. Stephanie sat huddled against the base of a huge tree, clasping something against her with one arm. Her clothing was torn and bloody, but her head rose as he looked at her. She stared back into the lights, and even from his seat in the air car, he saw the bottomless relief on her bruised and bloody face. Yet even as he recognized that, and even as his heart leapt in joy so sharp it was anguish, stunned surprise held him frozen, for his daughter was not alone.

A grisly ruin of white bone and mangled tissue lay to one side. Richard had done enough anatomical studies of Sphinxian animal life to recognize the half-stripped skeleton of a hexapuma, but neither he nor any other naturalist had ever seen or imagined anything like the dozens and dozens and *dozens* of tiny "hexapumas" who surrounded his daughter protectively.

He blinked, astonished by his own choice of adverb, yet it was the only one which fitted. They were *protecting* Stephanie, watching over her, and he knew—as if he'd seen it with his own eyes—that they, whatever *they* were, had killed the hexapuma to save her.

But that was all he knew, and he touched Marjorie's arm gently.

"Stay here," he said quietly. "This is my area, not yours."

"But—"

"Please, Marge," he said, still in that quiet voice. "I don't think there's any danger—now—but I could be wrong. Just stay here while I find out, all right?"

Marjorie Harrington's jaw clenched, but she fought down her unreasoning surge of anger, for he was right. He was the xeno-veterinarian. If the problem had been plant life, he would have deferred to *her* expertise; in this case she must defer to his, however her heart raged at her to rush to her daughter's side.

"All right," she said grudgingly. "But you be careful!"

"I will," he promised, and popped the hatch. He climbed out slowly and walked very carefully towards his daughter, carrying the emergency medical kit. The sea of furry, long-tailed arboreals parted about his feet, retreating perhaps a meter to either side and then flowing back in behind him, and he felt their watchful eyes as he stepped into the small clear space about Stephanie. A single creature crouched by her side—smaller and more slender than the others, with a dappled brown and white coat instead of their cream and gray—and he felt its grass-green eyes bore into him. But despite the unnerving intelligence behind that scrutiny, his attention was on his daughter. This close, the bruises and bloodstains—few of the latter hers, thank God!—were far more evident, and his stomach clenched at the evidence of her injuries. Her left arm hung beside her, obviously badly broken, and her right leg was stretched stiffly before her, and he had to blink back tears as he dropped to his knees.

"Hello, baby," he said gently, and she looked at him.

"I messed up, Daddy," she whispered, and tears welled in her own eyes. "Oh, Daddy! I messed *everything* up! I—"

"Hush, baby." His voice quivered, and he cupped the right side of her face in his palm. "We'll have time for that later. For now, let's get you home, okay?"

She nodded, but something in her expression told him there was more. He frowned speculatively— and then his eyebrows shot up as she opened her jacket to reveal another of the creatures hovering all about them. He stared at the badly mauled animal, then jerked his eyes to his daughter's.

Stephanie read the question in her father's gaze. There wasn't time to explain everything—that would have to come later, when she also accepted whatever thoroughly merited punishment her parents decided to levy—but she nodded.

"He's my friend." Her voice trembled, heavy with tears—the voice of a child begging her parents to tell her the problem could be fixed, the damage mended . . . the friend saved. "He . . . he saved me from the hexapuma," she went on, fighting to keep that fraying voice steady. "He *fought* it, Daddy—fought it for *me*—and he got hurt so *bad*. I—" Her voice broke at last, and she stared at her father, white-faced with exhaustion, pain, fear, and grief. Richard Harrington looked back, his own heart broken by her distress, and cupped her face between both his hands.

"Don't worry, baby," he told his daughter softly. "If he helped you, than I'll help *him* any way I can."

❖   ❖   ❖

Climbs Quickly floated slowly, slowly up out of the blackness. He lay on his left side on something warm and soft, and he blinked. He felt the pain of his hurts and knew they were serious, yet there was something strange about the *way* they hurt. The pain was distant and far away, as if something were making it less than it should have been, and he turned his head. He looked up, seeking what he knew was there, and made a soft sound—a weak parody of his normal, buzzing purr—as he saw the face of his two-leg.

She looked down quickly, and the brilliant flare of her joy and relief at seeing him move blazed through the odd, pleasantly lazy haziness which afflicted his thoughts. She touched his fur gently, and he realized the blood had been cleaned from her face. White bits of something covered the worst of her cuts and scratches, and her broken arm was sheathed in some stiff, white material. He tasted an echo of pain still coloring her mind glow, but the echo was almost as muted as his own. She opened her mouth and made more of the sounds the two-legs used to communicate, and he rolled his head the other way as another, deeper voice replied.

His person was seated on one of the two-legs' sitting things, he realized, but it took several more breaths to realize the sitting thing was inside one of the flying things. He might not have realized even then, without his link to his person, but that same link—and the haziness—kept him from panicking at the thought of tearing through the heavens at the speed at which the flying things regularly moved.

Two more two-legs—his two-leg's parents—sat in front of them. One looked back at his two-leg, and he blinked again as their link helped him recognize her as *his* two-leg's mother. But it was the other adult—his two-leg's father—who spoke. The deep, rumbling sounds still meant nothing, and Climbs Quickly decided vaguely that he really must start learning to recognize their meanings.

"He looked at me, Daddy!" Stephanie cried. "He opened his eyes and *looked* at me!"

"That's a good sign, Steph," Richard replied, putting as much encouragement as he could into his voice.

"But he looks awfully weak and groggy," Stephanie went on in a more worried tone, and Richard turned his head to exchange glances with Marjorie. Despite the painkillers, Stephanie still had to be suffering fairly extreme discomfort, but there was no concern at all for herself in her voice. Every bit of it was for the creature—the "treecat"—in her lap, and it had been ever since they'd found her. She'd insisted that her father examine the "treecat" even before he set her arm, and given the vast, silently watching audience of *other* treecats—and the fact that Stephanie, at least, was in no immediately life-threatening danger—he'd agreed. Neither he nor Marjorie could make much sense of the bits and pieces of explanation they'd so far heard, but they'd already concluded that Stephanie was right about one thing: whatever else they might be, these treecats of hers were another sentient species.

God only knew where *that* was going to end, and,

at the moment, Richard and Marjorie Harrington didn't much care. The treecats had saved their daughter's life. That was a debt they could never hope to repay, but they were quite prepared to spend the rest of their lives trying to, and he cleared his throat carefully.

"He looks weak because he *is*, honey," he said. "He's hurt pretty badly, and he lost a lot of blood before you got that tourniquet on him. Without that, he'd be dead by now, you know." Stephanie recognized the approval in his voice, but she only nodded impatiently. "The painkiller I used is probably making him look a little groggy too," he went on, "but we've been using it on Sphinxian species for over forty T-years without any dangerous side effects."

"But will he be *all right?*" his daughter demanded insistently, and he gave a tiny shrug.

"He's going to live, Steph," he promised. "I don't think we'll be able to save his forelimb, and he'll have some scars—maybe some that show even through his fur—but he should recover completely except for that. I can't guarantee it, baby, but you know I wouldn't lie to you about something like this."

Stephanie stared at the back of his head for a moment, then swiveled her eyes to her mother. Marjorie gazed back and nodded firmly, backing up Richard's prognosis, and a frozen boulder seemed to thaw in Stephanie's middle.

"You're *sure*, Daddy?" she demanded, but her voice was no longer desperate, and he nodded again.

"Sure as I can be, honey," he told her, and she

sighed and stroked the treecat's head again. It blinked wide, unfocused green eyes at her, and she bent to brush a kiss between its triangular ears.

"Hear that?" she whispered to it. "You're gonna be all right. Daddy said so."

Yes, Climbs Quickly thought fuzzily, he really *did* have to start learning what the two-leg sounds meant. But not tonight. Tonight he was simply too tired, and it didn't matter right now, anyway. What mattered was the mind glow of his two-leg, and the knowledge that she was safe.

He blinked up at her and managed to pat her leg weakly with his good arm. Then he closed his eyes with a sigh, snuggled his nose more firmly against her, and let the welcome and love of her mind glow sing him to sleep.

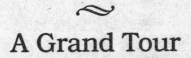

A Grand Tour

David Drake

Edith Mincio waited as her friend and employer, Sir Hakon Nessler, Fourteenth Earl of Greatgap, stepped from the landing shuttle hatch onto the soil of Hope. He stumbled. The earl was a good spacer, so good that his body had adjusted to the rhythmic fluctuations of the artificial gravity during the five-day journey aboard the battered shuttle's equally battered mother ship.

"Oof!" he said. The doubled sound reminded Mincio they still wore the plug intercoms they'd needed to speak to one another over the noise of the small freighter. She took hers out of her left ear canal and returned it to its protective case.

Hope had little to recommend it as a planet, but at least its gravity remained at a constant level. The earl's quick adaptation was now playing him false, though Mincio knew he'd be back to normal in a few hours. Not for the first time she envied the tall youth. She was only twenty years older than her pupil, a mere eyeblink for a society with prolong, but sometimes he made her feel ancient.

Mincio disembarked with only a little more dignity than the luggage the crew began to toss through the hatch as soon as she'd cleared it. She wasn't a good spacer by any stretch of the imagination, and almost anyone would have been made queasy by conditions aboard the sorts of vessels Earl Greatgap—

Mincio made herself pause, reminding herself that her employer had decided to travel at least partly incognito. His accession to his father's title was almost as recent as it had been unexpected, and in areas as prone to lawlessness as this it was only common prudence to appear no more ransomable than one must. It was a point which irked his valet immensely, and there was no point in trying to hide the fact that he was at least wealthy. But admitting membership in the aristocracy seemed to make one even more appealing as a potential source of income, and so he traveled as simple Sir Hakon Nessler.

And the best way to support that was for his travel companions to remember his official name, Mincio thought. She gave herself a mental shake, collected the small case which contained her personal computer and journal from the growing heap of bags, and turned to survey her surroundings.

Her breath caught. On the distant horizon winked a line of six crystal pylons, just as Kalpriades had described them in his *Survey of the Alphane Worlds*—written five hundred years ago and still the most comprehensive work on the vanished prehuman star-travelers. If dizziness and a stomach that would take days to settle down were the prices required to see the remnants of the Alphane civilization in person, then Mincio would pay willingly.

The landing field was plain dirt, blackened by leaked lubricants where landing craft had hammered low spots into the ground. Half a dozen other vessels were present, most of them cargo tenders for intrasystem freighters without Warshawski sails. At the far end of the field sat a large cutter with worn hints of gold-leaf decoration. A dozen men and women in baggy gray uniforms got up from the cutter's shade and slouched toward Nessler and Mincio.

Hope's planetary capital and the League Liaison Office were here at Kuepersburg. From the field all Mincio could see in the way of civilization were houses roofed with heavy plastic a kilometer to the north.

The remainder of Nessler's party had waited to disembark until the shuttle's crew had dumped the luggage in a large pile. Beresford, Nessler's personal servant, was green rather than his ruddy norm; Rovald, the recording technician, looked as though she'd been disinterred after a week of burial. Mincio was queasy, but at least she could tell herself that she was a better traveler than those two.

Nessler extended his imaging goggles to view the Six Pylons. Kalpriades claimed the towers had once been connected by a bridge of gossamer crystal, but there were no signs of it from this distance. The pylons stood in the middle of a plain with no obvious reason to exist.

"Hope!" muttered Beresford. He was a stocky little man, forty years older than his employer and a dependent of the Nesslers of Greatgap as every male ancestor of his back to the settlement had been. "Damned little of that here that I can see."

"It was originally named Salamis, I believe, but the Teutonic Order renamed it Haupt when they

made it their capital," Mincio explained. "The pro-
nunciation decayed along with everything else
associated with the Order."

"And a good thing, too," Nessler said, closing his
imager with a snap. He was twenty-two T-years old
and had a good mind as well as a fierce enthusiasm for whatever he was doing. When he took up
his tutor's interest in the Alphanes, that enthusiasm
translated itself into a tour of the Alphane Worlds
for both of them. On their return Sir Hakon would
enter into the stewardship of one of the greater
personal fortunes of the Manticore System, as well
as one of its oldest titles. "Quite a knot of vipers,
that lot. Although . . ."

His eyes drifted toward the plastic-roofed shacks
of Kuepersburg and toyed with the imager, though
he didn't reopen it. "I wouldn't say League membership has done a great deal for any of the worlds
we've visited in this region."

Rovald found the cases holding her equipment,
but she didn't have the strength or enthusiasm at
the moment to lift them from the pile. She was a
slight woman, at least Beresford's age, with an
intuitive grasp of electronic circuitry but no pre-
tensions.

There was nothing wrong with Rovald's health,
but events had shown that she wasn't really mentally resilient enough for the rigors of travel here
at the edge of the settled universe. Mincio was
afraid that they'd have to send the technician home
soon, and there wasn't a chance they'd find anyone
as good to replace her.

"Region Twelve's been a backwater ever since the

Alphanes vanished," Mincio agreed. "The League uses it as a dumping ground for personnel who might do real harm if they were anywhere important."

Beresford spat. "Which this sandbox sure ain't," he said.

The planet Salamis had received one of the earliest generation ship colonies. After its brief spell as Haupt under the Teutonic Order early in the Warshawski period—"flowering" was too positive a term to describe the era during which those psychopathic brutes ruled four neighboring star systems—the planet had sunk to near barbarism before rediscovery.

As Hope, it had joined the Solarian League in the belief that this would aid its advancement, but nothing much had changed. Hope had no unique mineral or agricultural resources. The soil and climate permitted growing Earth-standard crops with ground-water irrigation, so Hope fed the small-scale mines and manufacturing complexes in neighboring systems. The whole region was singularly devoid of wormhole junctions, and since it was on the edge of the human-settled sphere there wasn't even the chance of through-trade stopping over.

The Alphane civilization was the only reason anybody from the advanced worlds would be interested in Hope, and the difficulties of travel to the region meant that such interest normally remained a distant one. No one knew what the Alphanes had looked like; even the name was one coined by Kalpriades because he believed they were the first star-traveling race in the Milky Way galaxy.

Alphanes had built in crystal on at least a score of worlds known to humans, vast soaring structures which survived only as shattered remnants. Lava that overflowed an Alphane city on Tesserow had been dated to 100,000 T-years ante Diaspora. How much older the ruins might be was anybody's guess.

Besides their structures, the Alphanes had left nut-sized crystals which formed holograms in the air above them when subjected to alternating current. Kalpriades claimed the crystals were books, and most scholars following him had agreed. Few of the crystals thus far found were whole, and the patterns varied according to the frequency and intensity of the current.

To decipher the patterns a scholar first had to determine the correct input, and there were as many theories about that as there were scholars. Books the crystals might be, but they gave no more information about the Alphanes than did the gleaming skeletons of Alphane cities.

The four-man crew of the Klipspringer freighter's shuttle began to walk away. They'd secured their vessel by running a heavy chain around the hatch release and through a staple welded to the hull, then padlocking it. Even so they eyed the people shambling from the cutter askance.

"Captain Cage?" Nessler called sharply to the owner, who had accompanied them down. "Can we expect port officials to arrive shortly?"

"Naw, you have to see the League boss yourself," Cage mumbled. He'd filled his mouth with a wad of chewing tobacco as soon as the shuttle touched ground and he had a place to spit. "There's a merchant named Singh who looks after folks like you from the Inside Worlds. I'll tell him there's a Manticoran arrived at the field, and he'll send somebody out for you."

"Sod that for a lark," Beresford muttered, his hands on his hips as he faced the people from the cutter. "Who're you?" he demanded of the squat, gloomy woman in the lead.

"Please, Good Sir," she said. "Can you give us food? We are very hungry."

"All right, here's the plan!" Beresford said. "Sir Hakon could buy this whole planet if he felt like it. If you pick up his baggage and take it to Mr. Singh's, you won't be the worse for it." He clapped his hands. "But hop to it!"

"One moment, Beresford," Nessler said with a slight frown. "Madam, are you League officials?"

The woman patted her eyes, her ears, and finally her mouth with both hands in a gesture of abject submission. "Good Sir," she said, "I am Petty Officer Royston. We are Melungeon spacers from the *Colonel Arabi*. Please, we will carry your bags. Mr. Singh is a good man. He gives us food often."

"Were you shipwrecked?" Nessler said in growing puzzlement.

The Grand Duchy of Melungeon lay to the galactic south of the Solarian League. Melungeon was an occasional tourist destination for wealthy Manticorans, particularly those who liked to hunt wild animals in conditions in which all the comforts were available to those who could pay for them, but from everything Mincio had heard it was an exotic rather than a really civilized place.

The petty officer started to repeat her salute. Mincio caught her hand to prevent a degradation she found creepy.

"No, Good Sir," Royston said with a worried look to be sure Nessler wasn't going to strike her. "The ship is in orbit. We are to stay with the cutter while the rest of the crew digs for Lord Orloff, but there is no food for us."

Nessler grimaced. "Yes, all right," he said. "Take our luggage to Mr. Singh and I'll see to it you're fed."

With a glance toward Mincio to make sure they were together, Nessler set off for Kuepersburg at his usual long-limbed saunter. Mincio kept up easily though her legs scissored at three strides to Nessler's two. She proceeded through life with a fierce drive that contrasted with her pupil's apparent relaxed ease, but both of them managed to reach their goals.

"I was hoping to see growlers," Nessler said. "Kalpriades said they were common on Hope. Of course, five hundred years . . ."

"Relatively common," Mincio corrected judiciously. "I wouldn't expect to find them near the landing field. They seem to dislike petroleum smells, and small craft like those"—she twitched a thumb at the field behind them—"always leak oil and hydraulic fluid."

Nessler sighed. "I suppose," he agreed grudgingly. "And I don't suppose they can really be the Alphanes, much as I'd like to believe they are."

Growlers were scaly, burrowing herbivores with an adult weight of about thirty kilograms. They were found on most of the worlds with Alphane material remains—and vice versa. Growlers were sweet-tempered and fairly sluggish, with no means of defense. That they were able to survive was due to the fact that no carnivore larger than a dachshund remained on any world where growlers lived. That wasn't an accident, because in many cases the fossil record contained major predators.

Kalpriades took as an article of faith that the growlers were themselves the descendents of his Alphanes; other scholars—almost everybody else who'd visited the Alphane worlds—believed that the growlers had been pets or even food animals rather than the Alphanes themselves.

Mincio had kept an open mind on the question until she'd seen the creatures herself for the first time. If the growlers were the offspring of star-traveling builders in crystal, then the process of descent had been going on for much longer than a hundred thousand years.

Nessler looked over his shoulder to be sure the rest of the entourage was behind them. The dozen Melungeons clomped along stolidly with the luggage while Royston called cadence.

Rovald was at the end of the line. The technician still looked wan, but she managed a smile when Nessler called, "We're almost there!" in encouragement.

To Mincio in a low voice Nessler said, "We'll be spending a little time here on Hope. If she doesn't get her feet back under her, though, I'm afraid I'll have to arrange her return home."

Beresford trotted up to Nessler and Mincio, pumping his arms in time with his strides. "It's a

crying shame the way those poor devils is treated,"
he said as he came abreast. "Royston says Lord
Orloff, that's the captain, just left them to fend for
themselfs and they're six months behind in their pay.
They've been begging. Can you imagine it? What
kind of navy puts its spacers to begging on a dirtpile
planet like this one?"

"Navy?" Nessler said in surprise. "The *Colonel
Arabi* is a Melungeon naval vessel?"

Beresford nodded briskly. "It surely is," he said.
"A light cruiser, though I don't know what that
means where they come from. The captain's a great
curio fancier, Royston says, and he's come out here
to haul an Alphane building back to the Duke's
museum on Tellico."

Mincio missed a step in surprise. "Take a building?" she said. "Good God Almighty! Surely they
can't do that?"

Beresford shrugged. "She says Orloff's got most
of the crew digging around one of them towers on
the horizon," he said. He hooked his thumb in the
direction of the Six Pylons. "They didn't bring any
equipment, just bought shovels and picks here
because that's all there is to be had on Hope."

He spat dismissively into the blowing dust. "Some
expedition, huh? Orloff sounds like a thick-headed
barb to me, for all he's got 'lord' in front of his
name."

"Watch your tongue, Beresford," Nessler said with
what was for him unusual sharpness. "Persons may
be gentlemen even though they don't come from
the Manticore system."

"Indeed they may, Sir," the servant said in a chastened voice. He bobbed his head. "I beg your pardon."

"I can't believe that someone would try to move one of the pylons," Mincio murmured. "And to Tellico, of all places."

"Not exactly a galactic center of scholarship, is it?" Nessler said in a tone of quiet disapproval. "The Melungeon nobility is given to whims, I'm told. It's perhaps rather unfortunate that Lord Orloff seems to have a whim for Alphane artifacts."

He wouldn't stand for his servant calling a fellow nobleman a thick-headed barbarian, but Mincio suspected that he privately agreed with Beresford's assessment of someone trying to move one of the largest and finest surviving Alphane structures. Certainly Mincio agreed.

They'd reached the outskirts of Kuepersburg. Up close the buildings were more substantial than they looked at a distance. They were built of sandy loam stabilized with a cellulose-based plasticizer, a material as permanent as lime concrete and a great deal easier to shape before it set. Many of the locals had brightened the natural dun color with dyes or exterior paint.

Children played in the street among the pigs, chickens, and garbage. They came crowding around with excited cries as soon as they saw that the travelers were well-dressed strangers. The heavily-laden Melungeons and Rovald were far to the rear.

"Half a Solarian credit to the child who leads Sir Hakon to Merchant Singh's!" Beresford called, holding high a plastic coin with a coppery diffraction grating at its core. "Hop it, now! Sir Hakon's too important a person to wait."

Nessler met Mincio's eyes with a wince. He didn't call Beresford down since the boast was already spoken. Mincio shrugged and chuckled.

The children screamed and leaped for the coin like so many starving rats desperate for a tidbit—though in fact none of them looked undernourished. Beresford chose a tall girl with an exceptional willingness to elbow clear the space about her. With the guide strutting in the lead and Beresford obsequiously in the rear, the party turned right on a cross-street nearly as wide as the track from the landing field.

The girl halted in front of a compound. Wind-blown dirt dimmed the wall's white paint and several patches had flaked away, but somebody'd recently cleaned the surface with a dry broom.

The gate was open, but a husky servant sat across it polishing scale off a screen of nickel filigree. He rose when he saw the mob of children and strangers coming toward him.

"Here's the Singhs!" the girl caroled. "Give me the money! Give me the money!"

A middle-aged man stepped out the front door of the largest of the three buildings within the compound. He had a full beard and wore a dark velvet frock coat of the type that was almost a uniform for respectable small businesspeople in the League's hinterlands.

"Yes?" he called in a resonant voice. Two women, one his own age and the second a twenty-year old of exceptional beauty, looked out the door behind him.

"I'll handle this, Beresford," Nessler said with quiet authority. "Mr. Singh? I'm Sir Hakon Nessler, traveling with a party of three from Manticore to view Alphane sites. I was given to understand that you might be able to help us to accommodations and supplies here on Hope?"

The gatekeeper immediately lifted his bench from the passage. He watched his master out of the corner of his eye to be sure that he wasn't misinterpreting his duty.

He wasn't. Singh strode forward and clasped hands with Nessler. "Yes, please," he said. "I am consular agent for Manticore on Hope." Singh grinned. "Also for a dozen other worlds. The duties don't take much time away from my own export business, you understand, and I take pleasure in the company of travelers from more settled regions. I like to believe that I am able to smooth their path on occasions. You will stay with me and my family, I trust?"

"We would be honored, but you must permit me to pay all the household expenses during the time we're imposing on you," Nessler said. "In particular—"

He glanced down the street to call attention to the arriving baggage carriers.

"—I've promised these persons that I'd feed them in exchange for carrying our traps. I'd like to fulfil that promise as soon as possible."

"Morey," Singh said to the gatekeeper, "go to Larrup's and tell her to ready . . ." He glanced out the gate to check the count. The gray-clad spacers halted, standing as silently as so many beasts of burden; which indeed they were. ". . . twelve dinners on my account. The parties will be along as soon as they have brought Sir Hakon's goods into the house."

"I'll direct them, dear," the older woman said. In a tone of crisp command she went on, "Come along, Ms. Royston. I'll show you where to put the parcels and then you can go to Larrup's for a meal."

She went inside. Beresford trotted in also. The servant began introducing himself to the woman of the house in terms that indicated he'd decided the Singhs were gentry to be flattered instead of common folk he could badger on the strength of his connection to Nessler. Mincio sighed. Sir Hakon's father and grandfather had never forgotten that they were Nesslers of Greatgap, and their wealth and Conservative Association political connections had let them enjoy—and project—an old-fashioned aristocratic arrogance which had long since become passe for most Manticorans. Sir Hakon himself held rather different views, much to the disgust of Baron High Ridge and the other Conservative party elders, but neither he nor Beresford were immune to the conditions under which they had been raised. Mincio knew the servant's insistence on his master's primacy in all things often irritated Sir Hakon, but she also knew the little man wouldn't have been nearly as useful a servant here in the back of beyond if he'd been less pushy.

"Are they really from the Melungeon Navy?" she asked Singh in a low voice as the last of the spacers disappeared into the house.

"Yes, indeed," Singh agreed. He gave a faintly

rueful shrug. "Maxwell, Lord Orloff, arrived in a warship three weeks ago. He and his cronies as well as most of his crew are at the Six Pylons twenty-five kilometers from here. You've seen the pylons, no doubt?"

"From a distance," Nessler said. "We hope to visit the site ourselves tomorrow, if transport can be arranged. But why doesn't his crew have food?"

Singh shrugged again. "You'd have to take that up with Lord Orloff, I'm afraid," he said. "I've had very little contact with him. He pays quite well for the needs of his immediate entourage, but the common spacers appear to be destitute. Kuepersburg isn't a wealthy metropolis—" He and the two Manticorans exchanged tight smiles. "—but we can't very well let fellow human beings starve. We've been providing basic requirements to the poor fellows, and they sometimes find a taker for a bit of their vessel's equipment."

"They're stripping their own ship to buy food?" Mincio said in surprise. "Surely that costs Melungeon more than it would to pay their crews properly—or at least to provide rations?"

"Sometimes what officials think are pragmatic decisions seem remarkably short-sighted to others," Singh said. "That was as surely true when I was home on Krishnaputra as it appears to be among the Melungeons. And certainly—"

Before continuing he glanced both ways down the street, empty except for the playing children again.

"Certainly it is true of the way the League deals with all the worlds of this region, particularly in the choice of officials the League sends here."

"There's also the matter that the cost of the policy is generally borne by a department other than the one which makes that policy," Nessler said drily. "The phenomenon isn't unique to the Melungeon Navy."

His eyes narrowed. Mincio had found her pupil to be a generally cheerful youth, but he had the serious side to be expected in a responsible heir to a great fortune. "Though I must say," Nessler added, "I might wish that we had the Melungeon Navy to fight rather than that of the People's Republic of Haven."

The Melungeon spacers filed from the house, moving more briskly than Mincio had seen them do previously. Royston was in the lead; she held a chit written on a piece of coarse paper. Singh's wife shepherded them out with a proprietary expression.

The younger woman remained beside the doorway. She gave Mincio a shy smile when their eyes met. She was clearly Singh's daughter, though the greater delicacy of her similar features made her strikingly attractive.

"From what the Manticorian captains on Klipspringer and Delight told us," Mincio said, "the ships of the Expansion Navy of the People's Republic aren't a great deal better."

Nessler nodded, a placeholder that wasn't really an agreement. To Singh he explained, "Once an assembly line's set up it's actually easier to build ships than it is to provide crews for them. The Peeps thought to get around the problem by drafting ablebodied personnel from the Dole list to crew what they call their Expansion Navy. As Mincio says, the result was less than a first-rate combat fleet. *But*—"

He turned his glance toward his tutor.

"You'll recall that the freighter captains who sneered so enthusiastically at the 'Dole Fleet' were nonetheless holding their own vessels in League sovereign space. Expansion Navy ships are quite adequate for commerce raiding, and they provide the Peeps with a presence in far corners from which our very excellent navy lacks the numbers to sweep them."

"You speak like an expert, Sir," Singh said. The Krishnaputran merchant had to be a sharp man to have created a comfortable life for himself and his family in a location that didn't encourage commercial success.

"Scarcely that," Nessler said with a deprecating smile. "I spent a year as an ensign of the Royal Manticoran Navy, and a less than brilliant example of that very junior rank. I resigned my commission when my father and elder sister drowned in a boating accident and I became perforce head of the family. While I regret the death of Dad and Anne more than I can say, I'm better qualified as an estate manager than I was as a naval officer."

He grinned at Mincio. "And I like to think I'm a gentleman scholar."

"Certainly a scholar to have come so far for knowledge, Sir," Singh said. "And a gentleman, also certainly, for that I see with my own eyes." He looked toward his wife and said, "My dear?"

"The rooms will be ready in a few minutes," she replied, "and water for the bath is heating. Will you introduce me, Baruch?"

Singh bowed in apology for forgetting the lack of introductions. "Dear," he said, "this is Sir Hakon Nessler. Sir Hakon, may I present my wife Sharra and our daughter—"

The younger woman came down from the open porch to stand at her father's side.

"—Lalita, of whom we're very proud."

Nessler bowed and took Lalita's fingertips between his. "May I in turn present my friend Edith Mincio?" he said. "She tutored me through university and has kindly consented to accompany me on my travels before taking up a post as Reader in Pre-Human Civilizations at Skanderbeg University on Manticore."

A post which only Sir Hakon's influence gained me, Mincio thought as she touched fingertips with father and daughter. *For all that I was the most qualified applicant.*

Sharra Singh smiled but didn't offer her hand. While she was clearly a person of independence and ability, her idea of a woman's place in society was not that of Manticore or of her own daughter.

"Father, can we have a dance tonight?" Lalita said with kittenish enthusiasm as she hugged Singh's arm close. The girl might well be two T-years younger than Mincio had first judged; she was at that point in physical development where the prolong treatments always made age estimates difficult. "Please father? They'll have all the most exciting new music, I just know it!"

She looked up at the Manticorans. "Oh, you will let me invite my friends to meet you, won't you? They'll be ever so excited!"

"I'm sure our guests are exhausted from their journey," Singh said with a serious expression. "Dear—"

"Oh, not at all," Nessler rejoined cheerfully. "As soon as I've had a bath and a bit of dinner, there's nothing I'd like more than some company that isn't ourselves and a quartet of spacers from Klipspringer. Isn't that so, Mincio?"

"Yes indeed," Mincio agreed. She wasn't nearly as social a creature as her pupil, but his statement had been basically true for her as well. In any case, it was the only possible answer to make to Lalita's desperate longing.

Rovald and Beresford came out the side door. Beresford held a bun and a glass of amber fluid. Rovald wasn't to the point of being ready to eat and drink yet, but at least her face had color and animation again.

"As for music, though," Nessler continued with a frown, "I'm afraid I've brought only a personal auditor with me on my travels. You're more than welcome to listen to the contents, Ms. Singh, but I'm afraid we won't be able to dance to it."

"They have an amplifier and speakers, Sir," Rovald said unexpectedly. "With your permission, I can run the auditor's output through their system."

"Your equipment will fit ours?" Singh said. "Really, I don't think . . . My set is very old and came from Krishnaputra with me, you see."

"I can couple them, I think," Rovald said with quiet assurance. "It'll help if you have a length of light-guide, but I can make do without it."

"Rovald's the best electronics technician on

Manticore," Nessler said. "If she says she can do it, consider it done."

Rovald beamed with pardonable pride as she and Lalita went inside. The technician had been an object of pity through the uncomfortable voyage and after landing; now at last she was able to show herself as something better than a queasy wreck.

"Would our guests care to come in, now?" the older Ms. Singh said, ostensibly to her husband. "The bath water should be hot."

"Go ahead, Mincio," Nessler said. "I took the last of the warm water on Klipspringer, as I recall."

"Well, if you don't mind . . . ?" Mincio said. Regular hot baths were the one luxury that she really missed in these hinterlands of human habitation.

"You know . . ." Nessler said. Mincio paused, thinking for a moment that he was responding to her immediate question rather than returning to a subject they'd been discussing earlier. "There isn't any complicated difference between the Royal Manticoran Navy and the Dole Fleet or even the Melungeons. It's just a matter of constant effort by all those concerned, the officers even more than the men. If my sister had inherited as she should have, I would have been one of those officers—and I'm very glad I'm not. I'd much rather do something I was good at."

Wearing formal dress that—except for the footgear—would have passed muster at a royal levee on Manticore, Nessler and Mincio approached the League Liaison Office. Their boots were a concession to streets whose sandy muck would have swallowed the iridescent slippers which should have completed their outfits.

Singh had given them directions, but relations between League officials and the commercial elite of most worlds in this region were about as bad as they could be. The League personnel were the dregs of a very advanced bureaucracy; the merchants tended to be the most dynamic citizens of the tier of worlds marginally more developed than, say, the systems once controlled by the Teutonic Order.

Singh's native Krishnaputra was a typical example. The planet had a local electronics industry, but half the people didn't have electricity in their homes.

League officials could sneer at the local elites as being unsophisticated products of dirty little worlds: mushrooms springing from dungheaps. The local population in general regarded most of the liaison officers sent to them as dense, grasping failures with an overdeveloped sense of their own importance. From everything Mincio had seen or heard, the League Liaison Officer on Hope, the Honorable Denise Kawalec, fell into the expected category.

The League offices on Hope comprised three rectangular buildings touching at the corners like dominoes spilled on a table. They were flat-roofed modular constructions cast from cold-setting ceramic.

Each slab was a different saturated color. Though the structure was probably a standard bureaucratic design from the generation in which Hope first became a League protectorate, Nessler and Mincio hadn't seen anything like it before on their travels.

It wasn't something one would forget. The corner where walls of lime green and royal blue met was particularly eyecatching.

The offices were intended for total climate control. The only original opening on this side was the double main door, though there were probably emergency exits in the rear as well. Plastic panes in frames of native wood now covered window openings crudely hacked through the walls to provide light and ventilation during power failures. Mincio guessed that outages were more probable than not, given Hope's technological level and the quality of the League personnel who'd have to maintain a separate generator.

"Will you show us in to Officer Kawalec, lad?" Nessler said to the urchin sprawled in the building's doorway. He'd been watching them approach with an expectant sneer.

"Why should I?" the boy said without getting up. His clothing was cut down from pieces of Liaison Service and Gendarmerie uniforms.

Nessler flipped him a small coin. The boy jumped to his feet and ran around the building. "Sucker!" he called over his shoulder. "Find her yourself!"

"I suppose we'd better do that," Nessler said without expression, pushing open the door.

The hallway was dim but the room at the east end had a light which pulsed at the cyclic rate of the current feeding it. They turned in that direction. Two men wearing black Gendarmerie uniforms walked out of one room and into another, ignoring the visitors.

The Gendarmes were supposed to uphold

League regulations on the less-developed worlds which had a Liaison Officer instead of a League High Commissioner. Every contact with Gendarmes during this tour had convinced Mincio that the service attracted people who did little for the reputation of the League, or for law and order more generally.

"Carabus!" a woman shouted from the lighted room. A paper placard tacked to the half-open door read CLO2 DENISE KAWALEC. "Damn you, what have you done with the bottle?"

Mincio entered the room on Nessler's heels. Kawalec glared up from her search in the bottom drawer of a cabinet for filing hardcopy. When she saw strangers rather than whoever she'd expected, her expression quivered between fear and greed. While Kawalec wasn't precisely ugly, Mincio had never met a human being for whom the word "plain" was a better fit.

"Who are you?" Kawalec demanded, sliding back behind her desk. Its surface was littered with orange peel and fragments of less identifiable food; local scavengers the size of a fingerbone wriggled their single antennae at the newcomers, then went back to their meal.

"Officer Kawalec," Nessler said, "we're Manticorian citizens touring Alphane sites. My name is Nessler, and my friend is Ms. Mincio."

Mincio handed Kawalec the travel authorization from the League's Ministry of Protectorate Affairs both in the form of a read-only chip and a stamped and sealed offprint. The hardcopy had generally proven more useful in Region Twelve, where chip readers—particularly working chip readers—were conspicuous by their absence.

Kawalec flicked the hardcopy and said, "It doesn't cover Hope by name."

"It covers the whole of Region Twelve—" Mincio began hotly.

"A moment, Mincio," Nessler said. "May I see that again, Officer?"

He took the document from Kawalec's hands, folded it over a gold-hued coin he'd palmed from his purse, and handed it back. "I believe you'll find the mention if you check now."

Mincio stared stone-faced at the wall-hung hologram of the League Palace in Geneve. Bribes were only to be expected when dealing with officials on undeveloped worlds, but *League* officials shouldn't be pocketing them. Nessler could easily afford the expense, but when the representatives of developed civilizations were on the take, then the barbarians were truly at the gates.

"Right, I see it now," Kawalec said with an approving nod. She returned the authorization to Nessler, but her right hand remained firmly closed over the coin. When her eyes narrowed, she looked even more ratlike than before. She continued, "Now of course there'll be fees for any antiquities you discover. Port duties as well if you ship them out."

"Of course," Nessler said blandly, as though he were unaware that League regulations specifically forbade private traffic in Planetary Treasures—a category covering Alphane artifacts as well as the vestiges of early human settlements. "Payments should be to your office rather than to the government of Hope?"

"There *is* no government of Hope except for me!" the liaison officer snapped. "These savages can't wipe their own bums without help!"

"I was wondering about the arrangements you've made with the Melungeon expedition," Mincio said. "Are they really going to take one of the Six Pylons offworld with them?"

"That bastard Orloff!" Kawalec said. "He's going to take any damn thing he pleases, it seems like, and not so much as kiss-my-hand to me!"

"Because he has approval from the Ministry of Protectorate Affairs on Old Earth?" Nessler asked.

"Because he's got a bloody cruiser in orbit!" snarled the League official. "I'd complain to Geneve, but Orloff'll be long gone by the time a courier gets there and back. And that's *if* anybody on Earth gives a hoot whether I starve here on this pisspot planet."

She glared at Nessler with transferred fury. "But you, boyo," she said. "You're going to pay!"

"I'm sure we will, if we choose to remove any artifacts," Nessler said calmly. He tipped his beret to Kawalec. "Thank you for seeing us, Madam," he said.

Mincio was out of the office ahead of him. People like Denise Kawalec made her angry in a quite unscholarly fashion, but an insult to the bureaucratic highwayman wouldn't help matters.

Besides, it was unlikely that there was anything Mincio could say that Kawalec hadn't already heard.

Edith Mincio finished her third *estampe* of the

evening with a pirouette that she couldn't have managed in a million years if she'd paused to think about it. Usually she danced merely as a social obligation: mating rituals weren't one of her interests in either the abstract or the specific. This party at the Singhs was genuinely pleasant, though; not least because she was a center of attention instead of a wallflower as usual.

The dance steps that had been current on Manticore when she and Nessler left were years ahead of anything the young people of Hope had seen. At least one man had cut in every time Mincio was on the floor, and the belles of Kuepersburg society stared at her with undisguised envy.

A servant handed Mincio a glass of punch; she downed it in three quick gulps. The room was hot despite the open door. This was the most exercise Mincio had gotten in the weeks since she and Nessler climbed the Bakersfield Cordillera on muleback in search of the Crystal Grotto.

Somebody offered her another glass. She started drinking before she realized that the Singhs' daughter, not one of the servants, had given it to her.

"Oh!" Mincio said. "I'm sorry, I've been spinning around so fast that my head hasn't settled down yet. I do apologize, Lalita."

"Oh, please," the girl said with a blush. "We are so honored to have you here."

Mincio eyed the line of men circling just beyond Lalita, preparing to pounce on the Manticoran guest. Across the room Nessler stood at the center of a similar bevy of local girls, visible only because he was a full head taller.

"Lalita," Mincio said, "would you care to get some fresh air for a moment? I'm not up to another dance just now, and I'm afraid I'll be trampled if I try to sit one out inside here."

Lalita turned. To the largest of the young men she said brusquely, "Carswell, Ms. Mincio and I will be taking a turn outside. She would prefer not to be bothered. See that everyone understands, please."

Carswell nodded with a look of grim determination. The men and boys around him were already backing away. Lalita acted like a ten-year-old when dealing with the visitors from Manticore, but her authority among her fellows was as assured as Sir Hakon Nessler's own.

The two women walked out of the sliding doors. A group of men stood near the entrance, talking and chewing tobacco, but Lalita's steely glance parted them.

Inside the sound system broke into a spirited *gavotte*. Rovald presided proudly over the jury-rigged apparatus. The link between the amp and Nessler's personal auditor worked perfectly, and Mincio was willing to bet that in addition the Singhs' speakers had never sounded better.

The dance was being held in a warehouse which Singh's laborers had emptied during the afternoon. There wasn't a hall on the planet large enough to hold the crowd, all the "best people" who could reach Kuepersburg in time. Some of them had arrived by mule-drawn carriage, but there were motorized vehicles also and half a dozen air cars—perhaps all the private air cars on the planet.

The breeze was dry and cool, at least compared

to the atmosphere inside the warehouse. The grit it picked up as it sailed between the town's dingy, ill-lit buildings was an acceptable price to pay.

"I so envy you," Lalita said wistfully. "I don't see why someone as rich and wise as you are would want to come here, Ms. Mincio."

"Call me Edith, please," Mincio said, a little more forcefully than the number of times in the past she'd made the same request. "I don't claim to be wise, Lalita, though I'm knowledgeable about a few things that don't matter in the least to most other people. As for rich, though—your father could buy or sell me a dozen times over, I suspect. I'm here very much at Sir Hakon's expense. Don't let the fact that we're friends mislead you into thinking that we're equals in the economic or even social spheres."

"Oh, you can say that," Lalita said dismissively. "You have the whole galaxy at your fingertips and you don't know what it's like for us living on a pile of . . . of dirt."

The warehouse was on the east side of town, at a distance from the landing field but perhaps more secure for being near the Singh dwelling. The two women walked along the sidewalk of stabilized earth a handsbreadth above the cracked mud of the street proper. Lalita picked her way over the irregular surface without a skip or stumble, despite pools of shadow which the lights of neighboring buildings didn't reach. Hope's three moons were scarcely brighter than planets.

Three people approached from up the street in the direction the women were walking. There was laughter and a snatch of song in which Mincio recognized Beresford's voice.

"Lalita," Mincio said, "it's never a good thing to feel trapped. Believe me, poverty is just as confining as . . . as a planet which is a long way from the centers of development. After this tour I'll have a position that will provide for me all the rest of my life without any need for concern on my part. That security is as close to paradise as I ever expect to come."

She smiled faintly. *And if I die before returning to Manticore, then that's security of another sort.*

"But don't let the fact that you feel trapped make you blind to the beauties of Hope," Mincio went on fiercely. "And to the beauties of your life here. There are many, many women on Manticore who'd trade their lives in a heartbeat to be as lovely and *central* as you are here."

"Ah, Ms. Mincio?" Beresford said. A lamp over the adjacent house cast its light through the bars of the fenced courtyard in front of the dwelling. The servant stepped close while his two companions kept a little behind in the shadows.

"Good evening, Beresford," Mincio said coldly. Beresford was with a pair of female spacers from the Melungeon vessel; they were carrying bottles. Mincio assumed their association with Beresford was a mercenary one. She didn't approve, but it wasn't her place to object; anyway, that would be a waste of breath.

"I've arranged to borrow an air car for you and the master tomorrow," Beresford said. "A farmer named Holdt's staying in town and lent it. I was coming to tell him that, but I wonder if you'd . . . ?"

"Yes, all right," Mincio said. There was no telling when Beresford would get back to the Singh compound, and there was no need for him and his presumed whores to come any closer to the party in his master's honor.

"Thank you, Ms. Mincio," Beresford said, tipping his hat and returning to his companions. "We'll be off, then."

Beresford seemed to like Mincio well enough, and he never failed to treat her as the gentlewoman she was by birth. There was always an undercurrent of amused contempt when he spoke to her, though. Beresford knew *his* status; Mincio was neither fish nor fowl. As she'd said to Lalita, poverty was as surely a trap as any backward planet could be.

"We should get back anyway," Mincio said. "Though I don't know that I'm going to be ready for anything faster than a saraband."

They turned together, putting the breeze behind them. It felt cool now. Snatches of Beresford's song reached them; Mincio hoped that the girl couldn't understand the words, though she didn't suppose anyone on Hope could be described as "delicately brought up."

Two figures came up the alley just ahead of them. *A man and a boy*, Mincio first thought; then realized she'd been wrong in both identifications. The first growler she'd seen on Hope was following an old woman who wore a cloak and floppy hat as she plodded steadily toward the dance.

"Oh, it's Ms. deKyper," Lalita said, her lips close to Mincio's ear so as not to be overheard. The old woman was only a few steps ahead. "She's from

Haven. She's been here oh! so many years, studying the Alphanes like you. She used to be rich, but something happened back home and now she just scrapes by."

"I'd like to meet her," Mincio said. "If she's as expert as you say, she'd be a perfect guide for the time we're on Hope."

"Ms. deKyper?" Lalita called. "May I introduce our guest, Ms. Mincio of Manticore?"

"Oh my goodness!" deKyper said. She swept her hat off as she turned; a thin, tired woman, showing her advanced age despite prolong, whose eyes nonetheless sparkled in the area light flooding from the compound across the street. "I'm honored I'm sure. I came as soon as I heard that scholars touring the Alphane worlds had arrived."

Her face hardened in wooden disapproval. "You're not, I trust," she said, "associated with Lord Orloff and his fellow savages?"

"We are not," Mincio said, her tone an echo of the older woman's. They touched fingertips. "While my friend and pupil Sir Hakon Nessler may gather a small souvenir here or there, for the most part we view and record artifacts with the intention of recreating some of them on his estate."

The growler stuck out a tongue almost twenty centimeters long and licked Mincio's hand. The contact was rough but not unpleasant, something like the touch of a dry washcloth. It was completely unexpected, though, and Mincio jerked back as if from a hot burner.

"Oh, I'm very sorry!" deKyper said. "She's quite harmless, believe me."

"I didn't know what it was," Mincio said in embarrassment. "I was just startled."

The growler's broad forehead tapered abruptly to the nose and jaws from which the tongue had snaked. Its skin was covered with fine scales; they showed a sheen but no particular color under the present dim light. According to images and travelers' descriptions, growlers were generally gray or green.

Mincio reached tentatively to stroke the beast's head; it began to purr with the deep buzzsaw note that had gotten the creatures their common name. The sound was a shock to hear even though she knew it was friendly, not a threatening growl.

"Does he have a name?" Mincio asked. The growler licked her wrist as she petted it. The tongue was remarkable, virtually a third hand in addition to the four-fingered appendages on the ends of the arms.

"She, I believe," deKyper said, "but I don't know her name."

She straightened and added with the emphasis of someone who knows she's making an insupportable statement, "There's no doubt that growlers are the real Alphanes. I can tell by the way she attends when I play Alphane books."

"Can you read Alphane crystals, Ms. deKyper?" Lalita said. "Oh, that's wonderful! I didn't know that."

"Well . . ." the old woman temporized. "I've discovered the frequency at which the crystal books are intended to be played, but I haven't deciphered the symbology as yet. I'm sure that will come in time."

And so will Christ and His angels, Mincio thought. *Another enthusiast who's discovered the key to the universe by studying the site of the Great Sphinx of Giza; or here, its Alphane equivalent.*

Aloud she said, "Would you care to meet my companion, Sir Hakon Nessler? We like to have a guide knowledgeable about local sites when we visit a planet. Of course there'd be a special honorarium for a scholar like you, if you wouldn't be embarrassed."

The growler stopped licking Mincio and shuffled close to deKyper again. Though its hind legs were short, the beast was fully bipedal. It leaned its head against deKyper's chest and resumed its thunderous purr.

"I long ago stopped being embarrassed at honest ways to receive money," deKyper said with a wan smile. "And it doesn't happen so frequently that I'm apt to get bored with the experience, either. In any case, I'd be proud to accompany real scholars."

Her resemblance to her pet went beyond a degree of physical similarity that itself was surprising in members of such different species. They both shared a dreamy harmlessness, and neither really belonged—here or perhaps anywhere. Mincio could empathize with the lack of belonging, but she herself was unlikely ever to be mistaken for a dreamer.

Perhaps deKyper understood Mincio's guardedly neutral expression; wistful the old woman might be, but she certainly wasn't stupid. "It's of particular importance that we translate Alphane books," she said. "The knowledge and the public *excitement* that will generate in the developed regions will bring tourists to the Alphane worlds in large numbers."

"You want mass tourism?" Mincio said. "I would have thought . . ."

"Ms. Mincio," deKyper said, "if only scholars like you and your companion toured the Alphane worlds, I would be delighted. But for every pair like yourselves there's a party which knocks chunks off the pylons with a hammer—and now we have the unspeakable barbarians from Melungeon who plan to spirit a pylon clean away! Only large-scale interest among civilized peoples will permit arrangements that will save the remaining artifacts for future generations."

"I see," Mincio said. She fully empathized with the old woman's hopes, but wishful thinking about the translation of Alphane books wouldn't bring those hopes to fruition. "Let's go see Nessler, Ms. deKyper. And perhaps tomorrow while the three of us visit the Six Pylons, our technician Rovald can stay behind to take a look at the crystals in your collection. She has an absolute genius at anything to do with electronics."

The three women walked toward the music and the fan of light spilling through the warehouse doorway. The growler followed with a rumble of soft contentment.

Nessler dropped the air car skillfully downwind of the long tent with its sides rolled up. The dozen people sitting at cards in its shade turned to watch the vehicle land. A few of them got up.

Hundreds of workers with hand tools continued

to toil. Some dug away the ground at the base of the tallest pylon while others carried loosened earth from the pit in baskets to pour in a heap a hundred meters away. The men wore shorts; the women sometimes as little. Mincio frowned at thought of what the sun and gritty wind must be doing to their skin. The burrows in the gully wall east of the site must be housing for the laborers.

"Oh, the barbarians," deKyper whimpered from the back seat. The pylon was the easternmost of the line of six. Almost the entire length of the shaft was covered by countergrav rings like those used for moving heavy gear aboard a warship. Several of the rings were dark, obviously dead, while others shimmered nervously with a surface discharge that implied incipient failure.

The party—the officers under the tent at least— had arrived on an ornate air car big enough to carry all of them together. A cutter had landed nearby in the recent past. Despite the skirling wind, the scars from its lift jets remained as pits in the soil.

Nessler shut down the air car, smiling vaguely in the direction of the Melungeon officers. In a tone much more grim than his expression he said to Mincio, "I really don't believe those grav rings will take the pylon's weight, not unless the ones that haven't failed are all at a hundred percent. But I don't suppose Orloff would thank me for telling him."

"I doubt there are any additional rings available on Hope," Mincio said. "As you say, it's their business." The whole Melungeon operation disturbed her profoundly, but focusing her mind on the details of it wouldn't do any good.

She turned to help deKyper out of the back of the open vehicle. The door was wired shut so the passenger had to step over the side. The older woman was gray with silent despair.

They walked to the tent, Nessler slightly in the lead. The Melungeon officers wore ornate uniforms, but their jackets were mostly unbuttoned and the garments weren't clean enough for Mincio to have imagined putting any of them on. The officers carried sidearms in flap holsters. Navy ratings, probably thankful that they weren't at the backbreaking labor of the pit, acted as servants.

The half dozen civilians present were obviously prostitutes, though Mincio wasn't sure they were all Hope residents. Four were women, two men.

Nessler approached the big man who'd been sitting at the head of the table. He wore an open white tunic with gold braid most of the way to the elbows. The fellow was completely bald, but he had a full mustache and a mass of chest hair so black that it looked like a bearskin gorget.

"Good morning," Nessler said. "I've been told this is the camp of Maxwell, Lord Orloff. If I may take the liberty of introducing myself, I'm Sir Hakon Nessler of Manticore. I'm a student of Alphane sites, as I see you are as well."

Orloff's face split in a broad grin. "I'm Orloff," he said. He ignored the hand Nessler raised to touch fingertips in Solarian League fashion and instead embraced his visitor in a great hug. "Come, have a drink!"

He glanced at Mincio and deKyper and added, "Two women, hey? You Manticorans know how to travel—though I like them with a little more meat myself."

He gave a bellowing laugh and banged Nessler on the back. A servant poured faintly mauve liquid into beakers.

"Permit me to introduce Edith Mincio, my tutor and superior in the study of Alphane remains," Nessler said in a tone of cool unconcern, as though he hadn't heard the last comment, "and Ms. deKyper, a Havenite scholar who's studied the Alphanes here on Hope for many years."

"What you're doing is unspeakable!" deKyper said angrily. "You're desecrating a site that's older than mankind!"

"Oh, you're the crazy lady," Orloff said with an amused chuckle. "Sure, I've heard of you. Well, have a drink anyway, my dear. We're only taking one pillar, you see. That'll leave five right here for you, but mine will be the only one on Tellico."

There'd been a poker game going on when the visitors arrived. The seven or eight players were using cash rather than chips. The denominations Mincio recognized—the currency of a dozen worlds was on the table—were large ones. Melungeon officers were nobles and either wealthy or at least addicted to the vices of wealth, of which high-stakes gambling was the most common.

Mincio knew the type very well. She shivered. *Sheep for the shearing*, she thought as she glanced at the half-drunk, none-too-bright, faces around the table. She hadn't realized how deeply she'd been infected as a child.

Orloff's officers talked among themselves, not so

much deferential to their commander as disinterested in the visitors. One of the men walked to the end of the tent and began to urinate on the dry sand.

Servants filled two more beakers. Mincio took hers; deKyper ostentatiously turned her back and walked toward the pylon fifty meters away. Orloff's face darkened in a brutal scowl before he said, "Maybe you'd like to take a pillar yourself, Nessler? There's plenty for all, it seems to me."

Nessler lowered the beaker from which he'd been sipping. "I'm afraid it'd cost half my fortune to ship home something so huge. My heirs will be disturbed enough at the amount their crazy forebear spent to recreate copies of Alphane artifacts from imagery."

A Melungeon crewman who wore tunic and trousers in token of his higher status—he was however barefoot—clumped up to Orloff. When he caught Orloff's eye he gave the degrading Melungeon equivalent of a salute.

"Please Sir," the crewman said. "There's a problem. We can't get the pillar loose."

Orloff rumbled a sound of disgust. "No more brains than monkeys," he said. "Let's straighten them out, Nessler, and then we'll talk about cards."

He strode toward the pit, pushing the crewman aside as he might have kicked a dog that got in his way. Mincio and Nessler traded expressionless glances as they followed. The remainder of the Melungeon officers trailed after, though Mincio noticed that all the card players put their money in their pockets before leaving the table.

The diggers had lowered the ground at the pylon's

base by a distance of three meters, laying bare the natural substrate. Though most of the crystal shaft was hidden behind countergrav rings, the tip forty meters in the air caught the sun and wicked it down through the base. Light spilled in dazzling rainbows across the pit and those laboring in it.

"It appears that the Alphanes didn't set their pylons on the bedrock, Lord Orloff," Ms. deKyper said with dispassionate clarity. "They fused them *to* the rock. I dare say your peons here will be some while chipping away at the granite, don't you think?"

Orloff ripped out a series of oaths that were both blasphemous and disgusting. Mincio kept her face studiously blank and her eyes focused on the pylon. It would be ill-bred to let Orloff know what she thought of him. There was enough ill-bred behavior here already.

She wondered how the Alphanes had managed the attachment. Crystal had flowed down into the dense rock, but streaks of granite wove upward into the pylon's base as well. The zone of contact looked as though colored syrups had been stirred into a mixture, then frozen.

In a mood swing as abrupt as sun after a rainsquall, Orloff draped his big arm over Nessler's shoulders and walked the Manticoran back to the tent with him. "Well, I'll have to get some equipment from the ship, but tomorrow will be time enough for that. Shall we have a friendly game of poker?"

Orloff pointed to one of the servants and said, "Alec! The new cards in honor of our visitor!" His index finger jerked from the man to an ornate wooden storage chest which showed the marks of hard traveling.

"And one of you dogs bring some more liquor!" he added in a bellow. In a friendly, almost wheedling, voice he went on to Nessler, "It's Musketoon. Have you had it before? It's our Melungeon national drink, brandy distilled from the wine of the Muscadine grapes our ancestors brought from Earth."

Mincio had sipped at her beaker and hoped to avoid further contact with the fluid within. Musketoon's cloying sweetness tried to conceal an alcohol content sufficient to strip paint. She tipped the remaining contents onto the roots of a spiny bush.

"I think I've got enough in my glass for now," Nessler said mildly. His host had brought him to the card table with as little ceremony as a policeman conducting a drunk. The servant handed Orloff a flat case from the storage chest. "And as for cards—"

Orloff opened the case; Mincio felt her face harden. Inside were two decks with mottled designs on the back: one vaguely blue, the other a similarly neutral green. They were made of thin synthetic, not paper, and looked pristine.

Pocketed incongruously with them in the case was a meerschaum tobacco pipe whose stem was of black composition material. The intricately-carved bowl of porous stone was white, unused.

"—I think that'll have to wait for another time," Nessler continued. Mincio's muscles relaxed, though she still felt cold inside.

Nessler rotated himself out of Orloff's grasp; the motion seemed intended only to let him gesture toward the line of pylons. "We'd like to see the remainder of this site yet during daylight. Tomorrow we'll come back with our imaging equipment to record them, this pylon in particular, and perhaps we'll have time for cards."

He handed his beaker—still full—to a servant, bowed to the Melungeon captain, and said, "Good day, Sir!" He turned on his heel before the other could respond.

Orloff stood with a slight frown. He'd taken the pipe from its case and was twiddling the stem with his powerful fingers. "Yes, all right, tomorrow," he called to Nessler and Mincio. Ms. deKyper was already in the air car, sizzling in fury at the Melungeon sacrilege.

The next pylon was almost half a kilometer away, sufficient distance to free their party from the Melungeons' presence. Nessler landed, downwind as before, though sand spurting from beneath the air car wouldn't do any significant harm to the crystal shaft.

Mincio got her breath. She found she was more angry, not less, now that her conscious mind had processed the information to which she'd reacted instinctively on first receipt.

"Nessler," she said, breaking into deKyper's litany of displeasure, "under no circumstances should you play cards with that man. The deck he brought out is fixed. The cards broadcast their values. Orloff picks up the signals in clicks through the stem of his pipe."

Nessler raised an eyebrow as he got out of the

air car. "Cheating at cards would be in keeping with the rest of the man's character, wouldn't it? I, ah . . . I'm glad you recognized the paraphernalia. I wouldn't have done so."

Mincio tried to stand. She failed because her muscles were trembling. She covered her face with her hands.

Nessler helped deKyper from the vehicle. The two of them spoke for a moment in low voices; then deKyper said, "I'll be on the other side of the pylon," and her feet crunched away.

Nessler cleared his throat. "Ah, Mincio?" he said.

Mincio lowered her hands. Without meeting Nessler's eyes she said, "I never talked about my father. He was a professional gambler. My earliest memories are playing cards with my father. He punished me when I made a mistake. I was three years old, maybe not even that, and he whipped me for drawing to an inside straight."

"I'm sorry that this matter arose," Nessler said quietly. "We needn't go anywhere near the Melungeons tomorrow. Perhaps Rovald can get some imagery."

"It doesn't bother me to see people play," Mincio said. She smiled wanly in the direction of the far horizon. "Really what it does is excite me. My father taught me very well, but I haven't touched a deck of cards since the day he died."

She stood and looked directly at her friend and employer. She smiled again, though the corner of her lips wobbled. "He was shot dead when I was sixteen. It wasn't a duel—merely a murder, a contract killing. Given that several of the victims he cheated had committed suicide, I suppose justice was done."

Nessler shook his head slowly. "I'm sorry about your father's death, Mincio," he said. "Also about the way he chose to live his life. But that wasn't your choice. I'm honored to have been your pupil in the study of the Alphane culture, and I remain in awe of your learning."

"I hope you're not so great a fool to be awed by mere knowledge," Mincio said tartly. "Any more than I am by mere wealth. Let's take a look at this pylon, shall we? I want to see whether all six are the same molecular composition."

They'd dropped deKyper off at the pair of storage sheds in which she lived on the edge of Kuepersburg. Nessler brought the borrowed air car down in Singh's courtyard. Generator-powered electric lights were on all over the complex of buildings, and dozens of people had to crowd out of the way to permit the vehicle to land.

"Sir!" Beresford said as soon as Nessler shut off the turbines. "There's a Jathan freighter in orbit that's brought in a pinnace from a Manticoran navy ship that a Peep cruiser blasted in the Air System. They're hoping that, you know, you being a gentleman—"

Nessler rose with a subtly changed expression. "A gentleman I hope," he said, "and a reserve naval officer beyond question. May I ask who's in charge of this party?"

Singh stood at his front door but didn't interfere in what he hoped was no longer his business. Mincio moved from the car to a corner where she'd be out of the way while she observed what was happening.

The people who nearly filled the courtyard wore either utility uniforms of the Royal Manticoran Navy or loose, locally-made garments which must have been provided by the consular agent. Some of the castaways had been injured; most had sallow, hollow-eyed expressions which were more than a trick of the low-voltage lights that illuminated them. From the looks of them, they must have been forced to subsist on the life support capability of their pinnace/lifeboat to avoid overloading the limited capacity of the hyper-capable freighter which had picked them up.

"Sir!" said a powerfully-built woman who planted herself in front of Nessler and threw a crisp salute. "Leona Harpe, Bosun, late of Her Majesty's destroyer *L'Imperieuse*. There's thirty-seven of us, everybody who survived."

"Stand easy, Harpe," Nessler said in a tone of calm authority very different from that of his normal discourse, and different even from his dealings with servants like Beresford. "Now, what are your primary needs?"

"Mr. Singh fed us right after we landed in the pinnace," Harpe said. She rubbed her eyes. "He doesn't have tents for shelter, and I don't know how long we're going to be stuck here."

"We need a way to get to a Navy ship big enough to serve out the Peep bastards who whacked us!" somebody called from a rear rank.

"Belt up, Dismore!" Harpe snapped without

turning her head. "Though I'm looking forward to that too, Sir. They hit us without warning in League territorial space—we didn't even know there was a war on . . . if there is! All we knew was that someone started jamming us, then opened fire. We did our best—I think we may even've got a lick or two in—but the Peeps had a heavy cruiser." She shook her head. "The old *Imp* was like a puppy up against a hexapuma, Sir."

She paused for a moment, then inhaled sharply. "After a hit sent the fusion bottle climbing toward failure, all the survivors got off in the two cutters and the pinnace . . . and that's when the bastards opened up all over again. They lasered the blue cutter under Mr. Gedrosian, the XO. Ms. Arlemont, she was Engineering Officer, tried to ram them with the red cutter. They lasered them too."

Harpe swallowed. "The Captain got *us* clear before he died," she said. "I couldn't have evaded the bastards myself. He'd lost his legs from the hit on the bridge but I don't think it was that what killed him. He just gave up." She swallowed again.

"We knew the Peeps were on Air, so we couldn't go back there. It was just luck the *Jerobahm* was bound out-system and her skipper was willing to let us ride her hull. We'd be dead for sure otherwise, Sir. Those bastards don't want any witnesses left."

"Yes, all right," Nessler said. "Wait here for a moment while I consult with Mr. Singh."

Nessler stepped toward Singh on the porch. The shipwrecked spacers parted with mechanical precision. They'd lost everything but the clothes they stood in—and clothes as well in some cases—but

their discipline held. Mincio had always considered
herself a scholar and above petty concerns of nation-
ality, but in this moment she was proud to be a
citizen of the Star Kingdom of Manticore.

"Excellent!" Nessler said after a brief conversation. Mr. Singh disappeared into the house, calling
half-heard orders.

"Bosun Harpe," Nessler continued, still on the
porch which put him a head higher than the spacers
he was addressing. "You and your people will be
billeted in a warehouse and provided with rations
during the period you're on Hope. I'll defray Mr.
Singh's expenses and be repaid on my return to
Manticore. Mr. Singh is summoning a guide right
now."

Mincio doubted that Nessler would even request
reimbursement for an amount that was vanishingly
small in comparison to his annual revenues. Government paperwork was a morass, and she suspected
that the Navy was worse even than the Star Kingdom's civilian bureaucracy. The comment was his
way of not seeming to boast about his wealth.

"We really do want to get back for another crack
at those Peeps, Sir," Harpe said. "They took us
down, that's war. But the lifeboats . . ."

"We'll deal with that, Bosun," Nessler said
sharply, "but first things first." Nodding toward the
servant who'd appeared at the door behind him he
continued, "You're to report to your new quarters
until seven hundred hours tomorrow. A delegation
of petty officers will wait on me here at that time.
Dismissed!"

"Hip-hip—" called a rear-rank spacer.

"Hooray!" shouted the whole body, sounding to Mincio like many more than thirty-seven throats in the echoing courtyard.

As crewmen filed from the courtyard behind Harpe and the servant guiding the party, Mincio moved to where Nessler was talking to Beresford. "This is horrible," she said.

"The other side of the Dole Fleet not being very competent at waging war," Nessler said without emphasis, "is that they're willing to commit acts that would be unthinkable to a professional force. Like destroying lifeboats."

Mincio nodded. "I'd think that any war was bad enough without people trying to find ways to make it worse," she agreed, "but as you say—failed people are desperate to have *anyone* else in their power."

"I was just pointing out to the master," Beresford said, "that with the Peeps being the sort they is, and Air being so close by to Hope, maybe it'd be a good idea if we cut things short in this sector and got back to systems where the Navy shows the flag with something more impressive than a destroyer." He spat. "To take on a heavy *cruiser*, for chrissake!"

"The normal problem in League Sector Twelve is piracy," Nessler said in a voice as flat and hard as a knifeblade. "But I agree that it might have occurred to someone in the Ministry that when the Peeps began sending out cruisers for commerce raiding, our anti-piracy patrols should have been either reinforced or withdrawn. No doubt the Admiralty had other things on its mind."

Rovald came out of the house with a hologram projector, part of the extensive suite of equipment she'd brought on the voyage. She started to speak but stopped when she realized Nessler and Mincio, though silent, were focused on more important matters.

Beresford had no such hesitation. "So shall I see about arranging transport, say, to Krishnaputra?" he said. "Captain Cage hasn't broken orbit yet. It might be three months before another Warshawski ship touches down here!"

Nessler shook his head no. He said, "Yes, that's the problem. We can get out of the region, but the survivors of *L'Imperieuse* cannot—certainly not in their pinnace, and not with any likelihood on any of the small-capacity vessels which call on a world like Hope."

"Well, Sir . . ." said Beresford, looking at the ground and thereby proving he knew how close he was skating to conduct his master would find completely unacceptable. "It seems to me that when they signed on with the Navy, Harpe and the rest, they kinda . . ."

"Yes, one does take on responsibilities that one may later find extremely burdensome," Nessler said in a cold, distinct tone. "As I did when I took the oath as an officer in Her Majesty's Navy. Nothing that touches you, of course, Beresford. I'll send you and Rovald—"

"Sir!" Beresford said. With a dignity that Mincio had never imagined in the little man he continued, "I don't guess anybody needs to teach his duty to a Beresford of Greatgap. Which it may be to keep his master from getting scragged, but it doesn't have shit to do with leaving him because the going got tough."

Nessler made a sour face. "Forgive me, Beresford," he said. "This isn't a good time for me to play the fool in front of the man who's looked after me all my life."

"Sir?" said Rovald, perhaps as much to break the embarrassing silence as because she thought anybody cared about what she had to say. "As Ms. Mincio instructed, I've analyzed the damaged crystals in the deKyper collection to find a common oscillation freq—"

"A moment please, Rovald," Nessler said, raising his hand but looking at Mincio rather than the technician. "Mincio, would it be possible for you to win a great deal of money at poker from Lord Orloff? More money than he could possibly pay?"

"No," Mincio said, her words as clipped and precise as the click of chips on hardwood. She and Nessler were no longer tutor and pupil, though she didn't have the mental leisure to determine what their present relationship really was.

Ignoring the chill in Nessler's expression she continued, "He wouldn't play with me for amounts in that range. If I have the complete cooperation of Beresford and Rovald, however, I think I might be able to arrange for you to—" she smiled like a sharp knife "—shear him like a sheep yourself in a day or two."

Beresford guffawed. "Who d'ye want killed, boss?" he asked; not entirely a joke from the look in his eyes, and the sudden tension in Rovald's thin frame.

"Just a matter of borrowing a deck of cards from Orloff's camp," Mincio said. "It shouldn't be difficult, given your contacts with the Melungeon crew; and perhaps a little money, but not much."

She turned to the technician. "As for you, Rovald," she continued, "I'll want you to reprogram the deck's electronic response. I could probably do the job myself with your equipment, but I couldn't do it as quickly and easily as I'm sure you can."

Rovald let out her breath in a sigh of relief. "I'm sure it won't be a problem, Ma'am," she said.

"I'm going to win at poker?" Nessler said. "That'll be a change from my experience at school, certainly." He chuckled. "But you're the expert, of course. And Beresford? Before I surrender your services to Mincio, be a good fellow and find my alcohol catalyzer. Orloff's bound to be pushing his horrible brandy at me, and I wouldn't want him to think I had a particular reason to keep a clear head."

It was midmorning before Reserve Midshipman Nessler finished his meeting with the ranking survivors of the *L'Imperieuse*. That suited Mincio much better than an early departure for the pylons. She was still feeling the effects of the dance two nights before.

Besides letting her muscles work themselves loose, the delay permitted Mincio to examine Rovald's work of the previous day. The technician had calculated the range of resonant frequencies for the four least-damaged Alphane "books" from deKyper's collection. The next step would be to calculate the frequency of common resonance, then finally to determine the factor by which that prime had to be modified to properly stimulate the crystals in their present damaged state.

If Rovald was successful—and that seemed likely—the breakthrough in Alphane studies would be the high point of Mincio's scholarly life. She wasn't really able to appreciate it, though, because for the first time since her father died Edith Mincio wasn't primarily a scholar.

Nessler lifted the air car. He and Mincio were in the front seats; Beresford and Rovald shared the back. There was space for a fifth passenger, but none of them cared to chance adding even deKyper's slight additional weight. The drive had labored just to carry three the day before.

They'd barely cleared the walls of Singh's courtyard before they saw the Melungeon air car curving down toward the landing field. Lord Orloff's vehicle had a fabric canopy with tassels which whipped furiously in the wind of passage.

"Ah!" said Nessler as he leaned into the control yoke to turn the car. "I think we'd best join them before going on. You may have to drive Rovald to the site yourself, Beresford."

"I guess I can handle that," the servant said. "Seeing as I've been driving air cars since I was nine. And *didn't* your father whip my ass when he caught me, Sir."

Orloff and his entourage were about to enter the Melungeon cutter when Nessler settled his borrowed car nearby. Orloff beamed at them and cried, "Nessler! Come and see my *Colonel Arabi*. Then the two of us can go back to the camp and play cards, not so?"

"Mincio and I would be delighted to visit your ship, Captain Orloff," Nessler said cheerfully. He strode to the Melungeon and embraced him enthusiastically. Mincio noticed that this time Nessler's arms were outside Orloff's instead of being pinned to his chest by the Melungeon's bear hug. "There's no problem with my servant and technician going to your camp to record the pylon before you remove it, is there?"

"Foof!" said Orloff. "Why should there be a problem? Alec, go back to camp with my honored guest's servants and see to it that the dogs there treat them right. It's only the other ranks there now, you see."

"And perhaps tomorrow when we've had a chance to rest," Nessler added, "I'll be in a mood for some poker. I hope you don't have a problem with high stakes?"

Lord Orloff's laughter thundered as he patted Nessler ahead of him into the pinnace.

Mincio had no naval experience, so the view of the approaching cruiser wouldn't have meant anything to her even if the cutter's view screen had been in better condition. If the fuzzy image was an indication of the *Colonel Arabi*'s condition, however, the cruiser was in very bad condition indeed.

"Why, if I didn't know better," Nessler said as he looked over the coxswain's shoulder, "I'd have said that was a *Brilliance*-class cruiser of the People's Republic of Haven! That's *very* good. Did the Grand Duchy purchase the plans from the Peeps, or . . .?"

"Not plans, no," Orloff said from the command seat to the right of the coxswain. "We bought the very ship! Nothing is too good for Melungeon, and nothing on Melungeon is too good for Maxwell, Lord Orloff." He pounded his broad chest with both fists. "My very self!"

The cutter passed into the cruiser's number two boat bay and settled into the docking buffers. The mechanical docking arms clanged rather more loudly than Mincio had expected, and the personnel tube ran out to the cutter's lock.

The sale of warships to minor states would be a useful profit center for a government like that of Haven, which needed massive production capacity for its own purposes. Post-delivery maintenance wouldn't be part of the deal, however.

"We bought the *Colonel Arabi* not twenty years ago," Orloff continued as crewmen manually opened the cutter's hatch. The powered system didn't work. "Direct from the yard on Haven, not some dog of a castoff. Have you ever seen so lovely a ship in your life, Sir Hakon Nessler? *My* ship!"

The view of the boat bay gallery beyond through the personnel tube didn't strike Mincio with anything but an awareness of squalor, but Nessler seemed genuinely impressed as he followed Orloff down the tube. "This is much more than I'd expected," he said. "Lord Orloff, I'll admit that I didn't think the Melungeon navy had so very modern a vessel in its inventory."

Orloff's officers were obsequious to both him and Nessler, but they showed no such reserve toward Mincio or one another. After Mincio had been pushed aside by a woman with three rings on her sleeves and a dueling scar across her forehead, she waited to disembark after all the ship's officers.

"Get to work on the forward lasers, Kotzwinkle," Orloff said. "Whichever one you think. And I don't want to spend all day here, either! A drink, Nessler?"

"So . . ." Mincio said as she caught up with the others as they left the boat bay. The Melungeons were intent on their own business; she was in effect speaking only to Nessler, though without any suggestion of secrecy between them. "This ship is actually the equal of the Peep vessel on Air?"

"Oh, good God, no!" Nessler said in amusement. "This is a light cruiser. The ship on Air is a heavy cruiser, quite a different thing, and newer as well. Though—" in a lower voice, still amused "—there may not be a great deal to choose between the professional standards of the crews. And it *is* a great deal better than I expected."

Orloff turned and thrust one of the two beakers of brandy he now held into Nessler's hand. "Come! Look at my lovely ship."

Mincio followed the pair of them, glad not to have more Musketoon to deal with. Nessler had swallowed a catalyzer before boarding. It converted ethanol to an ester which linked to fatty acids before it could be absorbed in the intestine. So long as Nessler had a supply of suitable food—the bowls of peanuts on the Melungeon card table would do fine—nobody could drink him under the table.

The catalyzer didn't affect the *taste* of Musketoon,

however. If Mincio had a choice, she'd prefer to drink hydraulic fluid.

Several of the officers went off on the business of the ship, shouting angry orders at the enlisted personnel still aboard. With Nessler at his side, Orloff led the rest of his entourage on a stroll through the vessel. Mincio followed as an interested though inexpert observer.

The voyage from Melungeon to Hope was long and presumably a difficult piece of navigation, so the officers and crew had to have at least a modicum of competence. More than a modicum, given the *Colonel Arabi*'s terrible state of repair.

No expertise was needed to notice the ropes of circuitry routed along the decks, sometimes to enter compartments through holes raggedly cut in what had been blast-proof walls. Equipment didn't fit the racks and was interconnected by exposed cables. Sometimes a replacement unit was welded *onto* the case of the original.

Above all, everything was filthy. Lubricants and hydraulic fluids had obviously won their battle to bleed over every surface within the closed universe of any starship. Only constant labor by the crews could remove the slimy coating. There was no sign that anybody aboard the *Colonel Arabi* even made the effort. Mincio saw 20-centimeter beards of gummy lint wobbling everywhere but in the main traffic areas.

They entered an echoing bay. For the most part the *Colonel Arabi* had given Mincio the dual impressions of being very large and simultaneously very cramped. This was the first time she had the feeling of real volume. Crewmen flitted half-seen in the shadows; only a fraction of the compartment's lighting appeared to function.

"Here we will store the pillar," Orloff said, gesturing expansively with both hands. "Three months it took to open the space! Our dockyard on Melungeon, it's shit!"

He spat on the deck at his feet. "Cheating crooks, just out to line their pockets!"

"That bulkhead separated the forward missile magazine from a main food storage compartment, did it not?" Nessler said. "Removing the armor plate from a magazine would have been a serious job for any dockyard, Lord Orloff. And I wonder . . . don't you have flexing problems as a result of the change? That was the main transverse stiffener, I believe."

"Faugh!" Orloff said. "We had to have room for the pillar, did we not? What use would it be to come all this way if we couldn't carry the damned pillar?"

As Mincio's eyes adapted to the lack of lighting she made out the forms of two huge cylinders, each nearly the size of the *Colonel Arabi*'s cutter. They were missiles, sublight spaceships in their own right, each with a nuclear warhead as its cargo.

Perhaps a nuclear warhead. Based on the rest of what she'd seen of the Melungeon navy, the warhead compartment might be empty or hold a quantity of sand for ballast.

"You've had to remove most of your missiles to make room to store Alphane artifacts, I gather, Lord Orloff?" Mincio said. In fact she didn't think anything of the sort. Close up she could see that the cradles which should have held additional missiles were pitted with rust. It had been years if not decades since they'd last been used for their intended purpose.

"This is just the forward missile magazine, Mincio," Nessler said quickly. "There's the stern magazine as well, and it hasn't been affected by these modifications."

"Faugh!" Orloff repeated. "What do we need missiles for? Are the Alphanes going to attack us, my friend?"

He whacked Nessler across the back and laughed uproariously. "Besides, do you know how much one of those missiles costs? Much better to spend the naval appropriations on pay for deserving officers, not so?"

A bell chimed three times. A voice called information that Mincio couldn't understand: the combination of loudspeaker distortion, echoes, the Melungeon accent, and naval jargon were just too much for her.

"Hah!" Orloff cried. "Kotzwinkle is ready so soon. I'll have to apologize for calling him a lazy dog who'd rather screw his sister than do his duty, will I not?"

His laugh boomed again as he shooed both Manticore visitors ahead of him toward the hatch by which they'd entered the bay. "Another drink and we go back to the camp and play poker, not so?" he said.

"Another drink," Nessler agreed. "And tomorrow I'll come out to your camp and we'll play poker, yes."

✧   ✧   ✧

It had rained at the campsite during the night, a brief squall that seemed to have done nothing to lay the dust. Tiny shoots sprang up from what had been bare soil. The vegetation was an unattractive gray hue and it had spikes capable of piercing the fabric sides of Mincio's utility boots. She'd need to get tougher footgear if they were to stay on Hope any length of time.

Beresford was erecting a small tent beside the Melungeons' own shelter. Rovald carried her gear to the spot, making a number of trips rather than chance dropping a piece and damaging it. Mincio had offered to help, but the technician didn't trust anybody else with the equipment. They hadn't been able to bring the protective containers in which the pieces normally traveled. Even now the borrowed air car was only marginally flyable with four people aboard and the minimum additional weight.

"So," said Orloff cheerfully. "You didn't bring your old fool deKyper to watch? I thought she'd want to say good-bye to her precious pillar."

"She wanted to stay home and check some values Rovald here has calculated for Alphane books," Nessler lied. His smile looked as bright and natural as sunrise. You had to know him as well as Mincio did to notice the vein throbbing at the side of his neck. "That would be a wonderful thing, wouldn't it, if we could actually decode their records?"

"Books are all well and good," Orloff said dismissively. He gestured toward the pylon in its wrapper of countergrav rings. "But this, *this* is what will knock their eyes out!"

Beresford had the tent up. It was of Manticoran manufacture, a marvel of compactness and simplicity. It would sleep four and even hold a portion of their personal property if necessary. Some of the lodgings Nessler's party had found on the tour were rudimentary, but this was the first time they'd actually used the tent.

Crewmen had unloaded the laser they'd stripped from the cruiser's defensive armament. Under Kotzwinkle's shrill commands they were manhandling it the ten meters from the cutter to the edge of the pit where it could point at the rock on which the pylon rested.

The weapon didn't have a proper ground carriage: it lay in the bed of an agricultural cart purchased from a nearby latifundium. Mincio supposed that was all right since a laser wouldn't recoil, but both Nessler and Rovald had warned her not to get near the power cable which connected the weapon to the cutter's MHD generator. Neither of them thought the wrist-thick cable would hold up to the current for long.

A Melungeon servant huddled for a moment with Beresford. The officers paid no attention; those who'd gotten bored with watching the preparations were playing a half-hearted game of snap. It wouldn't have mattered if they'd all been staring at the servants. Even knowing what to expect, Mincio couldn't tell when Beresford passed the reprogrammed deck of cards back to the Melungeon.

"I wonder, Lord Orloff," Nessler said loudly enough to be heard by most of the officers. "Might I borrow a pistol from one of your men to do a little target shooting? At one time I used to be pretty good."

"Sure, use mine," Orloff said, pulling a gleaming weapon from the holster on his belt. It was a little thing, almost hidden in Orloff's hand, a symbol rather than a serious weapon which would weigh the wearer down uncomfortably.

"But say," he added. "Don't shoot more than a dozen or so of my dogs of crewmen, will you? We still need to get the pillar aboard!"

Orloff doubled over with the enthusiasm of his laughter. Nessler chuckled also as he examined the borrowed pistol.

He turned and brought the weapon up. It *whacked*, an angry, spiteful sound, and the short barrel lifted in recoil. Dirt spewed fifty meters from where Nessler stood.

"What are you trying to hit?" Orloff asked genially. Several other officers walked over, some of them drawing their own sidearms in the apparent intention of joining in.

Nessler fired again. There was no flash or smoke from the muzzle so Mincio supposed the weapon used electromagnetic rather than chemical propulsion. A second geyser of dirt sprayed from the same bit of ground.

"Seems to group nicely," Nessler said. "If it was mine, I'd adjust the sights; but so long as it groups, I don't mind holding off."

He fired a third time: a fist-sized rock, half a meter from the original point of impact, sprang into the air. He hit the rock twice more before it disintegrated as it bounced across the landscape.

"You meant to do that?" a Melungeon officer said in amazement.

"Of course," said Nessler. He picked up a pebble with his left hand. Mincio noticed that despite Nessler's seeming nonchalance he never let the muzzle waver from the stretch of empty landscape toward which he'd been shooting. "Watch this."

He tossed the pebble skyward. It disintegrated at the top of its arc. The *whack* of the pistol and the *crack* of rock being hammered into sand were almost simultaneous.

"Hit *this*!" said Orloff. He hurled a pebble no larger than the first toward the horizon with all his strength.

Nessler's body swung onto the new target, the pistol an extension of his straight right arm. The pebble was a rotating reflection forty meters from Nessler when it vanished in a spark and a spray of white dust.

"Yes, very nice," Nessler said as he turned to the astounded Melungeons. He offered the pistol, its muzzle in the air, to Orloff between thumb and forefinger. "Haven't done any shooting in a very long time. Haven't dared to, really."

"Where did you learn to shoot like that?" Orloff said. Though he closed his hand over the pistol, he seemed completely unaware of what he held.

"Well, it wasn't my first love," Nessler said airily. "But after a while people refused to fight me with swords so I had to learn to shoot. I was a terror at school, I'm afraid. How many did I kill in duels, Mincio? It must have been near twenty, wasn't it?"

"More than that," Mincio said, shaking her head sadly. "It was quite a scandal."

Nessler nodded. "Yes," he agreed, "I was on the verge of being sent down. My sainted mother on her deathbed made me swear never to fight another duel. I've kept that oath thus far. But I must say, when I hold a weapon in my hand again it makes me wonder if a little hellfire for a broken oath would really be so bad."

He gave the Melungeons a bright smile. Orloff rubbed his mustache with his fist, trying to process the unexpected information.

"We're ready!" Kotzwinkle called from beside the laser. A crewman murmured a protest, his head abjectly lowered. "We're ready, I say!" the officer roared.

Everyone moved toward the edge of the pit. Orloff had his arm around Nessler's shoulders. He fumbled the pistol into its holster with his free hand.

"The best thing I could say about the master's mother," Beresford whispered into Mincio's ear, "is that after she ran off with the undergardener ten years ago she never troubled the family again. And Sir Hakon never fought a duel in his life."

"He never had to fight," Mincio whispered back. "He made sure that everyone at school knew he was as deadly a marksman as ever walked the Quad. He gave trick-shooting demonstrations to entertain the bloods. Nobody would have thought of calling him out."

She nodded toward Nessler, listening to their host's expansive boasting. "And he's just done the same thing again, Beresford."

The big laser was aimed at bare granite beside the pylon's crystal shaft. Some of the Melungeon crewmen were directly across the pit, itself less than thirty meters in radius.

"I wonder if we should be standing so close?" Mincio observed aloud. Everyone ignored her, though she noticed Nessler was covering his eyes with his left forearm. She did the same.

Kotzwinkle signalled a crewman, who switched on the cutter's MHD generator. Its roar overwhelmed any chance for further conversation.

The laser's oscillator whined up into the reaches of inaudibility. When the weapon fired, the sound of the beam heating the air was lost in the crash of granite shattered by asymmetric heating.

Bedrock exploded into secondary projectiles ranging in size from sand to head-sized rocks. Most of them flew into the side of the pit, but crewmen on the other side were down and the stone that howled past Mincio's ear could have knocked her silly if not worse.

At the same time as the bedrock disintegrated, a varicolored short circuit blew out the side of the laser. The cable had proved more durable than the weapon it fed. Kotzwinkle fell shrieking into the pit with his tunic afire. His roll down the gritty slope smothered the flames.

Mincio lowered her protective arm; Nessler had done the same. Everybody was shouting, mostly in delight and wonder. The fireworks had been the most entertainment the Melungeons, officers and spacers alike, had seen in a long time.

The pylon wavered, then started to tilt. The rock

to one side of the crystal was broken into fragments but the granite shelf on the other side remained whole; the base was partly supported, partly free.

The shaft tilted minusculely farther. Then the entire pylon disintegrated into shards no bigger than a fingernail with a trembling roar like that of ice breaking in a spring freshet.

The countergrav rings flew loose, freed when the shaft they bound dribbled out of their grip. Glittering ruin filled the pit with the remnants of an object that had survived longer than men had used fire. Kotzwinkle had started to climb up the sandy slope. The crystal flowed over him. The Melungeon's screams continued for a little longer than even his outstretched arm was visible.

Mincio swallowed. Her eyes were open, but tears blinded her. From her side Nessler said in a low voice, "I'm glad we didn't bring Ms. deKyper. It'll be bad enough that she has to hear about it."

The last fragments tinkled down. In the silence to which even his own personnel had been struck, Orloff said, "Well, shall we play poker, Sir Hakon? Let's see if things go right for at least one of us this day!"

"Yes," said Nessler. "I think we should play cards."

"I've always loved poker, but I'm afraid I'm not very good at it," Nessler said as he sat in the indicated chair to Orloff's left. Two other Melungeon officers took their places at the table; the remainder watched with greedy expressions, some of them toying with the prostitutes as they did so. Enlisted personnel drifted to their burrows or sat stolidly around the glittering wreck.

Mincio stood at the flap of the Manticoran tent. She heard Nessler's voice through the intercom in her left ear canal and, a half-beat later, via the air in normal fashion.

"Hah, don't worry," Orloff said, taking the deck of special cards from his servant. He put the pipe in his mouth. "We teach you to play good today, not so?"

"If you can hear me," Mincio said softly, "lace your fingers against the back of your neck and stretch."

Nessler laced his fingers and stretched. "Well, so long as we play for table stakes," he said, "I don't guess I can get into any serious problems. Can we stipulate table stakes?"

"Well . . ." Orloff said.

"I don't mean small stakes, necessarily," Nessler added. He brought a sheaf of credit vouchers from his purse and laid them on the table. Each was a chip loaded by the Royal Bank of Manticore, with an attached hardcopy of the terms and amount of the draft.

Orloff picked one of the printouts at random and looked at the amount it represented. "Ha!" he bellowed. "I should say not! Table stakes indeed! Let us play, my friends. Sir Hakon thinks he can buy all Melungeon, or so it seems!"

"I'm going to check the imagery, Nessler," Mincio called. Everyone ignored her; Orloff was shuffling the cards.

She went into the tent; Beresford walked over

to stand in front of the flap, his eyes on the card game in the adjacent tent.

Rovald had a receiver set up inside. It already displayed the deck's arrangement in the form of an air-projected hologram. The glowing layout shifted instantly every time Orloff mixed the cards.

"All he's got is a code signal through his teeth on the pipestem," Rovald explained proudly as Mincio seated herself before the display. "It tells him what the top card in the deck is. You see the whole thing."

"Yes," Mincio said. "Now, don't move till I tell you, and don't talk."

The technician jerked as though slapped. Mincio, though wholly immersed in the job at hand, knew she'd sounded very like her late father. Well, she could apologize later.

Play started with Orloff dealing. Nessler plunged deeply on two pair, losing the hand to another of the Melungeons with three queens.

Mincio said nothing during that hand or any of the scores of hands following. She'd instructed Nessler to bet heavily and to bluff frequently— precisely the sort of mistakes that came naturally to someone rich and unskilled. Mincio needed to get the measure of the opposition, and Nessler had to lose a hefty amount before he could move in for the kill anyway. There was no need to force the pace.

"Another drink!" Nessler's voice snarled through the intercom. "Goddammit, isn't it enough that my cards are all shit? Do I have to die of thirst as well?"

He was a good actor; she could almost believe the anger and frustration in her pupil's tone were real. Maybe they were: even though he knew that losing was necessary to the plan, it couldn't be a great deal of fun for somebody like Sir Hakon Nessler. He prided himself on being extremely good at the narrow range of categories in which he chose to compete.

The shifting display was all Mincio's life for the moment. The Melungeons played five-card draw, nothing wild; an expert's game, and Edith Mincio was the greatest expert on Hope.

"Goddammit, I've got to sign over another of these drafts," Nessler's voice snarled. "You'll have my shirt before I leave here, Orloff. And where's that damned bottle? Can't a man get a drink in this place?"

A youth with more money than sense. A bad player growing even wilder as he gulped down brandy . . .

It took three hours before the deck broke the way Mincio needed it. Orloff was dealing. Even before the second round of cards pattered onto the table, Mincio turned to Rovald. "Switch the signals from these two cards," she ordered.

The technician touched the keyboard. The minuscule cue reprogrammed the chosen pair of cards.

The deal finished. Nessler's hand contained the ten, nine, seven, and six of spades, and the king of clubs. So far as Lord Orloff knew, the top card remaining in the deck was the jack of diamonds.

"Nessler, this is it," Mincio said crisply. The bone-conduction pickup was part of the bead in her ear canal. "Bet as high as you can. There won't be another chance. Discard the king and take one card on the draw."

"By God, I'm tired of this penny-ante crap!" Nessler's voice rasped in her ear. "What's the pot? Well, let me sign this over and we'll have a real pot!"

"God and holy angels!" one of the Melungeons said, loud enough to be heard through the tent's insulating walls.

Mincio got up from her chair and wobbled outside. Her legs were so stiff they threatened to cramp. She was dizzy, thirsty, and sick with fatigue. She had nothing more to do, so she might as well watch. Beresford stepped aside to give her room, but he kept his eyes on the game.

The two officers who'd been makeweights for the game folded their hands immediately. By luck or design the big pots had all gone to their captain. Table stakes meant they had to show the money they were betting, and they simply didn't have it.

"So, we put another of your little chits in to match you," Orloff said genially. "You must have very good cards, my friend. Still, God loves a brave man, not so?"

"From the cards I've been getting, He doesn't love me today," Nessler grumbled. He drank off the rest of a beaker of Musketoon and slapped the king of clubs facedown in the center of the table. "One card!"

Orloff slid the top card to his opponent, then set the deck down. "The dealer stands pat," he said. "Perhaps I have very good cards too, or perhaps . . ."

He laughed loudly to imply he was really bluffing. He wiped spittle from his mustache with the back of his hand. Orloff was nervous despite what must be his certainty that everything was in his pocket. The amount the fool from Manticore had already lost would make Orloff one of the wealthiest men on Melungeon.

"So, are they this good?" Nessler said. He thrust three more drafts onto the table, equalling the full amount of Orloff's winnings and original stake. "Brandy! Somebody give me a glass of damned brandy, won't you?"

A Melungeon officer instantly handed over the full beaker which he'd been holding for the purpose.

"I will see you, yes," Orloff said. His voice was no longer confident. He stared for a moment at the remainder of the deck, but he pushed out the matching bet.

Melungeon officers whispered among themselves; Beresford was as taut as an E-string. Mincio was relaxed as she watched events roll to their inevitable conclusion.

Nessler slammed down the beaker, empty again. "Then by God I'll raise!" he said. "I'll double the damned pot!"

He pulled another draft from his purse. The printout had red wax seals and the face amount was five times that of any document already on the table. "Do you see me now, Orloff?"

Orloff's bare scalp glistened with sweat. "I see you," he said. "But I call. We would not have it seem that you bought the pot."

"I accept your call," Nessler said. He laid his cards faceup on the table.

Orloff displayed his hand with a great sigh of relief. "A full house, jacks over fives," he said. "Which beats your busted flush, I'm afraid, Sir Hakon!"

"It's not a busted flush," Nessler said. "It's complete to the ten of spades. A straight flush to the ten, which beats a full house. My pot, I believe."

"Holy Savior!" a Melungeon officer said, crossing herself. "He's right!"

Orloff's face went from red to a white as pale as if he'd been heart-shot. "But I thought . . ." he gasped. He raised the top card on the deck. It was the jack of diamonds which he'd thought was in Nessler's hand.

Nessler stood up and stretched lithely. He didn't look drunk, or young, or foolish, any more. Mincio walked toward the card players, her face calm.

"I don't intend to break the game up now that I'm ahead," Nessler said mildly. "I'll give you a chance to win your money back, of course. But first we'll settle this pot. Table stakes, you'll remember."

Orloff remained in his chair. The other two players rose and stepped quickly away, as though they'd been thrust back by bayonets.

"I'll give you my note," Orloff whispered. He was staring at the cards on the table rather than attempting to meet the Manticoran's eyes.

"No, Sir," Nessler said in a voice like a whiplash. "You will settle your debt immediately like the gentleman I assumed you were. If you choose instead to affront my honor—"

He left the threat hanging. Half of Orloff's officers stared toward the scarred sand where Nessler had proved he could put a whole magazine through his opponent's right eye if he so chose.

"Actually, My Lord," Mincio said, "this may be all to the good. Why don't you rent Orloff's ship for a month or two in settlement of the debt?"

Orloff looked up, blinking as he tried to puzzle out the meaning of words which seemed perfectly clear in themselves.

"A good thought, Mincio," Nessler said in easy agreement. They hadn't worked out the details of this exchange, but they knew one another well. "That'll serve everybody's purpose."

"But . . ." Orloff said. "The *Colonel Arabi*? I cannot—the *Colonel Arabi* is a Duchy ship, I can't rent her to you, Sir Hakon."

"As I understand it, Lord Orloff," Mincio said musingly, "your government put the ship at your disposal to facilitate your collection of Alphane artifacts. Is that so?"

Orloff swallowed. "That is so, yes," he said. His officers were all at a distance, staring at their captain as if he were a suicide beneath a high window.

"I'd say that renting the ship to Lord Nessler here was well within the mandate, then," Mincio said. "After all, old man, you can't collect many artifacts after your brains are splashed over a hectare or so of sand."

Orloff lurched to his feet. Mincio thought he was going to say something. Instead the Melungeon turned and vomited. He sank to his knees, keeping his torso upright only by gripping the card table with one hand.

"Yes, all right," he said in a slurred voice. "The *Colonel Arabi* for a month. And we are quit."

Nessler looked behind him to be sure that Rovald was recording the agreement. "Very good," he said. He picked up his winnings before Orloff managed to tip the table into the pool of vomit beside him. "I suppose the cutter should be part of the deal, but I won't insist on that."

He grinned brightly around the awestruck Melungeons. "I think I'll use the pinnace from *L'Imperieuse* instead."

A few artificial lights were already on in Kuepersburg as Nessler flew them home at a sedate pace. Days were short on Hope, but this one had vanished almost without Mincio's awareness.

She turned to the servants in the air car's back seat. "Rovald," she said, "this was your win. A child could beat professionals at cards with your help."

"Thank you, Ma'am," Rovald said. The technician had been unusually stiff and withdrawn ever since Mincio silenced her so abruptly at the start of the game. At last she relaxed—to her usual stiff, withdrawn personality.

"You were both splendid," Nessler said. He sighed. "Now all I have to do is figure out how to get a light cruiser from Hope to Air with thirty-seven spacers and a very rusty astrogator."

Mincio twisted around suddenly in her seat. Stabbing pains reminded her of how tense she'd been as she watched the progress of the card game. "Surely you don't need to go to Air?" she said. "I thought you were going to use the cruiser to frighten away the Peeps if they came here?"

"If we give the Peeps the initiative as well as all the other advantages . . ." Nessler said. He raised the air car to clear the walls of Singh's courtyard. "Then they'll certainly destroy us. Based on what we've heard of the Dole Fleet, I'm hoping that if we attack and then retreat, they'll make an effort to avoid us thereafter."

The air car wasn't stable enough to hover. Nessler brought them down in a rush, doing his best to control the bow's tendency to swing clockwise.

They hit and bounced. As the turbines spun down he added, "The problem is getting there with a tenth the normal crew, of course."

"You can have all the Melungeons working for you if you like, Sir," Beresford said. "Barring the officers, of course, which I *don't* think is much loss. I'll pass the word that they'll get a square meal every day. They'll trample each other to come along."

Lalita and several household servants came into the courtyard to help if required. Nessler had started to climb out of the vehicle; he paused with his right leg over the side.

"Are you serious?" he said. "I'll certainly do better than a meal a day if you are!"

"Sure you will, Sir," Beresford said with a satisfied smirk. "But I won't tell 'em that, because they wouldn't believe me. You just let me handle this, Sir."

He hopped out of the air car and strolled to the

front gate, his hands clasped at the back of his plump waistline. He was whistling.

Nessler watched the little man leave the compound. "I'll be damned," he muttered to Mincio as he finally got out of the vehicle. "There's actually a chance this might work!"

The two ranks of Manticoran spacers in the Singh courtyard looked more professional than they had the last time Mincio had seen them. It wasn't just that they were well-fed and rested; those who'd lost their clothing with the *L'Imperieuse* had now turned local fabric into garments closely resembling the issue uniforms their fellows wore.

"This is a private venture," Nessler said in a carrying tone. "In a moment I will ask those of you who volunteer to board the *Colonel Arabi* with me to take a step forward."

He spoke with the exaggerated precision that Mincio knew meant her pupil was nervous. It was easy even for her to forget that Sir Hakon Nessler, the self-assured youth with all the advantages, had never really felt he belonged anywhere except in his dreams of the distant past.

"I can't order anyone to come," Nessler continued, "because so far as I know my reserve commission is still inactive. Also, I'd like to say that we were going to Air to sort out the Peeps who murdered your fellows, but I can't honestly claim I see any great likelihood of success. The ship at our disposal is in wretched shape and has been virtually disarmed besides."

Nessler cleared his throat. The spacers were silent

and motionless, their faces yellowed by the court-yard lighting. Naval discipline, Mincio knew, but it still gave her a creepy feeling. It was like watching Nessler declaim to a tray of perch at a fish-monger's.

"Still," Nessler said, "a gentleman of Manticore does what he can. I'll make arrangements for those of you who choose to stay and—"

"*Attention!*" Harpe said from the right front of the double rank. "On the word of command, all per-sonnel will take one step forward!"

"Wait a minute!" cried Nessler, taken completely aback. "Harpe, this has to be a free choice."

"And so it is, Sir," the Bosun said. "Mine, as senior officer of this contingent until we put our-selves under your command."

She turned to the spacers. "Now *step*, you lousy bastards!"

Laughing and cheering, the thirty-six spacers obeyed. Harpe stepped forward herself, threw Nessler a sharp salute, and said, "All present and accounted for, Captain."

"Begging your pardon, Sir," said a brawny spacer. "But what did you think we were? A bunch of fucking Peeps who were going to argue about orders?"

"No, Dismore," Nessler said as if he were answering the question. "I don't think that at all."

"All right, ten minute break!" Beresford called from the adjacent compartment. "You're doing good, teams. Damned if I don't think I'll be buying beer for both lots of you come end of shift!"

Nessler slid out from beneath a console which he'd been discussing with a Melungeon and a Manticoran yeoman who'd crawled under from the opposite side. Mincio had to hop clear. She was standing nearby in a subconscious attempt to seem to have something useful to do. In fact she didn't know the purpose of the console, let alone what problem it was having.

"Mincio, do you know where Rovald is?" Nessler said as he noticed her. His face and clothing were greasy; there was a nasty scratch on the back of his left hand. "The damned intercom system doesn't work, of course."

"I don't—" Mincio began.

"Fetch her here, will you?" Nessler continued without waiting for an answer. "I think she's in Navigation Two. All the levels check, but there's no damned display!"

Mincio nodded and trotted into the passage, thinking of the curt way she'd acted toward Rovald during the card game. Nessler was focused on putting the *Colonel Arabi* in fighting trim for perhaps the first time since the vessel was delivered to the Grand Duchy of Melungeon. He didn't have time for what anybody else might want.

Work parties—generally a group of Melungeons under the direction of one or two survivors of *L'Imperieuse*—were busy all over the ship, readying her for action. Beresford had no naval or technical experience, but he'd proven to be a wonder in these changed circumstances. Not only was he acting as personnel officer, he'd formed unassigned

Melungeons into teams to clean up the vessel's squalor.

Rovald's help was even more crucial. Third-rate navies like the Grand Duchy's train their personnel to use their ship's equipment, but they don't as a general rule care whether anybody *understands* that equipment. First-rate navies like that of the Star Kingdom *do* train their people to understand it so that they can do more than by-the-book maintenance, but no fleet has time to train its personnel to understand everyone *else's* equipment. In a ship like the *Colonel Arabi*, where so much was jury-rigged and none of it was of standard Manticoran design, Rovald's ability to troubleshoot unfamiliar systems was invaluable.

Mincio had no useful skills whatsoever. She'd thought of joining Beresford's custodial teams, but she decided that she wasn't ready to humble herself completely to so little purpose. She couldn't convince herself she'd be much good at wiping oily scum off the walls.

She stepped aside for six spacers grunting under the weight of a three-meter screwjack. All the cruiser's countergrav rings were down at the pylon site. Nessler hadn't sent for them because he didn't want to discuss with Orloff what he knew about the desertion of the entire enlisted complement of the *Colonel Arabi* and the sabotage of the Melungeon air car.

"Have you seen Ms. Rovald?" she called to the Manticoran rating at the head of the gang.

"Navigation Two!" the man shouted back. "Next compartment to port!"

Which didn't mean "left" as Mincio assumed; it meant "left when you're facing the ship's bow" which she was not, but she found Rovald by a process of elimination. The technician sat cross-legged in front of a bulkhead. Before her an access panel had been removed to display a rack of circuitry. The compartment felt cold and musty; the air was still.

"Good day, Rovald," Mincio said. "Sir Hakon needs you in, ah . . . I'll lead you."

Rovald didn't stir. Mincio blinked and partly out of curiosity said, "You're fixing the environmental system here?"

"I can't fix that," the technician said in a dead voice. "They used the power cable for the laser, and it's still on the ground at the Six Pylons. Five Pylons."

"Well," Mincio said. "Sir Hakon—"

Rovald sucked in a great gulp of air and began to cry.

Mincio knelt beside the older woman. "Are you . . ." she said. She didn't know whether to touch Rovald or not. "That is . . ."

"I'm not a soldier, Ma'am!" Rovald sobbed. "I don't want to die! He doesn't have a right to make me be a soldier!"

"Ah!" said Mincio, glad at least to know what the problem was. "Dear me, Nessler had no intention of taking you with him to Air," she lied brightly. "You'll be landed as soon as he's ready to, ah, proceed. No, no; you're to continue your work on Alphane books. If worse comes to worst, our names as scholars will live through your work, you see?"

"I don't have to come?" Rovald said. Her tears had streaked the dirt inevitable on anybody working aboard the *Colonel Arabi*. "He just wants me while we're in orbit here?"

"That's right," Mincio said. That would be true as soon as Nessler learned how the technician felt. She stood and gestured Rovald up. "But I think there's some need for haste now."

"Of course," said Rovald as she rose. "They'll be in Generator Control, I suppose."

She stepped briskly off the way Mincio had come to fetch her. Mincio followed, thinking about people. It was easy to understand why Rovald would want to avoid this probable suicide mission. It was much harder to explain why Mincio planned to go along. . . .

"The pinnace just docked, Sir," Harpe said. "She'll be dogged down in five minutes, and then we're ready."

Mincio completed the statement in her mind: *Ready to depart.* Ready to voyage to Air. Ready to die, it seemed likely. She couldn't get her mind around the last concept, but it didn't seem as frightening as she'd have assumed it would.

"Thank you, Bosun," Nessler said. "I'll hold a christening ceremony, then we'll set off."

As if he'd read her thoughts, Nessler turned to Mincio and said, "I don't think we'll have a great deal of difficulty with the drive and astrogation equipment. Orloff managed a much more difficult voyage than this little hop to Air, after all. The problem is that the closest thing to an offensive weapon aboard is a broken-down cutter that we've re-engined and hope will look like a missile to the Peeps."

"But there *are* missiles," Mincio said in puzzlement. "Two of them, at least."

"Ah, yes, there were," Nessler said. "But those we've converted to decoys since there weren't any decoys aboard. Have to think of our own survival first, you know."

He smiled.

If we were thinking of our own survival, we wouldn't any of us be aboard, Mincio thought; but perhaps that wasn't true. History was simpler to study than to live.

Beresford trotted through the armored bridge hatch, holding a suit bag high in his left hand. "Rovald's all happy and digging into them crystals with deKyper," he said cheerfully. "And the folks in Kuepersburg, they sent these up for you and Ms. Mincio. All the ladies in town worked on them with their own hands."

"You were supposed to stay on Hope too, Beresford," Nessler said in a thin voice.

"Was I, Sir?" said the servant as he opened the bag's zip closure. "Guess I musta misheard." He looked at his master. "Anyhow, I want to make sure these Navy types treat my wogs right. Since I recruited them, I figure they're my responsibility."

Mincio winced to hear the Melungeon spacers called wogs; but on the other hand, it was hard to fault the sentiment.

Beresford flicked the bag away from the garments within. "For you, Sir," he said, handing one of the hangers to Nessler. "They worked from pictures of you when you was a midshipman."

"Good God!" Nessler said. "Royal Manticoran Navy dress blacks!"

"Close enough, Captain Nessler Sir," Beresford said with a smirk. He turned to Mincio. "And for you—"

"I'm not a naval officer," she protested.

"You are now, Commander Mincio," Beresford said as he handed over the second uniform. "What's a ship as don't have a second in command, I say?"

Mincio rubbed a sleeve of her uniform between thumb and forefinger. The cloth was of off-planet weave but clearly hand-sewn as Beresford said. Nessler stared at his collar insignia.

"Those started out as Gendarmerie rank tabs," the servant explained. "A little chat with a barracks servant and a little work with a file, that's all it took."

A three-note signal pinged from the command console. "All systems ready, Sir," Harpe said.

"Then I'll have my little ceremony," Nessler said. He started to drape his uniform over the back of a seat; Beresford took it from his hand instead.

Nessler rang a double chime, then touched a large yellow switch. Mincio heard carrier hum from the intercom speaker above the hatch.

"This is the Captain speaking," Nessler said. His voice boomed from the intercom but it didn't cause feedback. The *Colonel Arabi*'s internal communications system worked flawlessly again. "In a moment we'll get under way, but first I wish to take formal possession of this vessel for the Star Kingdom of Manticore."

He took a 100-milliliter bottle from the breast pocket of the jacket he was wearing. "With this bottle of wine from the Greatgap Winery," he said, "I christen thee Her Majesty's Starship *Ajax*."

He flung the bottle to smash on the steel deck. The intercom managed to pick up the clink of glass.

"May she wear the name with honor!" Harpe cried.

There was frenzied cheering from neighboring compartments. From the volume, most of it must be coming from the Melungeons.

"The course is loaded," Nessler said. "Get us underway, Bosun."

Nessler looked a little embarrassed as he walked over to Mincio at the rear bulkhead. There should probably be a squad of officers at the empty consoles; instead the two of them, Beresford, and Harpe with a pair of Melungeons were the entire bridge crew. In a dozen other compartments enlisted personnel did work that officers would normally have overseen. . . .

Though on the *Colonel Arabi*, perhaps not overseen as closely as all that. The present crew was up to the job, of that Mincio was sure. A Melungeon had already sponged up the splash of wine and thin glass without being told to.

"I was never much of an astrogator," Nessler muttered.

"If Orloff can find Hope," Mincio said, "then you can find Air. You've got proper spacers aboard, besides. A few of them."

"You know," said Nessler, "that's an odd thing.

The Melungeons are working harder than I've ever seen spacers do. I think they're trying to prove to the fancy folk from Manticore that they're really good for something. And our people are working doubly hard to prove they *are* fancy folk from Manticore, of course."

The *Ajax* shuddered as systems came on line. An occasional drifting curse, and clangs that might be hammers on balky housings, indicated that not every piece of equipment was being cooperative. Nevertheless, a panel of lights on the main console was turning green bit by bit.

Beresford walked over to them. "Shall I hang the Captain's uniform in the Captain's cabin?" he said.

"I . . . yes, that would be a good idea," Nessler said. To Mincio he added, "We should probably sit down. This may be a bit rough. That—" He gestured at the console across the bridge. "—is the First Officer's station while cruising. Though I don't suppose it matters."

"Of course," Mincio said. She wondered what a First Officer did. Wear a black uniform, at any rate.

"I was wondering, Nessler," she said aloud. "How did you happen to pick that name for the ship? *Ajax*, I mean."

"Well, actually, I'd been given orders to take up the sixth lieutenancy aboard *Ajax* when I got word of my father and sister," Nessler said without meeting her eyes. "Instead I resigned my commission, of course."

He cleared his throat. Still looking at the deck he continued, "Three weeks later *Ajax* was lost with all hands. Funny how things work out, isn't it?"

A bell rang three slow peals. Mincio strode to what was apparently her station, the new uniform in her hands. "Yes, isn't it?" she said.

And wondered if Fate was planning to pick up the last of the former *Ajax*'s crew, along with all his present associates.

The Plot Position Indicator showed the *Ajax* in close conjunction with Air, at least if Mincio understood the scale correctly. Harpe and her Melungeon aides muttered cheerfully as they adjusted controls on a console with a curved bench seat holding three, and Nessler himself was whistling as he eyed the various displays with his hands in his pockets.

In theory the crew of the *Ajax* was at battle stations, but ever since the vessel entered the Air system Beresford had been leading a stream of Melungeons through the bridge to gape at the optical screen. Mincio knew she was of less use in a battle than the Melungeons were, so she felt free to stroll over to Nessler and say, "I'm not an expert, but it seemed to me to be a nice piece of astrogation."

"Yes, it rather was," Nessler said, beaming. "I'm leaving the pilotage to Harpe and her team, though. The largest craft I've piloted was a pinnace, and my deficiencies then didn't encourage me to try my luck with a cruiser."

He chuckled, embarrassed at being so proud of the dead-on positioning he'd achieved as the *Ajax* reentered normal-space. "It may have been luck, my failures cancelling out those of the equipment, of course."

"Stop that, Mr. Nessler!" Mincio said. "You'll find no lack of people to criticize your performance unjustly. You should not be one of them."

Nessler straightened and smiled faintly. "Yes, tutor," he said.

A large warship filled the main optical display. Even Mincio could identify the ominous row of gunports and extrapolate from them to the serious weaponry within the hull. The Melungeon crewmen continued to babble to one another at the clarity of the image even as Beresford shooed them out to make room for another group of sightseers.

"Have they never seen a ship?" Mincio said. Surely they'd at least have seen the *Colonel Arabi* from the lighters that ferried them aboard. . . .

"The software for this screen was misinstalled," Nessler explained with a grin. "It had never worked until Rovald fixed it—in about three minutes. The equipment is actually brand new and very good, though not of quite the most current design."

He cleared his throat and added, "I hope Rovald's having equal fortune with the artifacts. That's really more important, of course. I've made arrangements for our findings to be returned with her in the event . . ."

Mincio nodded to the optical screen. "I gather we're still out of range?" she said.

"Oh, goodness no!" Nessler said. "But we can't attack them within the Air System—that's League sovereign space and would be an act of war against the League."

"But *they* attacked *L'Imperieuse* here!"

"Of course they did." The chill smile Nessler gave

her belied the lazy humor of his tone. "But no one *knows* they did, you see. By now, they have to assume Harpe and all her people are as dead as the rest of *L'Imperieuse*'s crew. They didn't planet on Air, after all, and their pinnace's life support would be long since exhausted. In fact, that's probably why they massacred the survivors in the first place—to keep them from making any embarrassing allegations about violation of League neutrality. I doubt they'll try anything this close to the planet, though. If they do—" he twitched a shrug "—our defenses are all on line."

Beresford guided what appeared to be the last dozen Melungeons off the bridge. "I hope they are, at any rate," Nessler muttered. In a louder voice he said, "Any sign of life from the Peeps, Harpe?"

"Dead as an asteroid, Sir," the grizzled woman replied. "I'll bet they're all asleep. Or drunk."

She looked up from the console. "You know, Captain," she added diffidently, "what with the condition of our ship, nobody'd be surprised if there was a short-circuit in the fire-control system . . .?"

"Carry on, Bosun!" Nessler snapped. "If we're not in the plotted orbit in three minutes, I'll want to know the reason why."

He turned. Softly he went on to Mincio. "They may all be asleep, but we can't expect them to have disabled their automatic defense systems. And absolutely nothing that could happen to us would be worth the risk of bringing the League into this conflict on the Peeps' side."

Beresford sauntered over to them, his duties as tour guide completed. "I was wondering, Sir," he asked. "Why did they name the place Air? Did they come from a planet that didn't have any?"

"It was 'Ehre,' Honor, when the Teutonic Order named it," Mincio explained. "The League has a sub-regional headquarters here, so it's probably a little more lively than Hope. For the same reason there's not much in the way of Alphane remains, though."

"I'll go down and give the League commander notice to order all combatant vessels to leave League sovereign territory within forty-eight T-hours," Nessler said. "That's proper under interstellar law, but heaven only knows what'll actually happen. Between the Dole Fleet and the sort of people the League sends to these parts . . ."

"No," Mincio said. "I'll deliver the notice; I dare say it's my duty as First Officer, isn't it? It'll give me a chance to wear my pretty new uniform."

"Well, if you're sure, Mincio . . ." Nessler said.

"I'll set it out for you in your cabin, Commander," Beresford said with an obsequiousness she'd never before heard from the man who was very clearly *her employer's* servant.

The *Ajax* shuddered as her impeller wedge went down. "Braking into final orbit, Sir," Harpe called loudly.

"Besides," Mincio said. "If the Peeps react the wrong way, the *Ajax* can much better spare my expertise than it can yours, Captain Nessler."

Air's landing field was a little more prepossessing than that of Hope. The vessels sat on cera-macrete hardstands—most of them cracked to little more than gravel, but still better than Hope's dirt—and a solid-looking courtyard building stood on the field's western edge. The town of Dawtry, the planetary capital, lay in the near distance to the north and west. Mincio didn't see any air cars, but there was a respectable amount of motorized transport running on paved—mostly paved—roads.

The pinnace cooled with a chorus of pings, chings, and clanks that might even have been pleasant if Mincio hadn't been so nervous. One of the four Manticoran spacers escorting her muttered, "*That* cutter's Peep, and *that* one's Peep, and I figure that big lighter—"

"Belt up, Dismore!" said Petty Officer Kapp, the detachment's leader. She added with a sniff, "And you notice there's not an anchor watch on any of them? That's Peeps for you. Bone idle."

"Right," said Mincio. "Two of you come with me while the others guard the boat."

She strode toward the truck parked beside a cargo shuttle from an intrasystem freighter. A man in greasy coveralls was working on tubing exposed when a panel was removed from the vessel's stern.

"Excuse me, Sir!" Mincio called. If Kapp hadn't spoken she wouldn't have known to leave anyone with the pinnace. Dismore would probably have told her even if the petty officer had been too polite. "Will you drive us to the League Liaison Office? We'll pay well."

The mechanic turned with a puzzled expression. "Why d'ye want to ride there?" he said. He gestured toward the building adjacent to the field. "You could just about spit that far, couldn't you?"

"Ah," said Mincio. "Thank you."

"I figured the damned thing was Port Control," Dismore muttered, immediately making her feel better. "I guess these hicks don't have anything so advanced as that."

"Right," Mincio said, turning on her heel and striding toward the building with what she hoped was a martial air. Dismore was on one side, Kapp on the other.

The spacers were armed. The guns were hunting weapons found while ransacking the Melungeon officers' compartments, but fortunately hunting on Melungeon involved weapons that would have been military-use-only in most other societies. Certainly no society Mincio found congenial would hunt goat-sized herbivores with heavy-caliber pulse rifles firing explosive projectiles like those which now equipped her escort.

A squad of Protectorate Gendarmes guarded the headquarters entrance. They didn't look alert, but they at least stood up when they saw an armed party approaching.

"Commander Mincio, Royal Manticoran Navy, to see the liaison officer ASAP!" Mincio said in her driest tone. She'd used it only once on Nessler, the time he translated a Latin passage referring to twenty, *viginti*, soldiers as "virgin soldiers."

"I don't have orders to admit anybody to see Flowker," the leader of the gendarmes said. "Maybe we'll mention it to him when we go off shift."

Several of the underlings snickered. Mincio couldn't tell whether the fellow was angling for a bribe or simply being difficult because his own life wasn't what he wanted. A lot of people seemed to feel a need to pass the misery on. Nessler had filled her purse as she embarked in the pinnace. She didn't dare offer a bribe, though, because it would be out of keeping with her claimed authority.

"Listen, slime." Mincio didn't shout, but her voice would have chipped stone. "There's a dreadnought in orbit over you. Every moment you piss away is one less moment Officer Flowker has to make up his mind—and believe me, he's going to know who's responsible for that!"

The guard commander backed a step from what he thought was fury. Mincio would have described her emotion as closer to terror, fear that she'd fail in this crucial juncture and destroy the chances of those depending on her. She'd willingly accept a misunderstanding in her favor.

"Allen, take the Commander to Flowker's suite," the fellow said to one of his underlings, this one female. He glared at the spacers. "These other two stay, *and* they give up those guns."

"Wanna bet, sonny?" Dismore said pleasantly.

Allen led Mincio across the courtyard at a brisk pace. She seemed to want to put as much distance as she could between herself and the two armed groups at the gate. Mincio didn't let herself think about that. Kapp and Dismore were more competent to handle their situation than she was, and she had enough concerns of her own.

The building—another League standard design, presumably—showed Moorish influences in its arches and coffered ceilings. Mincio could see people in offices to either side of the courtyard.

Only half the desks were occupied, and nobody seemed to be doing any work.

There was only one door in the wall facing the outer gateway, and the pointed windows to either side were curtained. Allen opened the door; another gendarme looked up from the chair where she watched a pornographic hologram.

"Sarge says let this one see Flowker," Allen said. "But it's your business now."

She turned and walked away, letting the door slam behind her. The interior guard hooked a thumb toward the portal beside her. "Why should I care?" she said and went back to watching the imagery. One of the participants seemed to be an Old Earth aardvark.

Mincio thought of knocking on the door. It was plastic molded to look—when it was newer, at least—like heavy, iron-bound wood. She discarded the idea and simply shoved her way through.

Five people lounged on cushions in the room beyond. Three were women in filmy harem suits. They were pretty enough in a blowsy sort of way and were most probably locals. The heavy man being fed grapes by one of the women wore a sleeveless undershirt and the khaki trousers of the Protectorate Liaison Service: Officer Flowker by process of elimination.

The wasp-thin woman against the other wall was in a black Gendarmerie uniform with Major's collar insignia; like Flowker, she was barefoot. She jumped up when Mincio appeared but remained tangled in the baggy trousers of the girl who'd been entertaining her.

The third girl was by herself, but the green uniform jacket on the cushion didn't belong to her. A commode flushing in the adjacent room explained where the garment's owner was. The coat sleeves had gold braid, cuff rings with the legend *Rienzi*, and the shoulder flashes of the People's Republic of Haven. As elsewhere in Region Twelve, the Peeps were on very good terms with local League officialdom.

Mincio drew herself up to what she hoped was "Attention." "Sir!" she said. She threw Flowker a salute as crisp as she could make it after fifteen minutes' coaching from Harpe—all there'd been time for.

It was a *terrible* salute, just terrible; her right elbow seemed to be in the wrong place and she couldn't for the life of her remember what her left hand was supposed to be doing. The saving graces were that the present audience might never have seen a Manticoran salute delivered properly, and that they couldn't have been more dumbfounded by the situation if the floor had collapsed beneath them.

"Who the hell are you?" Flowker said. He tried to stand but his legs were crossed; he rose to a half-squat, then flopped down on the cushion again.

"Commander Edith Mincio," Mincio said, shifting her legs to something like "Parade Rest." "First Officer of Her Majesty's Ship *Ajax*, on patrol from our Hope station. I'm here as representative of Captain Sir Hakon—"

A man burst from the commode, one hand holding up the uniform trousers he hadn't managed to close properly.

"—Nessler, Earl of Greatgap."

"What's she doing here!" the Peep demanded, looking first to Flowker and then at the Gendarmerie major. "You didn't tell me there was a Manticoran ship operating on Hope!"

"How the hell would I know, Westervelt?" said the liaison officer peevishly. "Do I look like I know what she's doing here?"

As Flowker struggled to his feet—successfully this time—Mincio said, "Sir, by long-established interstellar law, the armed vessels of belligerent powers are to leave the sovereign territory of neutrals within forty-eight T-hours of notice being given by one party to the conflict. I'm here to deliver that notice to you as the representative of the neutral power."

"This is League territory!" Westervelt said. He was a tall, stooping man; soft rather than fat. His hair was impressively thick, but it didn't match the color of his eyebrows. "You can't order me out of here!"

"Of course not," Mincio agreed. The three girls in harem costumes had moved close together and were watching avidly. They'd unexpectedly become the audience rather than the entertainment. "But Officer Flowker will do so under the provisions of interstellar law, and *Ajax* will most certainly attack your vessel upon the expiry of that deadline whether or not you've obeyed the League authorities."

"Now see here . . ." said Flowker. He bent to grope at the cushion where he'd been sitting. His tunic lay crumpled against the back wall where he couldn't have located it without taking his eyes away from Mincio.

He straightened and continued, "You can't attack the *Rienzi* in League space, and I'm *not* going to order them away. Look, go fight your war—"

"I beg your pardon, Officer Flowker," Mincio said with no more emotion than the blade of a band saw. "If you refuse to give the required notice, Air is no longer neutral territory. If your legal officer can't explain the situation to you, I'm sure your Ministry of Protectorate Affairs will do so in great detail during its investigation."

She drew a chronometer, flat as a playing card, from the outer breast of her tunic. The timepiece was a useful relic of Nessler's naval service, and she entered the present time, then put the chronometer back.

"Good day to you, Officer Flowker," she said, wondering if she ought to salute again.

"We don't need an investigation, Flowker," the Gendarmerie major said, the first time she'd spoken. "If they start looking at the staff payrol . . ."

"Goddammit, what do you expect me to do?" Flowker shouted. "Does this look like it was my idea? I—"

"Look, Flowker—" said Westervelt with a worried expression.

"You get your ship out of here!" Flowker said. Turning his furious glare toward Mincio he went on, "You *both* get your damned ships out of League space! Forty-eight hours, forty-eight minutes—I don't care, I just want you out!"

"I'll report your cooperative attitude to Captain

Nessler, Sir," Mincio said. Deciding not to risk another salute, she turned on her heel and strode from the office.

Westervelt spat at her back. He missed.

On the *Ajax*'s main optical screen a cutter maneuvered to dock with the *Rienzi*; it was the third in the past hour. The image appeared to rotate slowly because the two cruisers were in different orbits. The *Rienzi*'s pinnace edged toward the bottom of the display as it dropped for another load of spacers.

Mincio sighed. "I'd begun to think they were going to ignore the deadline," she said to Kapp. "I wondered what would happen then."

"The Peeps never manage to do anything to schedule," the petty officer said, her eyes scanning ranks of miniature displays. She'd set her console to echo all the bridge screens; the other positions had only a Melungeon on duty. "The Dole Fleet, they're even worse than usual. Thirty hours to do what'd take us twelve, that's about right."

She and Mincio were the only Manticorans on the bridge. The others and most of the Melungeons were readying more anti-missile missiles for use.

At the moment only thirteen countermissiles were fully operable. Since a Peep heavy cruiser could launch more missiles than that in a single broadside, the pragmatic reality was more chilling than superstition could be.

The total stock of countermissiles aboard *Ajax* was fifty-six. Nessler said they might cannibalize enough parts from the junkers to add fifteen or sixteen more to the thirteen. After that, defense was up to the laser clusters. Mincio had already seen the vessel's lasers in operation.

"Well, at least we can make it look like a fight," Kapp said. Somebody reliable had to be on the bridge; Nessler, as Captain, had decided it was her. She'd obviously prefer to be getting her hands dirty in a place she didn't have to watch the hugely superior Peep warship preparing for battle.

"Nessler . . ." Mincio said. "That is, Captain Nessler says we're just going to launch one, ah, missile and run. Launch our pretend missile, that is. And hope the Peeps choose to give us a wide berth in case we might do better the next time."

Kapp snorted. "Right, the next time," she said caustically.

She caught herself with a cough. "That is, I think there's a damned good chance it'll work. It's quite, well, possible. Anyway, it's better than what happened to the cutters, and better than what those bastards'd do to us if they found us on Hope." She gave Mincio a lopsided grin. "Besides, it's our job, ain't it?"

"Yes," said Mincio, "it is."

It was the job of every decent human being to fight evil; people who destroyed lifeboats were evil. It was a simple equation.

Unfortunately, Mincio was too good a historian to believe that evil always lost.

Ajax shuddered in dynamic stasis. The planet rotated beneath while the cruiser's reaction thrusters lifted her nose before her impeller wedge carried her into a higher orbit. The *Rienzi*'s impeller nodes were hot but the Peeps weren't underway yet. The "Manticoran" ship's wedge came up, boosting her clear of the planetary parking patterns at a leisurely two hundred gravities. Hopefully, it looked like the leisure of the totally confident rather than the concession to a less than fully reliable inertial compensator which it actually was.

Behind them, *Rienzi* began to move at last. She climbed away from the planet, following roughly in *Ajax*'s wake, and Mincio licked her lips. By interstellar law, a system's territorial limit extended half a standard light-day from its primary. Technically, then, neither belligerent could attack the other within twelve light-hours of Air's primary . . . but *Rienzi* had already violated that law once, and every sensor *Ajax* boasted watched her carefully as she cracked on a few more gravities of acceleration.

"Hold the roof of the wedge towards her," Nessler said. His voice over the ship's address system sounded cool, almost bored. Mincio watched from her console on the other side of the bridge as his long, aristocratic fingers moved, then glanced at Kapp with a raised eyebrow.

"We're in energy range, Ma'am," the petty officer explained quietly, "but the bastards can't shoot through an impeller band. They want to try ambushing us again, they'll have to use sublight weapons that can maneuver after us."

Mincio nodded thanks and returned her attention to her own display.

"Captain, we're picking up radar and lidar!" Harpe announced sharply. "Looks like their fire control's trying to lock us up."

"In that case, you may launch the decoys, Bosun," Nessler said in the same disinterested tone. He touched another control.

The *Ajax*'s hull twitched minutely, then rang again in a note that syncopated harmonics of the first. "Decoys away!" the Bosun reported from the Combat Information Center.

That armored citadel at the center of the ship was properly the First Officer's station during combat. Harpe was there instead of Mincio because Harpe knew what she was doing. Edith Mincio might as well have been on the ground for all the good she was now.

She could have stayed on Air when the pinnace lifted Kapp and the spacers back to the cruiser. She would have survived that way, but she wasn't sure she could have lived with herself afterward. It didn't matter now.

Twenty-one seconds to the expiration of the deadline. Twenty . . . nineteen . . . eighteen . . .

"Enemy is launching missiles!" reported Petty Officer Bowen, who manned the console nearest Mincio's. His voice was higher than it had been when he showed her how to adjust the scale of her display.

Two, six, eight, fifteen miniature starships, reaching for the *Ajax*'s life with laser heads. . . .

Because the ships were still within easy optical range of one another, the decoys that mimicked the cruiser's electronic signature were of no defensive value: Peep missiles could guide on the visual image of their target. Nessler had kept the *Ajax* close instead of gaining maneuvering room before the deadline as a calculated risk. This way the missiles would be at the start of their acceleration curves and so more vulnerable to *Ajax*'s point defense lasers.

If the lasers worked, that is.

"Engaging with lasers," reported a laconic female voice that Mincio didn't recognize. The buzz of high-energy oscillators added minute notes to the vibration of a cruiser underway with all her systems live. Five missiles, then five more, tore apart or diverged in vectors from the smooth curve they'd been following. Vaporized metal expanded behind the missiles at the point they went ballistic and therefore harmless. Two more disappeared, but they only had to get to within twenty or thirty thousand kilometers and the lasers weren't going to stop them all after all and . . .

Ajax rang with a quick shock as a single bomb-pumped laser smashed at her sidewall. The over-aged, under-maintained Melungeon sidewall generators were no match for the power of a modern laser head, but the angle was bad. The laser smashed through the passive defenses and thread-bare radiation shielding like a battering ram, but it was an ill-aimed ram that somehow missed her hull completely. Simultaneously the remaining Peep missiles failed, one in a low-order explosion instead of mere loss of guidance.

"Bosun, lock them up," Nessler ordered. "Radar and lidar both. I want a lock so hard you can give me a hull map."

"Aye, aye, Sir!"

Despite her own tension, Mincio recognized the

glee in Harpe's reply and darted another glance at Kapp.

"Skipper wants the Bosun to hit 'em hard enough with our fire control to burn out their threat receivers, Ma'am," the petty officer whispered. "Don't know if it'll do any—"

"Number Four battery down!" a voice with a Melungeon accent said. "Five minute, five minute only say Ms. Lewis! We back in five minute!"

"Enemy launching—" said Bowen. His voice changed. "Holy shit! Those are people! They're throwing out bodies!"

"The crew tried to mutiny!" Nessler said, at last sounding excited. "They're throwing out mutineers!"

"Christ, that one's *moving*!" Bowen said. "They're alive!"

Mincio instinctively increased her display's magnification. She blinked at the bodies falling astern as *Rienzi* continued to accelerate away from them. The victims had been alive when they left the airlock without suits. It seemed very unlikely to Mincio that any of them were still alive by the time Bowen spoke. She felt a little nauseous at the thought, but this was war.

The countdown had reached zero without her noticing it. She reduced the magnification so that the drifting corpses were merely specks lost against the immensity of the *Rienzi*'s hull.

"Enemy launching!" Bowen said once more.

"Stand by point def—" Nessler said, professionally calm again.

"They're abandoning ship!" Bowen screamed. "That's their boats! That's not missiles!"

"Do not fire!" Nessler said. "I repeat, do not fire point defense!"

Ajax continued to drive outward. On the optical screen the *Rienzi* lost detail as *Ajax*'s enhancement program segued slowly from sharpening the image to creating it.

"Sir!" called Harpe. "Sir! Those weren't mutineers going out the lock, those were the officers! Those worthless dole-swilling bastards killed their officers when we locked them up rather than fight!"

"Yes," Nessler said. "I rather think they did."

Six smaller craft—pinnaces and cutters—and two great cargo lighters had left the *Rienzi*. As they braked away under reaction thrusters, fighting to clear the safety perimeter of their mother ship's impeller wedge, the cruiser's image started to swell, losing definition. Mincio thought something had gone wrong with her display.

Rienzi brightened into a plasma fireball. A front of stripped atoms swept inexorably across the fleeing light craft, catching them without even the protection of their own impeller wedges, buffeting them from their intended courses for a few moments before the boats' structures and all aboard them dissolved into hellfire.

The bubble of sun-hot destruction continued to expand. Air's upper atmosphere began to fluoresce in response.

"One of the officers survived long enough to scuttle her," Nessler said. He sounded either awestruck or horrified; Mincio wasn't sure of her own emotions, either.

Bowen stood at his console. "Guess our buddies

from the *Imp* have an escort to Hell, now," he said. He gave the optical screen a one-finger salute. "And a bloody good thing it is!"

Hope was a blue-gray jewel in the main optical screen. Because *Ajax* was in clockwise orbit, the planet's apparent rotation was very slow. The survivors of *L'Imperieuse* were drawn up in a double rank across the forward bulkhead.

Nessler handed the Melungeon petty officer her wages in currency—a mixture of League and Melungeon bills, the incidental fruits of the poker game that gained him the use of the cruiser. They exchanged salutes, which in the Melungeon's case meant the eye, ear, and mouth gesture that Mincio still found unsettling.

"That's the last one, Nessler," she said, then to be sure double-checked the database she'd created during the return from Air. The vessel's computers hadn't contained a crew list when the Manticorans took over. Mincio couldn't pretend that she thought anybody would use the records she was leaving behind, but she'd done what she could.

"Very good," Nessler said. To Mincio his smile looked forced. "Well, I suppose . . ."

"Excuse me, Sir," Harpe said. "We'd like to say something. Ah, the crew, that is."

Nessler raised an eyebrow. "Certainly, Bosun," he said. He caught Mincio's eye; she shrugged a reply of equal ignorance.

Harpe bent over the intercom pickup of the command console. "The crew of *L'Imperieuse* would like to thank the crew of the *Colonel Arabi*," she said, her voice booming into every compartment of the ship. "May you someday get officers as good as you deserve."

She straightened and faced the double rank of Manticoran spacers. "Hip-hip—" she cried.

"*Hooray!*"

"Hip-hip—"

"*Hooray!*"

"Hip-hip—"

"*Hooray!*"

From deep in the ship, permeating it, the throats of four hundred Melungeon spacers growled, "*Urrah!*" It was like the sound of the engines themselves.

"Time to board the pinnace, I believe," Nessler said. He'd swallowed twice before he could speak. Mincio blinked quickly, but in the end she had to dab her eyes with the back of her hand.

"I'd almost like to . . ." Nessler continued. "But then, a light cruiser wouldn't be much good to me back on Manticore, and she probably isn't up to the voyage anyway."

"Don't you say that about *Ajax*, Sir!" Dismore said. "She'd make it. She's got a heart, this old bitch has!"

"Dismore—" the bosun snarled in a tone all the more savage for the fact she didn't raise her voice.

"That's all right, Harpe," Nessler said, raising his hand slightly. "Yeoman Dismore is quite correct, you see. I misspoke."

One of the spacers began to whistle "God Save the Queen" as the Manticorans marched off the bridge. By the time they'd reached the pinnace that would take them to the ground they were all singing; every one of them, Edith Mincio included.

Because League officials in this region favored the Peeps, Hope's native population was loudly pro-Manticore. The party filling the streets of Kuepersburg had started before the pinnace touched down. It looked to be good for another six hours at least.

Mincio wasn't good for anything close to that. The only thing on her mind now was bed, but the Singh compound was the center of the festivities. She edged her way with a faint smile past people who wanted to drink her health. *She* hadn't taken an alcohol catalyzer, and anyway she was barely able to stand from fatigue.

Chances were there'd be a couple having a private party in her room. If Beresford was involved, "couple" was probably an understatement. Mincio hoped that by standing in the doorway looking wan, she might be able to speed the celebrants **on** their way.

The door was ajar; a light was on inside and she heard voices. Sighing, Mincio pushed the panel fully open.

The growler moved aside with grave dignity. Rovald jumped up from the bed on which she'd been sitting; deKyper started to rise from the room's only chair though Mincio waved her back quickly.

"Congratulations on your great victory, Ma'am!" Rovald said. The technician spoke with a little more than her normal animation, but there was a tinge of embarrassment in her voice also. "We didn't want to intrude during the celebrations, but we hope you'll have a moment to see what we achieved while you were gone."

She nodded toward the equipment she'd set up on the writing desk. DeKyper was standing despite Mincio's gesture. She squeezed against the bed so that Mincio had a better view. The growler wrapped its tail around its midsection and licked the old woman's hand.

"Yes, of course," Mincio said. Actually, this reminder of her real work had given her a second wind. She'd collapse shortly, perhaps literally collapse, but for the moment she was alert and a scholar again.

Gold probes as thin as spiderweb clamped the sharp-faceted "book" into the test equipment. The crystal was one of Rovald's reconstructed copies, not an original from deKyper's collection. Not only was it complete, its structure was unblemished down to the molecular level where the Alphanes had coded their information. Even apart from gross breakage, real artifacts all had some degree of surface crazing and internal microfractures.

An air-formed hologram quivered above the equipment. It was as fluidly regular as a waterfall and very nearly as beautiful.

"That's Alphane writing, Ma'am," Rovald said. "This is *precisely* the frequency the books were meant to be read at. I'm as sure as I can be."

Mincio bent for a closer look. The crystal was a uniform tawny color, but the projected hologram rippled with all the soft hues of a spring landscape. She could spend her life with the most powerful computers available on Manticore, studying the patterns and publishing weighty monographs on what they meant.

It was the life Mincio had always thought she wanted. She straightened but didn't speak.

"The frequency should be much higher," said deKyper sadly. "I'm sure of it. But it really doesn't matter."

The control pad contained a keyboard and dial switches as well as a multifunction display which for the moment acted as an oscilloscope. She rested her fingers at the edge of it while her free hand caressed the growler's skull. The beast rubbed close to her and rumbled affectionately.

"Ma'am," Rovald said. "I've calculated this frequency, not simply guessed at what it might possibly be. This is the base frequency common to all the books in your collection. When they were complete, that is."

Mincio thought of the tomes she had read in which the scholars of previous generations translated Alphane books to their own satisfaction. She would create her own translations while she taught students about the wonders of Alphane civilization. Later one of her own students might take her place in the comfortable life of Reader in Pre-Human Civilizations, producing other—inevitably different—translations.

Rovald and deKyper faced one another. Neither was angry, but they were as adamantly convinced of one another's error as it was possible for a professional and an amateur to be.

DeKyper sagged suddenly. "It doesn't matter," she repeated. "More Orloffs will come to Hope and will go to the other worlds. In a few generations the Alphanes will be only shards scattered in museums. Everyone but a handful of scholars will forget about the Alphanes, and we'll have lost our chance to understand how a star-traveling civilization vanishes. Until we vanish in turn."

Fireworks popped above Kuepersburg. A dribble of red light showed briefly through the bedroom's window. The hologram in the test rig danced with infinitely greater variety and an equal lack of meaning.

Mincio touched the old woman's hand in sympathy. She knew deKyper was right. Destruction didn't require strangers like Orloff and his ilk. Mincio herself had seen worlds where the growing human population broke up Alphane structures that were in the way of their own building projects. People would blithely destroy the past unless they had solid economic reasons to preserve it.

That would require either political will on the part of the Solarian League—a state which hadn't for centuries been able to zip its collective shoes—or mass tourism fueled by something ordinary humans could understand.

They couldn't understand a pattern of light quivering above a crystal. Edith Mincio could spend her life in study and she wouldn't understand it either, though she might be able to delude herself to the contrary.

"I'm very sorry," she said to deKyper.

"Say!" said Rovald. "Don't—"

The growler touched one of the pad's dials, a vernier control, moving it almost imperceptibly. The beast took its four-fingered hand away.

Instead of a cascade of light in the air above the Alphane book, figures walked: slim, scaly beings wearing ornaments and using tools.

The three humans looked at one another. None of them could speak.

Fireworks popped with dazzling splendor in the sky overhead.

AUTHOR'S NOTE: readers may be amused to learn that both the climax of this story and the archeological methods described therein are closely modeled on real events which took place in the Eastern Mediterranean in 1795.

A Whiff of Grapeshot

S. M. Stirling

The Committee of Public Safety of the People's Republic of Haven rarely met in full session. There were security reasons, for one thing; for another, since the purge of the Parnassian faction, the rivalries had gotten too savage. Two dozen men and women sat stiffly along the long table the new regime had inherited from the old Legislaturalist government. The room had a restrained elegance of dark wood and creamy panelling that spoke of that older era, as well. Say what you liked about the Hereditary Presidency and its elitist flunkies, they'd had good taste. Much good it had done them when the jaws of his trap closed on them.

Well, at least we're not shooting at each other, Chairman Robert Stanton Pierre thought wearily. *Yet.* There were times when he wondered who was worse, the profiteers who swarmed over the State like flies, or Cordelia Ransom and her grim incorruptibles.

Out at Trevor's Star the navies of the People's Republic and the Star Kingdom of Manticore *were* shooting at each other. Men and women were dying by the thousands to buy the Committee more time. By *God*, he was sick of these cretins wasting it!

"Citizens," the Chairman of the Committee of Public Safety said coldly.

That brought silence. He gave a wintry nod. Those rivalries were not helping the war effort of the People's Republic, but they *were* making it less likely that enough of the other Committee members would combine against him . . . and he knew with a leaden certainty that none of his possible replacements would do as well. His eyes slid of their own volition to the head of State Security. Saint-Just's face was calm as always, his appearance so utterly unremarkable that the only thing noticeable about it was its own extreme inconspicuousness. *Oscar could do it.* But State Security had inspired too much hatred along with the fear, not least among the People's Navy. Nobody would accept the head executioner of the purges as head of state. More, the first move of any new head of the Committee would be to purge Security, which meant that Security had no choice but to keep supporting him.

And Oscar knows better. We've been in this together too long. The paranoia was getting to him. Oscar Saint-Just was as reliable a friend as he had on the Committee.

I hope, he thought. *When you're riding the tiger, you can't dismount.* He had no choice but to bring himself and Haven through and out the other side of the crisis. Cordelia Ransom smiled back at him and nodded. *And I need her too.* Ransom was the one who'd built up the Committee's propaganda machine, who'd lashed the Dolists out of their apathy. She'd overseen the public carnival of blood as they fed the Legislaturalists and their families to the People's Courts, and then convinced the masses that the Star Kingdom of Manticore was their deadly enemy.

It was blind, it was stupid—it was beyond stupidity, it was self-contradictory—and it tied his hands completely. His power was unassailable, but only as long as he took the great billion-headed beast in the direction it wanted to go. *And she has helped me mobilize the Dolists.* The vast parasitic horde that had dragged the old regime down with their incessant demands for more and more of the BLS—Basic Living Supplement—were thronging into the People's Navy and Marines, into the shipyards and war-factories. Giving up their bread and circuses. Begging, *demanding* to work, willing to really learn, which was something the People's Republic hadn't been able to get them to do in what passed for an educational system in generations. The sheer power of it was exhilarating and terrifying all at once; it was the only force he could imagine destroying the huge mass of social inertia that had been dragging down his nation all his life. If only they could win the war . . .

Then they could relax, then he could do something *positive* with the power he'd bought at the cost of so much of his self and the capacity to sleep without hauntings. Yet if he hesitated for an instant, it would all come down on him. Ransom's True Believers were waiting, and behind them factions whose fanaticism was so grotesque it chilled even the golden-haired Cordelia. LaBoeuf and his Conspiracy of Equals, for instance, the Levelers.

We've woken the Beast, he thought. *Well enough,*

as long as we can ride it. But what if it begins to think as well?

"We're here," he went on bluntly, "to consider a major change in our overall policy. As you know, we've reinvigorated our armed forces with a policy of meritocratic egalitarianism."

Meaning we killed everyone we thought wasn't reliable and everyone who showed any sign of incompetence.

"But we've reached a point of diminishing returns with the . . . austere policy instituted immediately after the Coup."

Meaning we've got a young, energetic, competent, utterly terrified officer corps. And the latter is beginning to outweigh the benefits of the former.

The departed Legislaturalist scions who'd run the Navy before hadn't been any loss. It was time for the Committee and its political officers to remember that the new breed owed everything to the new regime. For that matter, the professionals and conscripts who'd provided the rank-and-file of the old regime's navy were being diluted by the tidal wave of revolutionary volunteers pouring out of accelerated training courses.

"We *have* to alter—" he began, then looked up in astonishment as a door burst open.

"Sir!" the Committee Security Force officer said. "Sir, we've got an emergency."

Citizen Admiral Esther McQueen didn't particularly like the Committee of Public Safety. Not that it hadn't done her a good turn or two; it had swept the Legislaturalists out of her way, and without a patron she'd never have risen far in the Navy of the People's Republic under the *ancien regime*. Killing all the Legislaturalist ruling families, and shooting everyone else who didn't give a convincing imitation of loyalty, *and* anyone who lost a battle to the Manties, had created very rapid promotion for the survivors.

The problem was that most of the Committee, as far as she could see, were pig-ignorant about naval affairs, which was bad enough, and absolutely unwilling to *admit* that they were ignorant, even to themselves. That was potentially deadly. Not to mention their habit of shooting anyone who lost, anyone related to anyone who lost, anyone who was a friend of anyone who lost, and all *their* relatives as well. That sort of thing could get alarming, and it certainly didn't encourage a bold, daring command style. The Committee evidently thought you could win victories without taking any risks.

She looked across the waiting room at her Citizen Commissioner—translated, political watch-beast—Erasmus Fontein. He was waiting patiently himself, looking out the hundred-and-fifth floor window over the towerscape of the People's Republic of Haven's capital city. Nouveau Paris had a certain tattered beauty still, even after generations of decay under the Legislaturalists' grotesque economic policies and the strain of the long war with Manticore. From this height all you could see was the grandeur of her towers. Not the empty windows and broken lights, not the curdled rage and suspicion, the terror of the mass arrests and the cold fear of midnight disappearances. Or the worse nightmare of the People's Courts and mob vengeance that outdid even the old gangs. Worst of all were the ones who came back from "Re-Socialization Centers." Very quiet people who talked seldom and worked like machines. Usually they had no teeth.

Well, I'm fairly *sure they aren't going to shoot* me, *at least*. They'd gotten her out of that debacle at the front ahead of time, at least. Although you never knew . . . and that left the question of why they'd parked her here in this out-of-the-way tower full of bureaucrats. It made her invisible; if there was one thing that Haven was well-equipped with, it was towers full of data-shufflers. *Our sensor equipment isn't all that great, the Manties have better inertial compensators, but when it comes to producing bureaucrats, we're cutting edge. Bah, humbug, bullshit.*

Fontein had been dropping cryptic hints and half-statements about an "important interview," possibly with the Chairman himself. It was about time to cut to the chase. She opened her mouth to speak. A quiver in the fabric of the huge building beneath her halted the words.

Fontein looked around; he was a mild-faced man, and most of the time he looked like a complete fool, albeit one whose position made him dangerous. Right now his face was liquid with shock, and the intelligence in his eyes startled her.

"What is it?" she said. "Earthquake?"

Another quiver shook the tower, stronger this time. McQueen pushed past the Commissioner and looked out herself. The bright actinic flash made her whip her head aside in reflex and throw up a hand, then blink back tears of pain as afterimages chased themselves across her retinas. Nobody needed to tell a veteran of space combat what that blink of light in the night sky had been. *Nuke*, she thought. *Fairly big one.* A warhead burst, not the type that pumped X-ray lasers for ship-to-ship combat.

The thought came from some insanely logical, dispassionate part of her mind. The rest of it was gibbering. Haven itself *couldn't* be under attack—

"The Manties," she said. "They could have decided to go for broke . . . throw everything through at us . . ."

Their eyes met in mutual appalled horror. The staff studies of the People's Navy said the risk was far too high for any sane commander to take. But White Haven, the Royal Manticoran Navy commander, had been taking a *lot* of chances lately.

Their shoulders bumped against each other as they dove for the waiting room's communications terminal. McQueen ruthlessly shouldered the older Havenite aside as her fingers danced on the keys. She ignored the public news channels; they wouldn't know anything, and they wouldn't be allowed to say it if they *did* know. There was a surreal quality to watching bits and pieces of *news* about aquaculture, the glories of the New Republic, and happy Dolists taking accelerated learning courses—at least that was more or less true, they were finally getting substantial numbers of the idle Prole bastards to volunteer to do something useful, namely enlist for the war effort. More light blinked in through the window, and static cut through the reports. *EMP is getting to the relays.* Quite a lot of it, if it was getting past the digital noise filters. She cut through to the Naval emergency channels.

"Uh-oh," she said quietly.

"Uh-oh?" the Commissioner repeated.

"Logic bomb," McQueen said. "Look." She extended the screen and pivoted it. "Hash. Rerouting, cross-connections, garbled text, crossed order-response loops, spontaneous memory core dumps . . . *Nothing* working the way it should."

"Impossi—" Fontein began.

They looked at each other again. Every military service in the human-settled galaxy depended on information systems; every service had unbreakable protection against logic bombs from the outside. Every ship had an emergency response, too; cut all connections to the net to guard against infiltration if the system was compromised.

Which meant someone had done it from the *inside*, and that they'd effectively cut the Home Fleet into so many isolated units for as long as it took to bring the system back up. Hours, at least, and a good deal could happen in a couple of hours. Any commander would hesitate to act without orders or hard data. Particularly in the People's Navy, where exercising independent initiative without orders tended to get you stood up against the nearest convenient wall.

"Citizen Commissioner," McQueen said slowly. "I think you'd better try the Security Service net. And find out what the hell is happening."

"This is the best I can do, Citizen Admiral," Erasmus Fontein said, fifteen minutes later.

He was acutely conscious of the sweat running down under the collar of his uniform. In a man so precisely controlled, one who'd spent decades perfecting the art of emitting no signal of voice or body except those intended, it was humiliating.

"My clearance is being recognized," he said at last. "But that's triggering some subroutine that shunts my calls—some sort of viral AI parasite living in whatever open memory it can find. Whoever did this is damned clever, it's like having hostile ghosts loose in the machine."

"Can you get *anything*?"

"I've got a one-way bleed on the Security net. The contacts last about six to twelve seconds, and then the AI kicks me out. Take a look."

McQueen did. The first was a helmet pickup, showing ground level. The Admiral blinked; she'd never seen that many people all at once. Dolists, from their shabby-colorful clothes. They carried signs—*Purge the Traitors* and *Victory to the People*, liberally sprinkled with *Equality Forever, Equality Now*—but what bothered her was the sound they were making. It was nothing like a chant; more like a storm she'd seen once, on another planet. One where long slow waves crashed into a cliff in endless gray ranks, and made the solid rock vibrate beneath her feet. The sound of the crowd was like that, but it was alive. And it hated. The Committee had set out to prod the Dolists out of their apathy into revolutionary fervor, and it had succeeded. Succeeded all too well.

"Fire," she said. "Come on, whoever's in charge, give the order to—"

The helmet camera did a quick glance right and left. A long line of Public Order Police stood there, two deep, armed with riot shields and clubs; a slab-sided vehicle floated behind them, its dorsal turret loaded with soundbombs and stickgel.

"Citizen Admiral, the police can't use deadly force without political authorization. And right now, that detachment can't get authoriz—"

The crowd surged forward, throwing a surf-wave of bottles and rocks before it. McQueen had stood on her bridge without undue difficulty in engagements where tens of thousands died . . . and a flagship was *not* invulnerable to weapons that could turn it into a ball of expanding plasma. The thousands of snarling faces racing towards the pickup still made her draw back in the seat, the way the sudden appearance of a lion might. It spoke to instincts far older than spaceflight—older than fire or chipped flint.

Just before the screen blanked the pickup slammed forward to the ground. She could see boots going by, and the helmet juddered as the crowd stampeded across it. *And across,* she realized, *the body wearing the equipment.*

The screen blanked and then jumped. Another helmet pickup, but this time the scene was a little more familiar; a tac display table, but the groundside model. It carried a holo-schematic of the city, but the information markers were mostly amber blinking lights, signifying "no data."

"Citizen Lieutenant," a voice said testily—the voice of the person wearing the helmet.

"Citizen Captain!"

The lieutenant was wearing chameleon fatigues and the torso portion of a set of infantry armor. The branch-of-service flashes on her collar were red-on-black, and only State Security used that *waffenfarbe*.

Intervention Battalion, McQueen thought. State Security goon squads, but heavily armed.

"Citizen Lieutenant, *something* is going on, but we're getting no intelligence at all. Take a floater, get out there, and *eyeball* the situation. Then report directly to me. Understood?"

"Yes, Citizen Captain!"

The lieutenant put on her helmet, face vanishing behind the facemask, and trotted towards a vehicle park on the outer rim of the tower-top. Then a voice screamed: "Incoming! *Incoming!*"

McQueen saw figures around the tac display table begin to dive for cover, and the pickup went black with a finality that was different from the system switch she'd seen before. A few seconds later, like an echo, a distant drawn-out *booooommm* came through the window.

"That's enough," she said crisply to the Commissioner. "We're not going to do anything useful here. There's obviously some sort of attack on the government."

The Committee's watchdog nodded. "Exactly. But we don't have any more information than—" he twitched his hand towards the screen, which showed a bored Security officer sitting sipping coffee before a bank of screens "— they do."

McQueen met Fontein's eyes. "In your professional estimation, Citizen Commissioner, what the hell is going on?"

Fontein was silent for a long moment. Then his face moved slightly, as if he was biting into a bitter fruit. *Deciding he has to tell the truth,* McQueen thought. That would be unpleasant.

"Citizen Admiral, I think it's an attempt to overthrow the government, through a coup disguised with a popular uprising. As to who . . ." he hesitated again. "I can't say. I'd *guess* it was LaBoeuf's Levelers. Total crazies, a breakaway faction of the CRP, but they have a small core of very smart people in their inner cadre."

"Pity the Committee hasn't shot *them*," McQueen answered.

"Perhaps, although they were useful against the Parnassians. In the meantime, we still have no information at all."

"No, Citizen Commissioner, we don't," McQueen answered. "But let's say I made previous arrangements for things that couldn't be handled through channels. Citizen Sergeant Launders! Execute Tango Three-Niner!"

Fontein's face went pale as the door burst open and a dozen Marines in full battle armor showed beyond it. Every one of them had a pulse rifle or energy weapon deployed . . . and every one of them was pointing it right at him.

Their eyes met again. *Right, watchbeast. I wasn't going to go quietly if getting me dirt-side was a maneuver to arrest me.* State Security had already learned that trying to arrest an admiral on the bridge of her flagship wasn't the most economical way to go about things.

"Citizen Admiral?" the noncom said politely.

"We're getting out of here, and now," she said. "Move it."

"Neufer," the sergeant said.

One of his squad raised a weapon. McQueen and Fontein both turned and shielded their eyes automatically. The light still shone through their hands, leaving the finger-bones in stark relief for an instant, just before the heat and pressure struck their backs like huge warm pillows.

They turned, blinking, and a pinnace was hovering outside the window. "Well, I knew you don't believe in half-measures," Fontein murmured.

"Let's go," she said. Two Marines gripped her by the arms, and another pair took Fontein; their powered armor and thrusters took them from shattered window to open hatch in a precise, mathematical curve.

"Citizen Ensign," McQueen was saying even before her feet touched the decking. "Take us out of here on a spiral over the city. Full scanners."

"Citizen Admiral, that's—"

"—highly illegal, do it nonetheless," McQueen said dryly.

The ensign's face was sweating as his hands moved over the control board. "Yes, *Ma'am!*"

Better watch that. Sir and Ma'am are counter-revolutionary, she thought dryly. "Do you have a secure line to the *Rousseau?*" she said.

"Yes, Ma—Citizen Admiral."

"Good. Full data-dump, and I want the staff on hand in my ready room as soon as we dock. Move it, and don't be shy about breaking windows. Visual feed to this screen."

She was conscious of Fontein's silent presence at her elbow as the pinnace rose with a howl of cloven air. Only a slight vibration and the tug of acceleration told of the wild corkscrewing path the craft was following, or of the dozens of near-collisions it left in its wake. *Of course, with a fleet to pick from, I was rather careful about who flew my own personal pinnace.*

"Sir," she said to Fontein—you *were* allowed to call a Commissioner by honorifics. "If we're going to pull through this, I'm going to need your *full* cooperation. Do I have it?"

"Citizen Admiral, you do," Fontein said quietly, looking at the screen.

"Here's the picture," McQueen told her staff.

A quick glance at the readout in the corner of the big display tank told her that it was an incredible mere half-hour since she'd felt that telltale quiver in the soles of her feet. Time enough for the world to turn upside down again, certainly. The men and women around her inched forward instinctively. The superdreadnaught *Rousseau* had been intended as a fleet flagship, and there was plenty of room—far too much, with the skeletal cadre she'd brought back with her, and their losses at Trevor's Star. A faint smell of ozone still hung in the air, underlain with scorched synthetics and despite all the cleanup crews had done, a slight smell of rotting blood. Only the shipyard would get that out.

"The Home Fleet and Nouveau Paris military and Security com nets are down for the foreseeable future—hours, at least, and that's all that's needed."

She gestured towards the tank. It had been designed to show ship dispositions together with coded schematics. The projection of the city below them was almost eerie in its detail. The ship's scanners were picking up enough tactical information to show raw numbers and weapons-types with some accuracy. At least there hadn't been any more mininukes, not after the first salvo.

"As you can see, there's considerable fighting going on down there. Nothing in space yet, thank God, but at a guess I'd say that the compromised com system was used to disinform the various police and Security forces to the point where many of them are fighting *each other*, under the impression that the next man over is part of the insurrection. At the same time, very large numbers of—" she stopped herself just short of saying "Proles" "— popular elements are in the streets. Initially that was directed by partisans of the coup leaders, but it spread, and right now there may be a *million* rioters out there, killing and looting under the general impression they're defending the Revolution. Those Security forces that aren't distracted by false messages *are* spending most of their efforts trying to keep the mob out of the governmental towers."

"Oh, beautiful," her flag captain said. A relatively junior officer spoke: "Citizen Admiral . . . there's the entire Capital Fleet in orbit here, several Marine brigades in transit, hell, there's the equivalent of a division in the Marine parties on ships alone. What's stopping them putting this lunacy down?"

McQueen cleared her throat and looked at

Commissioner Fontein. He nodded bleakly. *We've shot everyone in the Navy who even looked like they might intervene in politics.* The whole revolt against the Legislaturalists had started with an action that made the Navy appear to be launching a coup.

"Due to . . . various circumstances . . ." Fontein began. "It is unlikely that any of the Capital Fleet's captains or higher officers will undertake any *immediate* action." The Capital Fleet had been purged with more than usual severity; after all, they were closest to the Committee. "At least not for some time. The conspirators are undoubtedly counting on this. They must plan to complete their actions before any counterattack can be organized."

"As you're all aware, Citizens," McQueen said neutrally, "there are advantages and disadvantages to an extremely centralized decision-making structure."

And right now, one of the disadvantages has reared its ugly head and bitten the Committee of Public Safety on its sorry ass, she thought.

The same logic train was running through every face looking at her. The *Rousseau* might very well be the only remotely independent actor in a position to save the present Committee.

Which left only one question: should they? She could feel the *let them swing* pouring out from better than half the officers present, and that didn't count the ones skillful enough to keep their faces completely blank. McQueen looked up at Fontein's face, and watched it go pale as he realized that all she had to do was wait. McQueen was far too self-controlled to smile; she wouldn't have lived this long if she wasn't. It wasn't necessary, anyway.

"In fact, due to coincidence, I am probably the only ranking officer who has a real idea of what's happening. Now, I will say nothing critical of the Committee." Heads nodded unconsciously; only a complete idiot would do *that*. "Let me put it hypothetically, then; even someone who *didn't* approve of the Committee's heroic efforts to save the People's Republic would be wise to come to its aid at this juncture, on the basis of the old principle that one should always consider the alternative. Citizen Commissioner, perhaps you could fill us in on the background of LaBoeuf's Levelers."

Fontein did. The calm control of his voice and the dispassionate terms he used made the description all the more effective. The fall of the Legislaturalists had taken the cork out of the bottle, and some extremely odd ideological scum had floated to the surface. McQueen nodded thanks when he finished, noting the looks of horror on the faces of the officers around the plotting tank. What LaBoeuf had in mind for the People's Republic made Rob S. Pierre look like a humanitarian.

"It's certainly true that we have no orders," she began. "Just as an exercise, however, let's consider—"

Rob S. Pierre, Chairman of the Committee of Public Safety, looked down the table. In theory, and until about forty-five minutes ago in practice, the men and women sitting here had power of life and death over every single individual in the People's Republic. The Republic's power extended over hundreds of light-years and scores of planets, scores of billions of human beings.

"But right now, we hold this building and not much else," he said. "We don't even know *who* is attacking us. The only thing we know is that they're winning."

Some of the people sitting at the table jerked as if he'd pressed a button and sent a shock charge through their chairs. *There are times . . .* he thought bitterly. Even under the airscrubbers you could . . . not quite smell . . . sense the anger and the fear. Then: *Back to present business.*

"I retract that statement. We also know that they've penetrated our ranks, because otherwise this wouldn't have occurred just when I'd called a plenary emergency meeting. You realize, Citizens, that our entire leadership cadre, *and their staffs,* are in this building right now? That that circumstance hasn't happened more than once in the last year and a half?"

Some of them evidently hadn't; the temperature in the long bare room seemed to drop another degree or two, and the glances they'd been sneaking at each other went from furtive speculation to glares. He turned to the nervous-looking technical officer Security had brought in to explain things. The man was standing at a stiff brace, looking as if he was willing his vital functions to stop.

I'm beginning to thing we've reached the limits of what can be accomplished with terror, he thought with a detached corner of his mind, the part that wasn't concerned with his own probable death in the next hour or two.

"Report, please, Citizen Major," he said.

"Citizen Chairman, we will have the net available

again—the high-priority sections—in not more than two hours forty-five minutes. Possibly as little as two hours, but I couldn't guarantee that."

Somebody broke in: "Not good eno—"

"Silence!" Pierre shouted, and slapped his hand down on the table. The gunshot crack cut through the rising babble. "Panic will not help!" He turned to the officer. "Please do the best you can, Citizen Major. The Republic's future is in your hands."

And in the hands of the uncoordinated efforts of four separate and distinct guard forces, two of which are fighting each other, he thought.

They'd taken very careful precautions against all the armed forces close to the Committee. The problem seemed to be that the precautions had destroyed most of the ability of those forces to deal with anyone except each other.

At this moment, Rob S. Pierre wished very much that he believed in God. Because right now, there didn't appear to be anyone else he could get in touch with.

"Citizen Admiral," the Marine brigadier said. "There are four problems—four interlocking problems here."

Citizen Brigadier Gerrard Conflans was short but trim and broad in the shoulders, with long-fingered hands that gave an impression of strangler's strength. His face was set now, but you could see smile-marks at the corners of his eyes, and he had an unusual and flamboyant mustache.

His cursor moved over the streets of the city. "First, there are the mobs. Many of them are armed, and there are simply so many of them attacking so many targets that they make any movement impossible.

"Second, there are the Presidential, Capital, Committee and State Security forces. Many of them are actively engaged against each other, and all of them are out of effective communications with the Committee, unless someone's sending runners with hardcopy messages. They're unlikely to believe that a naval force appearing suddenly and without warning is anything but another threat.

"Third, there're the actual conspirators, and *they've* overrun the last Security Intervention units blocking them from attacking Committee HQ.

"Fourth and most serious, while the other units of the Capital Fleet don't know what the hell's going on and are apparently sitting this out, they'll certainly know *we're* doing something and may not believe us when we say that we're acting to protect the Committee. It'll certainly *look* like we're involved in whatever's going on down there. And they certainly have standing orders to prevent any People's Navy unit from undertaking offensive action against Nouveau Paris!"

McQueen nodded. The other officers and the Commissioner were utterly silent, their eyes fixed on her like so many laser links, scanning for information. The destiny of Haven balanced on a sword's edge.

"Thank you for that accurate summation, Citizen Brigadier," she said. "I will remark again that the insurrection seems to have been started by LaBoeuf's Levelers, and that they make Cordelia Ransom look like a benign moderate. As Citizen Brigadier Conflans has outlined, frustrating their attack presents us with multiple problems. I believe, however, that we can kill a number of birds with one stone here."

"Citizen Captain Norton," she said. The commander of *Rousseau* came to attention. "I want you to take this ship down. As far down as you safely can, in a stable circuit over the capital. That may—should—make anyone else hesitate about firing on us. Because anything that misses will go straight down into the built-up area."

There were a few winces. A fifty-megaton explosion in space was no great matter, unless it happened to be near the pinprick dot of a ship. A fifty-megatonner going off on a planetary surface didn't bear thinking about, and an X-ray warhead would be like driving the red-hot poker of God into the surface over and over again.

"You will also," she went on, "rig for planetary bombardment—kinetic energy strikes."

"Within the city limits, Citizen Admiral?"

"That's where the potential targets are. You will of course commence strikes only on my explicit order." Her voice had the mechanical precision of an industrial forging hammer as it went on: "Citizen Brigadier, you will prepare to embark the *Rousseau*'s full complement of Marines in everything that will get to the surface. You are tasked with securing the perimeter of Committee HQ and holding it against all comers."

"Citizen Admiral," he said quietly. "As I said, there are over a *million* rioters attacking the Government district."

"That will also be taken care of," McQueen said, her face like something carved from crystal. She looked up at Fontein. "I assume that you will authorize all necessary measures, Sir?"

The silence stretched. "All necessary measures, Citizen Admiral," Fontein said. "Any and all measures necessary are hereby authorized in advance at your discretion. I will so record it."

"Excellent," McQueen said. "Most excellent, Sir." She turned to her staff. "This is now a purely military operation."

"Ah . . . Citizen Admiral," the Marine officer said. "With a million citizens in the streets, how can the situation be considered purely military?"

McQueen's face showed expression for the first time in the meeting. The gesture that drew her lips back over her teeth was not in the least like a smile.

"Don't think of it as millions of citizens, Citizen Brigadier Conflans," she said. "Think of it as having a very, very large target selection." She met his eyes. "This is essential to the future of the People's Republic. Am I understood?"

He nodded, and her eyes went back to the display. *And when it's over, a good many of the imbeciles who've kept Haven from having a rational domestic policy will be . . . no longer a factor in the equation.*

"Citizen Captain Norton, in the event of any People's Navy unit firing on you, you will respond vigorously in such manner as to best defend this vessel. I will personally command this operation from a forward HQ on one of the pinnaces. Now let's get cracking on the planning side, because we have about ten minutes to do it."

The HQ building's internal net was still functioning. Rob S. Pierre watched the display monitor on the wall with a show of clinical detachment as a massive armored door blew a hundred and fifty stories below them. The muted roar over the sound membranes came a perceptible instant sooner than the feeling beneath his feet.

"Why don't they just blow the building?" Cordelia Ransom asked.

"Decapitation," the Chairman said absently. "If someone else is sitting here and giving orders when the system comes back up—particularly if they have a familiar face or two—"

Nobody looked much more guilty than anyone else. *Pity*. But then, everyone at this level had first-rate acting ability.

"— nearly everyone will go right on obeying orders on sheer reflex. If there's nothing but a large glowing hole in the ground, the admirals will fight it out with each other for who gets to pick the bones. You know, we've got to do something about all this, presuming we survive the next couple of hours."

The glow died down on the pickup. Plasma bolts were coming through the door, and figures in body armor. Pulser darts tore into them, turning the entrance into a mist of blood and body parts. Then something flashed through and there was a blaze of white light and the pickup went dead. When the screen came back on, it showed Chairman's Guards piling up office furniture in an undamaged corridor further up from the sub-basement. A harassed-looking officer turned for an instant as the pickup indicated somebody with a command override was taking the transmission.

"They're loaded for bear, Sir," she said. *Must think it's her CO,* Pierre realized. "And there's a lot of them. We can't get out to ground level to cut them off because of the crowds. But we'll make them pay for every foot they take as long as we've got anyone standing."

Pierre felt himself nodding, and an uncomfortable tightness in his chest. They were selling their lives to buy *him* time.

"You know," he said aloud—the unit wouldn't carry anything back— "I don't think we could have gotten this sort of performance from the Guard by holding their families hostage, even if they *are* an elitist remnant of the old regime. And equipped only with light personal weapons."

Various expressions rippled across the knots of Committee members scattered through the room. He saw with a faint nausea that they were still divided into the usual factional clusters. How relevant those would be when the attackers burst into the room and started shooting them down was moot. Of course, if they waited long enough to put on show trials, at least half the Committee would be clamoring to switch sides.

I wanted to help *Haven, make it great again,* he whispered in the back of his mind. *I had to act, the Legislaturalists were riding us right down the river of entropy in a ship with engines dead. I had to do it.*

That was the problem. Every single step had seemed inevitable and inescapable all along the way. And it had brought them to this.

"Let 'em have it!" the officer on the other end of the pickup said. "Let 'em—"

Pulser rifles snarled. A plasma gun answered them, and droplets of burning metal and plastic scattered backward. A man rolled past the pickup's lens, beating at the molten stuff that coated his legs. Another rose to fire over the burning barricade and toppled backward with his helmet and brains splashing away from his headless trunk. Pierre forced back the hand that would have turned off the input. He *deserved* to have to watch this. They all did, but he suspected that most of his dear friends and associates would never know why.

"This is going to require careful coordination," McQueen said, in the pinnace's co-pilot seat.

The figures in the screens nodded at her. She smiled at them; it was rare, unexpected, and had just the effect she was looking for.

"Actually, it's going to require a fucking miracle, but we're going to do it anyway, people. Now let's go."

The pinnace rolled and dived. The huge white-and-blue shield of the planet grew before her, swelling with alarming speed. The pinnace had been made for high-speed atmosphere transits, and the scanners compensated for the growing ball of incandescent air around it. Her mouth quirked. One side-benefit of the confusion the Leveler coup attempt had created was that Traffic Control was completely screwed up, along with the ground-based point defense systems.

"Orbital Fortresses *Liberty* and *Equality* are signalling." That was a relayed voice from *Rousseau*. "Citizen Captain, they demand we vacate prohibited space immediately."

Norton's voice came through, harsh and authoritative. "Record. *Rousseau* is acting in aid to the civil power, under the direct instructions of the Committee. Any interference in her mission will be treated as treason to the People's Republic. End."

"Wait," McQueen said over the relay. *Good man,* she thought. Not imaginative, but extremely solid. "Sir, would you please sign off on that for the transmission as well, as Citizen Captain Norton's Commissioner?" Fontein nodded and added his voice.

He'd insisted on coming down with her. He hadn't asked aloud, but . . . she leaned towards him. "Because *I'm* going to be the one who handled this situation," she said softly. "Not commanded it from orbit, not ordered it done, but the one who *did* it."

Fontein nodded. That would also make her the one who'd saved the Committee . . . if, that was, she intended to save the Committee and not complete its execution, possibly as a "mistake" in the strike that took out the Levelers. He knew her people would follow her *whatever* decision she made.

"Speed down to Mach Seven and dropping," the pilot reported. "Nothing so—acquisition! We're being painted!"

McQueen nodded to herself as the shock cages clamped around them and the world outside spun with crazed, chaotic viciousness. Something whined past, dark and solid for a fleeting instant. *Close enough to see it, by God,* she thought. That meant really inspired piloting. The pinnace juddered in its path as a warhead blew up behind them, and static hashed an electromagnetic pickup.

"Maniacs," she said softly. They were using nuke warheads within the atmosphere. Not total fools, though. They hadn't put all their faith in the logic bomb to keep the Navy from intervening while their coup went on.

Rob S. Pierre kept his eyes on the wall display, hands kneading at the gray streaks over his temples. Everyone else was looking now too, and the fighting was close enough that the building shuddered continuously with the outrages being done to its structural members. Anguish shouted from the speakers: *"Don't, George, don't!"*

The pickup showed a wounded man slumped back against a ceramacrete-armored door. He looked up, his face knotted into a rictus, and worked doggedly at the hose connector that lay across his lap. A fumbling grip undid it at last, and the man's head slumped back in exhaustion against the metal. His tongue licked lips gone paper-dry with the thirst that blood-loss brings, but his eyes opened again as cautious steps sounded in the corridor outside. The battered, scorched furniture had been luxurious once, and the floor was covered in a pile of deep sea-green carpet. It sopped up the rather thick liquid that gouted out of the armored cable, leaving it an inconspicuous spreading stain rather than the slippery mass it would have been on bare pavement or metal.

Body-armored figures swarmed forward down the corridor, groups forming fire-parties and then leap-frogging forward. Pulser rifles whined as they "checked" the rooms to either side with fire, and an occasional grenade blasted fragments and dust out into the corridor itself. The view narrowed as the man leaning against the door let his head droop; all they could see then was the circle of sopping carpet, and the dead bodies scattered across it, insurrectionist and Chairman's Guard.

"We need the access code, traitor," a voice said, cold with hate.

The man looked up again, seeing his own bloody face reflected in the visor-shield of the enemy standing over him. Boots kicked away weapons.

"Don't, George! Don't do it!" Evidently the attackers could hear that clearly too, and they looked up and around. The one with the visored helmet laughed.

"Don't be brave, George—be smart." He ground his foot down on the prone man's shattered leg, bringing a convulsive moan of agony. "The access code! Give it to us, *now!*"

"I'll . . . give . . ." the man wheezed.

The visored face nodded, bent to hear. At that range Pierre could see through the visor, see the flicker of horror as the wounded man's fingers dropped the lighter to the carpet and he realized what was about to happen.

"Don't George, don't—it's useless, don't—"

An instant's searing flame showed through the

pickup, and then the rippling bubble of melted plastic. A long hollow *boooomm* sounded through the fabric of the building, echoing up through ventilators and elevator shafts. Two dozen pairs of eyes swivelled to the exterior view, and halfway up the tower they saw windows punched out in an echoing bellow of flame.

Saint-Just was busy at his console. "That was part of the automated defenses," he said, in his colorless bureaucrat's voice. "Inoperable. George Henderson led a party back down through the shafts to enemy-held floors to try and activate it manually." The pale, passionless eyes rose for a second. "He succeeded."

"How long until we have the systems back?"

"One hour forty-five minutes," the head of Security said. "Captain Henderson has bought us some time; besides their casualties, they'll have to wait for that level to cool, or bring in firefighting equipment. On the other hand, we've also suffered very severe losses. It's going to be a tossup."

Not for the first or last time that day, Rob S. Pierre wished that he could pray.

Liberty and *Equality* massed fourteen million tons each, more than twice the weight of a superdreadnaught like the *Rousseau*, and they were armored and armed to match. Ordinarily a close-range engagement would crush the ship like a food pack under a power-armor boot. Their problem was that they couldn't approach the planetary surface as closely as a mobile ship. Everything they could throw towards *Rousseau* would also be thrown towards the planetary surface where their families lived. Even fanatics would hesitate at that prospect.

"Hesitate, but not forever," Captain Robert Norton muttered to himself, leaning back in the command chair. Aloud: "Hold station."

"Citizen Captain." His Tac officer spoke, and Norton glanced at the appropriate repeater.

Goddammit, Citizen ThisandthatRank not only sounds ridiculous, it's cumbersome when you're in a hurry, some distant part of his mind fumed. Probably the irritation was comforting because it was so familiar. Few of the officers who'd served before the Revolution were comfortable with the new titles.

"They're launching their LACs," he said, watching the display's schematics indicate small vessels swarming out of the fortresses' holds. "Logical."

Light Attack Craft were designed for close-in point defense. They had no armor to speak of, no sidewalls, and only a single light energy gun and strap-on pods of single-shot missiles. Putting them up against a superdreadnaught was like sending ants against an elephant. But ants could sting, and enough of them . . . and he was a stationary target, too.

"Launch," he said. "Let's try and close up the net."

The huge ship shuddered as her broadside batteries went to salvo, and scores of heavy missiles streaked across the screens. Engagement ranges were insanely close; the forts would have cut him into drifting wreckage if they'd dared use their laser and graser batteries, but *Rousseau* was shooting *up*. They might still blast him, if they were desperate enough. He glanced around. Point defense was active, treating the LACs as if they were missiles themselves. *Insane*. Nobody was going to have time to react to anything.

"Closing," the Tac officer said. "Ten point two seconds to launch. Mark."

Spots of brilliant light began to flare silently against the blackness and unwinking stars of space; the tank listed them as nuke warheads, the stabbing flicker of bomb-pumped X-ray swords, the fuzzier explosions of fusion bottles rupturing under the massive fists of *Rousseau's* energy batteries. Machines were dueling with machines, and men and women died.

And here I am a sitting duck, he thought bitterly. Nothing for a captain to do; the ship couldn't maneuver.

He looked to another screen, this one showing his assigned targets for bombardment. That made him lick dry lips. *Insane*, he thought again. Kinetic energy bombardment, warheadless missiles fired straight down at—literally—astronomical velocities. When they met the surface, mass in motion would be converted into heat. They didn't *need* warheads. The thought of that type of strike on a populated area, on *Nouveau Paris*, for Christ's sake, made his testicles try to crawl up back inside his abdomen.

"We didn't start it," he reminded himself. The gang of madmen who did start it had used *nukes* in a populated zone, and that showed you the sort of thing they'd do and order him to do if they got their hands on the levers of power.

He still tasted vomit at the thought of what he

had to do, and what the Admiral was going to order herself. *McQueen, when I'm fighting the Manties, I'd trust you to the limit.* She was a hard CO, but she got the job done and she didn't flinch herself. *Can I trust you here?*

Rousseau's eight million tons leaped and shuddered as an energy lance went through her sidewalls and blasted into her armor.

"Damage control," he said in a metronome-steady voice.

"Compartments twenty-six through eight open to vacuum. Graser one down."

"Reconfigure—"

There was no need to look at the display screens anymore, though some still did. Rob S. Pierre sat with his hands on the table, looking ahead, ignoring the worried glances and whispers where Oscar Saint-Just and Cordelia Ransom had their heads together.

Everyone looked up as a couple of Security noncoms came through the door, their arms full of pulse rifles.

"Citizens," one of them said. "It's time."

They began handing the weapons out.

"Hit them," McQueen said.

They were coming in over the city of Nouveau Paris at twenty-five thousand meters, and even from here the pillars of smoke were obvious. One or two of the huge towers must have *fallen* to create the gaps she saw. There was an ominous-looking crater, and her skin crawled as she watched the readout. Oh, it wasn't really a very large weapon—subcrit squeeze job—and it was designed to be relatively clean, but "relatively" was the operative word there. She remembered an old, old grisly joke: *A tactical nuclear weapon is one that explodes a thousand kilometers downwind of you.*

"That used to be Regional Intervention Battalions HQ, didn't it?" she said.

"Yes." Fontein's voice was flat.

Fourteen thousand people, she thought. *More than a good-sized fleet engagement usually killed.*

"Status on the crowds," she said.

"They've thinned out. Everyone must have gotten the idea that something serious is going on, and the fun-seekers have gone home," one of her staffers said. "We estimate that *only* two hundred thousand are still out."

Still a fairly substantial number, even in a city with a population of thirty-two million.

"These must be the real Leveler militants. They're all in or near Committee HQ and adjacent parts of the Government district. No particular organization, but plenty of arms."

"Citizen Brigadier Conflans."

"Citizen Admiral, I can't proceed until the . . . mob . . . is cleared out of my way. Dropping ground troops into that would be like throwing a handful of buckshot into a barrel of snot."

"And I can't do that until the airspace over the Avenue of the People is safe," she said thoughtfully. Then on another channel: "Citizen Captain Norton, execute."

"Ma'am—" there was an edge of desperation in his voice. "Ma'am, those are *government* units."

McQueen throttled an impulse to shout. She couldn't *force* Norton to obey her; all bets were off, and everyone was proceeding on personal convictions and loyalties. Norton had been with her all through the fighting around Trevor's Star; he'd stayed calm when the *Rousseau*'s bridge was blown open to space and they were slugging it out with Manty superdreadnoughts at energy-weapon range and a main fusion bottle started to go critical. . . .

"Bob," she said quietly, "we can't spare the time to convince them of our bona fides, and they'll fire on us. There's no *time*. Clear our way, but whatever you do, we're going in."

The voice that answered might as well have been a robot's. "Affirmative, Citizen Admiral. Initiating."

Someone gasped as a solid bar of white light stretched down from heaven; air riven to ionized gas, and fragments of ablative shielding. The bar touched earth, and a pattern of shocked-white fury reached out from that point. The shock wave moved after it, and buildings rippled and blew away like straw around it.

"God have mercy on anyone within half a klick of any of those."

"Civilians," she said to nobody in particular, "call this sort of thing a *surgical strike*. Sort of like surgery with a chain-saw."

"Two," someone murmured. Another bar of light; she looked away, blinking at the after-images behind her eyelids. "Three. Four. Five. Six. Seven." A pause. "Eight."

"Citizen Admiral," Norton's voice said. "*Liberty* and *Equality* have opened fire with their energy armaments." Another pause, and surprise in his tone: "*Fraternity* is opening fire on *them*."

"Get out of there, Bob. You've done all you can." She switched channels. "Prepare to execute, Citizen Brigadier Conflans." To her own tiny flotilla of pinnaces: "Let's convince the Leveler militants they're in the wrong line of work. *Execute Grapeshot*."

Many of the crowd that filled the Avenue of the People for two kilometers were in a holiday mood; the police officers hanging from the streetlamps on either side, or twitching on the points of the decorative wrought-iron fences around gardens added to the festive air. There was still fighting going on towards the three-hundredth floor of the Committee's tower, but they didn't have to do anything in particular. A few of the more energetic were amusing themselves by dragging out civil servants from the lower floors of the towers on either side, and giving them impromptu People's Justice. Others passed bottles around, sang the war-chants of the Conspiracy of Equals, or simply stood or sat and waited. It wouldn't be long now.

Many of them looked up at the turbine wail. Police vehicles had tried overflights an hour ago, and a few of them had even gotten away, but the falling debris from the others had been dangerous. Leveler cell-leaders at the fringes of the street barked into their communicators.

Some of the mob might have had time to realize the nature of the pepper-flake tiny loads the pinnaces were dropping. None of them had time to run before the tens of thousands of fragmentation loads from the cluster munitions reached their preprogrammed height and exploded in a long surf-wall of white fire. Each of them threw *thousands* of pieces of jagged ceramic shrapnel into the air, cutting across the crowd at chest-height at thousands of meters per second. Where they struck blood and flesh and bone *splashed*, divided into a spray of damp matter as liquid as the blood alone.

The crowd was huge, more than eighty thousand on this avenue alone. The laws of probability and various obstacles assured there were more than enough left alive to scream as the pinnaces began their second run.

One man managed to stagger back to his feet and fumble at the load across his back. Blood was running down into his eyes, and there was a wetness when he tried to breathe, but his hands still functioned.

"They're running, Ma'am," the pilot begged, forgetting himself and the presence of Citizen Commissioner Fontein. "They're *running*."

"And I want them to keep on running for a long, long time," McQueen said softly. "All their lives, in their heads. How do you think those bodies got to hanging from those lamp-posts, son? We'll make another pass, with the pulsers, slow and level. All pinnaces, one more pass. Citizen Brigadier Conflans, we've cleared your way for you. Now go in there and make it worth something."

The pinnace screamed up in a near-vertical turn, passing near the scarred, smoking side of the Committee tower, then looped over again and began another run down the Avenue of the People. This time she was working from the rear of the crowd forward, towards the building the mob had hoped to overrun. To either side of her nose heavy tri-barrel pulsers raved in long spears of white light, sending thousands of heavy explosive projectiles down into the street below. Bodies living and dead blew apart, and the ground-cars and pavement below them offered little more resistance as they erupted into volcanoes of shredded metal and stone. Lime in the concrete burned white under the howling lash of projectiles driven to thousands of meters a second by the impeller coils. Wrecks trailed the clean blue flame of burning hydrogen in the pinnace's wake.

"Target acquisition!" the pilot shouted as an alarm shrieked and blinked red from his control panel. He rammed his throttles home.

The pinnace leapt forward. Something slammed into its side, and one of the massive air-breathing turbines lurched free and pinwheeled away. Admiral Esther McQueen watched it slam into the side of a tower. Her last thought was an angry impatience. She wouldn't even get to see if her gamble had succeeded or failed.

"Citizen Chairman," the Marine said, saluting. "I am pleased to report that this building is under control. I must ask you all to remain here until we've—"

"Got it!" someone shouted. "Sir, the net's back up! We killed the fucking ghost!"

"Excuse me," Rob S. Pierre said to the Marine brigadier. He turned and took two steps to the terminal, sat, and began giving orders. It was twenty minutes before he sat back.

"Citizen Committeeman Saint-Just," he said. "Perhaps you could tell me exactly what happened, at this point?"

Saint-Just swallowed; he'd just allowed the most massive Security breach in the new regime's history. *Of course,* Pierre thought behind the mask of his face. *He knows I know everyone makes mistakes. But he can't really be certain of that.* A wry smile tugged at one corner of his mouth; it would be an odd start to his New Look policy to have his second-in-command shot, anyway.

The head of State Security had the Marine officer in tow; the man was looking guarded, which any sensible officer would at being in this close contact with the Committee.

"Now, Citizen Brigadier . . . Conflans?" The officer nodded. There were scorchmarks and rusty-looking dried fluids across the arm and chest of his combat armor. "Perhaps you could explain exactly how your most *timely* assistance came about?"

The Chairman's brows rose until he felt his forehead ache. "Timely indeed," he murmured when the man was finished. "Esther McQueen, eh?" He looked at Saint-Just; the Security chief nodded. *And I was supposed to interview her this afternoon.* He looked at a screen; three hours almost to the minute since this began. He felt as if it had been that many decades . . . and where had he managed to get that bruise, or tear his jacket?

"Well, where is the lady?" he said. "I gather from you and Citizen Captain Norton that she isn't on *Rousseau*?"

"No, Citizen Chairman," the Marine said. The fierce, handsome face behind the sweeping mustaches suddenly looked pinched. "Her pinnace went down while it was directing the final operations. We haven't . . ."

Rob S. Pierre looked at his Security chief. "Find her for me, Oscar. I think the lady has gone from a *possibility* to a certainty, and it would be excessive irony if she were dead."

The calm, pale bureaucrat's face nodded. "Of course, Citizen Chairman. At once."

Esther McQueen realized that death was much like space; very dark, with flashes of light in infinite depth.

After a second she realized she was dangling upside-down and watching electronic equipment self-destruct. The battle steel hull of the Naval pinnace had withstood a collision that would have left a civilian vehicle travelling at its velocity smeared across the side of the tower. The remains of the pinnace were sticking into the side of it now, like a knife thrust halfway into a giant cheese. A gaping rent directly below her showed the three hundred and fifty story drop to the pavement of the People's Avenue . . . and if the buckled shock harness gave way, she'd drop straight down to make her smeared remains one with the multi-thousand victims of her strafing run.

That made her laugh. The tearing pain of *that* brought her fully back to consciousness with an involuntary whimper, enough to feel the pinnace shifting in its stony cradle. More lights danced behind her eyes as she froze; intellectually she knew that a seven-hundred-ton pinnace wasn't likely to shift and fall because a short, slight woman moved, but her gut was harder to convince. Carefully, slowly, she raised one hand to her face and wiped her eye, then pushed back the flap of scalp that was hanging loose. Coagulating blood held it in place.

Ribs, she thought. She wasn't actually coughing blood, so the splintered ends weren't likely to kill her in the immediate future . . . unless she moved vigorously. *Which, since I'm hanging upside-down over a long, long drop, I probably will have to do.* All the other figures she could see were immobile, either unconscious or dead.

All except People's Commissioner Fontein. His shock harness had broken even more thoroughly than hers, but it had broken away as a unit. The last fastening point had held, so far, and it swung him out over the gap in the pinnace's hull. As she watched he tried to reach for a dangling piece of wreckage, and the fastener gave a small, tooth-gritting wail.

"Fontein," she said—whispered, rather.

"You're alive?" he blurted.

"Temporarily." She grinned. The expression was

ghastly in the bloody mask of her face. "Let's see how temporarily . . . how badly are you hurt?"

He *looked* terrible, his face and what she could see of his body a mass of bruises and dried blood; tear-tracks cut half-clean runnels through the matter on his face, except where the skin had been abraded away and oozed raw. She was almost glad that her nose was broken and swollen shut; she had no wish to smell this charnel-house of her own making.

"I'm . . . no broken bones except for this." He twitched his left hand, and she saw that the little finger was at right angles to the others and swollen to sausage-size.

"Good . . . for . . . you," she wheezed painfully. *Christ, but this* hurts. *No matter. Get going, bitch.* "Is the release catch on your shock harness working?"

"I think so. I'd really rather not find out, though, Citizen Admiral."

Fontein looked down. An acrobat in high training might be able to catch something in the half-second before he fell clear and down a long, long way. A middle-aged man of sedentary habits with serious injuries might as well flap his arms hard on the way down, for all the good it would do him.

"Here's my plan," McQueen said, and laughed again, stopping herself with a shudder of agony as things moved and grated in her torso. "Sorry, classical reference. Getting a little light-headed. You swing across and grab my hand with your right. Then, *as soon as I've got you*, you hit the release—do it fast, so you don't lose momentum. I'll swing you on across to there," she said, indicating a section of wall plating with dangling cables festooned across it. "Then you can go and get help for the rest of us."

Fontein looked at her blank-eyed for a moment. Then he spoke: "You don't give up very easily, do you, Citizen Admiral McQueen?"

"White Haven didn't think so."

He nodded. "On the count of three."

"One." The Commissioner heaved his weight backward, like a child on a swing.

"Two."

She closed out everything except the hand she would have to grasp.

"*Three.*"

It jarred into hers, and she heard a *click-snap* and falling clatter as her fingers clenched. Then she was screaming, screaming and tasting iron at the back of her throat as Fontein's weight came onto her out-stretched arm and wrenched her savaged body against the unyielding frame of the shock harness. Blackness surged over her, welcome as the memory of her mother's arms, then receded into a red-shot alertness. She spat to clear her mouth; that *was* blood this time. A steady trickle of it, if not an arterial gusher. The bone spears had hit something.

"See," she said to Fontein's shock-white face where he clung to the wreck's wall not more than an arm's length away. "We really do accomplish things when we cooperate, Citizen Commissioner."

Then the blackness returned.

Rob S. Pierre looked down at the stretcher. "Will it endanger her life?" he said.

"No, Sir," the medtech said unwillingly.

"Then I insist." He stepped back.

Esther McQueen's eyes opened, and she sighed once in blissful relief; the stretcher's lights blinked as it swept away her pain. Her eyes moved.

"Gerrard?" she said, her voice faint but steady. The Marine went to one knee and looked at her, his face warring between relief and revulsion. "The butcher's bill?"

"Light, Skipper," he said. "By the time we hit them they were running on empty; the Chairman's Guard bled them bad."

"Ship?"

"Some damage, but Citizen Pierre called them off in time."

She nodded again, and the Chairman of the Committee of Public Safety stepped forward. "Citizen Admiral McQueen," he said. "The People's Republic, the Committee, and I myself are in your debt. Your prompt action . . . we'll talk more about this later. I already intended to have an interview with you today, but tomorrow will do just as well."

"Thank you . . . Sir," she said. The eyes began to wander again, and he stepped back and motioned the techs to take her away.

He looked around the wreckage of the Committee's tower. The other members were dispersing about their various tasks; it would be some time before they got this mess cleaned up and returned to the agenda he'd intended to spend the day on.

"But we *will* get back to it, by God," he whispered, and looked out the gaping windows over his city.

They were his people out there; weak and foolish and stupid and short-sighted, but they were as others made them. *He* would remake them, and give them back their pride. If he had the right tools.

He looked after McQueen's stretcher. Any good tool kit needed a knife, a sharp one. If you cut yourself using it, that was your fault, not the tool's.

The Universe of Honor
Harrington

David Weber

Honor Harrington was born on October 1, 1859 Post Diaspora, at Craggy Hollow (the Harrington family homestead), County Duvalier, in the Duchy of Shadow Vale, Sphinx. In general, one might say that she was born at the twilight of what had been a long, relatively stable and peaceful period of galactic history. Her native Star Kingdom of Manticore was widely respected as one of the wealthiest star nations in existence (probably *the* wealthiest, on a per capita basis), and its carrying trade dominated the interstellar freight lines outside the Solarian League itself. The galaxy had not seen a major war in over a century, although there were always places (like the Silesian Confederacy) where ongoing low-level conflicts were the norm rather than the exception. Aside from rumblings out of the economically devastated People's Republic of Haven, which had recently forcibly annexed a half dozen neighboring systems, there seemed little reason to expect that to change.

But by 1901 PD, (the time of *On Basilisk Station*) it *had* changed, and changed drastically. The PRH's steady economic collapse had driven its expansionism to heights unseen since pre-space days on Old Terra, and the Star Kingdom of Manticore lay squarely in the Peeps' path. The last century's "golden age" was coming to an end with the approach of an interstellar war which would, before it ended, see virtually the entire human-occupied galaxy choosing up sides, with military operations on a scale no one had ever previously contemplated.

This appendix sketches in some of the salient points of the galaxy into which Honor was born . . . and which she, willingly or not, was to play a major part in changing forever.

(1) Background (General)

The first manned interstellar ship departed the Solar System on September 30, 2103. Although no other ship followed for almost fifty years, 2013 CE, became accepted as Year One of the Diaspora, and January 1 of that year became January 1, 01 PD for purposes of interstellar dating.

For over seven centuries after the *Prometheus* became the first manned starship, FTL movement remained impossible, leaving generation ships (followed in the fourth century PD by the development of practical cryogenic hibernation vessels) as the only means of long-distance interstellar expansion. The original starships used fairly straightforward reaction drives with hydrogen catcher fields to sustain boost after the initial onboard reaction mass was exhausted. Later generations attempted more esoteric propulsion systems, but though they graduated to fusion and photon drives, they remained locked into the sublight reaction principle until 725 PD, when the first crude hyper drive was tested in the Solar System.

The interface between normal and hyper-space was speed-critical, for if velocity at hyper translation exceeded .3 c, the translating starship was destroyed. In addition, a hypership had to reach the hyper limit of a star's gravity well before it could enter hyper, and the hyper limit varies with the spectral class of the star, as shown in Figure 1.

The original hyper drive was a man-killer. The casualty figures over the first fifty years of hyper travel were daunting. Worse, vessels which were destroyed were lost with all hands, which left no record of their fates and thus offered no clue as to the causes of their destruction. Eventually, however, it was determined that most had probably been lost to one of two phenomena, which became known as "grav shear" (see below) and "dimensional shear" (violent energy turbulence separating hyper bands from one another). Once this was recognized and the higher hyper bands were declared off limits, losses due to dimensional shear ended, but grav shear remained a highly dangerous and essentially unpredictable phenomenon for the next five centuries. Despite that unpredictability and continuing (though lower) loss rates, hyperships' FTL capabilities made them the vessel of choice for survey duties and other low-manpower requirement tasks. Crews of highly paid specialists willing to accept risky employment conditions were enlisted for survey work and for the early mail packets, but the loss rate continued to make any sort of interstellar bulk commerce impractical and insured that most colonists still moved aboard the much slower but more survivable cryogenic ships. As a consequence,

Star	Hyper Limit	Star	Hyper Limit	Star	Hyper Limit
O	49.60 LM	G2	21.12 LM	K7	14.52 LM
B	33.42 LM	G3	20.68 LM	K8	14.08 LM
A	28.75 LM	G4	20.24 LM	K9	13.64 LM
F0	25.42 LM	G5	19.80 LM	M0	13.20 LM
F1	25.98 LM	G6	19.36 LM	M1	12.76 LM
F2	25.54 LM	G7	18.92 LM	M2	12.32 LM
F3	25.10 LM	G8	18.48 LM	M3	11.88 LM
F4	24.66 LM	G9	18.04 LM	M4	11.44 LM
F5	24.20 LM	K0	17.60 LM	M5	11.00 LM
F6	23.76 LM	K1	17.15 LM	M6	10.56 LM
F7	23.32 LM	K2	16.72 LM	M7	10.12 LM
F8	22.88 LM	K3	16.28 LM	M8	9.68 LM
F9	22.44 LM	K4	15.84 LM	M9	9.24 LM
G0	22.00 LM	K5	15.40 LM	RedGiant	5.64 LM
G1	21.56 LM	K6	14.96 LM		

Figure 1

the rate of advance of colonization did not increase terribly significantly during the period 725-1273 PD, although the ability to pick suitable targets for colonization (courtesy of the FTL survey crews) improved enormously.

The best speed possible in hyper prior to 1273 PD was about fifty times light-speed, a major plus over light-speed vessels but still too slow to tie distant stars together into any sort of interstellar community. It *was* sufficient to allow establishment of the oldest of the currently existing interstellar polities, the Solarian League, consisting of the oldest colony worlds within approximately ninety light-years of Sol.

The major problem limiting hyper speeds was that simply getting into hyper did not create a propulsive effect. Indeed, the initial translation into hyper was a complex energy transfer which reduced a starship's velocity by "bleeding off" momentum. In effect, a translating hypership lost approximately 92% of its normal-space velocity when entering hyper. This had unfortunate consequences in terms of reaction mass requirements, particularly since the fact that hydrogen catcher fields were inoperable in hyper meant one could not replenish one's reaction mass underway. On the other hand, the velocity bleed effect applied equally regardless of the direction of the translation (that is, one lost 92% of one's velocity whether one was entering hyper-space from normal-space or normal-space from hyper-space), which meant that leaving hyper automatically decelerated one's vessel to a normal-space velocity only 08% of whatever its velocity had been in hyper-space. This tremendously reduced the amount of deceleration required at the far end of a hyper voyage and so made reaction drives at least workable.

Since .3 c (approx. 89,907.6 km./sec.) was the maximum velocity at which an "upward" translation into hyper-space could be made, the maximum initial velocity in hyper-space was .024 c (or 7,192.6 km./sec.). Making translation at speeds as high as .3 c was a rough experience and not particularly safe. The loss rate at .3 c was over 10%; dropping translation velocity to .23 c virtually eliminated ship losses in initial translation, and, since the difference in initial hyper velocity was less than 1,700 KPS, most captains routinely made translation at the lower speed. Even today, only military commanders in emergency conditions will make upward translation at .3 c. There is no safe upper speed on "downward" translations. That is, a ship may translate from hyper-space to normal-space at any hyper-space velocity without risking destruction. (Which is not to say that the crews enjoy the experience or that it does not impose enormous wear and tear on hyper generators.) Further, translation from one hyper band to a higher band (see below) may be made at any velocity up to and including .6 c. No vessel may exceed .6 c in hyper (.8 in normal-space) because radiation and particle shields cannot protect them or their passengers at higher velocities.

Once a vessel enters hyper, it is placed in what might be considered a compressed dimension which corresponds on a point-by-point basis to "normal-space" but places those points in much closer congruity. Hyper-space consists of multiple regions or layers—called "bands"—of associated but discrete dimensions. Dr. Radhakrishnan (who, after Adrienne Warshawski, is considered to have been humanity's greatest hyper-physicist) called the hyper bands "the back-flash of creation," for they might be considered echoes of normal-space, the consequence of the ultimate convergence of the mass of an entire normal-space universe. Or, as Dr. Warshawski once put it, "Gravity folds normal-space everywhere, by however small an amount, and hyper-space may be considered the 'inside' of all those little folds."

In practical terms, this meant that for a ship in hyper, the distance between normal-space points was "shorter," which allowed the vessel to move between them using a standard reaction drive at sublight speeds to attain an *effective* FTL capability. Even in hyper, ships were not capable of true faster-than-light movement; the relatively closer proximity of points in normal-space simply gave the *appearance* of FTL travel, which meant that as long as a vessel was dependent on its reaction drive and could not reach the higher hyper bands, its maximum apparent speed was limited to approximately sixty-two times that which the same vessel could have attained in normal-space.

Navigation, communication, and observation all are rendered difficult by the nature of hyper-space. Formed by gravitational distortion, hyper-space itself acts as a focusing glass, producing a cascade effect of ever more tightly warped space. The laws of relativistic physics apply at any given point in that space, but as a hypothetical observer looks "outward" in hyper-space, his instruments show a rapidly increasing distortion. At ranges above about 20 LM (359,751,000 km.) that distortion becomes so pronounced that accurate observations are impossible. One says "about 20 LM" because, depending on local conditions, that range may vary up or down by as much as 12%—that is, from 17.6 LM (316,580,880 km.) to 22.4 LM (or 402,921,120 km.). A hypership thus travels at the center of a bubble of observation from 633,161,760 to 805,842,240 km. in diameter. Even within that sphere, observations and measurements can be highly suspect; in effect, the "bubble" may be thought of as the region in which an observer can tell something is out there and very roughly where. Exact, precise observations and measurements are all but impossible above ranges of 5,000,000 to 6,000,000 km., which would make navigational fixes impossible even if there were anything to take fixes on.

This seemed to rule out any practical use of hyper-space until the development of the first "hyper log" (known as the "HL" by spacers) in 731 PD. The HL is analogous to the inertial guidance units first developed on Old Earth in the 20th century CE. By combining the input from extremely acute sensor systems with known power inputs to a vessel's own propulsive systems and running a continuous back plot of gravity gradients passed through, the HL maintains a real-time "dead reckoning" position. Early HLs were accurate to within no more than 10 LS per light-month, which meant that, in a voyage of 60 light-years, the HL position might be out by as much as two light-hours. Early hyper-space navigators thus had to be extremely cautious and make generous allowances for error in plotting their voyages, but current (1900 PD) HLs are accurate to within .4 light-second per light-month (that is, the HL position at the end of a 60 light-year voyage would be off by no more than 288 light-seconds or less than 5 light-minutes).

From the beginning of hyper travel, it was known that there were multiple hyper bands and that the "higher" the band, the closer the congruity between points in normal-space and thus the higher the apparent FTL speed, but their use was impractical for two major reasons. First, translation from band to band bleeds off velocity much as the initial translation. The bleed-off for each higher band is approximately 92% of the bleed-off for the next lowest one (that is, the alpha band translation reduces velocity by 92%; the beta band bleed-off is 84.64%; the velocity loss for the gamma band is 77.87%, etc.), but it still had to be made up again after each translation, and this posed an insurmountable mass requirement for any reaction drive.

The second problem was that the interfaces between any two hyper bands are regions of highly unstable and powerful energy flows, creating the "dimensional shear" which had destroyed so many early hyperships, and dimensional shear becomes more violent as band levels increase. Moreover, even the relatively "safe" lower bands which could be reliably reached were characterized by powerful energy surges and flows—currents, almost—of highly-charged particles and warped gravity waves. Adequate shielding could hold the radiation effects in check, but a grav shear within any band could rip the strongest ship to pieces.

Hyper-space grav waves take the form of wide, deep volumes of space, as much as fifty light-years across and averaging half their width in depth, of focused gravitational stress "moving" through hyper-space. Actually, the wave itself might be thought of as stationary, but energy and charged particles trapped in its influence are driven along it at light- or near-light-speed. In that sense, the grav wave serves as a carrier for other energies and remains motionless but for a (relatively) slow side-slipping or drifting. In large part, it is this grav wave drift which makes them so dangerous; survey ships with modern sensors can plot them quite accurately, but they may not be in the same place when the next ship happens along. The major waves in the more heavily traveled portions of the galaxy have been charted with reasonable accuracy, for sufficient observational data has been amassed to predict their usual drift patterns. In addition, most waves are considered "locked," meaning that their rate of shift is low and that they maintain effectively fixed relationships with other "locked" waves. But there are also waves which are not locked—whose patterns (if, in fact, they have patterns at all) are not only not understood but can change with blinding speed. One of the most famous of these is the Selkir Shear between the Andermani Empire and the Silesian Confederacy, but there are many others, and those in less well-traveled (and thus less well-surveyed) areas, especially, can be extremely treacherous.

The heart of any grav wave is far more powerful than its fringes, or, put another way, a "grav wave" consists of many layers of "grav eddies." For the most part, all aspects of the wave have the same basic orientation, but it is possible for a wave to include counter-layers of reverse "flow" at unpredictable vertical levels. Despite the size of a grav wave, most of hyper-space is free of them; the real monsters that are more than ten or fifteen light-years wide are rare, and even in hyper the distances between them are vast, though the average interval between grav waves becomes progressively shorter as one translates higher into the hyper bands. The great danger of grav waves to early-generation hyperships lay in the phenomenon known as "grav shear." This is experienced as a vessel moves into the area of influence of a grav wave and, even more strongly, in areas in which two or more grav waves impact upon one another. At those points, the gravitational force exerted on one portion of the vessel's structure might be hundreds or even thousands of times as great as that exerted on the remainder of its fabric, with catastrophic consequences for any ship ever built.

In theory, a ship could so align itself as to "slide" into the grav wave at an extremely gradual angle, avoiding the sudden, cataclysmic shear which would otherwise tear it apart. In practice, the only way to avoid the destructive shearing effect was to avoid grav waves altogether, yet that was well nigh impossible. Grav waves might be widely spaced, but it was impossible to detect them at all until a ship was directly on top of one, and with no way to see one coming, there was no way to plot a course to avoid it. It *was* possible to recognize when one actually entered the periphery of a grav wave, and if one were on exactly the right vector, prompt emergency evasion gave one a chance (though not a good one) of surviving the encounter, but the grav wave remained the most feared and fearsome peril of hyper travel.

Then, in 1246 PD, the first phased array gravity drive, or impeller, was designed on Beowulf, the colonized world of the Sigma Draconis System. This was a reactionless sublight drive which artificially replicated the grav waves which had been observed in hyper-space for centuries. The impeller drive used a series of nodal generators to create a pair of stressed bands in normal-space, one "above" and one "below" the mounting ship. Inclined towards one another, these produced a sort of wedge-shaped quasi-hyper-space in those regions, having no direct effect upon the generating vessel but creating what might be called a "tame grav wave" which was capable of attaining near-light speeds very quickly. Because of the angle at which the bands were generated relative to one another, the vessel rode a small pocket of normal-space (open ahead of the vessel and closing in astern) trapped between the grav waves, much as a surfboard rides the crest or curl of a wave, which was driven along between the stress bands. Since the stress bands were waves and not particles, the "impeller wedge" was able, theoretically, at least, to attain an instantaneous light-speed velocity. Unfortunately, the normal-space "pocket" had to deal with the conservation of inertia, which meant that the effective acceleration of a manned ship was limited to that which produced a g force the crew could survive. Nonetheless, these higher rates of acceleration could be maintained *indefinitely*, and no reaction mass was required; so long as the generators had power, the drive's endurance was effectively unlimited.

In terms of interstellar flight, however, the impeller drive was afflicted by one enormous drawback which was not at first appreciated. In essence, it enormously increased the danger grav shear had always presented to reactor drive vessels, for the interference between the immense strength of a grav wave and the artificially produced gravitic stress of an impeller wedge will vaporize a starship almost instantly.

In the military sphere, it was soon discovered that although the bow (or "throat") and stern aspects of an impeller wedge must remain open, additional "sidewall" grav waves could be generated to close its open sides and serve as shields against hostile fire, as not even an energy beam (generated using then-current technology) could penetrate a wave front in which effective local gravity went from zero to several hundred thousand gravities. The problem of generating an energy beam powerful enough to "burn through" even at pointblank ranges was not to be solved for centuries, but within fifty years grav penetrators had been designed for missile weapons, which could also make full use of the incredible acceleration potential of the impeller drive. Since that time, there has been a constant race between defensive designers working new wrinkles in manipulation of the gravity wave to defeat new penetrators and offensive designers adapting their penetrators to defeat the new counters.

The interstellar drawbacks of impeller drive became quickly and disastrously clear to Beowulf's shipbuilders, and for several decades it seemed likely that the new drive would be limited solely to interplanetary traffic. In 1273 PD, however, the scientist Adrienne Warshawski of Old Terra recognized a previously unsuspected FTL implication of the new technology. Prior to her *Fleetwing* tests in that year, all efforts to employ it in hyper-space had ended in unmitigated disaster, but Dr. Warshawski found a way around the problem. She had already invented a new device capable of scanning hyperspace for grav waves and wave shifts within five light-seconds of a starship (to this day, all grav scanners are known as "warshawskis" by starship crews), which made it possible to use impeller drive *between* hyper-space grav waves, since they could now be seen and avoided.

That, alone, would have been sufficient to earn Warshawski undying renown, but beneficial as it was, its significance paled beside her next leap forward, for in working out her detector, Dr. Warshawski had penetrated far more deeply into the nature of the grav wave phenomenon than any of her predecessors, and she suddenly realized that it would be possible to build an impeller drive which could be reconfigured at will to project its grav waves at *right angles* to the generating vessel. There was no converging effect to move a pocket of normal-space, but these perpendicular grav fields could be brought into phase with the grav wave, thus eliminating the interference effect between impellers and the wave. More, the new fields would stabilize a vessel relative to the grav wave, allowing a transition into it which eliminated the traditional dangers grav shear presented to the ship's physical structure. In effect, the alterations she made to *Fleetwing* to produce her "alpha nodes" provided the ship with gigantic, immaterial sails: circular, plate-like gravity bands over two hundred kilometers in diameter. Coupled with her grav wave detector to plot and "read" grav waves, they would permit a starship to literally "set her sails" and use the focused radiation hurtling along hyper-space's naturally occurring grav waves to derive incredible accelerations.

Not only that, but the interface between sail and natural grav wave produced an eddy of preposterously high energy levels which could be "siphoned off" to power the starship. Effectively, once a starship "set sail" it drew sufficient power to maintain and trim its sails *and also for every other energy requirement* and could thus shut down its onboard power plants until the time came to leave hyper-space. A Warshawski Sail hypership thus had no need for reaction mass, required very little fuel mass, and could sustain high rates of acceleration indefinitely, which meant that the velocity loss associated with "cracking the wall" between hyper bands could be regained and that use of the upper bands was no longer impractical.

This last point was a crucial factor in attaining higher interstellar transit times. The maximum safe velocity in any hyper band remained .6 c, but the higher bands, with their closer point-to-point congruencies, added a significant multiplier to the FTL equivalent of that velocity. Prior to the Warshawski Sail, not only had dimension shear made translating into the upper bands dangerous, but the successive velocity losses had made it highly uneconomical for any reaction drive ship. Now the lost velocity could be rapidly regained and the higher, "faster" bands could be used to sustain a much higher average velocity. As a result, the dreaded grav wave became the path to ever more efficient hyper travel, and captains who had previously avoided them in terror now used their new instrumentation to find them and cruised on standard impeller drive between them.

Of course, there wasn't always a grav wave going the direction a starship needed, but with the grav detector to keep a ship clear of naturally occurring grav waves impeller drive could, at last, be used in hyper-space. In addition, it was possible for a Warshawski Sail ship to "reach" across a wave (which might be thought of as sailing with a "quartering breeze") at angles of up to about 60° before the sails began losing drive and up to approximately 85° before all drive was lost. By the same token, a hypership could sail "close-hauled," or into a grav wave, at approach angles of 45°. At angles above 45°, it was necessary to "tack into the wave," which naturally meant that return passages would be slower than outgoing passages through the same region of prevailing grav waves. Thus the old "windjammer" technology of Earth's seas had reemerged in the interstellar age, transmuted into the intricacies of hyper-space and FTL travel. By 1750 PD, however, sail tuners had been upgraded to a point which permitted the "grab factor" of a sail to be manipulated with far more sophistication than Dr. Warshawski's original technology had permitted. Indeed, it became possible to create a negative grab factor which, in effect, permitted a starship to sail directly "into the wind," although with a marginally greater danger of sail failure.

The Warshawski Sail also made it possible to "crack the wall" between hyper bands with much greater impunity. Breaking into a higher hyper band was (and is) still no bed of roses, and ships occasionally come to grief in the transition even today, but a Warshawski Sail ship inserts itself into a grav wave going in the right direction and rides it through, rather like an aircraft riding an updraft. This access to the higher bands meant the first generation Warshawski Sail could move a starship at an apparent velocity of just over 800 c, but an upper limit on velocity remained, created by the range capability of the vessel's grav wave detectors. In the higher bands, the grav waves were both more powerful and tightly-spaced due to the increasingly stressed nature of hyper-space in those regions. This meant that the five-light-second detection range of the original Warshawski offered insufficient warning time to venture much above the gamma bands, thus imposing the absolute speed limitation. In addition, the problems of acceleration remained. The Warshawski Sail could be adjusted by decreasing the strength of the field, thus allowing a greater proportion of the grav wave's power to "leak" through it, to hold acceleration down to something a human body could tolerate, but the old bugaboo of "g forces" remained a problem for the next century or so.

Then, in 1384 PD, a physicist by the name of Shigematsu Radhakrishnan added another major breakthrough in the form of the inertial compensator. The compensator turned the grav wave (natural or artificial) associated with a vessel into a sort of "inertial sump," dumping the inertial forces of acceleration into the grav wave and thus exempting the vessel's crew from the g forces associated with acceleration. Within the limits of its efficiency, it completely eliminated g force, placing an accelerating vessel in a permanent state of internal zero-gee, but its capacity to damp inertia was directly proportional to the power of the grav wave around it and inversely proportional to both the volume of the field and the mass of the vessel about which it was generated. The first factor meant that it was far more effective for starships than for sublight ships, as the former drew upon the greater energy of the naturally occurring grav waves of hyper-space, and the second meant it was more effective for smaller ships than for larger ones. The natural grav waves of hyper-space, with their incomparably greater power, offered a much "deeper" sump than the artificial stress bands of the impeller drive, which meant that a Warshawski Sail ship could deflect vastly more g force from its passengers than one under impeller drive. In general terms, the compensator permitted humans to endure acceleration rates approaching 550 g under impeller drive and 4-5,000 g under sail, which allows hyperships to make up "bleed-off" velocity *very* quickly after translation. These numbers are for military compensators, which tend to be more massive, more energy and maintenance intensive, and much more expensive than those used in most merchant construction. Military compensators allow higher acceleration—and warships cannot afford to be less maneuverable than their foes—but only at the cost of penalties merchant ships as a whole cannot afford.

In practical terms, the maximum acceleration a ship can pull is defined in Figure 2.

These accelerations are with inertial compensator safety margins cut to zero. Normally, warships operate with a 20% safety margin, while MS safety margins run as high as 35%. Note also that the cargo carried by a starship is less important than the table above might suggest. The numbers in Figure 2 use mass as the determining factor, but the *size* of the field is of very nearly equal importance. A 7.5 million-ton freighter with empty cargo holds would require the same size field as one with full holds, and so would have the same effective acceleration capability.

Note also that in 1900 PD, 8,500,000 tons represented the edge of a plateau in inertial compensator capability. Above 8,500,000 tons, warship accelerations fell off by approximately 1 g per 2,500 tons, so that a warship of 8,502,500 tons would have a maximum acceleration of 419 g and a warship of 9,547,500 tons would have a maximum acceleration of 1 g. The same basic curves were followed for merchant vessels.

| Ship | Normal-space | | Hyper-space | |
Mass in Tons	Warship	Merchantship	Warship	Merchantship
0-79,999(FG/DD)	550 g	253g	5,280 g	2,429 g
80-499,999 (CL/CA)	520 g	240 g	5,018 g	2,308 g
500,000-1,499,999 (BC)	500 g	230 g	4,825 g	2,215 g
1.5-4,999,999 (BB)	470 g	215 g	4,536 g	2,085 g
4-6,999,999 (DN)	450 g	207 g	4,345 g	1,990 g
7-8,499,999 (SD)	420 g	190 g	4,053 g	1,860 g

Figure 2

In 1502 PD, the first practical countergravity generator was developed by the Anderson Shipbuilding Corporation of New Glasgow. This had only limited applications for space travel (though it did mean cargoes could be lifted into orbit for negligible energy costs), but incalculable ones for planetary transport industries, rendering rail, road, and oceanic transport of bulk cargoes obsolete overnight. In 1581 PD, however, Dr. Ignatius Peterson, building on the work of the Anderson Corporation, Dr. Warshawski, and Dr. Radhakrishnan, mated countergrav technology with that of the impeller drive and created the first generator with sufficiently precise incremental control to produce an internal gravity field for a ship, thus permitting vessels with inertial compensators to be designed with a permanent up/down orientation. This proved a tremendous boon to long-haul starships, for it had always been difficult to design centrifugal spin sections into Warshawski Sail hyperships. Now that was no longer necessary. In addition, the decreased energy costs to transfer cargo in and out of a gravity well, coupled with the low energy and mass costs of the Warshawski sail itself *and* the greatly decreased risks of dimensional and grav shear, interstellar shipment of bulk cargo became a practical reality. In point of fact, on a per-ton basis, interstellar freight can be moved more cheaply than by any other form of transport in history.

By 1790 PD, the latest generation Warshawskis could detect grav wave fronts at ranges of up to just over twenty light-seconds. A hundred years later (the time of our story) the range is up to eight light-minutes for grav wave detection and 240 light-seconds (4 light-minutes) for turbulence detection. As a result, 20th Century PD military starships routinely operate as high as the theta band of hyper-space. This translates an actual velocity of .6 *c* to an apparent velocity of something like 3,000 *c*. The explored hyper bands and their bleed-off factors and speed multipliers over normal-space are given in Figure 3.

In addition to his inertial compensator, Dr. Radhakrishnan also enjoys the credit for being the first to develop the math to predict and detect wormhole junctions, although the first was not actually detected until 1447 PD, many years after his death. The mechanism of the junction is still imperfectly understood, but for all intents and purposes a junction is a "gravity fault," or a gravitic distortion so powerful as to fold *hyper-space* and breach the interface between it and normal-space. The result is a direct point-to-point congruence between points in normal-space which are seldom separated by less than 100 light-years and may be separated by several thousand. A hyper drive is required to utilize them, and ships cannot maintain stability or course control through a wormhole junction without Warshawski Sails. Nonetheless, the movement from normal-space to normal-space is effectively instantaneous, regardless of the distance traversed, and the energy cost is negligible.

The use of the junctions required the evolution of a new six-dimensional math, but the effort was well worthwhile, particularly since a single wormhole junction may have several different termini.

Band	Translation Bleed-Off	Velocity Multiplier	Effective Times *C* Warship	Effective Times *C* Merchant
Alpha	92%	62	37.2	31.0
Beta	85%	767	460.2	383.5
Gamma	78%	1,473	883.8	736.5
Delta	72%	2,178	1,306.8	1,089.0
Epsilon	66%	2,884	1,730.4	1,442.0*
Zeta	61%	3,589	2,153.4	1,794.5*
Eta	56%	4,294	2,576.4	2,147.0*
Theta	52%	5,000	3,000.0	2,500.0*
Iota	48%	6,000	currently unattainable	

*Merchantmen do not normally use these bands. This represents maximum theoretical speed for them if they *did*. Q-Ships and merchant cruisers with reworked drives and compensators sometimes can reach these bands.

Figure 3

Wormholes remain extremely rare phenomena, and astrophysicists continue to debate many aspects of the theories which describe them. No one has yet proposed a technique to mathematically predict the destinations of any given wormhole with reliable accuracy, but work on better models continues. At the present, mathematics can generally predict the total number of termini a wormhole will possess, but the locations of those termini cannot be ascertained without a surveying transit, and such first transits remain very tricky and dangerous.

There are other ambiguities in the current understanding of wormholes, as well. In theory, for example, one should be able to go from any terminus of a wormhole junction directly to any other. In fact, one may go from the central nexus of the junction to any of its other termini and vice versa but cannot reach any secondary terminus from another secondary. That is, one might go from point A to points B, C, or D but could not go from B to C or D without returning to A and reorienting one's vessel.

Despite their incompletely understood nature, the junctions opened a whole new aspect of FTL travel and became focusing points or funnels for trade. There were not many of them, and one certainly could not use them to travel directly to any star not connected to them, but one *could* move from any star within a few dozen light years of a wormhole terminus to the terminus then jump instantly three or four hundred light-years in the direction of one's final destination with a tremendous overall savings in transit time.

In addition, of course, the discovery of wormhole

junctions and a technique for their use imposed an entirely new pattern on the ongoing Diaspora. Theretofore, expansion had been roughly spherical, spreading out from the center in an irregular but recognizable globular pattern. Thereafter, expansion became far more ragged as wormhole junctions gave virtually instantaneous access to far distant reaches of space. Moreover, wormhole junctions are primarily associated with mid-range main sequence stars (F, G, and K), which gives a high probability of finding habitable planets in relatively close proximity to their far termini.

Once initial access to the far end of a wormhole junction had been attained, the habitable world at the far end (if there was one) tended to act as the central focus for its own "mini-Diaspora," creating globular quadrants of explored space which might be light-centuries away from the next closest explored star system.

(2) Warshawski Sail Logistics

By their very natures, the impeller drive and Warshawski Sail had a tremendous impact on the size of spacecraft. With the advent of the impeller drive, mass as such ceased to be a major consideration for sublight travel. With the introduction of the Warshawski Sail, the same became true for starships, as well. In consequence, bulk cargo carriers are entirely practical. Transport of interplanetary or interstellar cargoes is actually cheaper than surface or atmospheric transportation (even with countergrav transporters), though even at 1,200 *c* (the speed of an average bulk carrier) hauling a cargo 300 light-years takes 2.4 months. It is thus possible to transport even such bulk items as raw ore or food stuffs profitably over interstellar distances.

By the same token, this mass-carrying capability means interstellar military operations, including planetary invasions and occupations, are entirely practical. A starship represents a prodigious initial investment (more because of its size than any other factor), but it will last almost forever, its operational costs are low, and a ship which can be configured to carry livestock and farm equipment can also be configured to carry assault troops and armored vehicles.

Hyperships come in three basic categories: the low-speed bulk carrier; the high-speed personnel carrier; and warships.

The maximum acceleration and responsiveness of a Warshawski Sail starship is dependent upon the power or "grab value" of its sails and the efficiency of its inertial compensator. The more powerful (and massive) the sail generator, the greater the efficiency with which it can utilize the power of the grav wave; the more efficient the compensator, the higher the acceleration its crew can endure. Moreover, it requires an extraordinarily powerful sail, relative to the mass of the mounting ship, to endure the violent conditions of the upper hyper bands. This means that larger ships, with the hull volume to devote to really powerful sails, have greater inherent power and maximum theoretical average velocities (transit times) because they ought to be able to pull more acceleration from a given grav wave (thus reaching their optimum velocity of .6 *c* more rapidly) and to access the higher hyper bands (where the "shorter" distances effectively multiply their .6 *c* constant velocity by a quite preposterous factor).

There are, however, offsetting factors. The more powerful a Warshawski Sail, the slower its response time in realigning to a shift in the grav wave. This is potentially disastrous, but is, once more, offset to some extent by the ability of the more powerful sail to withstand greater stress. That is, it isn't as necessary to the starship's survival that it be able to reset or trim a sail to survive fluctuations in the grav wave about it. Put another way, a bigger ship with more powerful generators can "carry more sail" under given grav wave conditions than a smaller vessel and, all other things being equal, run the smaller vessel down.

But, of course, things aren't quite that simple. For starters, a smaller, less massive vessel gains more drive from the same sail strength. Because it is less massive, it accelerates more quickly for the same power. And the inertial compensator, marvelous as it may be, becomes more effective as its field area grows smaller and the mounting vessel's mass decreases, which means that a smaller ship can take advantage of its acceleration advantage over a larger vessel riding the same grav wave (and hence having access to the same "inertia sump") without killing its crew. If the smaller vessel can accelerate to .6 *c* (the highest survivable speed in hyperspace) before the larger ship, the larger ship's theoretical speed advantage is meaningless, as it can never overhaul. Under extreme grav wave conditions, the larger ship can maintain a greater effective acceleration, compensator or no, because the smaller ship's lighter sails are forced to "reef" (reduce their "grab factor") lest their generators burn out. This is particularly true in and above the zeta band, and few merchant ships ever venture that high. Even fairly small warships tend to have extremely powerful sails for their displacement, so that they can reach those higher bands, but smaller ships are simply unable to match the mass of a large ship's sail generators. This means that in some circumstances the larger ship can climb higher in the hyper bands and/or derive sufficiently more usable drive from a grav wave to offset its lower compensator efficiency.

In addition, smaller ships with less powerful sails can trim them much more rapidly and with greater precision. In wet-navy terms, smaller ships tend to be "quicker in the stays," able to adjust course with much greater rapidity and to take the maximum advantage of the power available to them from a given sail force. This means that a smaller ship with an aggressive sail handler for a captain can actually turn in a faster passage time over *most* hyper voyages than a bigger ship. There are, however, some passages (known to starship crews as "the Roaring Deeps") where exceptionally powerful, exceptionally steady grav waves operate. In these regions, the bigger ship, with its more powerful sails, is able to make full use of its theoretical advantages and will routinely run down smaller vessels.

In *sublight* movement, the larger vessel's more powerful sails (which equate to a more powerful impeller drive, as well) *do not* give it a speed advantage because of the nature of the inertial compensator. The curve of the compensator's most efficient operation means that a smaller vessel (with a smaller area to enclose in its compensator field) can pull substantially higher accelerations, and no amount of brute impeller power can create an *artificial* grav wave with a sufficiently deep inertial sump to overcome this fundamental disadvantage of a large ship. Capital ships thus are as fast as lighter warships in *sustained* flight but tend to be slower to accelerate or decelerate.

The tuning or trimming components of a Warshawski Sail generator are its most expensive and quickest wearing parts, and they wear out much more rapidly on more powerful generators with their higher designed power loads. Because of this, bulk carriers tend to use relatively low-powered sails and the lower hyper bands, which limits their practical speeds to perhaps 1,000-1,500 c. Passenger ships and those vessels specializing in transport of critical cargoes accept the higher overhead cost associated with more powerful sails and run in the range of 1,500-2,000 c. For the most part (though there are exceptions) only warships are designed around the most powerful sails and compensators their displacement will permit, giving speeds of up to 3,000 c. A bulk carrier's tuning components may last as long as fifty years between replacements and those of a passenger ship up to twenty years, but a warship is likely to require complete tuner overhaul and replacement as frequently as once every eight to ten years. On the other hand, a warship may spend decades "laid up" in orbit, making no demands at all upon its sails, so the actual life span of a given set of tuners may vary widely between ships of the same class, depending upon their employment history.

(3) The Mechanics of the Diaspora

It was discovered early in the Diaspora that the maximum practical safe speed for a sublight ship was approximately .8 *c*, as radiation and particle shields can not protect the vessel above that velocity.

The generation ships were built as complete, life-sustaining habitats oriented around the smallest practical self-sustaining population and designed to boost to that velocity at one gravity. In the long term, onboard gravity was provided through centrifugal force. In addition to their human passengers, the generation ships also had to provide for all terrestrial livestock and plants which would be required to terraform the colonists' new home for their survival. Even aboard these huge ships, space was severely limited, and many early colonial expeditions reached their destinations only to come to grief through the lack of some essential commodity the settlers had not known to bring along. This sort of disaster became less common after about 800 PD, when the original, crude hyperships made it possible to conduct extensive surveys of potential colony sites before the slower colony ships departed, but by that time the generation ships were a thing of the past, anyway.

In 305 PD, cryogenic hibernation finally became practical. It had long been possible to cryogenically preserve limbs and organs, though even the best anti-crystallization procedures then available were unable to prevent some damage to the preserved tissues. But where minor damage to an arm or a liver was acceptable, damage to a brain was not, and the early cryogenic pioneers' enthusiastic predictions about indefinite suspension of the life processes had proven chimerical.

It was Doctor Cadwaller Pineau of Tulane University who, in 305, finally cut the Gordian knot of cryogenic hibernation by going around the crystallization problem. He found that by lowering the hibernator's temperature to just barely above the freezing point he could maintain the physiological processes indefinitely at about a 1:100 time ratio. In other words, a hibernating human would age approximately one year for every century of hibernation, and his nutritional and oxygen requirements were reduced proportionately. Over the next several decades, Pineau and his associates further refined his process, working to overcome the problem of muscular atrophy and other physiological difficulties associated with long comatose periods, and eventually determined that optimum results required a hibernating individual to rouse and exercise for approximately one month in every sixty years (ie., after six physiological months), which remained a fixed requirement throughout the cryogenic colonization era.

What this meant was that the life support capabilities of a cryo ship could be vastly reduced in comparison to those of a generation ship. Moving at .8 c, the colonists experienced a 60% time dilation effect; in other words, each sixty-year period of hibernation used up one century of voyage time by the standards of the remainder of the universe. Thus an entire one-century voyage could be made without a single "active" period and would consume only 7.2 apparent months of the traveler's life span. Longer voyages would require periodic awakenings, but they could be staggered, permitting the currently roused crew to use only a fraction of the life support the entire crew would require. The result was to permit far larger numbers of colonists to travel on a given sized ship with a far lower subjective time passage.

A further boost to colonization came about in 725 PD with the advent of the first hyper drive. The casualty rates among early hyperships were so severe that it took a rather daredevil mentality to go aboard one, and colonists weren't normally noted for that sort of personality. To claim a new home world they would take risks, yes, but not risks they could avoid.

But what the hyperships provided was a survey vehicle which could travel more than sixty times as fast as a sublight ship, and the people who went in for discovering and exploring (as opposed to settling) new worlds had just the sorts of mentalities to risk hyper travel. A situation thus arose in which survey ships, generally operated by private corporations, undertook the high-risk job of locating potential colony sites which were then auctioned to prospective colony expeditions. Even with the hyper drive, this required that everyone involved take a very long view of things, but humanity adjusted to that just as it had once adjusted to the novelty of instant communication to any point on a single planet.

It is believed that the first Warshawski Sail colony ship was the *Icarus*, which departed Old Earth on September 9, 1284 PD, under the command of Captain Melissa Andropov (and, despite its name, provided over two centuries of dependable, reliable service before it was finally scrapped in 1491 PD), but for well over five hundred years, the dichotomy of FTL hypership survey expeditions and sublight hibernation colony transports remained the standard.

When the transition finally occurred, there were several very unfortunate instances in which unscrupulous operators used the new hyper sail technology to pass hibernation ships en route to their new homes. When the original colonists arrived, it was only to find well-established (and armed) claim-jumpers already squatting on their planned home worlds. If there was an already established colony in the vicinity, it might take a hand to assist the original colonists, even to the extent of lending military aid to eject the claim-jumpers, in order to discourage such unsavory elements from ruining the neighborhood. If there was no such well-inclined planet in the vicinity, the original colonists were out of luck, particularly since their technology might be several centuries less advanced than that of the thieves they confronted. In some cases, this created a domino effect. Expeditions which found themselves dispossessed of their colony sites often lacked the resources to return whence they had come (even if they had the inclination) and many opted to risk settling an unsurveyed world if there were stars with habitable planets (or which were likely to have such planets) in the vicinity. Many of them came to grief as the old generation ship colonies had in attempting to settle worlds other than the ones they had planned their original expedition's equipment list to meet, and those which did not often wound up displacing yet another group of legitimate colonists. Other such instances ended far more happily, with the second group of settlers discovering a world which was already partly settled and a group of "squatters" who paid their own way with the improvements they had already made and were integrated peaceably into the ranks of the "legitimate" colonists.

With the advent of *Icarus* and her later sisters, however, the entire pattern of colonization shifted. It was now possible to make a 500 light-year voyage in barely two-and-a-half years, an interval which dropped steadily as improvements in Warshawski technology became available. Hibernation was still used on most colony ships, but now it was simply to cram in the largest possible number of passengers, not a necessity. Indeed, as higher and higher speeds became possible, the hibernation features began to fall by the wayside.

(4) The Star Kingdom of Manticore
(A) FOUNDING AND EARLY HISTORY

The original colony expedition to Manticore departed Old Earth on October 24, 775 PD, aboard the sublight hibernation ship *Jason* for the Manticore Binary. Manticore, approximately 512 light-years from Earth, was a G0/G2 distant binary first confirmed to have planets in 562 PD, by the astronomer Sir Frederick Clarke. Its distance from Sol was such that the voyage would take 640.5 years (just over 384 subjective years), requiring that each colonist be waked for exercise seven times. Accordingly, the colonists were investing about 4.5 years of their lives (and all of their money) in the voyage.

Sixty percent of the colonists were Western Europeans, with most of the remainder drawn from the North American Federation, the Caribbean, and a very small minority of ethnic Ukrainians. The total expedition consisted of 38,000 adults and 13,000 minor children, and the "rights" to the system had been purchased at auction from the survey firm of Franchot et Fils, Paris, France, Old Earth. "FF" (as it was known) had a high reputation, and its survey ship *Suffren* had made the same voyage in just twenty years. *Suffren*'s crew had done FF's usual, professional job, although, of course, all data was accompanied by the caution that it would be 650 years out of date when the colonists arrived, and FF sold its rights in the Manticore System to the Manticore Colony, Ltd., for approximately 5.75 billion EuroDollars. As part of the transfer of rights, FF expunged all data on the system from its memory banks, transferring the information to the Federal Government of Earth's World Data Bank's maximum security files. This was a standard safeguard to protect Manticore Colony against the occupation of the planet by later expeditions with faster ships, as it was already apparent that advances in hyper travel might well make such protection necessary, yet it was also recognized that there was no way to guarantee that faster, more capable hyperships would not beat the colonists to Manticore. Accordingly, Roger Winton, President and CEO of Manticore Colony (already elected first Planetary Administrator) opted to establish the Manticore Colony Trust of Zurich.

The MCT's purpose was to invest all capital remaining to the MC after mounting the expedition (something under one billion EuroDollars) and use the accrued interest to watch over the colonists' rights to their new home. It was a wise precaution, for when *Jason* finally arrived in the Manticore System on March 21, 1416 PD, her crew discovered a modest settlement on the planet they christened Manticore, but it was staffed by MCT personnel who also manned the four small Earth-built frigates protecting the system against claim-jumpers. Indeed, so well had the Trust done in the last six centuries that Manticore found itself with a very favorable bank balance, and the frigates became the first units of the Manticoran System Navy (later the Royal Manticoran Navy). Moreover, the small MCT presence on Manticore included data banks and carefully selected instructors assigned to update the colonists on the technical advances of the last six centuries. This last was a feature even Winton had not anticipated, and he had very good reason to be pleased both with his own decision and the diligence, foresight, and imagination with which a succession of MCT managers had discharged their duties.

It was as well that the colony had such unusual support and off-world financial strength, however, for after almost forty years in which things went perfectly, disaster struck Manticore in 1454.

The initial bid for Manticore had been so high for two reasons. One was that the G0/G2 binary was highly unusual—indeed, unique—in having no less than three planets suitable for human life. The second was that Manticore and Sphinx, the two Earth-like planets orbiting the G0 stellar component, were extremely Earth-like. Although each had its own unique biosphere, survey reports indicated that terrestrial life forms would find it unusually easy to adapt to all three, and so, indeed, it proved. Terran food crops did well, and while the local flora and fauna could not provide all essential dietary elements, much of it was digestible by the terrestrial visitors. Terraforming requirements thus were extraordinarily modest, consisting of little more than the need to seed food crops and selected terrestrial grasses to support imported herbivores. Unfortunately, that very ease of adaptation had a darker side, and Manticore proved one of the very few extra-terrestrial systems to possess microorganisms which could (and did) prey on humans.

The culprit was a virus—or, rather, a small family of viruses—which had been missed by the original survey team. Some virologists argue that it was not, in fact, missed but rather evolved in the six centuries between the initial survey and the arrival of the colonists. Still others suggest that it was actually the mutated descendant of a virus the colonists had brought with them from Old Earth. Whatever the truth of the matter, the virus was deadly, producing a condition analogous to virulent influenza and pneumonia simultaneously in its victims. Worse, it proved resistant to all existing medical technology, and ten years were to pass before a successful vaccine was found.

In that decade, almost sixty percent of the original colonists died. Their Manticore-born children fared better against the disease, experiencing a generally less violent manifestation of it, yet without the cushion provided by the MCT funds on Old Earth and the evolution of the Warshawski Sail hypership, the entire expedition would no doubt have come to grief.

As it was, the colony found itself in urgent need of additional homesteaders. These were recruited from Old Earth (yet another process made much easier by the existence of the MCT), but the original colonists, concerned about retaining control of their own colony, adopted a radically new constitution before opening their doors to emigration.

Roger Winton had been reelected continuously to the post of Planetary Administrator, serving superbly in the position throughout the early settlement period and the plague crisis. He was now an old man (over eighty) whose wife and two Terra-born sons had died of the plague, but he remained vigorous and his Manticore-born daughter Elizabeth showed promise at least equal to his. At fifty-three, she was President of the Board of Directors (effectively vice-president of the colony) and one of Manticore's preeminent jurists. Since she had a large and thriving brood of second-generation Manticoran children and her family had served so outstandingly, a convention of colony shareholders converted the Corporation's elective board into a constitutional monarchy and crowned Roger Winton King Roger of Manticore on August 1, 1471.

It was a post he was to enjoy for only three years before his death, but his daughter succeeded him as Elizabeth I in a smooth and popular transfer of power, and the House of Winton has ruled the Star Kingdom of Manticore ever since. Simultaneously, the surviving "First Shareholders" and their descendants, who held title to vast tracts of land (including most of the richest mineral resources of Manticore and Sphinx) and/or to extra-planetary resources in the Manticore System, acquired patents of nobility to go with their wealth, and the hereditary aristocracy of Manticore was born.

The new wave of immigrants arriving in the wake of the Plague comprised three distinct classes of citizen. Each immigrant received a credit whose value precisely equaled the cost of a second-class passenger ticket from the Solarian League to Manticore. That credit could be converted, at the holder's option, into a land credit on a planetary surface or into a share of equivalent value in any of several orbital and deep space industrial concerns. Most of the new immigrants, faced with virgin planets on which to live, opted for homestead rights there, although some of the sharpest among them made careful investments in the Star Kingdom's industrial infrastructure which later proved of enormous worth, instead.

Any individual capable of paying his own passage received the full credit upon arrival, whereas those incapable of paying their passage could draw upon MCT for a dollar amount equal to their credit to cover the difference between their own resources and the cost of passage. In addition, an immigrant whose resources were greater than the cost of his passage could invest the surplus, paying 50% of the "book" price for additional land and/or investment. The most affluent immigrants thus became "Second Shareholders," with estates (whether in terms of land or industrial wealth) which, in some cases, rivaled those of the original shareholders and entitled them to patents of nobility junior to those of the existing aristocracy. Those immigrants who were able to retain their base land right or perhaps enlarge upon it slightly became "yeomen," free landholders with voting rights beginning one Manticoran year (1.73 Terran Standard Years) after their arrival. Those who completely exhausted their credit to buy passage to Manticore were known as "zero-balance" immigrants and did not become full citizens until such time as they had become well-enough established to pay taxes for five consecutive Manticoran years (8.7 Terran Standard Years). While all Manticoran subjects are equal in the eyes of the law, whether enfranchised to vote or not, there were distinct social differences between shareholders, yeomen, and zero-balancers, and even today there is greater prestige in claiming a yeoman as a first ancestor than in claiming a zero-balance ancestor. And, of course, direct descent from a full shareholder is the most prestigious of all.

The constitutional system prospered over the next five hundred years, blessed by a series of strong monarchs and a steadily growing population base. The constitution contains a strong "Declaration of Fundamental Rights," but the franchise is limited to citizens who have paid taxes for at least five consecutive years. (The policies encouraging emigration with credits were ended after a period of fifty years, having served their purpose most effectively, and it is no longer possible for an immigrant to become an instant shareholder or gain the franchise immediately upon arrival.)

The Constitution created a two-house Parliament, a Royal Council, and a Crown Judiciary. The Parliament consists of a House of Lords and a House of Commons with mutual veto power, and the Crown has the rights of both initiation and veto. According to some constitutional scholars (though not all, by any means), the Framers intended for the executive power to be exercised by the Royal Council, which, by law, consists of the Prime Minister, his subordinate executive ministers, and certain hereditary members, such as the Keeper of the Seal, the heir to the throne (as a nonvoting member), and the monarch. In fact, however, the Royal Council, now commonly referred to as the Cabinet, became the instrument through which the monarch acts as head of Government as well as head of State. Although the Prime Minister, who (traditionally) is from the House of Lords but must be able to command a majority in the Commons, manages the Cabinet, he may be dismissed by the King or Queen at will and acts in most ways as the monarch's executive officer. At the same time, it is only a foolish monarch who capriciously or willfully ignores the advice of his or her ministers and, especially, *prime* minister.

The Crown retains the power to pardon and commute, appoints ministers and judges with the advice and consent of the House of Lords, and, unless overruled by a majority in both houses, possesses the power to interpret constitutional law through its appointees to the King's (or Queen's) Bench. The Crown cannot, however, create new peers without the consent of a majority of the House of Commons.

In cases of disagreement between the Crown and both houses of Parliament, the Lords serve as the supreme judiciary without right of veto by Crown or Commons. The strongest safeguards of the common population lie in (1) the Commons' power to approve or disapprove budgets, (2) the Constitutional requirement that the Prime Minister command a majority in the Commons, and (3) the right to remove the monarch.

It is up to the Crown (actually, the Cabinet), and not the Commons, to initiate economic policy and propose budgets, and the Crown has an additional discretionary fund drawn from the extensive Crown lands and industrial holdings, but the Crown and Lords both know that they cannot long defy the Commons if the lower house decides to withhold budget approval. The fact that the Prime Minister, although serving at the Crown's pleasure, must also be able to poll a majority in the House of Commons (a similar majority in the House of Lords is *not* a constitutional requirement, although most PMs who cannot generally resign their office), also helps to insure that the viewpoint of the Star Kingdom's commoners will always be heard at the highest level. Finally, the Manticoran monarchy is one of the very few hereditary forms of government with a specific provision for the removal of a monarch for reasons other than incapacitation or criminal action. A monarch may be impeached *for any reason*, including but not limited to "high crimes and misdemeanors," by a two-thirds majority vote of the House of Commons. Impeachment proceedings may not begin in the House of Lords, and a three-quarters vote of both houses is required to actually remove a monarch. Although this constitutional provision has never been used and is now regarded by many constitutional authorities as a vestigial holdover from pre-monarchy days, it has never been removed, and the possibility of its exercise remains.

As a final safeguard intended to prevent the monarchy from losing touch with the non-aristocratic majority of the Star Kingdom's population, Roger I and Elizabeth I insisted that the Constitution include one additional provision. The heir to the throne is required by law to marry a commoner. Other members of the royal family may marry whomever they wish, but the Crown Prince or Crown Princess must marry outside the aristocracy.

The only real challenge to the Manticoran monarchy came in 1721 PD in the so-called "Gryphon Uprising," which remains the most internal excitement the Star Kingdom has been forced to confront. Gryphon, the least congenial of the three habitable planets of the Manticore System, has by far the smallest share of First Shareholder families, as its first outpost was not placed until fifteen years after the Plague. The bulk of its aristocracy came from the Second Shareholders, who, for the most part, had substantially less credit than First Shareholders and, accordingly, received smaller "Clear Grants" (that is, land to which clear title was granted prior to improvements by the owner/tenant). The Crown, however, had established the principle of "Crown Range" (land in the public domain and free for the use of any individual) to encourage emigration to Gryphon, and by 1715, the population of Gryphon had grown to the level set under the Crown Range Charter of 1490. At that point, as the charter required, the Crown began phasing out the Crown Range, granting title on the basis of improvements made, and the trouble began. Yeomen who hoped to become independent ranchers, farmers, or miners claimed that the planetary nobility was using strong-arm tactics to force them off the land—indeed, something very like a shooting war erupted between "squatters" and "the children of shareholders," and after two years of increasingly bloody unrest, a special commission was established with extraordinary police powers and a mandate to suppress the violence and reach a settlement.

The Gryphon Range Commission's final finding was that there was sound foundation to the yeomen's original complaints, and the Manticoran Army, having pacified and stabilized the situation, then oversaw a closely regulated privatization of the Crown Range. A degree of dislike between small landholders and certain of the noble families continues to this day, but it has become something of a tradition rather than a source of active hostility.

(B) MANTICORAN TIME-KEEPING:

All of the above dates are given in Terran Standard (Post Diaspora) Reckoning. Like all extra-Solar systems settled during the Diaspora of Man, the Manticore System found it necessary to create its own calendar to reflect the axial and orbital rotations of their new home, but in the Manticorans' case the situation was complicated by the fact that whereas most star systems are fortunate to have a single habitable world, their distant binary system possessed three of them, each with its own day and year.

As the rest of humanity, Manticorans use Standard Seconds, Minutes, and Hours, and Old Earth's 365.26-day year serves as the "Standard Reckoning Year," or "T-year," the common base to which local dates throughout known space are converted for convenience in dealing with inhabitants of other star systems. Like most extra-Solar polities, the Star Kingdom of Manticore's history texts follow the convention of counting years "Post Diaspora" (ie., in T-years from the year in which the first interstellar colony ship departed Old Earth) as well as in terms of the local calendar.

The Kingdom's Official Reckoning of dates is based on the rotational and orbital periods of Manticore-A III, the planet Manticore. This calendar is used for all official records, but doesn't really work very well for the seasons of any planet other than Manticore itself. Accordingly, both Sphinx (Manticore-A IV) and Gryphon (Manticore-B IV) have their own, purely local calendars, which means that a single star system routinely uses no less than four calendars (including Standard Reckoning). Needless to say, date-conversion software is incorporated in virtually every Manticoran computer.

The Kingdom's planetary days and years are:

Planet Name	Day In T-Hours	Year In Local Days	Year In T-Days	Year In T-Years
Manticore	22.45	673.31	629.83	1.73
Sphinx	25.62	1,783.28	1,903.65	5.22
Gryphon	22.71	650.46	615.51	1.69

The clocks of each planet count time in full 60-minute Standard Hours (or T-hours), with an additional, shorter "hour" called "Compensate" (or, more commonly, simply "Comp") to make up the difference. Thus the Planet Manticore's day consists of 22 hours (numbered 01:00 to 22:59) plus a 27-minute-long Comp, while Sphinx's day consists of 25 hours (numbered 01:00 to 25:59) plus a 37-minute Comp. The planetary week is seven planetary days long in each case, and Manticore's day is used aboard all Royal Navy vessels.

The official year of the Kingdom is 673 days long, with a leap year every third year. It is divided into 18 months, 11 of 37 days and 7 of 38, alternating for the first 6 and last 8 months, named (simply, if rather unimaginatively) First Month, Second Month, Third Month, etc., with a leap year (1 extra day in 4th Month) every third year. The Gryphon local year is also divided into 18 months (16 of 36 days and 2 of 37 days) with the extra days in Ninth

and Tenth and one extra day in Eleventh Month
every other local year. The Sphinxian year, however,
is divided into 46 months, 35 of 39 days and 11 of
38 days (the shorter months fall in even-numbered
months from Twelfth to Thirty-Second), with a leap
year every 7 years with an extra day in 15th Month.
All of these calendars are reckoned in "Years After
Landing" (abbreviated AL), dating from the day
(March 21, 1416 PD) the first shuttle from the
colony ship *Jason* touched down on the present-day
site of the City of Landing. Obviously, this means
that each planet's local year is a different "Year After
Landing" from any of the others. Thus Honor
Harrington's orders to *Fearless*, dated Fourth 25,
280 AL (using Official Manticoran Reckoning, or the
Manticore planetary calendar), were also written on
March 3, 1900 PD (Standard Reckoning), and on
Second 26, 93 AL (using the local Sphinxian calendar). This plethora of dates is a major reason
Manticorans tend to convert time spans into T-years
even in domestic matters.

(C) THE HOUSE OF WINTON:

Roger I .... 1471–1474 PD (32–34 AL)
Elizabeth I .... 1474–1507 PD (34–53 AL)
Michael .... 1507–1539 PD (53–72 AL)
Edward I .... 1539–1544 PD (72–74 AL)
                 (boating accident; succeeded by sister)
Elizabeth II .... 1544–1601 PD (74–107 AL)
David .... 1601–1642 PD (107–131 AL)
Roger II .... 1642–1669 PD (131–147 AL)
Adrienne .... 1669–1681 PD (147–154 AL)

William .... 1681–1690 PD (154–158 AL)
(assassinated)
William II .... 1690–1741 PD (158–188 AL)
Caitrin .... 1741–1762 PD (188–200 AL)
Samantha .... 1762–1785 PD (200–214 AL)
George .... 1785–1802 PD (214–224 AL)
Samantha II .... 1802–1857 PD (224–255 AL)
Roger III .... 1857–1883 PD (255–270 AL)
Elizabeth III .... 1883 PD–present (270 AL–present)

(D) MANTICORAN DOMESTIC POLITICS:

Manticoran political parties began as factions in the House of Lords and, in the Lords, retain much of their original factional nature.

The Constitution adopted following the Plague intended to place government primarily in the hands of the aristocracy, who would dominate the House of Lords (the senior branch of the Parliament) and the Royal Council, but things actually worked out somewhat differently. Although Roger Winton had been a very strong planetary administrator, it is improbable that the drafters of the Constitution truly intended for the Crown to acquire a firm grip on the executive authority. Elizabeth I, however, was a *very* shrewd administrator, and she quickly observed that the original Manticoran peerage comprised a group of spokesmen for competing interests rather than statesmen. By playing the interests of the various factions within the Lords off against one another, Elizabeth was able to establish (among other things) that the Prime Minister and all non-hereditary members of the Royal Council served at her pleasure. The Lords had the right to advise and consent on initial appointments, but *she* had the power to dismiss them at any time, and she could not be forced to accept anyone else's choice for any of those positions. With that principle firmly enshrined in the unwritten portion of the Star Kingdom's Constitution, Crown dominance of the government was established.

As a ruling house, the Wintons have proven extremely capable. Indeed, their only realistic competition as a dynasty has come from the Andermani Empire, and for all its undisputed accomplishments, the Anderman Dynasty has always suffered from a potentially dangerous degree of eccentricity which has never afflicted the House of Winton.

Nonetheless, it eventually dawned on the members of the peerage that the Crown had assumed (some might say usurped) much of the political power the Shareholders had intended to reserve for themselves and their children. It also occurred to them that Elizabeth had enjoyed the strong support of the House of Commons in her maneuvers, for the Commons (elected primarily by the yeomen and zero-balancers imported after the Plague) had recognized that the Constitution stacked the deck against them. In particular, the fact that both houses enjoyed the mutual power of veto but that members of the Lords need not stand for election, gave the upper house enormous leverage in any dispute between them.

Once recognition set in—and once the immediate factional squabbles of the early settlement and post-plague period had been settled—the Lords began to evolve genuine parties. For the most part, they grew up around the old personal factions, but they were also differentiated by clear ideological differences, and as they solidified, they reached out to the Commons for allies. Because of their advantages in not needing to stand for reelection, members of the aristocracy continue to head most of the political parties to this day, but they have learned the hard way to listen to the Members of Parliament from the Commons, as well. Most (though by no means all) Manticoran aristocrats have a fairly strong sense of *noblesse oblige* (those who do not are among the most self-centered and intolerant of the known universe), but without the input of their allied commoner MPs, the aristocratic leadership of any of the parties would quickly lose touch with the majority of the Star Kingdom's population and suffer for it the next time the House of Commons called a general election.

Despite this, the Star Kingdom's political parties tend to be working alliances of individuals with the same basic interests rather than closed ideological systems even today. Party discipline is often impressive when close votes must be fought through, but there is no "collectivist discipline" in the sense that a member of a party must publicly endorse and support policies with which he disagrees simply because the rest of the party does. MPs are more likely than Peers to "vote the party line," but the tradition of "voting one's conscience" is the Manticoran ideal, and most of the Star Kingdom's political parties have their own distinct "left," "right," and "center" wings.

The more powerful parties are: the Centrist Party and its normal ally the Crown Loyalists; the Liberal

Party; the Conservative Association; the Progressive Party; and the so-called "New Men" Party.

The Centrists, led by Allen Summervale, Duke of Cromarty, the current PM, are the largest single bloc, though they do not quite constitute a majority in their own right. The Centrists pursue a rather conservative domestic policy of gradualism and fiscal restraint, opposed to sweeping social changes and determined to avoid deficit spending. More importantly, they have been absolutely committed to the defense of Manticore against the growing Havenite threat for over fifty T-years, having believed that an eventual military confrontation was inevitable and should not be postponed in hopes it would go away. In particular, they believed that waiting for the Republic to weaken, however attractive it might seem, constituted a supine surrender of the initiative to their enemies and so invited long-term defeat. Moreover, unlike certain other political groups, the Centrists believe Manticore can survive open warfare with Haven and that even if they are defeated, the final cost will not be much worse than a craven surrender. It was the Centrists who supported Roger III in instigating the Star Kingdom's pre-war naval build-up and pushing through the annexation of the Basilisk System (a G5 star with a single habitable planet) to forestall Havenite occupation of the Junction terminus in that system, which was at the time a highly controversial move. Some critics saw it as the first step in a deliberate policy of imperial aggrandizement; others saw it as an unnecessary challenge to Haven which could provoke the very war they feared. The majority of Queen Elizabeth's subjects, however, supported the annexation, whatever their representatives might think. Of all the aristocratic-led parties, the Centrists have the strongest support in the Commons, which gives them an added depth that affords rather more clout than simple numbers might suggest.

The Crown Loyalists, led by Henry McShain, Marquis of New Dublin, might be thought of as Manticoran Tories. Their fundamental article of political faith is that stability and prosperity for all Manticorans depends upon the power and authority of the executive in the person of the monarch. From time to time, the Crown Loyalists differ with the current monarch on policy, but in those instances they generally seek to remonstrate in private while preserving a public front of solid support. The Crown Loyalists are extremely weak in the Commons. They are perceived, with a certain degree of justice, as the party of the great nobles, and while they are accorded great respect and deference, there is a belief (even among many Centrists) that they are insensitive to current issues, subjecting all of them to the litmus test of their effect on the Crown's authority (and the nobility's influence). Those who believe this also believe that the Loyalists will oppose any policy, however beneficial its final effects may be in other ways, if it weakens the Crown. In general, the Loyalists share the Centrist view on foreign policy, but they are even more conservative in fiscal policy (they felt prewar taxation levels were excessive) and have always had difficulty resolving their contradictory support for a strong fleet and opposition to high military spending.

The Liberal Party, headed by Marisa Turner, Countess of New Kiev, advocates humanist reform and is relatively disinterested in foreign policy. They are larger than the Crown Loyalists but smaller than the Centrists and have less numerous but extremely loyal adherents in the Commons. Although disheartened by the current state of affairs in the People's Republic of Haven, the Liberals believe that the fundamental objectives of the Havenite Declaration of Economic Rights (see The Republic of Haven, below) were laudable. In their opinion, the pre-war Legislaturalist Havenite leaders were "bad liberals" who had become prisoners of the "mobocracy" of the Haven System. Their own concern is with "bringing the Star Kingdom into the main stream of modern galactic political thought" (ie., extending and enlarging the franchise, providing relief for the indigent, equalizing income, and promoting greater popular participation in government), and they do not pay much attention to the manner in which affairs beyond the borders may impinge upon Manticore. They regarded the Centrist Party's prewar concern over Haven as alarmist, believing that however expansionist Haven's current leadership might be, it would hesitate to try conclusions with Manticore (lest it rouse the Solarian League by threatening the Manticore Wormhole Junction) and would eventually reach satiation and cease expanding. Since they preferred to increase spending on human services, they begrudged every penny spent on the fleet, which caused them to lose a great deal of public support once active hostilities with Haven broke out. Nonetheless, they continue to believe that "war never settles anything," and of all Manticoran political parties, they remain most comfortable with the official pre-war ideology of the People's Republic.

The Conservative Association, headed by Michael Janvier, Baron of High Ridge, is the smallest of the traditional political parties and might charitably be termed reactionary. It advocates an isolationist foreign policy, argues that foreign adventures are dangerous, and decries the "steady, liberalizing rot threatening Manticore with anarchy." As might be surmised, the Association is something of a crackpot group which attracts the nobles who find the Crown Loyalists entirely too permissive in defense of privilege. Indeed, they advocate return to an "original Manticoran balance of power" which never actually existed outside the imaginations of their own theorists. Although they felt the Centrists' annexation of Basilisk was an act of madness, the very sort of adventurism which could plunge Manticore into disastrous confrontation with foreign powers, Roger III and Cromarty knew they could be counted upon to support fleet appropriations, as their isolationist bent required a powerful fleet to police their borders.

The Progressive Party, headed jointly by the Earl of Gray Hill and Lady Elaine Descroix, is the third largest party and, in general, endorses many of the objectives of the Liberal Party. The Progressives share the Centrist determination to avoid deficit spending (which the Liberals see as an acceptable, temporary evil), would like to see "a better and more beneficial balance between social spending and military appropriations," and share the Liberals' distaste for foreign policy. Unlike the Liberals, they have never regarded concerns over Haven (which they see as an example of deficit-spending liberalism run berserk and corrupted by power-seeking politicos) as alarmist. On the other hand, they also felt (and, apparently, still feel) that any belief that Manticore can survive a fight to the finish with the Havenite military machine is lunacy. (Since the beginning of actual hostilities, the Progressives have been very vocally and publicly confident of Manticoran victory, but their opponents believe this is camouflage. According to this theory, the Progressive's present posture is designed to make their fear-based desire for a negotiated settlement appear to stem from their complete confidence in victory, instead.)

Because their primary concern is with domestic issues, their traditional foreign policy has always tended to be extremely simplistic, believing that "honest negotiators" can reach a live-and-let-live arrangement. Their pre-war Centrist and Loyalist critics argued, not without justification, that this really amounted to advocating that Manticore sell out the rest of the galaxy to save its own skin, a policy which must ultimately result in disaster when there is no more galaxy to sell to Haven. Yet while this may well be a not-inaccurate reading of the effect of their policy, it is unjust to argue (as their critics do) that it was their intended object. The real problem with the Progressives' foreign policy is that they simply don't think about it very much, relying on platitudes and vague beliefs rather than a reasoned analysis, which left them with no structured thought upon which to base themselves once the Havenite Wars actually began.

The "New Men" Party, led by Sir Sheridan Wallace, is a relatively new group which believes that power is far too concentrated in the hands of existing cliques of the aristocracy and wealthy merchants/industrialists. They argue that the traditional Manticoran practice of co-opting capable and ambitious individuals into those two groups is a mistake. The Centrists and Loyalists believe that co-option assures a continuous flow of new ideas into the aristocracy and financial elites in a controlled, gradualist fashion, whereas the Liberals and Progressives argue that the very concept of aristocracy is anachronistic and anti-democratic. The New Men view the practice of co-option as a deliberate, undisguised mechanism to keep control firmly in the hands of traditional power groups, which is rather Liberal-sounding—until one realizes that their problem is less that there are traditional elites than that *they* don't control them. In a very real sense, the New Men are the lesser nobility's counterweight to the Conservative Association, mounting perennial assaults on the bastions of power and entrenched privilege. Unlike the Liberals and Progressives, however, they believe that the spoils belong to the victors and are not out to overturn the system, but rather to seize the levers of power for themselves. The New Men have only the most rudimentary fiscal policy and share the Conservative Association's fundamental isolationism, yet distrust the military as one more bastion of the Powers That Be. In general, the New Men might be said to be in opposition to everyone. They enjoy the least support in the Commons of any of the major parties, but their intense party discipline puts Wallace in a position to reliably deliver an organized block of votes essentially at will. This, coupled with his readiness to make deals with anyone on a purely pragmatic basis, gives him much more power within Parliament than simple numbers might suggest.

In addition to the parties listed above, there are several small, *ad hoc* factions which come and go, generally focused around a single charismatic leader. The real power struggle is between the Centrist/Crown Loyalist alliance and the Liberal/Progressive Alliance, with the former holding a slight edge in the Lords and a larger one in the Commons. The Liberals and Progressives tend to be allied on a stronger, deeper, and more permanent basis than the Centrists and Loyalists, helped by the fact that both of them regard foreign policy as a distraction from the real concerns of the day. The Centrists and Loyalists often find themselves divided over particular points of domestic policy, but maintain a fairly united front on foreign policy and military preparedness. Both enjoy the support of the Crown, which is a decided plus, though the Loyalists remain far from convinced of the wisdom of the Centrists' pre-war willingness to accept (some would say court) a confrontation with Haven. Traditionally, the Conservative Association has helped tilt the balance in favor of the two Crown parties because of its insistence on maintaining a powerful fleet, but the potential has always existed for the Association to strike a deal with the Liberals and Progressives on foreign policy, although the fundamental antipathy of their domestic policy positions makes it unlikely an alliance between them could last. The real joker in the deck is the "New Men." For all their relatively small numbers, they are concentrated in the Lords, where the Centrist/Crown Loyalist majority is thinnest. No one in any party believes that the New Men could work indefinitely with the Liberals or Progressives, whose domestic policy is fundamentally at odds with their own, but the possibility of a temporary alliance to break the "stranglehold" of the Centrist/Crown Loyalist group is not at all out of the question. It would be a cynical marriage of convenience on both sides, probably with the tacit understanding that once their common foes had been smitten hip and thigh the Liberals, Progressives and New Men would fight it out to a conclusion, and the real fear of Duke Cromarty and his inner circle is that the New Men may decide the Liberals and Progressives are so evenly matched that, once the "entrenched power brokers" have been toppled, the New Men would find themselves in a position to control the outcome by choosing whom to support.

(4) The Manticoran Wormhole Junction
(A) GENERAL WORMHOLE MECHANICS:

Wormhole junctions consist of a central wormhole (referred to as the "wormhole nexus") and its associated termini (referred to as "secondary termini"). The nexus is connected to each terminus by a unique pattern of gravity waves, one pattern outbound and one inbound, normally referred to as the "terminus route." Each junction has an absolute tonnage ceiling, the maximum mass which can be put through any given terminus (including the central nexus) simultaneously, but the limit applies individually to each terminus route.

Traffic may be routed from the central nexus to any terminus and from any terminus to the central nexus, but direct routing between secondary termini is impossible. The tonnage limit can be moved simultaneously over different terminus routes.

Each time a vessel or vessels move along a given terminus route, the route "destabilizes" for a brief period, during which it cannot be used by other vessels, and the destabilization time is proportional to the mass being moved along the route. Thus the more massive the transit (ie., the larger the number of vessels involved) the longer it is destabilized.

The central nexus is thus the most flexible but, in a sense, the most vulnerable (militarily speaking) of the junction termini. It may dispatch an assault force equal to its tonnage limit to any or all of its secondary termini virtually simultaneously, but will then be unable to send reinforcements until the route(s) used stabilize once more. By the same token, an adversary in possession of two or more secondary termini of the same junction may use each of the termini it controls to send the full tonnage limit of warships into the central nexus. Hence the Star Kingdom of Manticore's extreme sensitivity to the possibility that any hostile power (such as the People's Republic of Haven) might obtain control of more than one terminus of the Manticore Junction.

(B) THE MANTICORE JUNCTION:

The Manticore Wormhole Junction was discovered in 1585 PD (98 AL). The Manticore Junction lies 412 LM from Manticore A and has the distinction of being the largest so far discovered, connecting to no less than five other star systems: Sigma Draconis (Solarian League), Gregor (Anderman Empire), Trevor's Star (People's Republic of Haven), Phoenix (Phoenix Cluster), and the most recently discovered (1856 PD/254 AL) Basilisk System. In addition, the Star Kingdom's astrophysicists are currently working with the latest survey data in the belief that the junction connects to at least one and possibly more additional termini which have yet to be isolated.

The wormhole junction has been a bonanza for the Manticoran economy, attracting a huge concentration of shipping. Unfortunately, it has also made the kingdom a player, will it or won't it, on the galactic stage, as the imperialistic and military implications of the junction are quite clear to all concerned. For obvious reasons, the Navy budget has received considerable attention in the last 50-odd T-years, and the kingdom has laid claim to its first extra-system planet (Medusa, a thoroughly unpleasant, marginally habitable planet in the Basilisk System) to safeguard that terminus of the junction. (Prior to 1901 PD, Manticoran diplomats took great care to avoid saying just whom they were safeguarding it against, but Basilisk's relative proximity to the People's Republic of Haven made that fairly clear, and there is reason to believe the Kingdom got away with the annexation so easily only because Haven was occupied with other matters when the Basilisk terminus was first discovered.) As Medusa is inhabited by a sapient alien species, this embroiled the kingdom in questions of aboriginal rights and protection, and the increasing pressure of Havenite "merchants" there for "legitimate trade with the natives" (who have very little worth trading) further complicated an already complex situation.

(5) Planets of the Star Kingdom of Manticore

MANTICORE: (Manticore-A III) The capital planet of the Star Kingdom, Manticore's diameter is approximately 13,500 km., with a hydrosphere of 76% and an axial tilt of 5°. This planet is slightly less dense than Earth, with a lower percentage of

metals, but still boasts considerable mineral wealth.
Average temperatures are close to Earth normal, and
the climate is considerably moderated by the lower
axial tilt.

Major Manticoran on-planet industries are agri-
culture, aquaculture, mining, and a well-diversified
industrial sector and R&D base. Population as of
1900 PD (280 AL) was approximately 1.5 billion. The
major shipyards and space industry of the Star Kingdom of Manticore orbit the capital planet.

SPHINX: Sphinx (Manticore-A IV) is larger than
Manticore (diameter=16,500 km.) It is also more
massive and richer in metals than the capital world.
Sphinx is habitable only because an extremely active
carbon dioxide cycle effectively extends the liquid-
water zone by giving it considerably more "green
house" effect than its sister planets, and its hydrosphere is 68% with an axial tilt of 14°, which,
coupled with its considerably lower average temperatures, gives it a much more active and less
inviting climate than Manticore.

The major on-planet industries of Sphinx are mining, forestry, and animal husbandry (the planet has
vast herds of Terran-adapted cattle and native
prongbuck). Planet-side industry has been slow to
develop but has made considerable ground in the
last century. Planetary population as of 1900 PD was
1,048,000,000.

GRYPHON: With a diameter of 13,200 km.,
Gryphon (Manticore-B IV) is actually the most
Earth-like (in terms of size and mass) of Manticore's

three habitable planets, but its hydrosphere is only 51% and its axial tilt is almost 27°. Coupled with its orbital radius (it is almost as far from the cooler Manticore B as Manticore is from Manticore A), this gives it a rugged "continental" climate with extremely cold winters and (relatively speaking) scorching summers. The planetary biosystem is also the least Earth-like of the Star Kingdom's habitable worlds, and the colony's original cattle did not do well there, but a genetically-engineered variant of the Plains Buffalo, imported from Beowulf (Sigma Draconis) in 1612 PD (113 AL), adapted with phenomenal success, and two of the Star Kingdom's major exports to the older planets are buffalo hides and meat. In addition, the Gryphon Kodiak Maximus provides one of the known galaxy's premiere peltries, though the Manticore Charter of Settlement requires that a relatively low ceiling be placed on the pelts taken.

Gryphon is poor in metals (relative to Manticore or Sphinx), and developed planet-side industry is primarily agrarian. Its severe climate has made this planet the last choice for colonization within the system, but, by the same token, this means it has the largest unclaimed areas (particularly with its limited hydrosphere), and it has tended to attract the more adventurous of the last two or three generations, giving it a particularly vigorous population. In addition, it actually has more *total* industry than Sphinx, despite its limited planetary supply of metals, because of Manticore-B's extensive asteroid belts. The Unicorn Belt's asteroid extraction operations (dominated by the Hauptman Cartel's Gryphon

Minerals, LTD., subsidiary) produce the lion's share of the Star Kingdom's raw ores, and most Gryphons who don't want to herd buffalo end up employed in one part or another of their planet's sprawling near-space industrial activities. Perhaps because of this space-going orientation, Gryphon provides a quite disproportionate percentage of the Royal Manticoran Navy's personnel. Indeed, the backbone of the RMN's petty officers come from Gryphon and seem to feel a divine mission to keep the sissies of Manticore-A in shape.

As of 1900 PD, Gryphon had a planetary population of 575,000,000 and a belter population of 298,500,000.

(6) Interstellar Politics and Imperialism
(A) EMERGENCE OF MULTI-SYSTEM POLITIES:

Before the introduction of the Warshawski Sail, interstellar trade and warfare were impossible. The only practical uses for hyperships were those with a sufficiently valuable return to justify the high risk of the vessel's loss—i.e., survey work—which was carried out not by planetary or system governments but by private corporations, most based on Old Earth or the very oldest colony worlds, who paid their crews of specialists handsomely indeed. With his or her high salary pre-paid and invested throughout the duration of his voyage, a survey specialist could retire to a life of wealth after a single cruise, though there was never any real shortage of repeat surveyors. The lure of the unknown and the lust to explore produced survey crewmen who pressed their luck again and again—in many cases until it finally ran out—and the frontiers of explored space were pushed steadily back despite the casualties.

Nonetheless, the repeat voyages which would make an interstellar cargo-carrier profitable were extremely unlikely, and no freight carrier could afford to pay the salaries survey crews commanded. Further, the same pressures which caused colony expeditions to prefer cryo ships to hyper-capable transports applied to any military expedition, and the distance between star systems effectively limited warfare to intramural affairs within a given system.

The Warshawski Sail changed that, along with everything else. Transit speeds soared as higher hyper bands were entered and their predominant grav waves slowly charted, and a Warshawski Sail hypership with inertial compensator could be of almost any desired mass. Huge ships might be slower than small ones, but they were still far, far faster than cryo ships, and their cargo carrying capacity could be enormous.

The first interstellar warships were (probably inevitably) piratical. Hyperships were scarcely needed for system defense, as any attacker was required to reenter normal space and could then be engaged by sublight ships with normal impeller drives, and after centuries of being literally unable to get at one another, there were no such things as power struggles between rival star systems. Humans had not changed appreciably, however, and the emergence of latter day "vikings" to prey on newly established or weakly defended colonies was almost a forgone conclusion. Ownership of at least eleven colonies changed hands by force during the first half-century of Warshawski Sail capability, financed in many cases by "respectable" corporations formed for the express purpose of mounting filibustering expeditions. In time, particularly as interstellar shipping established itself and began to grow, actual squadrons of independent pirates came into existence. As always, threats to commerce provoked the creation of navies to police the trade lanes, and the first system navies of interstellar warships appeared.

These navies were remarkably successful in running down and eliminating outright pirates, but they themselves didn't go away once the threat abated. Having been created, they took on a life of their own, particularly as the Warshawski Sail began knitting the far-flung community of Man back together. Traditional sources of contention reappeared, and the discovery of wormhole junctions created a whole new source of rivalry, as these were of immense value to trade, expansion, and warfare alike.

Since the restoration of the precious gift of the ability to make war upon one's neighbors, several inter-system polities have been created. Most have grown relatively peacefully, on the pattern of the old Solarian League; others have been forged by more forceful means, and no political unit can afford to overlook its own security needs any longer.

Aside from the Star Kingdom, the other three major polities of concern to Honor Harrington are:

The Solarian League, the Anderman Empire, and the Republic of Haven. Although important as a trade partner and near-neighbor of the Star Kingdom, the Andermani have not (as yet) impinged as directly on Manticore's prospects of survival as have the League and the People's Republic, which are briefly described below.

(B) THE SOLARIAN LEAGUE:

Composed of the oldest colony worlds, the Solarian League extends for roughly ninety-eight light-years from the Solar System. Old Earth is the League's capital but is only first among equals, as her daughter colonies had enjoyed centuries (in some cases over a millennium) of independence from the mother world and were unwilling to surrender their sovereignty when the new star nation emerged.

As a result, every member world of the Solarian League exercises full local autonomy. That is, the League's Executive Council, its highest governing body, has no legal authority over the local policies of its member worlds. On the "national" level, the Executive Council consists of delegates from all member worlds, and each world holds a veto right. On the surface any central government ought to find it impossible under such circumstances to maintain any sort of sustained policy, but there are countervailing pressures.

First, most of these worlds are quite populous, wealthy, and content, and pursue a consensual domestic policy, both locally and for the League as a whole, in which disputes which might draw a veto are unlikely to arise.

Secondly, the League's member worlds work off a great deal of their contentiousness in foreign policy debates because they feel safe in treating foreign policy as an area in which to make "statements of principle." Most League statesmen realize that this attitude makes any coherent military or diplomatic policy impossible, but the League is enormous. With the greatest concentration of wealth in human history (and counting almost two-thirds of the total human race as its citizens), it feels unthreatened by external dangers. Its navy is the largest in the galaxy, and the idea that any foreseeable combination of foreign powers could threaten its security is unthinkable.

Third, although every member world has veto right, the Executive Council has a counter-weapon; a two-thirds vote of the Council can strip any planet of its League membership. This power has never been used, but the *threat* of its use has brought several obstinate delegates to see reason over the centuries.

Despite its lack of an organized foreign policy, the League has an almost uninterrupted history of gradual expansion. From time to time an independent world will request admission to the League, and these requests are almost always granted, but any form of organized League imperialism is virtually impossible. In a sense, the League is isolationist—willing to trade with anyone, still the greatest source of recruitment for new colonies, but content to stand aloof from the power struggles prevalent in other regions of the galaxy. For all that, however, the League's size, power, and historical record of attracting requests for admission have given it a sense of manifest destiny. Its view (which, so far, has been justified by events) is that *any* of its neighbors will eventually recognize the advantages of League membership and ask to join. There is thus no need for the League to conquer anyone, as passing time and the inevitability of peaceful expansion will take care of the problem.

There have, however, been two exceptions to the League's "non-imperial" policy. First, the League has a tradition of extending protectorate status to what might be called "third-world planets" along and beyond its current frontiers. This is justified on the basis that such worlds are vulnerable to piratical raids and/or economic exploitation by less principled interstellar powers. As such, they need looking after . . . which just happens to give the *League's* merchants the inside track and prepares the ground for the protectorate's eventual admission to the League.

The second exception is a consistent policy of extending the same protectorate status to wormhole junctions with termini in or near League space. Among those junctions was the Erewhon Junction roughly a hundred light-years from the People's Republic of Haven's "southern" frontier, but this effort failed. The Erewhon Republic rejected League "protection," despite the proximity of the threat of the PRH. Instead, Erewhon chose to place its reliance upon the Manticoran Alliance and the assistance of the Royal Manticoran Navy—probably because the League's lack of a coherent foreign policy failed to fill the Republic with confidence in the face of Peep expansionism.

The League itself contains no wormhole junctions, but at least five junctions have termini in League territory. Where possible, the League has secured control of the junction at the far end of the wormhole as a defensive measure, though the use of *force majeure* to do so remains contrary to League policy. Nor, for the most part, has force been required, as the League is well able to proffer economic and industrial incentives to encourage most colony worlds to accept League membership quite eagerly.

The most important junction not to pass under League control is the Manticore Junction. Historically, Manticore has enjoyed congenial relations with the League but has no desire to submerge itself within the League's bureaucracy, and the combination of the revenues generated by the junction and the sturdily independent, continually growing population of its three worlds make the League's traditional incentives less attractive to the Manticorans than to most struggling colonies. In the last thirty years, however, an undeniable edge of strain has crept into League-Manticoran relations due to the looming conflict with the People's Republic. The one thing the Star Kingdom most fears is a situation in which the Peeps would be able to purchase advanced technology from the League, thus redressing their tactical inferiority vis-a-vis the Royal Navy. In its efforts to prevent that situation from arising, the Cromarty Government was forced to resort to strong-arm economic pressure to get a technology embargo out of the Executive Council. The effort succeeded, but at the result of strained relations.

(C) THE PEOPLE'S REPUBLIC OF HAVEN:

Although the Haven System lies 667 light-years from Old Earth, 155 light-years further distant than Manticore, the first shuttle landed on its habitable planet (also called Haven) in 1309 PD, over a century before Manticore was settled. This was possible because of the fashion in which the introduction of the Warshawski Sail had revolutionized the logistics of colonization. Haven's day is 24.56 standard hours in length, and its year is 412.25 local days in length, divided into 13 months: 9 of 32 days each and 4 of 31 days each. The short months are the 3rd, 5th, 10th, and 12th. Every 4 years, the 3rd month is 32 days long.

Haven lay in a particularly attractive region, with an unusually high proportion of F, G, and K class stars, and the original expedition was extremely well financed as a joint venture by no fewer than eleven corporations based on member planets of the Solarian League. Moreover, the planet of Haven proved well-named, for terrestrial life forms adapted to its environment with a minimum of difficulty and its climate was very nearly idyllic. With a powerful PR organization to tout its attractiveness, it exercised a magnetic effect on the would-be colonists of the League and, with the availability of the new hypership technology, grew at incredible speed. By 1430 PD, the Republic of Haven already boasted a planetary population of almost a billion and was beginning to mount colony expeditions of its own in what became known (despite the fact that six other systems in the same region had been colonized before or almost simultaneously with Haven) as the Haven Quadrant.

By 1475, the Haven economy and government had proven themselves extremely efficient and effective. Politically, Haven was a representative democracy with a strong and politically active middle class, and its economic policy enshrined the principles of liberal capitalism with minimal government interference. Coupled with the "jump start" provided by the colony's highly favorable initial circumstances, this combination of market efficiency and flexible government created a planetary standard of living at least as high as that of most Solarian League member worlds, and it became the envy and the pattern for every other world in the quadrant.

For the next two centuries, Haven continued to fulfill its promise, rising to a system population of almost seven billion and becoming a sort of interstellar Athens. The Haven Quadrant, although composed of independent worlds and star systems, rivaled the Solarian League for economic power, and it remained a vibrant and expansive entity, unlike the essentially satisfied and content League. Although the quadrant contained no wormhole junctions, it had access to the Manticore Junction (and, later, to the Erewhon Junction) and thence to the League, and there was every reason to believe that its expansion and prosperity would continue.

It did not. Precise identification of a specific

event which caused the change within the quadrant is impossible, but in general terms it might be called over-achievement. The quadrant—and, in particular, Haven—had done too well. Its wealth was incalculable, and it began to seem unfair that that wealth was not more evenly distributed. In particular, capitalism, as always, had produced stratified classes, ranging from the extremely wealthy to the marginal and even sub-marginal, and if the members of Haven's "sub-marginal" class were immeasurably better off than, say the pre-Anderman citizens of New Berlin, they were *not* well off compared to their own affluent fellow citizens.

The Republic thus began to experiment, cautiously at first, with assistance and welfare programs to increase the opportunities of its less advantaged citizens. Unfortunately, what began as an experiment gradually became something else. Transfer payments became increasingly important for the maintenance of the industrial poor, requiring greater levies on the productive elements of society. Marginal industrial operations were shored up by protective tariffs, government loans, and outright grants to encourage full employment, which both undercut the overall efficiency and productivity of the industrial base and encouraged inflation. Inflation further worsened the condition of the poor, requiring still higher transfer payments—payments which were soon adjusted for inflation on a mandated basis—and, as the network of assistance proliferated, it came to be seen as a fundamental "right" of those receiving the aid. By 1680 PD, Haven had issued its famous "Economic Bill of Rights," declaring that all of its citizens had an "unalienable right" to a relative standard of living to be defined (and adjusted as inflation required) by statute by the legislature.

In the process, the government had initiated an unending spiral of inflation, higher transfer payments, and increasing deficit spending. Moreover, it had (quite unintentionally, at least at first) undermined the fundamental strength of its own democracy. The middle class, the traditional backbone of the Republic, was under increasing pressure both from above and below, caught in the squeeze between an increasingly less productive economy and ever larger levies against its earnings to support the welfare system. Whereas the middle class had once seen the upper class as (at worst) essentially friendly rivals or (at best) allies in their joint prosperity, they came to see the wealthy, like the poor, as enemies, fighting over a dwindling prosperity. Worse, the middle class's traditional aspiration to upward mobility had become an increasingly remote dream, and it was much easier to focus resentment on those who had more than the middle class than on those who had less—a tendency which became ever more pronounced as "enlightened" commentators and academics secured dominant positions in the media and educational system.

Perhaps worst of all, was the emergence of the "Dolist" blocs. The Dolists (so called because they were "on the dole," receiving government assistance in greater or lesser degree) were still franchised voters and, quite logically, supported the candidates who offered them the most. It was a case of self-interest, and the Dolists' self-interest interlocked with that of increasingly careerist politicians. A new class of machine politicians, the "Dolist managers," emerged, playing the role of king-makers by delivering huge blocks of votes to chosen candidates. Incumbent politicians soon realized that their continued incumbency was virtually assured with the managers' backing—and that the converse was also true. A politician targeted by the "People's Quorum" (the official term for the alliance of Dolist managers) was doomed, and as the leaders of the Quorum became aware of their power, they selected specific politicians to punish as an example to all politicos of the power the Quorum represented.

Finally, as if to complete the system-wide outbreak of mass insanity, most of those who recognized that something was wrong embraced a "conspiracy theory" which assumed that their problems must result from someone's hostile machinations—probably those of the domestic "monied classes" or foreign industries who "dumped" their cheap, shoddy products on the Haven economy. Almost worse, there was an entrenched element of "this wouldn't be happening to us if we weren't somehow at fault" in the vast majority of mid-18th century Havenite political and societal analysis and rhetoric, and this masochistic tendency only became more pronounced as the century wound to a close.

By 1750 PD, the Republic—no longer "The Republic of Haven," but now "The People's Republic of Haven"—had become the captive of a coalition of professional politicians (indeed, politicians who had never had and were not qualified for any other career) and the Quorum, aided and abetted by a morally and intellectually bankrupt academic community and a mass media philosophically at home with the Quorum's objectives and cowed (where necessary) by threats of blacklisting. That the Quorum could succeed in blacklisting journalists had been demonstrated in 1746 PD, in the case of Adele Wasserman, one of the last moderate journalists. Her moderation, which was actually a bit left of center by mid-17th century standards, was labeled "conservative" or, more frequently, "reactionary" by her 18th century contemporaries. She herself was called "an enemy of the common man," "a slave of the monied powers," and (most cutting slur then available on Haven) "a fiscal elitist," and her employer, one of the last independent news services, was pressured into terminating her contract (for "socially insensitive and inappropriate demagoguery") by means of an economic boycott, strikes, and governmental pressure. Her firing, followed by her subsequent relocation to the Kingdom of Manticore and a successful career as a leading theorist of the Centrist Party, was the writing on the wall for any who had eyes. Unless something quite extraordinary intervened, the current Havenite system was doomed.

The problem was one which had arisen as long ago as Old Earth's Roman Empire: when power depends on "bread and circuses," those in power are compelled to provide ever greater largess if they wish to remain in power. In effect, the politicos required a bottomless and ever-filled public trough to pay off the Dolists and provide the graft and corruption to support the lives to which they themselves had become accustomed, and after almost two centuries of increasingly serious self-inflicted wounds, not even the once-robust Havenite economy could support that burden. It became apparent to the political managers that the entire edifice was in trouble: tax revenues had not matched expenditures in over 143 T-years; R&D was faltering as an increasingly politicized (and hence ineffectual) educational system purveyed the pseudo-scientific mumbo-jumbo of collectivist economic theory rather than sound scientific training; and the decreasing numbers of truly capable industrial and technical managers produced by the system were increasingly lured to other star systems whose economies allowed them to use their talents and enjoy the benefits thereof. The "Technical Conservation Act" of 1778, which revoked emigration visas for all research and production engineers by nationalizing their expertise "as a resource of the Republic," was intended to put a stop to that, but it could not reverse the fatal trends.

Real economic growth had stopped—indeed, the economy was contracting—but ever higher Basic Living Stipend payments were politically inescapable, and the stagflation which had resulted was becoming a self-sustaining reaction. In 1771 PD, a highly classified economic report to the House of Legislators predicted that by the year 1870 the entire economy would collapse in a disaster which would make Old Earth's Great Depression and the Economic Winter of 252 PD look like mild recessions. The Chiefs of Staff, apprised of the degree of collapse to be anticipated, warned that it would precipitate pitched warfare in the streets as Haven's citizens fought for food for their families, for Haven had long since attained a population which could not feed itself without imports, and imports could not be paid for with a negative balance of trade.

The government saw only two ways out: to bite the bullet, end deficit spending, abolish the BLS, and hope to weather the resultant catastrophic reorganization, or to find some other source of income to shore up the budget. The possibility of admitting they could no longer pay the interest on Haven's mortgaged future was too much for them to stomach, which meant only the second solution was a real possibility, but there was no more money to be squeezed out of the economy. A panicked group of legislators suggested draconian "soak the rich" schemes, but the majority recognized that any such panacea would be purely cosmetic. Aside from their own hidden assets, the wealthy represented less than 0.5% of the total population, and the totally confiscatory taxes proposed would provide only a temporary reprieve . . . and eliminate both future private investment and the highest tax brackets (already taxed at 92% on personal income and 75% on investment income) as a long-term revenue source. A self-sustaining tax base could be produced only by a strong middle class, and the middle class had been systematically destroyed; what remained of it was far too small to sustain the government's current rate of expenditure and had been for almost a century.

That left only one possible way to find the needed revenue, and the government, with the cooperation of the Quorum, prepared to seize it under the so-called "DuQuesne Plan."

The first step was a "Constitutional Convention" which radically rewrote the Havenite Constitution. While maintaining a facade of democracy, the new constitution, by redefining eligibility requirements and office qualifications and giving the House of Legislators the right to refuse to seat even a legally elected representative if the House found him or her "personally unfit for public office," created a legislative dictatorship with hereditary membership. (It was not a strictly parent-to-child inheritance but rather a codification of the "adoption" process which had become the normal career route for Havenite politicians over the past century; true dynasties came later.) The second step was not to limit deficit spending but to increase it, this time with the enthusiastic support of the military, which underwent the greatest peacetime expansion in Havenite history. And the third step, launched in 1846 PD, was to acquire additional revenue from a totally new source: military conquest.

The initial attacks were almost totally unopposed. The quadrant was so accustomed to the idea that Haven represented the ideal to which all humanity aspired that its steady collapse had been sadly underestimated. Haven's problems were known, but their severity was misjudged, and the consensus was that all of them could be solved if Haven would only put its house in order. Indeed, the majority of Haven's neighbors felt that Haven was on the right track but had simply gotten temporarily out of control, and many of them were in the early stages of the same process in a sort of lemming-like emulation of disaster. The sudden expansion of the Havenite military caused some concern, but those who suggested that long-friendly Haven contemplated hostile action were viewed as hysterical alarmists. Besides, the quadrant's other systems found their own economies were becoming increasingly strapped, and warships and troops cost money which was required for their own welfare programs.

The result was a turkey shoot for the Peoples' Navy. Between 1846 and 1900 PD, a period of barely more than fifty years, the People's Republic of Haven had conquered every star system within a hundred light-years of it, incorporating them by force into a new, interstellar PRH ruled by the now openly hereditary "legislature" of the Haven System.

Unfortunately for the Legislaturalists, they soon discovered that conquest was not the solution they had hoped. True, they could loot the economies of conquered worlds, but unless they wanted servile insurrection, there was a limit to how badly they could wreck their subject economies. Worse, the military machine required to conquer and then police their new empire cost even more than they had anticipated, particularly as their alarmed and (so far) unconquered neighbors began to arm in reply. Despite all efforts, their budgets remained stubbornly in the deficit column; they simply could not pay for both their military and the support of their subsidized population out of available resources. There was an appearance of prosperity on the home front, but those in informed positions knew that it was only an appearance. In short, the "Republic" had only two options: continue to expand, or collapse.

And so, in 1900 PD, the People's Republic had no choice but to look for fresh fields to conquer . . . and found, directly in its path, between it and the additional worlds it had to have, a small but wealthy star system known as the Star Kingdom of Manticore.

DAVID WEBER

Honor Harrington (cont.):

Field of Dishonor

Honor goes home to Manticore—and fights for her life on a battlefield she never trained for, in a private war that offers just two choices: death—or a "victory" that can end only in dishonor and the loss of all she loves....

Other novels by DAVID WEBER:

Mutineers' Moon

"...a good story...reminds me of 1950s Heinlein..."
—*BMP Bulletin*

The Armageddon Inheritance

Sequel to *Mutineers' Moon*.

Path of the Fury

"Excellent...a thinking person's Terminator."
—*Kliatt*

Oath of Swords

An epic fantasy.

with STEVE WHITE:

Insurrection
Crusade

Novels set in the world of the Starfire ™ game system.

And don't miss Steve White's solo novels,
***The Disinherited** and **Legacy**!*

continued ☞

THE SHIP WHO SANG IS NOT ALONE!

Anne McCaffrey, with Margaret Ball, Mercedes Lackey, S.M. Stirling, and Jody Lynn Nye, explores the universe she created with her ground-breaking novel, The Ship Who Sang.

PARTNERSHIP
by Anne McCaffrey & Margaret Ball
"[*PartnerShip*] captures the spirit of *The Ship Who Sang*...a single, solid plot full of creative nastiness and the sort of egocentric villains you love to hate."
— Carolyn Cushman, **Locus**

THE SHIP WHO SEARCHED
by Anne McCaffrey & Mercedes Lackey
Tia, a bright and spunky seven-year-old accompanying her exo-archaeologist parents on a dig, is afflicted by a paralyzing alien virus. Tia won't be satisfied to glide through life like a ghost in a machine. Like her predecessor Helva, *The Ship Who Sang*, she would rather strap on a spaceship!

THE CITY WHO FOUGHT
by Anne McCaffrey & S.M. Stirling
Simeon was the "brain" running a peaceful space station—but when the invaders arrived, his only hope of protecting his crew and himself was to become *The City Who Fought*.

THE SHIP WHO WON
by Anne McCaffrey & Jody Lynn Nye
"Oodles of fun." — *Locus*
"Fast, furious and fun." — *Chicago Sun-Times*